HANDBOOK *of* **Community-Based Clinical Practice**

EDITED BY

Anita Lightburn and Phebe Sessions

HANDBOOK
of
Community-Based Clinical Practice

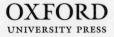

OXFORD
UNIVERSITY PRESS

2006

OXFORD
UNIVERSITY PRESS

Oxford University Press, Inc., publishes works that further
Oxford University's objective of excellence
in research, scholarship, and education.

Oxford   New York
Auckland   Cape Town   Dar es Salaam   Hong Kong   Karachi
Kuala Lumpur   Madrid   Melbourne   Mexico City   Nairobi
New Delhi   Shanghai   Taipei   Toronto

With offices in
Argentina   Austria   Brazil   Chile   Czech Republic   France   Greece
Guatemala   Hungary   Italy   Japan   Poland   Portugal   Singapore
South Korea   Switzerland   Thailand   Turkey   Ukraine   Vietnam

Published by Oxford University Press, Inc.
198 Madison Avenue, New York, New York 10016

www.oup.com

Oxford is a registered trademark of Oxford University Press

Library of Congress Cataloging-in-Publication Data
Handbook of community-based clinical practice /
edited by Anita Lightburn, Phebe Sessions.
p. cm.
Summary: "Bridges community practice and clinical practice by
collecting 33 chapters from social workers, psychologists, and
psychiatrists that outline and illustrate the state of the art.
Designed specifically for clinicians making the transition to
community-based work"—Provided by publisher.
Includes bibliographical references and index.
ISBN-13: 978-0-19-515922-6
ISBN: 0-19-515922-5
1. Community psychology.   2. Community psychiatry.   3. Community
mental health services.   I. Lightburn, Anita.   II. Sessions, Phebe,
1943–
RA790.55.H35 2005
362.2'2—dc22   2005010690

9 8 7 6 5 4 3 2 1

Printed in the United States of America
on acid-free paper

From Anita

For my parents, Kenneth and Ann Schimp
with love and admiration for your life of service.

For Kenneth Lightburn, wise consultant, invaluable support, and husband.

For Kara Elizabeth Lightburn, dearest daughter, as you embrace your global community.

From Phebe

Many thanks for "happy hearts and times together" to Dan, Jerri and Len, Bill and Abi, Dave and Betsy, Cathy and Frank, Hannah and Greg, Myra, Jonathan, Beth, Gillian and Michael.

In memory of Bud and Peg Sessions, and Jane and Flicka Rodman.

> We are caught in an inescapable network of mutuality.
> —Martin Luther King

And for this we are greatly blessed.

As a Lakota Indian activist once said, "If you think you're related to the stars, you'll have a different view of your responsibility." In isolation, it's easy for our vision to fail and our heart to grow cold. When we cultivate a sense of broader connection, however, we see further, we take more of existence into account. In short, we find our place in the world.

P. R. Loeb, *Soul of a citizen: Living with conviction in a cynical time*

Grandfather
Look at our brokenness.
We know that we are the ones
Who are the divided
And we are the ones
Who must come back together.

—Ojibway prayer

Preface

The Handbook of Community-Based Clinical Practice is inspired by and grounded in the experiences of pioneering clinicians, policymakers, and scholars who have developed new ways of working to meet developmental and mental health needs. Over the past two decades there has been considerable investment in developing comprehensive community-based services and systems of care to provide different answers for those coping with mental illness and acutely stressful family interactions. Promising approaches apply what is being learned from prevention science to guide programs aimed at primary prevention for children and adolescents.

In its Report on Mental Health in the United States, the New Freedom Commission on Mental Health (2003) entitled its findings "Achieving the Promise: Transforming Mental Health Care in America." The report begins by citing the World Health Organization's findings that mental illnesses rank first among illnesses that cause disability in the United States, Canada, and Europe, creating a major underrecognized public health burden (p. 3). The challenge in responding to this level of need involves assisting people to recover from mental illness in their communities. To this end, the commissioners recommend that mental health

services support recovery and build resilience instead of simply managing symptoms and accepting long-term disability. Accumulated evidence shows that a wide range of community-based alternatives are more effective than institutional care (p. 29). However, there is a considerable lag between what we know about providing community-based care and the way we continue to provide services, with half of mental health services still delivered in general medical settings (p. 59). To transform mental health services, theory, practice, and research need to be directed toward helping people recover in their communities.

Clinicians also have a critical role in contributing to mental health through developing early intervention and preventive programs. They need to work effectively with early childhood programs and family support centers, in comprehensive school-based mental health programs, in systems of care for children and adolescents, in community-based primary care, and in community care programs for adults and seniors. There is an urgent need for community-based clinicians to develop effective ways of integrating mental health principles into the fabric of community social life, in order to engage those who are hard to reach and not likely to use traditional mental health services. Clinicians have an important role in developing protective communities, such as sanctuaries and safe havens, supportive social networks, and communities in which those with mental illness can have an active part.

It is important to grasp the magnitude of the order of transformation that is needed. There is a long journey ahead to transform the current system, as change must include the structure and financing of services, the application and translation of research findings, the use of technology, and work with consumers and the public, while continuing to advance understanding of mental health problems and service delivery. Finally, there is a pressing need to attend to the workforce crisis in mental heath care (New Freedom Commission on Mental Health, 2003).

The challenge for clinicians is as formidable as it is exciting. Through professional training, clinicians and students should gain a foundation for mental health practice in communities. In part, this requires knowledge of evidence-based approaches to practice. It also requires competencies in community-based clinical work. Clinicians need to develop integrative models of practice to guide practice and research in and with community. These models will incorporate an understanding of trauma, recovery, resiliency, and cultural competence. We also need to enhance skills at working collaboratively with interdisciplinary colleagues, with a disposition that respects the rights, knowledge, and abilities of consumers, families, and natural helpers, all indispensable in the prevention and recovery processes. As we work together in community, we will benefit from building a community of care that enables us to work with commonly held values and beliefs that will have an important role in shaping service provision.

In concluding the bold vision for transforming existing mental health services, the commission observes that "local innovation under the mantle of national leadership can lead the way for successful transformation" (p. 86). We would add that there needs to be an appreciation and understanding of the innovations that are leading the way. To this end, we are pleased to have gathered in this volume many of the examples of innovations that are important mental health service transformations. Our authors introduce progressive work in early intervention initiatives and more comprehensive systems of care that has increased access to care in community and reduced the need for institutional care. These innovations counter stigma and offer culturally sensitive ways of supporting mental health and reaching vulnerable, underserved populations.

As these programs have become more established, it has been difficult to find a sufficient number of community-oriented clinicians. In a 2001 study of nine innovative programs in Massachusetts, we were surprised to learn of the challenges in locating clinicians who could work with system of care principles (Lightburn, Olson, Sessions, & Pulleyblank-Coffey, 2002; Pulleyblank-Coffey, Lightburn, Olson, & Sessions, 2002). Program leadership and consumers have expressed distress over the poor preparation of clinicians for working in community-based programs where consumer and families are partners, and strength-based, recovery-oriented empowerment approaches are needed. Teams in these innovative programs also observed that it was challenging to work with clinicians from traditional practice models not concerned about recovery, partnering with families, and connections to the community. This made it difficult to decrease service fragmentation and provide an effective system of care with an integrated collaborative service delivery plan.

As educators we are impressed with the responsibility that we have to prepare clinicians who can work in new ways. We know that this requires a multifaceted approach in the field and in our professional schools. Students and clinicians should be introduced to innovations in the field. Also needed are new models for community-based practice that integrate clinical knowledge and skill with knowledge and skill in community practice. Understanding recovery, cultural competence, trauma, resilience, the meaning of the culture of care, people's relationship with their communities, and communal practice approaches is necessary to support effective practice and research. We also need to understand program and practice evaluation to help us define and refine our work, so that we know if we are making progress in providing more effective services.

The recent mandate to transform mental health, set out by the New Freedom Commission on Mental Health (2003) will depend on community-based clinicians who take the lead in implementing the best practices that integrate evidence-based practice with meaningful application to different community situations and need.

The practice examples in this book offer insight into how innovative clinical practice has developed and continues to evolve as we understand more about the fundamentals of work in and with the community. The arena for community-based clinical practice will expand exponentially as state and national leadership support the commission's blueprint for transformation. It is our hope that this volume will contribute to the evolution of community-based clinical services.

About the Organization of This Book

This book is intended as a resource to support the ongoing development of community-based mental health care. In the first two chapters we introduce the changes that have brought to the forefront the need for this type of practice. We describe the many changes in our social order, knowledge base, and professional community that have contributed to the development of innovative practices. We look at our clinical practice traditions and the bridge to community that is being constructed through new ways of understanding development, and our relationship to the communities that nourish and support our lives with the challenges that we face in providing care in our society. Our authors examine our assumptions about the therapeutic relationship, considering the self in community, communal therapies, and the need for the reflective practitioner. We take a concerted look at anti-racist practice and the complexity of cultural competence, evaluating our current state of affairs and offer a guide for community-based clinicians work. To support this ongoing evolution in practice we also offer ways of using evaluation and teaching that are snychronous with work with the community.

We have brought together a diverse group of practitioners who share the evolution of their thinking and practice. Leaders who have made considerable contributions in the field share their insights about the public and personal journey to transform policy and practice. We value their personal stories. Their contributions show how transformation takes vision and courage to be different and challenge tradition, as well a long-term investment and an ability to develop new pathways. The practice examples that follow are drawn form four different practice areas, early childhood and family support, school-based mental health,

community-based child and adolescent mental health, and adult mental health. We provided a guide for authors as they developed these examples to include a definition of need, descriptions of program and practice, and research and evidence supporting the innovations, with lessons learned and a case example.

The History of This Book (Our Story)

This book began with presentations we did together at conferences integrating our work in school-based practice and family support in the context of our understanding of clinical knowledge. We greatly value the school-based and family support early intervention teams with which we have collaborated, and the students who have been an integral part of discovery with us. This work was always an adventure, with committed colleagues who worked hard to facilitate partnerships and find funding for the next year so that projects would stay alive. Work in community is often chaotic, never straightforward, as the interests of many are interwoven in the process of finding the best way to meet pressing needs. Work in community is also deeply gratifying, as each day brings unexpected challenges that stretch and pull you toward interdependence with others. There is nothing as rewarding as celebrating what everyone has accomplished.

We are thankful to Al Roberts, who was enthusiastic about our proposal to do a book that would bring to light the changes in practice we experienced and those we had observed in the field. He has a special gift for envisioning books and the rewards of collaboration and is most generous in sharing his wisdom. His introduction of us to Oxford University Press was fortuitous because the Press has been most supportive in seeing this project through from its inception. We are grateful for the enthusiasm of Joan Bossert, our editor at Oxford, and Maura Roessner, our associate editor, who have supplied consistent encouragement and have helped us see this through to completion.

Over the years we have benefited from a wonderful network of collaborators both in the field and in professional education. We have had the good fortune to expand our introduction to community-based practice through getting to know the work of our colleagues at some influential conferences such as the "Transforming Social Work" gatherings in Burlington, Vermont; the seminars of the International Association for Evaluation and Research in Children and Family Services, supported by the Zancan Foundation, Padua, Italy; "Systems of Care for Child and Adolescent Mental Health," sponsored by the University of South Florida; and the "International Narrative Therapy and Community Work Conference," in Australia, Atlanta, and Oaxaca. All these gatherings have made it possible to gain new perspectives that have expanded the boundaries of theory and introduced us to new ways of thinking and practicing. In important ways these groups are part of our communities!

Summer sessions at Smith College School for Social Work enabled colleagues to join in discussions on the potential of community-based practice. Edward Eismann has collaborated with us over the years as we developed principles of community-based practice drawn from our various experiences in the field. Mary Olson and Ellen Pulleyblank-Coffey generated our study on innovative practice programs in Massachusetts that substantively deepened our understanding of the challenges of innovation in community. Verba Fanolis brought to life and helped us understand the frontline work of school-based practice. Susan Donner and Joshua Miller brought us into important conversations about race and demonstrated what it means to live out commitment to social justice. Gerry Schamess has been an invaluable support and mentor in the journey, from joining us in community practice in the schools to supporting our writing about it. Catherine Nye has enlivened our understanding of culture through debates about how clinical theory and work can be integrated into community. Smith was also a place where different traditions have developed and influenced each other, as family therapists, psychologists, and social workers have learned each other's traditions and found common ground.

Personal Journeys

Important formative experiences in the field have brought us to this point, where community has become an integral part of clinical work. Some of the highlights of our personal journeys are shared here as the experiences and people who have inspired and contributed to our development and commitments to integrative practice.

For Anita, work in the 1990s with Hall Neighborhood House (HNH) administration, Pearl Dowell, and the family support team opened the door to new ways of thinking and working that demonstrated how powerfully community mediates help. As project evaluator of this Head Start demonstration, I benefited immeasurably from learning from all the parents who participated in the programs and from the staff at HNH. In particular, Jody Visage was an inspiration in innovative program development with her commitment to helping in ways that worked for the parents and staff. Ongoing conversations with Susan Kemp, a New Zealander and colleague at Columbia University, continued the process of liberating community from the background, as we thought about clinical work in a community center in the 1990s, integrating the clinical with empowerment and educational practice. In a similar way, our early work with Chris Warren-Adamson, with visits to the United Kingdom to share our experiences in family support, began a long and valued association that has brought an international perspective on the development of community-based practice. Our shared experiences and different traditions have enlivened our ideas, and our current work in cross-national research has moved our thinking forward with a theory of change that integrates clinical and community work for family center practice. Experience with the Safe Schools Healthy Student Initiative Early Childhood Team at the Hampshire Educational Collaborative, and the mental health advisory group that had the responsibility for mental health services in the Pioneer Valley school systems, has deepened my understanding of the considerable challenges and possibilities in providing community-based mental health.

When I think of the emergence of community-based clinical practice, I am reminded of conversations with Gisela Konopka, who long admired Eduard Lindeman (professor at the Columbia University School of Social Work), an early champion and developer of community and group practice methods in the 1930s and 1940s. Lindeman had a fervent belief in democracy and citizen participation in shaping services. He believed that mental health was supported through opportunity, becoming involved in community, lifelong learning, and receiving the benefits of community membership. Gisela herself was an inspiration, as she developed community in residential treatment and remand centers for adolescents, understanding the value of working with the center milieu. Her work was anchored in her deep belief in the dignity of every young person and their need for each other. Konopka was an early proponent of integration of mental health and child welfare services, and she actively worked for human service providers to invest in primary prevention. Our history of community-based practice has been evolving from the innovations of these pioneers and formidable leaders.

For Phebe, a passion for testing the relevance and utility of clinical theories and methods in communities where social oppression is met with creative resistance has informed my career. I was greatly supported in the early stages by Dr. Gerald Caplan and the Laboratory of Community Psychiatry at the Massachusetts Mental Health Center (MMHC), which encouraged both boldness in experimentation and caution about professional hubris. MMHC was also a place that supported rigorous exploration of theory and intensive learning of a range of clinical methods. Discovering the outreach efforts of the structural family therapists of the 1960s and 1970s helped me to integrate useful skills for family and community work at the Cambridge Youth Guidance Center (CYGC), with the help of the Family Institute of Cambridge. CYGC taught the values of community work by embodying them in its own organizational structure and teamwork.

I have benefited greatly from relationships with mentors and colleagues at the Smith College School for Social Work. Particularly significant in the evolution of my ideas and the ability to communicate them have been Connie Lemon, who saw more capacity in me than I did in myself, Ann Hartman and Joan Laird, whose fearlessness and passionate advocacy elicited a more public pursuit of my own commitments, and my "community-oriented compatriots," Gerry Schamess, Dorcas Bowles, Anita Lightburn, John Ehrenreich, and Cathy Riessman. My dissertation committee at the Heller School at Brandeis University, particularly Irving Zola and Janet Giele, challenged careless thinking and helped me to understand the values of the academy.

My collaborative relationship with Joan Rosenson and the South Shore Mental Health Center for over 20 years has been extremely important in my understanding of public mental health services and the adaptive permutations it must undergo to remain economically viable and committed to educating future generations of clinicians. I also deeply appreciate the creative energy of Lori Button-Szyzgiel and the Massachusetts Behavioral Health Partnership in forging innovative links with professional schools to change how trainees are prepared to work in community. Finally, collaborations with Verba Fanolis and Mary Olson have continually been sources of fresh insights and nourishing intellectual stimulation, as they both profoundly understand how to apply good ideas in relational contexts that encourage their use.

Thank you to the students who have come to my classes with open hearts and minds and passionately held commitments to excellence in clinical practice. Your values, experiences, and ideas are represented throughout this book.

Acknowledging the Contributors

We want to acknowledge the hard work of all our contributors. We are grateful for their generosity in responding to our questions and reviews. It has been inspiring to learn from their experience, tenacity, thinking, and ongoing work in the field. We are especially grateful for the insights and generosity of colleagues for their thoughtful reviews of earlier drafts of this work: Martha Dore, Katherine Gordy Levine, Lynn Hoffman, Mary Olson, and Sandra Scarry. We are thankful for the support of our deans, Carolyn Jacobs at Smith and Peter Vaughan at Fordham. We are most appreciative for the assistance of Michele Bala, who has been patient with details, grammar, and production, and who reminded us to breathe as we came down to the end. It is serendipitous that our journey with the book intertwined with her journey from Smith to New York and back. We are grateful to have fellow travelers to the end, acquainted with the many versions of this text. Thanks also to Angelica Hinjosa and Kathie Talbot, terrific research assistants, expert in finding lost references, developing tables, and detailing! This has been a major effort that could not have been accomplished without the support, intelligence, and abilities of many.

References

Lightburn, A., Olson, M., Sessions, P., & Pulleyblank-Coffey, E. (2002). Practice innovations in mental health services to children and families: New directions for Massachusetts. *Smith Studies in Social Work, 72,* 279–301.

New Freedom Commission on Mental Health. (2003). *Achieving the promise: Transforming mental health care in America. Final report* (DHHS Publication No. SMA-03-3832). Rockville, MD: Author.

Pulleyblank-Coffey, E., Lightburn, A., Olson, M., & Sessions, P. (2002). *Executive summary and report on selected Massachusetts innovative community mental family-based programs.* Northampton, MA: Smith College School for Social Work, Center for Innovative Practice and Social Work Education.

Contents

Contributors

Jean A. Adnopoz, MPH
Associate Clinical Professor
Yale University School of Medicine;
Director of Family Support Services
Yale Child Study Center
New Haven, CT

Jon G. Allen, Ph.D.
Professor of Psychiatry
Helen Malsin Palley Chair in Mental Health
   Research
Menninger Department of Psychiatry and
   Behavioral Sciences at the Baylor College of
   Medicine;
Senior Staff Psychologist at the Menninger Clinic
Houston, Texas

Borja Alvarez de Toledo, M.Ed.
Director of Mental Health Services
The Guidance Center Inc.
Cambridge, MA

Tom Andersen, M.D.
Professor in Social Psychiatry
University of (Trumsa) Tromsoe
Tromsoe, Norway

Paula Armbruster, MA, MSW
Associate Clinical Professor
Director, Outpatient Services
Director, Social Work Training
Yale Child Study Center
New Haven, CT

Lucinda Arnold-Whitney, RNC, B.S.N.
Baptist Lutheran Medical Center
Kansas City, MO

Susan C. Ayers, LICSW
Executive Director
The Guidance Center, Inc.
Cambridge, MA

Roni Berger, Ph.D. CSW
Professor
Adelphi University School of Social Work
Garden City, NY

Miriam Berkman. MSW
Assistant Clinical Professor in Social Work
Yale Child Study Center
New Haven, CT

Saglar Bougdaeva
Yale Child Study Center
New Haven, CT

Matthew J. Chinman, Ph.D.
Behavioral Scientist, Rand Corporation
Santa Monica, CA;
Health Science Specialist
West Los Angeles VA Healthcare Center
Los Angeles, CA

Ursula Chock
Clinical Instructor, Social Work
Yale Child Study Center
New Haven, CT

Joanne Corbin, Ph.D.
Associate Professor
Smith College School for Social Work
Northampton, MA

Maria D. Corwin, Ph.D.
Associate Professor
Bryn Mawr College Graduate School of Social
    Work and Social Research
Lawrenceville, NJ

Jane Crosby, MSW, LICSW
Clinical Supervisor
Holden School
Charlestown, MA;
Clinician and Supervisor
Child and Family Unit
South End Community Health Center
Boston, MA

Larry Davidson, Ph.D.
Associate Professor, Psychiatry
Yale University School of Medicine
New Haven, CT

Ruth Dean, Ph.D., LICSW
Professor
Simmons College School of Social Work
Newton, MA

Virginia DeCarennes, MSW
Yale Child Study Center
New Haven, CT

Susan E. Donner, Ph.D.
Professor
Smith College School for Social Work
Northampton, MA

Martha Morrison Dore, Ph.D.
Visiting Professor
Adelphi University School of Social Work
Garden City, NY

Edward Eismann, Ph.D.
Adjunct Professor
Smith College School for Social Work
Northampton, MA;
Faculty, The Alfred Adler Institute
New York, NY;
Clinical Director
Unitas Therapeutic Community
Bronx, NY

Laura Ewing, MSW
Yale Child Study Center
New Haven, CT

Verba Fanolis, MSW
Social Worker; School Counselor
Putnam School
Springfield, MA

Nancy Feldman, Ph.D.
Assistant Professor
Hunter College School of Social Work
New York, NY

Jennifer Frey, Ph.D.
Assistant Clinical Professor
Yale Program for Recovery and Community Health
Yale University School of Medicine
New Haven, CT

Jim Fultz, deceased
Statistician, Senior Staff
Menninger Department of Psychiatry
Menninger at Baylor Medical School
Houston, Texas

Amy Winnick Gelles, CSW
Deputy Director of Operations
Boys and Girls Harbor
New York, NY

AnnMarie Glodich, Ph.D., MSW
Private Practice
Lawrence, KA

Sandra Gossart-Walker, MSW
Clinical Instructor in Social Work
Family Support Service
Yale Child Study Center
New Haven, CT

James Griffith, M.D.
Professor of Psychiatry and Neurology
Director, Psychiatry Residency Program
Director, Psychiatric Consultation-Liaison Service
Department of Psychiatry and Behavioral Sciences
The George Washington University School of
    Medicine;
Member
Kosovar Professional Education Collaboration
    (KPEC)

Lynn Hoffman
Family Therapist
Eastworks
Easthampton, MA 01027

Katherine Gordy Levine, M.S.S., E.F.T.
Program Director
Visiting Nurse Service of New York Programs at
    F.R.I.E.N.D.S., Inc.
Bronx, NY

Anita Lightburn, Ed.D.
Associate Professor
Fordham University School of Social Service
Tarrytown, NY

Lisa Lochner
Postgraduate Fellow
Yale Child Study Center
New Haven, CT

D. Russell Lyman, Ph.D.
Chief Operating Officer
The Guidance Center, Inc.
Cambridge, MA

Steven Marans, Ph.D.
Harris Associate Professor of Child Psychoanalysis
    and Psychiatry

Yale Child Study Center and Department of Psy-
    chiatry;
Director
National Center for Children Exposed to Violence
New Haven, CT

Judith C. Meyers, Ph.D.
President and CEO
Children's Fund of CT
Child Health and Development Institute of CT
Farmington, CT

Joshua Miller, Ph.D.
Professor
Smith College School for Social Work
Northampton, MA

Chris Moody, MSW
Stormont-Vail Medical Center
Topeka, KS

Robert A. Murphy, Ph.D.
Executive Director
Center for Child & Family Health
Durham, NC

Catherine Nye, Ph.D.
Associate Professor
Smith College School for Social Work
Northampton, MA

Maria O'Connell, PhD.
Associate Research Scientist
Yale Program for Recovery and Community Health
Yale University School of Medicine
New Haven, CT

Mary Olson, Ph.D.
Associate Professor
Smith College School for Social Work
Northampton, MA 01063

Marcelo Pakman, M.D.
Director of Psychiatric Services
Behavioral Health Network
Springfield, MA;
Adjunct Professor
Department of Applied Social Sciences
Polytechnic Institute of Hong-Kong

Abigail Prestin
Senior Administrative Assistant
Yale Child Study Center
New Haven, CT

Ellen Pulleyblank Coffey, Ph.D.
Clinical Psychologist
Adjunct Faculty
Alliant University;
Co-Director
AFTNC Postgraduate Training Program in
    Couples, Families, and Community Practice
Berkeley, CA

Dennis Saleebey
Professor Emeritus
University of Kansas School of Social Welfare
Lawrence, KS

E. Martin Schotz, M.D.
Adjunct Professor
Simmons College School of Social Work
Newton, MA;
Consulting Psychiatrist
Family Services Clinic of South End Community
    Health Center
Newton, MA

Jaakko Seikkula, Ph.D.
Senior Assistant
Department of Psychology
University of Jyväskylä, Finland;
Professor (part-time)
Institute of Community Medicine
University of Tromso, Norway;
Psychologist and Family Therapy Trainer
Agder University College, Norway

Phebe Sessions, Ph.D.
Professor
Smith College School for Social Work
Northampton, MA

Martha Staedeli
Associate Research Scientist
Yale Program for Recovery and Community Health
Yale University School of Medicine
New Haven, CT

Carol R. Swenson, DSW
Professor
Simmons College School of Social Work
E. Falmouth MA

George Thompson, M.D.
Associate Professor
Department of Psychiatry
University of Missouri-Kansas City School of
Medicine
Kansas City, MO

Janis Tondora, Psy.D.
Assistant Clinical Professor
Department of Psychiatry
Yale University School of Medicine
New Haven, CT

Jusuf Ulaj, M.D.
Department of Psychiatry
University of Prishtina
Prishtina, Kosova

Cheri Varvil, MSW
Topeka 501 School District
Topeka, KS

Chris Warren-Adamson
Senior Lecturer
Department of Social Work Studies
University of Southampton
United Kingdom

Ann Weick, Ph.D.
Dean and Professor
University of Kansas School of Social Welfare
Lawrence, KS

Introduction and Model
of Practice

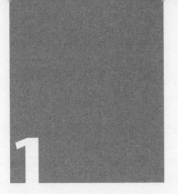

Phebe Sessions and Anita Lightburn

What Is Community-Based Clinical Practice?
Traditions and Transformations

Creative and responsive community-based clinical practice has emerged through a host of initiatives and programs that are now recognized as important means for meeting mental health needs. There is increasing evidence that these alternative approaches are an important addition to traditional practice and that they have a special role in meeting the needs of those whom traditional services have failed to help. In this book, we will be helping clinicians enter into the world of community-based clinical work in the diverse settings in which it is practiced.

To help orient the reader for the richly developed, detailed examples of this exciting area of practice, we will provide in these introductory chapters some succinct, preliminary answers to the following questions: What is community-based clinical practice? What social needs have propelled its development? How is it similar to and different from other traditions of community work, such as community mental health, system of care, community-oriented family therapy, and community organization and empowerment? Where is community-based clinical practice being practiced? What are the values, knowledge base, and skills that support it? What are some of the shared methods in contemporary community-based clinical

practice that differentiate it from traditional practice? Most important for the clinical practitioner, how are these ideas actually being implemented in real-world settings?

In this first chapter, we will focus on addressing what community-based clinical practice is, why it is reemerging now, what traditions it is building upon and expanding, and what significant ideas are fueling its development. In chapter 2, we will describe where it is being implemented and how it is influencing frontline clinical practices. In both chapters, we will prepare the reader for finding rich descriptions of these issues in the clinical applications that are located in part IV.

What Is Community-Based Clinical Practice?

Most commonly, the term "community-based clinical practice" refers to the location of mental health services beyond the walls of formal, medicalized clinics in settings where other kinds of services by other professions are delivered, in the neighborhoods of the client population whom clinicians are serving. This is an important defining characteristic of community-based services. Beyond the issue of the location of services, however, "community-based" also refers to practice grounded in a recognition of the profound interdependence of individual and community well-being, an understanding that the health of one is highly influenced by the health of the other. Community-based practitioners seek an infusion into clinical mental health practice of the values and perspectives of "community," an integration of interventions that build on the healing power of the collective, of belonging to a group that contributes to a social identity and provides opportunities for a meaningful, contributing social role. At the same time, community-based clinicians recognize that the highly specialized knowledge base developed in "the clinic" is extremely useful in "the community" as well, enhancing the capacity of individuals, families, and communities to support the health of all. Community-based clinicians work to render this knowledge usable within neighborhood and outreach settings, often hosted by professions in related disciplines.

There are some inherent tensions between the community and the clinic. An examination of the derivations and root meanings of these two words helps us to understand these tensions and ultimately, we believe, the complementarity of the two. The word "community" is derived from an Indo-European base, *kommein*, meaning "shared by all" (Brown & Isaacs, 1994), and from the later Latin word *communitas*, meaning "fellowship" (*American Heritage Dictionary*, 2000). Brown and Isaacs describe communities as "the most powerful mechanisms for creating human cooperation and reliable interdependence . . . where people learn the meaning of the common good" (p. 509). They discuss how healthy, well-functioning communities can promote collective capability through processes of mutual commitment, collaboration, and opportunities for contributions of diverse talent.

"Clinic" is derived from the Greek word *klinike*, the feminine form of *klinikos*, meaning bed or couch. A clinic is defined as a "facility often associated with a hospital or medical school devoted to the diagnosis and care of outpatients" or "a medical establishment run by several specialists working in cooperation." The adjective "clinical" carries the implications of "very objective, devoid of emotion, analytical, austere and antiseptic" (*American Heritage Dictionary*, 2000). Designation of mental health professionals as "clinical" links them to the histor-

ical traditions of formal diagnosis and treatment of medically linked conditions, interdisciplinary collaboration, and the development and application of theoretically based and scientifically validated knowledge. It implies removal of the patient from various social contexts for observation, study, and treatment of a particular medically defined condition.

In what ways can the community and the clinic enhance each other in pursuit of common goals? Knowledge generated by the scientific traditions and tested for its utility in the "antiseptic" interior of the "clinic" includes theories of human development; effects of trauma and other forms of violence; psychopathological syndromes; theories of risk and resilience; models of practice with individuals, families, and groups; and crisis theory, among many others. This knowledge base not only is profoundly useful for clinicians practicing within the four walls of the clinic but also can be empowering for people in multiple roles, living and working with each other in community settings. Furthermore, much of the knowledge base of the clinic can become desiccated and irrelevant if it is not opened to review and feedback on its utility in less removed, nonmedicalized settings. The clinic needs the exchange with its wider environment; the community needs the additional resources of the knowledge base to which scientific criteria have been applied in the clinic.

What Social Needs Have Propelled the Development of Community-Based Practice?

Recognition of the Toll of Poverty on Human Development

Community-based practice methods have been particularly well developed in contexts in which multiple risk factors create significant challenges to healthy development. Poverty is a major risk factor for poor outcomes in emotional health; this increased risk is due to cumulative rather than single sources of stress (Evans, 2004; Linver, Fuligni, Hernandez, & Brooks-Gunn, 2004; Luthar, 1999). In a review of both psychosocial and physical environmental risk factors, Evans (2004) documents greater exposure of poor children to family turmoil, violence, separation from families, poor air and water quality, more dangerous environments, and poorer quality schools and day care, among other variables. A major impetus for the development of community-based services has been the desire of clinicians to use their knowledge base to prevent poverty from exacting some of its toll in emotional stress through a range of interventions at multiple systemic levels, and extending access to services that lower-income populations might not otherwise seek, have available, or know how to utilize.

Trends Toward Increased Severity of Psychosocial Problems and Psychiatric Symptomatology Among Children and Youth

Reviewing the data from 30 years of research into the prevalence of significant symptoms of emotional disturbance in the American youth population, Achenbach, Dumenci, and Rescorla (2003) reported that the frequency and severity of such problems as reported by parents and teachers increased dramatically between 1973 and 1993. During the past decade, these increases have leveled off in some areas; however, the rates of disturbance remain unacceptably high. For example, suicide has become the third-leading cause of death for American youth, as suicide rates have risen 200% in the past 20 years (McWhirter, McWhirter, McWhirter, & McWhirter, 2004). Both exposure of children to violence and commission of violent acts by children continue at alarming levels (Garbarino, 1999; Jenkins & Bell, 1997). Recent studies (Herrenkohl, Chung, & Catalano, 2004) have shown that risk and protective factors that contribute to or mitigate against violence can be identified early in life. The complexity of the multiple stressors that generate these outcomes leads to increasing interest in integrating targeted clinical interventions with ecological understanding of problems and multitiered strategies to prevent and solve them.

Lack of Skills for Adapting to Increasing Diversity of American Population

The knowledge base and practice methods developed in clinical settings have tended to assume universal norms of human development and symptoms of psychological dysfunction across cultures.

This presumption of sameness has come under significant critique over the past 25 years from within and outside of the mental health professions. Knowledge of the diversity of developmental trajectories and preferred outcomes among cultural groups has increasingly been supported by research and clinical experience (Pumariega, 2003). At the same time, the demographics of the U.S. population, particularly among young families with children, show a marked growth in racial and cultural diversity, which will continue to increase dramatically in the future. These trends highlight the need for increased competence in providing mental health services cross-culturally (Sue & Sue, 2003; U.S. Department of Health and Human Services, 1999).

Erosion of the Centrality of Community Life in the United States and Rise of Communitarian Movement

Recent sociological studies have demonstrated the increasing removal of American citizens from participation in the public arena and community institutions. Etzioni (1993) and Putnam (2000) have been particularly influential in calling attention to the growing privatization of American life and the redirection of energy and engagement to the individualized concerns of family and vocational interests. Mutual aid and social support in times of vulnerability, as well as opportunities for meaningful participation in and contribution to community, are undermined by the demand for self-sufficiency. At the same time, there have been renewed calls for resistance to these trends, with explicit recognition of the social and cultural losses engendered by such deterioration in our social capital. Powerful voices in the social sciences, spiritually inspired visionaries, community advocates, and mental health clinicians speak to the need for community participation and integration in helping and healing (Cushman, 1995; Doherty & Beaton, 2000; Etzioni, 1993; Putnam, 2000). Advocates for attention to strong and supportive communities have cited recent developmental research that demonstrates that human beings are neurologically "hardwired to connect" with others in social relationships that are fundamental to biological, psychological, social, and spiritual development (Commission on Children at Risk, 2003). They seek to promote "authoritative" communities with reengagement of networks of caring and competent adults to support children at risk of poor developmental outcomes.

Dissatisfaction With the Limitations of Office-Based Clinical Practice in Engaging Vulnerable Populations

There is strong evidence that traditional office- or clinic-based mental health interventions do not succeed in serving a substantial percentage of the population in need of services. Historians of the community mental health movement indicate that without powerful advocacy by representatives of disenfranchised groups, services tend to evolve toward addressing the needs of those who are relatively culturally advantaged and who have less severe mental health problems (Cutler, Bevilacqua, & McFarland, 2003; Drake, Green, Mueser, & Goldman, 2003; Lourie, 2003). Office-based services can be delivered more efficiently, though not necessarily more effectively, without outreach efforts or modifications in technique from traditional clinical practices. At-risk populations with multiple challenges are less likely to view mental health interventions as potentially useful and may avoid clinics; clinic-based mental health professionals are often unwilling or unable to change their strategies to engage them, or to have the financial resources to provide the range of systemic interventions needed (Harrison, McKay, & Bannon, 2004; Madsen, 1999).

Service System and Professional Fragmentation Generates Need to Collaborate With Other Professions and Service Systems

Many individuals and families in need of mental health services are embedded in complex transactions with multiple service systems. The effort of clinicians to isolate one problem for intervention often leads to failure, as the conflictual enmeshment of clients in other systems complicates and undermines any single solution. In contrast, locating mental health services in communities promotes collaboration among service providers, enabling more complete understandings of client resources and difficulties to emerge, with complex plans for intervention.

Demoralization and Stress Affecting Human Service Workers With Need for Mutually Enhancing Collaboration

Human service workers in every area and at every level of professional preparation have been reporting increasingly stressful work conditions. They are confronted with more severe mental health problems in clients and community, have fewer resources to address them, and are required to produce and document successful outcomes with larger caseloads and less supervision. Many graduates of professional training programs feel they have been poorly prepared to function in the current contexts of their work (McGinty, Diamond, Brown, & McCammon, 2003). Many frontline nonprofessional workers similarly feel unprepared for and unsupported in their work. Professionals with specialized clinical knowledge and nonprofessionals with specialized local, community-based knowledge can collaborate in ways that renew and synergistically empower each other.

Undermining of Community Capacity Through Expert Knowledge

Clinical knowledge, informed as it is by research and infused with the prestige of its medicalized cultural context, can be used with great effectiveness to enhance the capacity of communities to care for their members. It can also, paradoxically, add another layer of disenfranchisement by undermining the beliefs within communities in their own indigenous sources of support and knowledge. The availability of a critical perspective on these social processes has helped to fuel a necessary humility about the superiority of knowledge that emerges exclusively from the clinical setting. Community-based clinicians have increasingly been motivated by respectful and appreciative curiosity about the resources of clients' cultures and communities (White, 1995).

How Is CBCP Similar to and Different From Other Traditions of Practice in Communities?

Community Mental Health

The development of contemporary forms of community-based clinical practice is occurring 40 years after the passage of legislation supporting the establishment of community mental health centers. The current surge in community-based clinical programs represents a renewal of the vision and goals of the original community mental health movement and an effort to infuse new knowledge into its programs and practices. It is being implemented both within and outside established community mental health centers.

The community mental health movement of the 1960s was inspired by energetic reformist ideals, including a desire to provide services and supports within communities for deinstitutionalized psychiatric patients and a commitment to extend services to underprivileged people in poor communities as part of the more general goal of reducing social inequity (Drake et al., 2003; Lourie, 2003). It was supported by advances in mental health knowledge and methods, particularly with the advent of more effective psychotropic medications, crisis intervention, and milieu and brief therapy approaches. Community mental health sought to apply a public health framework to mental health problems and services, based on a recognition of the need for primary (addressing the universal needs of a defined population), secondary (identifying people who are vulnerable to developing mental health problems at any early stage), and tertiary (intervening in problems with a lengthy history to prevent chronicity and institutionalization) levels of prevention.

The 40 years of experience with community mental health have seen marked successes in expanding access to mental health services for many Americans, and the movement has contributed to the enormous expansion of the mental health professions (Cutler et al., 2003). The goals of the original visionaries, however, have been only minimally fulfilled. Support for the chronically mentally ill through the development of a continuum of care to enable them to participate meaningfully in communities has been inadequate. The equity goals of bringing the resources of mental health knowledge and applying them to underresourced communities to prevent the development of emotional problems in at-risk populations have been repeatedly challenged and undermined. Full realization of the goals of community mental health encountered the roadblocks of erratic and parsimonious funding, lack of evidence of substantial effectiveness in its

early primary prevention efforts, conflict in some of its efforts to engage community boards, active resistance from mental health professional groups when their self-interest was challenged, and gravitation of mental health professionals toward clientele who were more satisfying to treat with their preferred models of intervention than were people with severe mental illness or with multiple psychosocial stressors. By the early 1980s, it was clear that major reform was needed. Jane Knitzer (1982) wrote an important exposé about the collective failure of the institutions serving children, including community mental health, to address the problems of the most vulnerable. In addition, advocates such as the National Alliance for the Mentally Ill and federal commissions inspired by the Carter administration began to decry the sorry state of resources available for the deinstitutionalized mentally ill.

Contemporary community-based clinical practitioners have continued to pursue the goals of the original community mental health act, and they continue to encounter modified forms of the same obstacles. However, they now have 40 years of trial-and-error experience, in addition to systematic study, in community mental health to learn from, as well as many new resources of knowledge and practice methods at their disposal. Greater attention has been paid to developing services that are "of" the community and not simply located "in" the community. This has been facilitated by what Pumariega and Winters (2003) have called "the new community psychiatry"—the system of care movement.

Systems of Care

The past 20 years have seen efforts to implement recommendations for the most vulnerable children and families inspired by the Child and Adolescent Service System Program principles developed in the mid-1980s (Meyers, this volume) and for the severely mentally ill by the community support and rehabilitation movements. Efforts to refocus services to address the needs of the most vulnerable within community mental health and between community mental health and other human service systems have led to innovations with "systems of care," which incorporate the following principles to guide program development:

1. access to a comprehensive array of services that address physical, emotional, social, and educational needs;
2. individualized services for children with emotional disturbance guided by an individualized service plan;
3. services in the least restrictive, most normative environment that is clinically appropriate;
4. full participation by families in all aspects of planning and delivery of services;
5. integrated services with linkages between child-serving agencies and mechanisms for coordinating services;
6. case management to ensure delivery of coordinated multiple services over time;
7. early identification of children at risk;
8. help with transitions from child to adult service systems;
9. promotion of advocacy efforts; and
10. nondiscrimination in access to services and responsivity to cultural differences and special needs (Stroul, 2003; Stroul & Friedman, 1996).

The system of care movement has substantially contributed to the reinvigoration of interest in community-based clinical practice and has affected practice methods in community mental health, as well as in other diverse practice arenas. These practice methods are based in community mental health goals of application of a public health perspective with a range of services from primary, through secondary, to tertiary levels of care; a continuum of integrated services for the most vulnerable clients; and recognition of the cultural location, strengths, and preferences of particular communities. The system of care movement has spelled out the necessary activities to make services accessible, targeted toward at-risk populations, and responsive to community concerns. At the same time, it has been criticized for focusing on a framework for the design of services without addressing the clinical theories and methods of intervention through which these services should be delivered (Fallon, 2003; Stroul, 2003). Stroul, who has been so influential in the development of system of care, has agreed that there is a need for greater attention to the clinical methods that are used to implement these principles. We hope that the "on-the-ground" clinical issues presented in this volume will help to fill this gap.

Family-Centered, Multisystemic Practice

A parallel movement to integrate clinical theory and interventions with systemic, community-based practice has occurred under the auspices of family therapy. Like the community mental health movement, family therapy had its intellectual roots in the 1950s but underwent substantial development beginning in the 1960s. Because it drew on systems and other social rather than psychological theories, family therapy has consistently had a "middle" position between the psychological and medical focus of individual work and the community network approaches. Beginning in the 1960s with Minuchin's groundbreaking work at the Wiltwyck School and extending through the 1970s and 1980s at the Philadelphia Child Guidance Clinic, one branch of family therapy, structural family therapy, particularly focused on experimentation with outreach work in poverty communities (Minuchin, Montalvo, Guerney, Rosman, & Schumer, 1967). The systemic orientation of family therapy succeeded in calling attention to the need to understand the meaning and intractability of any problem in its interactional and social contexts. Though many of the innovative programs of outreach into low-income neighborhoods were undermined by the wavering financial support and moral commitment for the War on Poverty, this systemic orientation has been consolidated in family therapy practice. Nevertheless, in more conservative times, most family therapists as well as individual therapists have gravitated toward practice with more reliable funding and support.

There have been repeated efforts to extend and renew the outreach tradition in family therapy in the ongoing work of the structural family therapists (Aponte, 1995); the narrative therapy practice of Michael White (1995); the reflecting team practices of Tom Andersen (1991, this volume); the important work of Hartman and Laird (1983) in making family therapy theories and methods relevant and applicable to a wide range of social work settings serving disenfranchised people; the culturally affirmative practices of Monica McGoldrick (1998), Nancy Boyd-Franklin (2003; Boyd-Franklin & Bry, 2000), and Celia Falicov (1998); the multisystemic therapy of Scott Henggeler and associates (Cunningham & Henggeler, 1999; Henggeler, Schoenwald, Bourduin, Rowland, & Cunningham, 1998; Henggeler, Schoenwald, Rowland, & Cunningham, 2002); efforts by William Doherty to integrate the communitarian critique into family therapy (Doherty & Beaton, 2000); the community family therapy of Ramon Rojano (2004); and the just therapy of the Family Centre team in New Zealand (Waldegrave, 1990). Some models have evolved to recontextualize their theory bases and methods to reflect postmodern influences. Whether from a modernist or postmodernist epistemology, the family therapy approaches, which have included outreach into community, have all included attention to the dynamics or discourses of social power and marginalization and their effects on people's lives. The practice models and detailed descriptions of skills developed over time by these family therapists provide a basis for implementation of the broadly defined practice principles of the system of care movement.

Community

Practice Traditions in Social Work

Though contemporary community practice is a multidisciplinary effort, the social work profession has contributed rich traditions with numerous models of practice that continue to evolve in response to need. These models seek to increase the capacity and efficacy of individuals through participation with others to improve the quality of life in their community. An unfortunate divide has separated community developers and organizers from clinicians, with strong differences in traditions, training, and ideology. Ten years ago, Specht and Courtney (1994), leaders in the community practice field, criticized the profession of social work for its overreliance on psychotherapy, based on individualistic solutions to social problems, when a community-based system of social care is needed. Social care, in contrast to psychotherapy, emphasizes prevention and normative interventions such as education, mutual aid, and support. The substantive innovations over the past 20 years in community-based services are moving us in the direction Specht and Courtney envisioned.

Over the past two decades there has been a robust conceptualization of community practice methods, including collaborative practice (Tourse & Mooney, 1999); capacity building and empowerment practice (Chaskin, Brown, Venkatesh, & Vidal, 2001; Delgado, 2000; Gutierrez, Parson, & Cox, 2000), community building (Naperstek, 1999; Poole, 2002; Saleebey, 2002); community

enhancement; and the development of urban sanctuaries (Delgado, 1999, 2000).

Collaborative Practice

These traditions emphasize the need to build partnerships with families, based on recognition of the exceptional contribution families make in caring for their relatives who are in crisis, have mental illness, or have other chronic disabilities. Capacity-building strategies in community complement such collaborations and honor family members' commitment and ability as caregivers and advocates. Such strategies enable clinicians to work more effectively with interdisciplinary teams, parents, and consumers to develop more accurate assessments, useful intervention plans, and valuable evaluations. Regardless of research documenting the necessity of collaborative work to achieve good outcomes, there is evidence that clinicians espouse this goal of collaborative practice but often do not fully realize it (see Ayers & Lyman this volume; Lightburn, Olson, Sessions, & Pulleyblank-Coffey, 2002). Nonetheless, collaborative work with families is central in system of care, wraparound approaches, community care for the adult mentally ill, family resource centers, and child welfare innovations (Chamberlin, 1996; DeChillo, Koren, & Mezera, 1996; Friesen, 1996; Kramer & Houston, 1999; Simpson, Koroloff, Friesen, & Grac, 1999). It is also recognized by the New Freedom Commission on Mental Health (2003) as fundamental to supporting mental health and providing community-based mental health care.

Empowerment and Strength-Based Integrative Practice

As indicated earlier, integrative social work practice models based on ecological theory strongly identify with and promote community practice traditions. Prominent among these social work models is empowerment practice (Cox & Parsons, 1994; Lee, 1994), the strengths perspective (Saleebey, 2002); the life model (Germain & Gitterman, 1996), and the person-environment practice model (Kemp, Whittaker, & Tracy, 1997). These integrative models ask that practitioners consider the dynamics of social forces and environmental stressors in our informal social networks, organizations, and communities as foci of practice. While emphasizing different strategies and priorities, each model promotes the development of nurturant supports and solid buffers in communities that are indispensable means for surviving destructive and toxic social realities such as racism, poverty, interpersonal violence, and abuse and neglect. This practice is about more than managing symptoms and coping; it is about liberation, hope, resilience, and transformation.

Of equal importance are the caring traditions of indigenous helpers in multicultural urban centers and the empowered helping that occurs in the nontraditional settings described by Delgado (1999). Clinical services have been translated and transformed through working with indigenous resources, honoring racial and ethnic heritage, and reinforcing collective values and traditional means of helping (Berger, this volume; Delgado, 1999; Gutierrez, Alvarez, Nemon, & Lewis, 1996; Parsons, 1989). An even longer tradition of empowerment in family support and resource center practice, derived in part from the settlement house models of social work, has supported parents' own development, increasing their self esteem and their personal and collective efficacy. Family centers have been described as beacons in the community, with a distinct role in social action (Jones, Garlow, Turnbull, & Barber, 1996; Joseph et al., 2001; Warren-Adamson, 2001; Warren-Adamson & Lightburn, this volume).

Sanctuary: Safe Havens in Urban Environments and Therapeutic Community

In these varied community practice approaches, a dominant theme is the "complex and abiding calculus of resilience," borrowing from Saleebey's (2002) apt summation of the findings from prevention science, "that community and individual or family resilience are inextricably bound together" (p. 229). People need to be part of a cohesive group and will benefit from a culture of care where they are accepted for who they are, often with special needs that must be met, whether this is to recover, gain strength, work out one's identity, or learn life skills. At the same time, there is reciprocity between persons who are in need of their community's help and their need and ability to help others, albeit in initially nascent ways. In this regard, there is a need for communities to have safe havens and sanctuaries where people belong, where they are protected, and where they can rest and find renewal. This can be in clubs, after-school programs, a spe-

cial circle on the street, a day care drop-in center, or a family center where community can be similar to a therapeutic milieu—all places to belong, with new opportunity and life-affirming experiences, respite, and connection (Delgado, 1999; see also Berger, this volume; Eismann, this volume; Levine, this volume; Warren-Adamson & Lightburn, this volume). It is through connection to each other that we nurture the resilience that protects, buffers, and brings forth the capacity to endure and recover from life's hardships and inequities. The potential of communal means for health and development can be realized through approaches that catalyze the creativity, resourcefulness, and commitment of people to each other in new and renewed communities.

Emergent Ways of Thinking

Recent efforts to reconceptualize and reenergize community-based clinical practice are grounded in significant developments in the base of social science knowledge available to it, as well as the social needs we have identified. These developments have, in turn, been profoundly influenced by shifts in the "metaperspectives," or fundamental philosophically based assumptions about what we mean by "knowledge," "reality," or "the self." Is the best and most reliable knowledge that which is derived from experiments to establish cause-and-effect relationships in order to develop abstract systems of knowledge, or are there multiple ways of knowing? Do we think of the "self" as a relatively autonomous "thing" in the interior of a person or as a way of describing a person's experience of continuity in identity? Do we think of language as reflective or constructive of what we experience as "real"? Over the past 30 years, powerful critiques have evolved, often presented under the rubric of "postmodernism," of the dominant assumptions generated during the Enlightenment period of the eighteenth century about what we know and how we know it. The epistemological challenges of postmodernism have infiltrated both the natural and the social sciences and have led to the questioning of such fundamental postulates as the ability of an observer to describe a phenomenon under study with complete objectivity, the ability to establish single cause-and-effect relationships in complex phenomena, the supremacy of abstracted knowledge over any other kind, the applicability of mechanistic models to explanations of human behavior, and the superiority of experimental models that hold constant or screen out the contextual variables affecting an object under study in knowledge production. Explicitly social theories such as social constructionism have developed out of the "postmodern turn" in the social sciences (Gergen, 1999). Social constructionism has been particularly influential in the evolution of ideas about the significance of community, reevaluation of the significance of relationship in human development, understanding of how linguistic practices shape the self in relation to others, shifts in family therapy toward community-inclusive theories and models, appreciation of the importance of culture in providing contexts for meaning, and the importance of understanding how discursive practices of power and privilege influence knowledge generation and therapeutic approaches. While not all clinicians choose to inquire deeply into these "metaperspective" developments, many who do are inspired by the kinds of creative and unexpected ideas that can emerge by exposure to transdisciplinary perspectives that link mental health ideas to broader intellectual themes.

Many contributors to this volume share postmodern assumptions about knowledge construction and have participated in the development of clinical theories and models for practice grounded in this critique. Nevertheless, it would be simplistic to dichotomize community-based from clinical theorists and practitioners simply on this basis. Postmodern theories and models have had a profound influence on practices in "the clinic" as well, but they have also indubitably provided new legitimacy to community-based values and practice priorities through promotion of alternative ways of knowing and healing. Social constructionism not only has developed new ways of thinking but also has brought forward and recontextualized traditional understandings, which were eclipsed by the dominance of beliefs in a narrowly defined scientific method.

In parts II and III of this text, contributors pose questions that attempt to get at how a more communal rather than individualistic orientation affects community-based practice theories, as well as design of essential components for practice that cross different domains.

What Do We Mean by "Community," and How Is It Related to Health and Well-Being?

Ann Weick and Carol Swenson provide rich, thought-provoking chapters on "care" and "community." Without the use of technical and distancing language, Weick engages us in a reflection on the meaning of "care" in this society, which, relative to other cultures, is so unbalanced in its overvaluing of individualism and self-sufficiency and devaluing of communal life. The need for care and caretaking is obviously fundamental to the survival of the species, as well as to the well-being of each individual person. Yet, in American culture, need for care has come to be connected with "deficiency," a stigmatized condition to be avoided or managed with the help of "strangers." The knowledge, skills, and values that enable care to happen within networks of intimate and ongoing relationships are taken for granted and assumed to require no particular acknowledgment or attention. This value stance removes dignity and skill from the important work of care that people are called on to perform all the time. Many functions of care have also been removed from their traditional locations in family and community and transferred to professionally designed services, delivered by technically managed systems. Weick calls for a rethinking of care, with attention to and respect for the informal networks or "webs" of care, as well as integration with the formal systems of service so that they can mutually enhance each other.

Swenson's chapter presents a rich description of various meanings of "community" and the "self" that goes beyond our "taken-for-granted" understandings of these familiar words. She draws on perspectives developed in several social science disciplines, as well as contemporary critical theories, which address how these understandings function in our culture. Teasing apart and elaborating these multiple perspectives helps to generate creative ideas for changing clinical practice interventions based on a richer understanding of community. Swenson reports on two qualitative research projects she conducted in collaboration with other instructors and master's-level social work interns to explore how their understandings of community affected practice. She discovered that the language available to clinicians to describe the meaning of community and work within it pales in comparison with the highly developed frameworks for thinking about the individual self. The process of discovering and uncovering the many different meanings of community then began to generate creative ideas about their clinical relevance and application.

How Does Human Development Occur?

Dennis Saleebey provides a powerful review and critique of academic traditions of understanding human development through the life span. He carefully evaluates what is useful in our ideas about stages of individual development and our emphasis on the role of parents in shaping their children's lives and what is omitted from these dominant theoretical models. Ideas that challenge the exclusivity of traditional developmental paradigms have come from several sources, including studies about resilience that document highly variable responses to exposure to similar adverse events; increased recognition of the significance of some biological givens, such as temperament; the profound influence of peers and cultural influences on children as they grow older; and, most significantly for this text, the differential access that children have to resources within communities that can provide opportunities for support, learning, and meaningful social roles. Saleebey draws on the perspectives of social constructionism to challenge the reality of an isolated and insulated "self" located inside the individual head, and he proposes that we attend to the need for a "developmental infrastructure" based on an appreciation for how multiple social contexts shape development.

How Do Our Linguistic Practices Construct Who We Are?

Lynn Hoffman takes us on a tour, perhaps even a "wild ride" of twisting turns and surprising developments, of different ideas and practices in family therapy that have broadly moved the field from efforts to overpower, instruct, or even trick families into change, to relationally based efforts to enter into conversations that open up possibilities for change. Hoffman describes the paradigm shift that occurred in family therapy as it reexamined its assumptions based on the larger cultural discourses of postmodernism. This shift has enabled clinicians to challenge some of the "elitist, remote, and un-

just" practices in which family therapists had firmly placed themselves in the driver's seat, conducting sessions from an expert view of how families should operate. Embracing uncertainty, engaging in reflexive consideration of one's own assumptions, and abandoning "blueprints" for structuring therapy has helped clinicians to generate conversations with families that more readily elicit their strengths and preferred solutions. From the earliest experiments with family therapy, Lynn Hoffman has been a powerful generator of ideas that have enabled this shift in priorities to occur, and she has been family therapy's most eloquent and insightful chronicler.

How Do Clinicians in Community-Based Practice Select Theories and Practices?

From a similar set of assumptions about the significance of the postmodern turn for community-based clinicians, Marcelo Pakman engages the reader in a challenging and very original discussion of the relationship between theory and practice for community mental health. He asserts that the current demoralization of many community mental health practitioners has been influenced by a disconnection between their "preferred" theories, selected on the basis of their graduate education, and their "theories in use," determined by a multitude of factors largely out of their awareness. Postmodern ideas allow clinicians to explore the relevance of different ways of thinking to the clinical tasks they must perform and to "unpack" assumptions that may be interfering with engagement with the work. Pakman provides a lengthy case example of consultation with a clinician about a particular family in which the deconstruction of these assumptions profoundly helped the clinician to move forward with the case.

How Does a Shift From Understanding Culture as a Static Set of Traits to a Set of Possibilities Influence Clinical Practice?

Catherine Nye begins her chapter with a series of penetrating questions about the meaning of cultural diversity for mental health practice, approaching the issue from a stance of inquiry. To avoid either simplification or dogmatism in this complex topic, she draws on the discipline of anthropology to elaborate multiple answers that have been proposed in response to these questions. She describes the perspective of "universalism" and the sociopolitical context, which supported this view that human beings are essentially the same across cultures so that differences need not be addressed. The perspective of "cultural relativity," in contrast, emphasized the variability in cultures, with the implication that understanding people of different cultural backgrounds in their differentness is challenging and hard to achieve but necessary. Polarization around extreme versions of these perspectives has more recently yielded to integrative positions of "cultural pluralism," which emphasize that cultures develop quite different priorities and worldviews out of a shared base of possibilities shaped by the human condition. The shared base of possibilities enables cross-cultural understanding to occur; the different priorities emphasized by different traditions make it challenging to achieve. Nye addresses the implications for mental health practice of the current demand for cultural competence in clinicians. Initial efforts to become culturally competent in mental health led to descriptions of cultural traits in different groups. More contemporary approaches advise clinicians to inquire actively into their own cultural assumptions and biases, recognizing the influence of the relativity rather than universality of their own frameworks. This kind of inquiry prepares the clinician for curiosity about the values and preferences of others and for a collaborative stance in practice.

Maria Corwin approaches the topic of cultural competence with more direct attention to the mental health and public policy literature. Nevertheless, she reaches some of the same conclusions. She observes that the advocacy of multicultural competence in Child and Adolescent Service System Program (CASSP) and system of care principles, as well as in recent Surgeon General reports (U.S. Department of Health and Human Services, 1999; U.S. Department of Public Health, 2000), has not led to a significant increase in skills in frontline mental health services. Brief trainings in broad principles for cross-cultural work do not penetrate deeply enough into practice delivery models to bring about sufficient preparation for work in an increasingly culturally diverse world. Corwin advocates adoption of a long-term commitment by agencies and the mental health professions, and a planned approach for operationalizing general concepts. She cites the limitations of previous efforts to educate professionals through static descriptions of

"other people's cultures," which led to stereotyping and a reduction in complex understandings. Multicultural competence requires a profound understanding of how culture shapes family life, priorities, and help-seeking behavior and an appreciation for the numerous cultural contexts in which people participate, out of which they forge complex identities. Corwin discusses the importance of clinicians' beginning with exploration of how they have been influenced by their own cultural experiences so that they develop the capacity to "see" and "hear" culture, rather than reducing difference to private, personal histories.

How Do Clinicians Gain Knowledge of the Dynamics and Effects of Social Oppression?

To prepare clinicians to practice cross-culturally demands greater knowledge not only of the meaning of their cultural contexts but also of the ways in which groups, based on race, ethnicity, religion, gender, sexual orientation, and health status, are exposed to different degrees of privilege or discrimination. Corwin's chapter addresses some of the social justice issues in mental health services and the need to ensure equal access, appropriate services, and equitable outcomes for all the cultural groups that agencies serve. This may require greater emphasis on strengths-based and culturally valid assessments, and skills oriented toward collaborative models of practice.

In their chapter, Susan Donner and Joshua Miller focus on preparing clinical practitioners to recognize and address issues of racism in themselves and in the organizations in which they practice. Drawing on their experiences in leadership in enhancing the knowledge base and skill level for antiracist activities in professional education and agency practice, they address questions about the significance of these activities, the strategies for implementing them, and the range of experiences that clinicians have as they engage in them. In their work, they push through resistance against acknowledging the ongoing significance of race in American society and in mental health practice. They point to the profound discrepancies in perceptions between many people of color and their white counterparts, both professional and nonprofessional, about cross-cultural dynamics. The inability to express and understand such differences contributes to dysfunctional and ineffective clinical encounters. Donner and Miller courageously step into this contested area to share their experiences as trainers and guides to prepare agencies and practitioners for more culturally informed practice.

How Would a Shift from Regarding Evaluation as an "After-the-Fact" Assessment of a Program to Thinking of It as a Generative Force in Program Development Affect Researchers, Program Developers, and Practitioners?

As an orientation for clinicians, program directors, and researchers, Martha Dore and Anita Lightburn present an overview of the form and phases of community-based evaluation, emphasizing the value of a constructivist approach. Program evaluators have appreciably broadened the scope of traditional outcome-based research as they have tackled challenging questions about the effectiveness of system of care and comprehensive community-based mental health care. We understand from their work the importance of grappling with the complexity of multisystemic programs, with widely varying perspectives on desired outcomes, and the need to account for the impact of community factors and the fidelity of planned intervention on the provision of care. And while we have learned important lessons from notable community-based studies, such as the Fort Bragg demonstration (Hoagwood, 1997), there remains considerable misunderstanding about evaluative methods, with a lasting misperception of what constitutes a useful evaluation of outcomes. In part, this misperception concerns the importance and place of process evaluations. Drawing from their evaluation experience, Dore and Lightburn illustrate how outcome evaluations can be significantly improved. They advocate for a developmental approach to evaluation, which contributes to the iterative process vital to refining programs and practice. Specifically, this helps community-based clinicians provide process information that is crucial in explaining outcomes of interventions and that enables them to identify interventions that can benefit from modification.

Dore and Lightburn show how a constructivist approach to evaluation involves a dance of learning and change toward a well-defined end: affecting systems change and refinement of both practice and outcomes that are more likely to be culturally rel-

evant and useful. Because a constructivist approach is collaborative, involving multiple perspectives from all stakeholders, including clinicians and consumers, there will be more productive avenues for understanding the meaning of "self in community" and the complex nature of community practice that is situated in and interdependent with community life. To manage all this with limited resources presents a prodigious challenge. Nonetheless, it is critical that we develop worthwhile evaluations of community-based clinical practice, with evidence that the outcomes measured are sensitive enough to show change, and therefore merit continued investment.

How Do We Prepare the Next Generation of Community-Based Clinical Practitioners Through Graduate Education and Postgraduate Training?

Mary Olson's chapter addresses these issues of education and training by presenting a richly developed curriculum for helping students and postgraduate professionals obtain the knowledge base and practice skills for collaborative models of practice. Beginning with the Batesonian premise that the self is a communal and linguistic construction, Olson examines four applications of postmodern family therapy, including the reflecting team practices of Tom Andersen, the Finnish Open Dialogue approach, the narrative therapy of Michael White, and the linguistic turn in feminist, multicultural, and social justice models. These approaches foster powerful relational connections in family and community to generate problem dissolution or transcendence. She carefully describes the principles of dialogue in clinical work as a conversational practice designed to generate new, previously unimagined possibilities for families and shows how these more collaborative models of practice are consistent with, and bring to the direct practice level, the broader principles of a system of care framework. Included are detailed examples of teaching methods and exercises to help the learner become deeply engaged in the learning process and to relate the more abstract theoretical principles to specific clinical interactions. Finally, she presents an in-depth case example of a young African American woman whose impending psychiatric hospitalization is prevented through family engagement.

How Does Innovation for Community-Based Clinical Practice Get Generated and Sustained?

Part III of this text, the "leadership journey," includes the contributions of four innovators in community-based practice who, without well-developed models to draw on, created new ways of bringing clinical understandings to community settings. Though all these innovators are firmly grounded in lengthy careers in clinical practice, their efforts to reform mental health services occur at the practice-policy interface. One innovator describes primarily her work in program development and policy formulation (Meyers); another in mental health administration (Ayers and Lyman); another in direct practice, teaching, and international network development (Andersen); and one in direct practice and program development (Eismann). Contributors were asked to describe the reforms they set in motion, the resistance they encountered, and some of the personal meaning that stepping out of their inherited disciplines had for them. Therefore, some of the chapters have included personal reflections, particularly when contributors' initiatives for reform engendered conflict, disappointment, and periods of professional isolation. Attending to the personal meanings and effects of innovation can help readers who are contemplating or already engaged in bold, but not fully supported, reform efforts.

Reforms initiated by Tom Andersen from an exquisitely beautiful but geographically remote part of Europe, above the Arctic Circle in Tromsoe, Norway, have had a profound influence on clinical practice theory and methods throughout the world. Andersen presents the development of a collaborative network of services and training programs that were initiated throughout Scandinavia, and now extend into Russia and the Baltic States of Eastern Europe, based on a profound shift in his understanding of how to think and talk about helpful collaboration in response to crises in families. Andersen describes his emergence from a successful and privileged career with full medical school teaching credentials into a more challenging relationship with the profession of psychiatry as he recognized the greater potential for healing in the recognition and enhancement of social networks. He began to advocate for community-based services, which drew people into the healing process instead of removing a targeted "patient" for individual intervention outside of his or her community of meaning. These changes had to be developed with little initial support, and sometimes active antagonism from professional stakeholders. Andersen describes his search for generative ideas and methods throughout Europe and the United States, as well as from within his own cultural traditions, which allowed him to begin an ongoing and open-ended process of formulating and reformulating practice theory, intervention models, and training programs, eventually leading to the development of an organized international network. One of the most striking aspects of Andersen's story is his stance of openness and inquiry in relation to ideas, methods, and practices, which enables him to be affected cognitively and emotionally in conversation with others. Though his work is based on firm commitments to principles of social constructionism, dialogue, collaboration, the use of "reflecting teams" in mental health practice, which he created, and the importance of networks in people's lives, his ability to allow himself to be "moved" by what he experiences in body, mind, and soul, in relationship to families and other coworkers, has enabled continuous evolution of his ideas over time. We are pleased to be able to bring his story forward.

Edward P. Eismann's story is similarly one of rebellion against the limited goals of traditional mental health services that utterly failed to engage a population of children in the South Bronx in need of an infusion of interest and resources to allow their capacity for reciprocal responsibility for each other to emerge. Few mental health providers have Eismann's courage to walk away from a securely defined job with salary, benefits, and other forms of protection and to allow himself through trial and error, as well as creative adaptation of inherited psychodynamic and social theories, to create a mental health service for children on the street. However, in every generation there are some who do, and this is an important story for those considering the costs and benefits of such a move. Eismann's story also helps to put those of us who are more risk averse, or who choose to work toward change from within established institutions, in touch with a particular moral compass and vision that is unyielding in the face of opposition, resilient after setbacks, and profoundly generative for the children with whom he engages.

Judith Meyers tells a story of struggles to implement mental health reform for children and families through her direct engagement in policy formulation and program implementation for an entire state. Meyers's story is one of powerful leadership to negotiate change in the midst of financial constraints and resistance from entrenched bureaucracies and stakeholders on multiple levels of government. It is also a description of a kind of leadership with which many women professionals will identify. Meyers, as a behind-the-scenes, obscure congressional aide, managed to "slip in" a brief provision into mental health legislation in the early 1980s that created the Child and Adolescent Service System Program. This act has revolutionized the principles to guide practice promoted by the subsequent commissions that have studied the state of child mental health, and it is currently influencing many programs of service attempting to implement system of care for children and families. Meyers's story includes both direct pursuit of goals and use of indirect means, always with carefully attuned awareness of the context in which she is trying to promote change.

The story of the Cambridge Youth Guidance Center, provided by Susan Ayers and Russell Lyman, describes the transformation over time of a traditional child guidance clinic into the child- and family-serving branch of an urban community mental health center and, finally, into a freestanding agency negotiating contracts with multiple funders. Terminating the integration with community mental health paradoxically enabled the agency to respond more flexibly to the mental health needs of children and families throughout the community. The agency leaders established a continuum of care based on a public health framework of primary, secondary, and tertiary levels of prevention. Ayers and Lyman present a case that helps to illustrate the impact of these philosophical, organizational, and programmatic changes on one family over time. They also address important issues of the impact on clinicians of efforts to implement system of care principles in a traditional mental health agency and the effects of using different funding streams.

Conclusion

In this chapter, we have tried to orient the reader to the field of community-based clinical practice and its increasing significance. We have grounded these practices in previous efforts to integrate clinical and community work and some of the more recent theoretical developments, which have infused these efforts with new energy. We now turn to the important questions of where these ideas are being applied in particular arenas for practice and how their application influences particular methods of practice.

References

Achenbach, T., Dumenci, L., & Rescorla, L. (2003). Are American children's problems still getting worse? A 23-year comparison. *Journal of Abnormal Child Psychology, 31,* 1–11.

American Heritage Dictionary (4th ed.). (2000). Boston: Houghton Mifflin.

Andersen, T. (1991). *The reflecting team: Dialogues and dialogues about the dialogues.* New York: Norton.

Aponte, H. (1995). *Bread and spirit.* New York: Norton.

Boyd-Franklin, N. (2003). *Black families in therapy* (2nd ed.). New York: Guilford.

Boyd-Franklin, N., & Bry, B. (2000). *Reaching out in family therapy: Home-based, school and community interventions.* New York: Guilford.

Brown, J., & Isaacs, D. (1994). Merging the best of two worlds: The core processes of organizations as communities. In P. Senge, A. Kleiner, C. Roberts, R. Ross, & B. Smith (Eds.), *The fifth discipline fieldbook* (pp. 508–517). New York: Doubleday.

Chamberlin, R. (1996). Primary prevention and the family resource movement. In G. Singer, L. Powers, & A. Olson (Eds.), *Redefining family support: Innovation in public-private partnerships* (pp. 115–134). Baltimore: Brookes.

Chaskin, R., Brown, P., Venkatesh, S., & Vidal, A. (2001). *Building community capacity.* New York: Aldine de Gruyter.

Commission on Children at Risk. (2003). *Hardwired to connect: The new scientific case for authoritative communities.* New York: Institute for American Values.

Cox, E., & Parsons, R. (1994). *Empowerment-oriented social work practice with the elderly.* Pacific Grove, CA: Brooks/Cole.

Cunningham, P., & Henggeler, S. (1999). Engaging multiproblem families in treatment: Lessons learned throughout the development of multisystemic therapy. *Family Process, 38,* 265–281.

Cushman, P. (1995). *Constructing the self, constructing America.* Reading, MA: Addison-Wesley.

Cutler, D., Bevilacqua, J., & McFarland, B. (2003). Four decades of community mental health: A symphony in four movements. *Community Mental Health Journal, 39,* 381–398.

DeChillo, N., Koren, P., & Mezera, M. (1996). Families and professionals in partnership. In B. Stroul (Ed.), *Children's mental health* (pp. 389–408). Baltimore: Brookes.

Delgado, M. (1999). *Social work practice in nontraditional urban settings.* New York: Oxford University Press.

Delgado, M. (2000). *Community social work practice in an urban context: The potential of a capacity enhancement perspective.* New York: Oxford University Press.

Doherty, W., & Beaton, J. (2000). Family therapists, community and civic renewal. *Family Process, 39,* 149–161.

Drake, R., Green, A., Mueser, K., & Goldman, H. (2003). History of community mental health treatment and rehabilitation for persons with severe mental illness. *Community Mental Health Journal, 39,* 427–440.

Etzioni, A. (1993). *The spirit of community: Rights, responsibilities and the communitarian agenda.* New York: Crown.

Evans, G. (2004). The environment of childhood poverty. *American Psychologist 59,* 77–92.

Falicov, C. (1998). *Latino families in therapy: A guide to multicultural practice.* New York: Guilford.

Fallon, T. (2003). Strengthening the clinical perspective. In A. Pumariega & N. Winters (Eds.), *Handbook of child and adolescent systems of care* (pp. 107–120). San Francisco: Jossey-Bass.

Friesen, B. (1996). Family support in child and adult mental health. In G. Singer, L. Powers, & A. Olson (Eds.), *Redefining family support: Innovation in public-private partnerships* (pp. 259–290). Baltimore: Brookes.

Garbarino, J. (1999). *Lost boys: Why our sons turn violent and how we can save them.* New York: Free Press.

Gergen, K. (1999). *An invitation to social construction.* London: Sage.

Germain, C., & Gitterman, A. (1996). *Life model of social work practice* (2nd ed.). New York: Columbia University Press.

Gutierrez, L., Alvarez, A., Nemon, H., & Lewis, E. (1996). Multicultural community organizing: A strategy for change. *Social Work, 41,* 501–508.

Gutierrez, L., Parson, R., & Cox, E. (2000). *Empowerment in social work practice: A source book.* Pacific Grove, CA: Brooks/Cole.

Harrison, M., McKay, M., & Bannon, W. (2004). Inner-city child mental health service use: The real question is why youth and families do not use services. *Community Mental Health Journal, 40,* 119–131.

Hartman, A., & Laird, J. (1983). *Family-centered social work practice.* New York: Free Press.

Henggeler, S., Schoenwald, S., Borduin, C., Rowland, M., & Cunningham, P. (1998). *Multisystemic therapy of antisocial behavior in children and adolescents.* New York: Guilford.

Henggeler, S., Schoenwald, S., Rowland, M., & Cunningham, P. (2002). *Serious emotional disturbance in children and adolescents: Multisystemic therapy.* New York: Guilford.

Herrenkohl, T., Chung, I., & Catalano, R. (2004). Review of research on predictors of youth violence and school-based and community-based prevention approaches. In P. Allen-Meares & M. Fraser (Eds.), *Intervention with children and adolescents: An interdisciplinary approach* (pp. 449–477). Boston: Allyn and Bacon.

Hoagwood, K. (1997). Interpreting nullity: The Fort Bragg experiment—A comparative success or failure. *American Psychologist, 52,* 546–550.

Jenkins, E., & Bell, C. (1997). Exposure and response to community violence among children and adolescents. In J. Osofsky (Ed.), *Children in a violent society* (pp. 9–32). New York: Guilford.

Jones, T., Garlow, J., Turnbull, H., III, & Barber, P. (1996) Family empowerment in a family support program. In F. Singer, L. Powers, & A. Olson (Eds.), *Redefining family support* (pp. 87–112) Baltimore: Brookes.

Joseph, R., Friedman, R., Gutierrez-Mayka, M., Sengova, J., Uzzell, D., Hernandez, M., & Contreras, R. (2001). *Final comprehensive report: Evaluation findings and lessons learned from the Annie E. Casey Mental Health Initiative for Urban Children.* Tampa: University of South Florida, the Louis de la Parte Florida Mental Health Institute, Department of Child Studies.

Kemp, S., Whittaker, J., & Tracy, E. (1997). *Person-environment practice: The social ecology of interpersonal helping.* New York: Aldine de Gruyter.

Knitzer, J. (1982). *Unclaimed children: The failure of public responsibility to children and adolescents in need of mental health services.* Washington, DC: Children's Defense Fund.

Kramer, L., & Houston, D. (1999). Hope for the children: A community-based approach to supporting families who adopt children with special needs. *Child Welfare, 78,* 611–635.

Lee, J. (1994). *The empowerment approach to social work practice.* New York: Columbia University Press.

Lightburn, A., Olson, M., Sessions, P., & Pulleyblank-Coffey, E. (2002). Practice innovations in mental health services to children and families: New direction for Massachusetts. *Smith Studies, 72,* 279–301.

Linver, M., Fuligni, A., Hernandez, M., & Brooks-Gunn, J. (2004). Poverty and child development: Promising interventions. In P. Allen-Meares & M. Fraser (Eds.), *Intervention with children and adolescents: An interdisciplinary approach* (pp. 106–130). Boston: Allyn and Bacon.

Lourie, I. (2003). The history of child community mental health. In A. Pumariega & N. Winters (Eds.), *Handbook of child and adolescent systems of care* (pp. 1–17). San Francisco: Jossey-Bass.

Luthar, S. (1999). *Poverty and children's adjustment.* Thousand Oaks, CA: Sage.

Madsen, W. (1999). *Collaborative therapy with multistressed families.* New York: Guilford.

McGinty, K., Diamond, J., Brown, M., & McCammon, S. (2003). Training of child and adolescent psychiatrists and child mental health professionals for systems of care. In A. Pumariega & N. Winters (Eds.), *Handbook of child and adolescent systems of care* (pp. 487–509). San Francisco: Jossey-Bass.

McGoldrick, M. (1998). *Re-visioning family therapy: Race, culture, and gender in clinical practice.* New York: Guilford.

McWhirter, J. J., McWhirter, B. T., McWhirter, E. H., & McWhirter, R. J. (2004). *At-risk youth: A comprehensive response* (3rd ed.). Pacific Grove, CA: Brooks/Cole.

Minuchin, S., Montalvo, B., Guerney, B., Rosman, B., & Schumer, F. (1967). *Families of the slums.* New York: Basic Books.

Naperstek, A. (1999). Community building and social group work: A new practice paradigm for American cities. In H. Bertcher, L. Kurtz, & A. Lamont (Eds.), *Rebuilding communities* (pp. 17–33). New York: Haworth.

New Freedom Commission on Mental Health. (2003). *Achieving the promise: Transforming mental health care in America.* Final Report (DHHS Publication No. SMA-03-3832). Rockville, MD: Author.

Parsons, R. (1989). Empowerment for role alternatives for low-income minority girls: A group work approach. In J. Lee (Ed.), *Groupwork with the poor and oppressed* (pp. 27–45). New York: Haworth.

Poole, D. (2002). Community partnerships for school-based services: Action principle. In A. Roberts & G. Greene (Eds.), *The social worker's desk reference* (pp. 539–544). New York: Oxford University Press.

Pumariega, A. (2003). Cultural competence in systems of care for children's mental health. In A. Pumariega & N. Winters (Eds.), *Handbook of child and adolescent systems of care* (pp. 82–107). San Francisco: Jossey-Bass.

Pumariega, A., & Winters, N. (2003). *Handbook of child and adolescent systems of care.* San Francisco: Jossey-Bass.

Putnam, R. (2000). *Bowling alone: Collapse and revival of American community.* New York: Simon and Schuster.

Rojano, R. (2004). The practice of community family therapy. *Family Process, 43,* 59–79.

Saleebey, D. (2002). Community development, neighborhood empowerment and individual resilience. In D. Saleebey (Ed.), *The strengths perspective in social work practice* (pp. 228–244). Boston: Allyn and Bacon.

Simpson, J., Koroloff, N., Friesen, B., & Grac, J. (1999). Promising practices in family-provider collaboration. In SAMHSA (Eds.), *Systems of care: Promising practices in children's mental health, 1998 Series* (Vol. 2). Washington, DC: Center for Effective Collaboration and Practice, American Institute of Research.

Specht, H., & Courtney, M. (1994). *Unfaithful angels: How social work has abandoned its mission.* New York: Free Press.

Stroul, B. (2003). Systems of care: A framework for children's mental health care. In A. Pumariega & N. Winters (Eds.), *Handbook of child and adolescent systems of care* (pp. 17–35). San Francisco: Jossey-Bass.

Stroul, B., & Friedman, R. (1996). The system of care concept and philosophy. In B. Stroul (Ed.), *Children's mental health: Creating systems of care in a changing society* (pp. 3–23). Baltimore: Brookes.

Sue, D. W., & Sue, D. (2003). *Counseling the culturally diverse: Theory and practice* (4th ed.). New York: Wiley.

Tourse, R., & Mooney, J. (1999). *Collaborative practice.* Westport, CT: Praeger.

U.S. Department of Health and Human Services. (1999). *Mental health: A report of the Surgeon General.* Rockville, MD: National Institute of Mental Health.

U.S. Department of Public Health. (2000). *Report of the Surgeon General's Conference on Children's Mental Health: A national action agenda.* Washington, DC: Author.

Waldegrave, C. (1990). Just therapy. *Dulwich Centre Newsletter, 1,* 6–47.

Warren-Adamson, C. (Ed.). (2001). *Family centres and their international role in social action.* Aldershot, UK: Ashgate.

White, M. (1995). *Reauthoring lives: Interviews and essays.* Adelaide, Australia: Dulwich Centre Publications.

2

Anita Lightburn and Phebe Sessions

Community-Based Clinical Practice
Re-Creating the Culture of Care

The culture of mental health care is being reshaped through community-based innovations, both across the United States and internationally, that are enabling healing and recovery in community. This chapter will present where the evolving traditions of community-based clinical practice have been most influential. As we preview the practice examples in this volume, the values and perspectives of community work come to life. We will see that mental health care is being transformed through clinicians' recognition that working *with* the resourcefulness and meaning of community is more than simply working *in* community.

Examples of some of these programmatic innovations include systems of care in child and adolescent mental health (Lourie, Stroul, & Friedman, 1999; Pumareiga & Winters, 2003; Stroul, 1996); the community care movement with assertive community treatment (Burns & Santos, 1995; Test, 1998); the family resource movement with family support and resource centers (Chamberlin, 1996; Joseph et al., 2001; Warren-Adamson, 2001; Weissbourd, 1987); community schools (Comer, 1995; Corbin this volume; Dryfoos, 1994) and school-family-community partnerships (McDonald et al., 1997); and social development initiatives with the "communities that care"

programs based on prevention research (Catalano & Hawkins, 1996). These programs honor the role that community has in people's well-being, as well as the clinical knowledge and skill needed to respond to serious mental health problems. Practice in these mental health, education, and child welfare arenas benefits from an infusion into clinical and community work of preventive, more normative and socially based interventions. These programs are largely based on ecosystemic thinking. The study of human ecology stresses that people are part of many different communities in which their reciprocal relationships shape how they learn, work, socialize, play, recover, care for one another, and create meaning in their lives. Ecosystemically oriented mental health interventions require involvement with the community as it supports families and as families, in turn, contribute to the development of more sustaining communities. Practice strategies that have evolved from these innovative programs are described as "promising practices" and guidelines for practice (see, e.g., Adelman & Taylor, 2000; Substance Abuse and Mental Health Services Administration (SAMHSA), 1998–2001; Singer, Powers, & Olson, 1996; Shore, 1997; Stroul, 1996). These guidelines support building capacity in communities through transferring knowledge and skill to families, to natural helpers, and across disciplines. An orientation to this new/old terrain follows, which for many is a new map for clinical practice in and with community.

Situating Community-Based Clinical Practice

The practice examples in this volume help to delineate the geography of this terrain. Our contributors challenge long-held ideas about the purpose, values, and assumptions that underpin traditional clinical knowledge and service delivery. They illustrate major developments in community-based clinical practice, with many authors providing integrated models of community-based care. Descriptions of lessons learned through research and innovative practice bring into focus the communal nature of practice, in which collaborative and integrated services generate systems of care, wraparound services, supportive social networks, sanctuaries, and communities of concern. Crucial to this work is providing continuity of care, supporting recovery through working with strengths, building capacity within the community and its caregivers, improving cultural competence, building alliances with consumers, and working for nonviolence and social justice. In deeply humane ways, these approaches call for building networks of concerned clinicians who assume collective responsibility for working with the needs that people have for each other. While much of their work in community responds to helping those who are seriously ill, distressed, and most vulnerable, community-based practitioners pay considerable attention to prevention to ensure strong developmental pathways and protection from violence and abuse.

Characteristics of Community-Based Clinical Practice

What follows is an overview of the principles, programs, and methods of community-based clinical practice in all the arenas described in this volume. As a means of describing the transformation of mental health care that is in process, we include three tables contrasting these evolving community-based principles and methods with many of the

limitations often experienced in traditional clinical settings. These tables, and the discussion of their contents, address changes that have taken place in the organization of community-based service, the community dynamic in service provision, and changes in clinical methods.

Community-Based Services

Table 2-1 lists basic characteristics of service provision. An overview of the major themes points to a transformation of services to be more expansive, inclusive, and responsive. They seek to ensure timely service provision, crisis response instead of waiting lists, continuity and a continuum of care, including individualized wraparound services, and the least restrictive option for care in the community.

Comprehensive Integrated Care

Intrinsic to all community-based services is the communal structure of service provision, which often integrates multiple services and includes the consumer in decision making. This communal structure stands in contrast to more traditional, fragmented services with their competing agendas and mandates rooted in a single solution tradition. Its development has been influenced by consumers who have been frustrated with and alienated by the minimal control they have had over their care, and their confusion over how to gain effective help with complex problems. Systems of care have been developed in recent years to provide comprehensive services based on multisystemic solutions that can occur with interdisciplinary teamwork and cross-professional inquiry and practice.

Accessible Care and the Development of a Continuum of Services

Traditional practice in the hospital, clinic, or office has provided limited options for working with the ecosystem. In contrast, colocating services in a school or neighborhood means that they are more accessible and can respond more flexibly to population needs. Through a web of relationships with human service providers and natural helpers, a continuum of care and wraparound services can be more readily developed and managed.

Outreach is a meaningful component of the continuum of care as a proactive way for community service providers to reach the most vulnerable

Table 2-1. Changes in the Organization of Clinical Services

Limitations of ineffective traditional clinical practice	*Efforts by CBCP to address limitations of traditional practice*
Fragmented, overlapping services competing agendas and mandates, single system solutions	Multi-systemic, comprehensive services that can include wraparound services, and a continuum of care
Patient-client treatment with clinician as director and expert; with inflexible design	Intensive service when needed with multiple modalities; an individualized plan that is flexible in design; interdisciplinary teams and cross-professional inquiry into practice and program solutions
Professionally conceptualized, organized, and delivered services	Consumer involvement in service design and plans (person-centered); families as partners
Institutional-based service provision (hospital, outpatient, residential treatment)	Co-located neighborhood based and accessible services in schools and community centers
Service determined by diagnosis (*DSM4*)	Developmentally responsive continuum of care; prevention to early intervention for high risk populations and at points of violence or trauma
Contract fee for service; autonomous and isolating practice	Intensive services and timely approaches for crisis management; use of service and natural networks
Waiting lists for service offered in a clinic	Crisis responses provided in the location
Institutional care removes individual from the community without transitional work to re-integrate back to community; clients trapped in long term institutional care	Use of institutional care for time limited crisis care; with integration plan for return to community; least restrictive care/solutions; maintain connections to community
Fee for service structure for outpatient services limits coordination of services	Integrated resources—mental health, juvenile justice; child welfare; education; and third party, foundation, and demonstration funding
Client's indigenous knowledge replaced by professional's theoretical knowledge	Diverse role responsibilities for clinicians who use clinical knowledge to guide outreach workers, advocates, mentors, natural helper and families

Adapted from A. Lightburn (2003). Systems of care: Expanding the response to school violence. In Miller, J., Schamess, G., & Martin, I. (Eds.), *School violence and children in crisis*. Denver, Co: Love Publications.

members of the community. There is a shift in where services are provided, which may be at home or in the street, a car, a local club, a police station, or a neighborhood program. Similarly, changes in the names of programs where help is received, such as the Neighborhood Place, Partners for Success, FRIENDS, Unitas, and the Family of Friends, signify a shift in the expectations for collaboration between professionals and consumers, reducing the stigma of mental health care in a clinic.

Intensive Services and the Benefit of Community Connections

Of utmost importance is the opportunity for emotionally vulnerable individuals to remain in their communities rather than becoming isolated and potentially trapped in long-term institutional care, at exceptional personal and financial cost. This requires services that are based in community that can provide intensive care "24/7," using multinodal approaches that are flexibly designed to meet individual need until stability is regained. This more expansive approach is rooted in different ideologies of helping, where professionals bring knowledge and skill to join with those of natural helpers and consumers. Expert knowledge makes a contribution but is not dominant. The onus is on practitioners to translate, educate, share, and collaborate with community members. Consumers are valued for their ideas and their capacity to be partners in the design, implementation, and evaluation of service.

The Community Dynamic in Service Provision

Table 2-2 introduces themes that characterize how communities provide protection and opportunities for growth and development, and are powerful resources for recovery and healing.

Table 2-2. Community Dynamics in Service Provision

Ineffective traditional clinical services	*Community-based clinical practice*
Clients receive services without contributing roles for others	Use of communal dynamic for healing, growth, development, and change; alternative and reciprocating contributions
Symptom reduction through individualized services	Recovery model; integration into community belonging and support
Clinical care separate from community care	Integrate clinical approaches with community care
Individual modality primarily; goal is symptom reduction, working through developmental arrest; interpretation leads to change	Family focused and family centered; enhance capacity through collectives, i.e., multi-family groups, psychoeducation/support
Care limited to therapeutic relationship	Milieu as a safe haven and developmental system; networks of relationships (kin, neighbors, natural helpers)
Individual target of change; capacity building of individual client	Enhances community and individual capacity; including capacity building activities in developing community resources
Mono-cultural based on universalistic theories and approaches	Culturally responsive professions and practice; bilingual; linguistic competence, integration of indigenous knowledge and preferred solutions
Privacy of services that are insulated from community	Focus on communities and neighbors as resources to draw upon and develop mutual aid; emphasizes belonging to community and citizenship
Therapist works with individual or family alone to resolve presenting problems	Collective focus, group; network-interconnections and interdependence
Social, contextual issues, including social power, are not addressed	Can address social justice issues (integration of policy and practice)

Adapted from A. Lightburn (2003). Systems of Care: Expanding the response to school violence. In Miller, J., Schamess, G., & Martin, I. (Eds.), *School violence and children in crisis*. Denver, CO: Love Publications.

Healing Communities

Multirelational bonds in community happen in sanctuaries, multifamily groups, and supportive alliances and partnerships. Through these community connections, friendships can flourish, and mentors and advocates provide guidance. Relationships with others support social learning through reciprocity, a learned helpfulness, which means that people are contributors to community as well as being recipients of all that community can provide. Participating in community reinforces belonging and identity, with shared goals, hope, and creative solutions. This type of belonging mitigates against social and physical isolation, which are known to contribute to depression, neglect, and alienation. In community, we experience compassion, being with others in their struggles, sharing one common humanity, finding our moral compass, and celebrating the meaning of brotherhood and sisterhood.

Building the Community of Service Providers

Communal approaches involve building formal and informal networks of service providers to support a system of care. The goal is to encourage participation and commitment to one another to function as a helping, caring community. Community building supports accountability and mutual appreciation and is a catalyst for resilience in service providers.

A Culture of Care and the Collective Power to Change Communities

Some of the limitations of individual solutions through traditional approaches become apparent when dealing with social problems such as violence and poverty, which contribute to stress and dysfunction. Our contributors demonstrate the importance of the strong associational community to ensure well-being. Associational communities are familiar places with culturally shaped traditions for giving and receiving help that honor indigenous knowledge and preferred solutions. Traditional services often use monocultural, universalistic theories and approaches and do not include ways of addressing social context and social power. With a communal focus, social justice concerns influence the understanding of problems and the development of solutions. Communal care depends on shared values that promote attachment, family, friendship, citizenship, nonviolence, mutual aid, acceptance, respect, forgiveness, and reconciliation. These values come alive in relationships that are both therapeutic and community-based.

Community-Based Clinical Work

The changes in the culture of care are based on widely varying assumptions about clinical practice and theories that explain recovery, growth, and coping. Some of our contributors have developed integrated models of practice, weaving together traditional and ecosystemic theories as guides for practice, while others have clearly set out in another direction, stating that traditional theories are inadequate to guide community-based practice and research. Contributors emphasize the need to adapt evidence-based approaches to meet the needs of consumers in diverse communities. Others emphasize the need to understand theories in action as a more realistic way of explaining and evaluating clinical work.

Clinical work in community means working in flexible ways, with interdisciplinary teams, and with consumers as partners. There is a new critical

perspective on knowledge and authority as indigenous knowledge and traditions are honored, and power is shared in decision making and in shaping and providing services. Table 2-3 summarizes clinical processes illustrated in the practice examples and is elaborated upon in the discussion that follows.

Ecosystemic Approaches

Community-based clinical work relies on a systemic, contextual, and transactional focus for defining problems and solutions, rather than on interventions that focus on internal psychology and personality change. This focus requires ecosystemic assessments, which are concerned with risk and protective factors in individual, family, culture, and community. Such assessments focus on strengths and assets that are identified as resources for solutions and recovery. The assessment process also can include diagnosis, which is considered as part of a more realistic picture of functioning, but not the sole criterion for defining problems and solutions.

Evidence-Based Approaches

Clinical work in the community is concerned with promoting resilience, buffering risk, and develop-

Table 2-3. Changes in Clinical Methods

Limitations of ineffective traditional clinical practice	Efforts by CBCP to address limitations of traditional practice
Assessment focused on diagnosis	Assessment based on risk and protective factors in individual, family, culture, community; strengths-focused
Intervention aims to correct or eliminate deficit in functioning; narrow focus on symptom removal, learning only to deal with problems	Intervention promotes resilience, buffering risk, developing protective factors Psycho-education, skill development, transformative learning, mastering life's curriculum
Focus on internal psychology and personality change	Systemic, contextual and transactional focus in defining problems and solutions; synergistic effects: sum is more than parts
Problem-solving, directive conversation	Emphasis on generative dialogue (reflexive process, intersubjective, open dialogue)
History reconstructive of "causative events"	Narrative construction of preferred solutions and identities, inclusive of local traditions and rituals
Therapist uses learned and preferred theories and models	Evidence based approaches (PACT, MST, social development) and community-based orientation emphasizing practice guidelines and principles that support system of care
Clinical knowledge applicable mostly in direct service to client	Indirect use of expert knowledge; use of clinical professional to coordinate care and as consultant, catalyst to develop culture of care

Adapted from A. Lightburn (2003). Systems of care: Expanding the response to school violence. In Miller, J., Schamess, G., & Martin, I. (Eds.), *School violence and children in crisis*. Denver, CO: Love Publications.

ing protective factors rather than primarily focused on eliminating deficits in functioning. Clinical work draws from the substantial findings of prevention science and from evidence-based individual, family, multisystemic, and community care approaches. Practice guidelines, protocols, and program evaluations contribute to refining practices so that they meet diverse needs in different communities and environmental contexts.

Proactive Family-Centered and Caregiver-Centered Strategies

The proactive work of community-based practitioners is family centered and, when appropriate, caregiver centered. This practice is in line with the family-centered practice movement's principles for practice, which recognize the family's central role in child development and caregiving, understand and work with systemic influences on families, build alliances with families and caregivers as colleagues and partners, emphasize their strengths, and work together with them and their community (Ronnau, 2001).

Narrative Approaches

Narrative means to therapeutic and communal ends provide increasingly valued ways to involve people in community. Narrative therapists are interested in the healing potential of dialogic process, stories, and coconstruction of solutions. Based on social constructionism, attention is given to how language shapes experience and to the deconstruction of professional discourses, so that they facilitate rather than constrict generative conversation. Strengths-based and empowerment-focused narrative works contribute to prioritization of interventions that tackle social justice issues.

Psychoeducation, Support, and Empowerment

Psychoeducation has emerged as an important staple of community-based clinical work. It is a tradition that has been productively coupled with supportive practices, including multifamily groups and other types of community groups. Collective learning opportunities are developed in response to serious needs to manage crises, traumatic life experiences, and illness. Strategic ways of advancing empowerment also include transformative and experiential learning approaches in adult education. The integration of these educational methods with clinical practice in the community offers normative

methods that are important catalysts for growth and development that move beyond traditional clinical work focused on symptom removal.

Integrating Mental Health Principles Into Social Life

Traditional use of clinical knowledge is most applicable in direct services with clients. While helpful, this approach does not take into account the potential of influencing the client/consumers' ecology through the integration of mental health principles woven into the social fabric that supports daily life. Integration of mental health principles is evident in the way that a community is developed through meetings, conferences, marathons, collaborations, and informal networks of consumers. It is also evident in program content in family support programs, school classrooms, after-school programs, and the workplace. Mental health principles are transported to the street where youth gather, and in neighborhood centers where drama, art, music, and recreation provide a rich medium for development and healing.

Capacity Building

Community-based clinicians also have important roles in enhancing the capacity of caretakers, service providers, consumers, and communities. Capacity building is a primary enabling intervention that makes it possible to achieve basic goals such as protection and safety, reduced barriers to learning in schools, support for parenting and caretaking, support for recovery of the mentally ill, and work for nonviolence and social justice. Capacity building involves developing mutually held commitments, resources, knowledge, and skill. Such goals, investment, and commitment to each other make it possible to set priorities, stay focused, and be accountable for follow-through with service plans and the use of resources. Capacity building is a proactive intervention that involves reaching out to interdisciplinary team members, such as teachers, nurses, and police officers, to develop collaborators in responding to interpersonal violence and racism, and to support inclusion of people with special needs and abilities.

This brief overview of the transformation in mental health care illustrates the changes in the way services are delivered, the importance of community to mental health, and the nature of clinical work that re-creates the culture of mental health care in community. Our contributors advance our understanding of the implications of these changes as they present the building blocks for practice in community and enrich this picture in their practice examples.

The Practice Arenas

In this volume we have organized practice examples around four major practice arenas: (1) early intervention and family support; (2) school-based practice; (3) community-based mental health services for children and families; and (4) community mental health for adults.

Early Intervention and Family Support

A Supportive Day Care Community

In this volume Martha Dore, Nancy Feldman, and Amy Gelles illustrate the benefits of a collaborative approach among parents, teachers, administration, and social workers within a day care community. Their work enhances the capacity (knowledge, skills, resources, and sense of efficacy) of providers and parents and increases the connections between caregivers and parents. Developed as a means for reducing child abuse and neglect based on research findings that identified community- and personal-level risk factors, the Family of Friends project drew on the concept of primary prevention with the goal of strengthening protective factors. This intervention was designed to enhance families' and children's experience in day care, build capacity in parents to parent and handle stress, and create a sense of community to provide social and emotional support for parents.

Program elements included parent chat groups led by professional social workers, a Parent Academy that provided peer educators to support parenting, and parent leadership development. Day care providers partnered with clinicians, learning together in the classroom, as they supported children's emotional and social development. Teachers' relationships with parents improved as they learned about parents' struggles and needs, and as they gained skill in child management. A new pattern of reciprocity was apparent: parents became more involved in the day care program, and teachers became involved in parent activities. Training and support enabled all to use knowledge about child

development and the special needs of traumatized children. This work requires nurturing, patience, and creativity, as well as knowledge of evidence-based curricula that can offer new avenues for supporting children's social, emotional, and cognitive development (see Yoshikawa & Knitzer, 1997; and the violence prevention curriculum of the Committee for Children, 2004).

Programs of Family Support for Fragile Families

The arena of family support in community-based programs includes intensive programs that are part of a continuum of care for families and children in crisis. These programs may target families' special needs, such as HIV/AIDS, domestic violence, substance abuse, and/or mental illness. As an underutilized resource for child welfare, family support centers often prevent out-of-home placement. When placement is necessary, centers help families to maintain attachment bonds through visiting until reunification can be supported. Most important, these programs integrate therapeutic work with a protective agenda to ensure that children and parents are safe. Clinicians in family support programs roll up their proverbial sleeves and grapple with life as it happens, during and between group sessions, standing in doorways, over cups of coffee, and in filial play groups, as well as when conflict between kin and friends spills over into center life. Mental health principles are integrated into the fabric of center life, blending educational and empowerment approaches with therapy. Authors in this volume describe the development of family support services and the complex clinical issues they address, with a growing research base affirming their value.

Chris Warren-Adamson and Anita Lightburn, drawing from their experiences in the United Kingdom and the United States, describe a model for integrated family center practice, which creates a caring culture of protection and nurturance in contrast to parents' experiences in disorganized and often dangerous neighborhoods and homes. Clinicians' varied responsibilities in the family center model include community-building activities within the center for staff and families in addition to individual, family, and group therapy and support. This integrative model of practice includes traditional and communal practice and works to provide needed services that support parents' development and ability to contribute to the life of the family center and to their personal communities. Professionals collaborate with natural helpers and parents to create the special synergy of these centers, where the total is more than sum of the parts. Warren-Adamson and Lightburn see this synergy as an important product of the family center that functions like a developmental system, similar to a family, that is both enabling and protective. This example is reflective of a generation of family center programs that integrate mental health services, with responsibilities for child protection, and grassroots community development (Canavan, Dolan, & Pinkerton, 2000; Hess, McGowan, & Bostko, 2000; Joseph et al., 2001; Lightburn & Kemp, 1994; Warren-Adamson, 2001; Weiss & Halpern, 1990).

Intensive Family Support Programs Within a Continuum of Mental Health Care for Troubled Children and Families

Family support programs can also be delivered through traditional mental health agencies that have explicitly modified their service delivery model to provide a continuum of care. Replacing histories checkered with institutional and foster care, families are helped to succeed in their communities. The family's needs, priorities, and abilities to partner become the focus for planning, support, and coordinating care, as illustrated in chapters by Susan Ayers and Russell Lyman, and Russell Lyman and Borja Alvarez de Toledo. These authors describe the revolutionary process of change in a traditional child guidance clinic as it moved from "agency-centered" and child-centered practice to family-centered and family-focused community practice. The Guidance Center's various specialized family support programs make it possible for it to work with young, stressed, and vulnerable families and those who are struggling with children and adolescents with serious emotional and behavioral disturbance. Creative outreach and after-school programs, investment in teamwork, and aggressive collaboration with schools and other community programs make it possible to integrate and fine-tune individualized treatment, weaving together services so that families receive the continuum of care with the level of intensity they need. The continuum of care also can extend over multiple generations of a family, ensuring stability through continuity in relationships.

In an era of managed care that tends to support mostly short-term treatment, it is critical to develop other means for meeting the needs of seriously troubled parents and children who need continuity in relationship, as well as time to heal and grow. The Guidance Center's community-based, "grassroots" system of care provides both ease of access and continuity of care. Its approach has prevented long-term residential care and hospitalization, kept families together, protected friendships, and provided opportunities to participate in normal community activities (Lyman, Ayers, Siegel, Alvarez de Toledo, & Mikula, 2001).

Family Support Outreach and Community Care

Outreach programs to strengthen at-risk families are vital for those who are stressed by HIV and AIDS. Community-based support flexibly responds to the needs of these parents and children wherever and whenever they occur—at home, in hospital rooms, traveling in the car to appointments, and at school. In this volume, Sandra Gossart-Walker and Robert Murphy provide a deeply humane description of the complex issues for parents as they manage an unpredictable illness while continuing to parent. Intimate knowledge of community resources, excellent connections with school personnel, and close work with child welfare services enable clinicians to foster understanding with all who can ease the trauma of suffering and loss.

Support means providing continuity for children from someone in the community who holds their history and can carry it forward on their behalf, so that it becomes part of their ongoing life with new caretakers. Clinicians support the web of community connections with advocacy and mediation to strengthen the often thin network of family and friends. This community-based work breaks through the isolation and loneliness in the final stages of illness, anticipates and works to meet complex emotional needs, and creates ways for parents and children to receive critical support. Clinicians weave together a caring community for children, parents, and their extended families who would otherwise have to manage on their own. Mental health needs are responded to as they emerge, anticipating loss, grieving, and mourning for what will never be, preparing children for new lives, and coping with the anger, suffering, and depression that are part of the roller coaster of illness that now may extend over many years.

Comprehensive Integrated School-Based Services

With the exponential development in school-based mental health services over the past 20 years, there has been a noticeable shift to a community-based model of clinical practice. Clinicians help school-based professionals think holistically about their students, to see social and emotional development as complementary and integral to cognitive development, academic achievement, and success in school. Adelman and Taylor (1997), from the UCLA National Center for School Based Mental Health, have championed the position that students experience "barriers to learning" and that all school programs should have an enabling component to address these barriers with interventions that include community-based clinical practice. They define six areas for intervention:

1. enhance classroom-based efforts to enable learning;
2. provide students and family assistance;
3. respond to and prevent crises;
4. support transitions;
5. increase home involvement in schooling; and
6. develop greater community involvement and support. (p. 416)

Partners for Success

In chapter 20, Phebe Sessions and Verba Fanolis introduce an example of a comprehensive program, Partners for Success, and the clinical work required to fully enable students to learn. They bring to life a 10-year collaboration of mental health providers and educators, illustrating how this multifaceted, multirelational work can develop in low-income urban elementary schools. Partnership and collaboration were the hallmarks of this multifaceted initiative for children, who otherwise would not have had access to mental health services. The evolution of this university–public school partnership illustrates how community-based practice transcends a narrowly defined individual focus and responds to the developmental and other pressing needs of the children and their schools. In an educational system encumbered by federal and state mandates to improve academic performance, it was essential for mental health providers to promote the emotional health of children to enhance learning through re-

moval of barriers to learning within the school environment. The unique structure of this partnership involved training sizable teams of clinical social work students so that there were sufficient resources to respond to the needs of teachers and students, have an impact in the school community, and evaluate innovative practice approaches. As a lively learning organization, this school partnership continued to change over time, responding to new needs, such as developing an early childhood consultation and prevention program.

System of care principles became guides for practice, so that an ecosystemic and strengths perspective shaped assessments and interventions, with priority given to culturally responsive services that worked with the African American and Latino heritage of the children. Outreach was supported to engage and partner with families. Classroom consultations, group work, and crisis intervention were dynamic components of the preventive work. Investment in capacity building enriched the knowledge and skill of administrators, teachers, and community providers to understand and help children who had been traumatized by continued exposure to violence. Partnerships extended to African American and Latino community centers, supporting center staff through training and program development to further benefit local children and families. These partnerships proved to enhance connections with the school.

Community Schools and the School Development Program

The focus on building protective factors that support learning for all students has also taken place in the context of school reform and comprehensive approaches to human services. Schools have become important centers for colocating services and integrating approaches to achieve an overall mission, such as a seamless web of services to support the needs of children and youth in low-income communities (Bix, Landergan, & Ford, 2000; Comer, 1995; Dryfoos, 1994). In her chapter, Joanne Corbin introduces one of the more prominent community school reform models, the Comer School Development Program (SDP), that has been instrumental in the development of community schools for more than 30 years. Developed in 1968 in New Haven, Connecticut, the SDP has supported schools in building partnerships between parents and the school community to work for equal opportunity in education for poor urban communities. The Comer SDP has been extensively researched, with reports of positive outcomes for students, including improved academic performance, school attendance, behavior, and self-concept, as well as school climate, and increased parent involvement. The Comer SDP has contributed significantly to the school's ability to effect change.

Corbin sees the professional challenge as one of leadership in helping a school build an effective community. The clinician's role is to support the development of relationships throughout the school community. The quality of relationships within the school is essential in building community. Ultimately these relationships determine improvement in the school climate that directly influences improvement in student learning. From her perspective, clinicians need to take on expanded roles that include environmental and resource assessment, mediation, and assisting the system with goal attainment and political action. Of equal importance is the clinician's educational role in helping the teachers and administration understand and respond to the developmental needs of the students.

Developing a Community of Concern Within a Public School

In a similar communal tradition, E. Martin Schotz, Ruth Dean, and Jane Crosby present their creative work in an inner-city school in Boston, Massachusetts, where children are treated as "beloved members" of the community. These authors, based in a community mental health clinic located in a public school, discuss how they revitalize the school community in addition to providing clinical work. They are guided by a philosophy of practice that emphasizes building a "community of concern" (to use Martin Luther King's phrase) for all members of the school community. They illustrate how this purpose shapes their work and transforms students', teachers', and parents' experience of alienation. They see social injustice at the base of students' social and psychological problems. This perspective leads them to use solutions that provide opportunity, acceptance, and inclusion. They advocate for long-term plans to support community change, counter injustice, and work on the shared goal of developing a culture of nonviolence. This

approach necessitates helping teachers and administrators understand oppression and how it affects their students and themselves. Their generative communal approach has drawn previously isolated and distrustful parents together to become involved in the school, which for this multiethnic and racially diverse school is a considerable achievement. Clinical work with individual students and in groups utilizes the strengths perspective, focusing on solutions that build capacity and emphasize the values of friendship and mutual aid.

Countering the Effects of Trauma for High School Adolescents

Ann Marie Glodich and her colleagues, a committed interdisciplinary team, are concerned with developing proactive ways of helping adolescents who have been traumatized by violence. In their chapter, they report on the development and refinement of a psychoeducational group for high school youth who are predisposed for recurrent risk-taking behavior. Because this problem can lead to substance abuse, violent acts, and dangerous thrill seeking, they have developed a dynamic collaboration with high school teachers and guidance staff, as well as the local police, to support their work. Like the community of concern, this approach brings together the resources of clinicians, teachers, administrators, and local police to help these young people understand the influence of early life experiences on current behavior and to learn how to act responsibly.

The psychoeducational program is shaped by an understanding of trauma and is guided by a protocol that includes facilitating dialogue about real feelings, fostering mentalizing capacity, and building compassion. Research continues to refine and validate how this approach works for individual students. As a nonstigmatizing prevention program, this intervention engages young people who would eventually endanger themselves and others, with long-term consequences. As community-based clinical practice, there is the added outcome of building capacity within the school and community (including the police) to understand trauma, and how the potential developmental sequelae of abuse and violence can be altered by preventive psychoeducation. This approach has also had the effect of building a network of advocates for traumatized adolescents.

Community-Based Mental Health Services for Children and Families

Systems of Care

Community-based clinical practice has been supported by systems reform in children's mental health, beginning with the Child Adolescent Service System Program (CASSP) in 1984 and now the current Comprehensive Community Mental Health Programs (supported by SAMHSA). These programs have been at the forefront of the development of a system of care for children and adolescents with serious emotional and behavioral disturbances. The success of these initiatives has led many states throughout the United States to develop systems of care at the state, county, or community level, or in some instances at multiple levels. This substantive change in the way services are delivered continues to challenge clinicians to develop models of practice that are congruent with the intent and philosophy of community-based care. There is much agreement that effective mental health practice requires adaptation of evidence-based approaches and theory-driven practice for use in community.

Federal, state, and foundation support has made it possible to create systems of care, such as the new developments in Connecticut's Community KidCare, described in this volume by Judith Meyers. Other community-based programs presented in this volume have creatively developed a system of care approach based on its philosophy and practice guidelines, including Yale's In-Home Child and Adolescent Psychiatric Services (IICAPS) family program described by Jean Adnopoz, Katherine Levine's example of a family-sponsored program that collaborates with a visiting nurse mobile crisis unit, and Russell Lyman and Borja Alvarez de Toledo's child guidance center's intensive community-based intervention. For these programs to accomplish an integrative approach, they must take responsibility for coordinating the various services (mental health, child welfare, education, and juvenile justice), as well as developing intensive, short-term services that ensure continuity in important helping and supportive relationships.

These systems-of-care approaches share the belief that changes in the environment will foster changes that persist over time for children, families, and communities (Burns, Schoenwald, Burchard, Faw, & Santos, 2002). They all share an ecological frame to guide assessment, intervention and culturally competent practice, office and home-based care provision (support and therapy), around-the-clock service provision when needed, a planned use of residential care and hospitalization with transition plans back to community, individualized wraparound services, and development of a continuum of care within the community. Interventions are typically strength based. Family therapy is based on systemic theory and is primarily solution focused, with support for family empowerment and natural supports integrated with therapeutic interventions. Substance abuse and violence are recognized as contributors to the clinical and social situation, so that interventions address safety, trauma, and recovery. Other service providers and parents are all valuable partners instead of adversaries or competitors in providing care. Each approach acknowledges that clinical knowledge and skill are critical to coordinating and ensuring quality care. Lyman and Alvarez de Toledo recognize the depth of knowledge and skill needed to do this work well; they advocate for the work of the "systems doctor," who works to draw together the web of services, melding the helping relationships for a unified approach.

These authors all integrate a wraparound philosophy and methodology, based on the model develop by Burchard, Vandenburg, and Dennis (Burchard, Bruns, & Burchard, 2002). The goal is to avoid institutional care through a plan that integrates services to meet the individual needs of a child or adolescent. Integration of fragmented services (child welfare, school, mental health) with friendly, normal supports such as parent advocates, mentors, big brother and sisters, after-school programs, recreation, and respite has reduced the need for institutional care and has maintained children and youth in their communities (Burchard et al., 2002; Santarcangelo, Bruns, & Yoe, 1998). Inside and outside knowledge of the community, with well-developed connections and ample use of creativity, ensure access to the multilevel services that are needed.

Both Adnopoz and Levine provide integrative practice approaches that address the complex, interrelated needs of the child, family, and community. The Yale IICAPS model draws from child development and family systems theory, developmental psychopathology, and a system of care perspective. Interdisciplinary teams work with family issues and communication and ensure that families are partners in the decision-making process and have the support they need. Multifaceted help is brought into the family home to improve family functioning. The FRIENDS tri-level care model requires that support and education are offered through home visits, as well as a neighborhood support program, entitled "Staying Strong," for families and their children. This program is based on multifamily group approaches and a 12-step model. Emotional stressors are seen as part of everyone's life; therefore, families need to gain strength and confidence through building their own emotional fitness, to enable them to cope with the stressful communications and erratic behaviors of family members with serious emotional disturbances. Nurturing a culture of care includes building a community for the family through multifamily groups and a drop-in center to mitigate isolation and stigma and to support the value and use of information and education about mental illness.

Outreach Programs for Targeted Populations of Vulnerable Children and Families

Nontraditional interventions reach out to meet children, families, and individuals where they are. For some, it is at the point in their lives when unimaginable violence or disasters cause serious crises and disruptions, challenging their ability to cope and in some instances survive. For other high-risk youth, it involves engaging them in relationships that will be a bridge to opportunities that enhance development and facilitate resilience. Our authors support engaging with those who might never seek or be able to access mental health services at critical junctures when they most need help.

The first example is the Child Development–Community Policing Program (CDCP), an innovative collaboration between police and child mental health professionals based in New Haven, Connecticut. This collaborative makes it possible to coordinate clinical work for children exposed to violence, using the crisis point as an opportunity to buffer its effects, help stabilize the situation, and make the connection to supportive community services as needed. The second program is a community mental health outreach program in Brighton Beach, New York, for Russian immigrant youth who are at high emotional risk because of traumatic experiences as refugees, continued social isolation, and economic hardship. The third practice example is the Neighborhood Place, designed as a prevention program to increase opportunities and provide supportive relationships for children and adolescents who were struggling with school and serious behavioral and emotional difficulties that had gone untreated. These collaborative services, which are linked with the police, schools, community centers, and community mental health clinics, are alternative programs that successfully engage traumatized children and youth and others who are alienated and marginalized from poor, disenfranchised communities. Based in their neighborhoods, using acceptable social and cultural avenues for engagement, these programs depend on imaginative use of relationships in nontraditional settings, such as a police station office or on the street, and through art, drama, activities, and recreation. These approaches enhance existing resources in the community and build capacity to enable more finely tuned, helpful responses from those involved in working in taxing and distressing circumstances. Clinical knowledge informs and guides decisions, shapes human interactions, and provides complex explanations for behavior and emotional responses.

Collaboration With Police

Steven Marans and Miriam Birkman, from the Yale Child Study Team, provided the leadership 10 years ago for a unique and productive collaboration with the New Haven police to provide an acute response to violence. They report that from 1998 to 2001, 2,443 children and youth have been seen through the CDCP consultation service. Built on the foundation of the community policing movement, this program is currently replicated in 12 communities across the United States. Special training programs create opportunities for police and clinicians to learn from each other. Training for police emphasizes understanding child development and the effects of traumatization, so that they can more readily recognize when intervention is needed. The 24-hour consultation involves complex issues about safety and psychological responses, and challenges in developing appropriate plans, which can include removing a child from an unsafe home. Plans are based on an integrated understanding of internal and external environmental factors affecting a child's experience, the need for safety, as well as environmental stability and psychological support.

The CDCP has enhanced the capacity of human

service providers to successfully collaborate with the police so that there are real alternatives for children who would have suffered from traumatizing events they could not control. The capacity to work with trauma victims is greatly enhanced with timely intervention, which often extends beyond the initial encounter to support ongoing therapy. The importance of working with the police's authority is highlighted as an integral means for accomplishing therapeutic goals Familiarity with the community enables police officers and clinicians to work together with neighbors, kin, and a wide range of supports that are instrumental in protecting children and helping troubled families.

Outreach to Immigrant Youth

Roni Berger introduces a mental health outreach program for adolescent immigrants that benefited from a decade of support from the Jewish Board of Family and Children Services. The considerable mental health needs of immigrant youth, who immigrated during their adolescent years and are considered at high risk for serious mental health concerns, are met through nontraditional, culturally sensitive, and culturally acceptable services. Berger presents these adolescents' need for support as they manage the double challenge of navigating adolescent development and acculturation to their new environment. Often caught between worlds, in conflict because of their obligations to their parents and new friends, these young people experience depression, anxiety, and suicidal preoccupation and become involved in substance abuse and delinquent activities. These youth need help as they struggle to find their niche within their new communities, where experiences of exclusion, coping with prejudice, and the development of a multicultural self influence their well-being.

Berger also reminds us to honor resilience, mindful of what she terms "PTSD growth," which acknowledges the strengths that often have developed out of refugee experiences. This strengths-based assessment needs to be balanced with a sensitivity to "PTSD risk" that has resulted from multiple losses of family, friends, homeland, familiar homes, and schools and the trauma of war. Because of these adolescents' unusual histories, it is also important to recognize unanticipated risk in their new communities. Innovative use of relationships helps to bridge the cultural divide that often requires challenging and reconciling the burden of exclusion and prejudice. This often begins with developing new respect for one's own cultural heritage and then fostering cross-cultural understanding to reinforce identity formation. The role of the community-based practitioner is often that of an interpreter, engendering understanding through presenting the complexity of their situation to teachers, other providers, families, and the youth themselves.

The Neighborhood Place

Paula Armbruster and her colleagues describe a multidisciplinary collaborative developed as an effective means of engaging and helping troubled youth. The entry point was the Neighborhood Place, an after-school program and a summer arts and athletics program. With a mission similar to that of the 21st Century After-School programs, which have been developed to increase academic success through mentoring and social activities, this program embeds mental health interventions within a creative arts and athletic program. The Neighborhood Place was designed as an alternative social experience with positive adult relationships. Activities were offered that broadened children's experiences into a world beyond their neighborhood. The arts and athletics provided a vehicle for self-expression and for the development of social skills, with clinicians collaborating with teachers and coaches to help youth indirectly with their emotional and behavior problems. A parent program augmented this work so that connections could be made and support given. Junior counselors provided mentoring, offering someone with whom to identify, respect, and trust.

This unconventional, 8-week, intensive mental health program was well received by all who participated. Parents were grateful for a safe environment that was a real alternative to life on the streets. There was the added benefit of enabling teachers, artists, and coaches to understand their students' particular struggles and to experience alternative ways of relating as they joined clinicians in helping youth become more competent in group situations, modify aggressive behavior, and increase their sense of achievement and self-worth. This intensive program created new pathways for growth and development, mitigating disadvantage through the arts and sports and providing youth with more relational experiences than an individual weekly therapeutic session.

Adult Community Mental Health

Three emerging models of community care are described by our contributors from their work in very different contexts, in the United States, northern Europe, and Kosovo. Each model re-visions community care, examining assumptions about recovery, exploring new use of language and the therapeutic process, and working with scarce resources to build capacity in support of the mentally ill and their families. These approaches respect an individual's capacity to be more than their illness, without long isolating periods in institutional care and with a good quality of life in the community. Each respects and collaborates with families, who are often caretakers, and optimizes natural supports. Foremost in this re-visioning of community care is the importance of relationship in the journey to recovery, with respect for the individual's right to self-determination. Some of these approaches are grounded in a profound recognition of how language and dialogue shape human connections through shared meanings that are elemental to new ways of coping and help to counteract the stigma associated with mental illness.

The Recovery Model

Larry Davidson and his colleagues in the United States advocate for a recovery model based on consumer direction, supported by professionals functioning as tour guides. In this volume, they describe recovery as a process that is mediated through supportive, collaborative relationships. Their integrated model of community-based care is based on a strengths perspective, with an emphasis on individual competencies in living, in contrast to the medical model's concern with deficits and prescriptions for treatment. The community-based clinician's goal is to enhance personal agency that enables the individual in recovery to take multiple paths to join in community.

Consumers learn to work with supportive services, develop life skills, and find personal direction. Supplanting traditional therapeutic models and case management, the clinician's role is to help consumers discover their abilities to participate in community for the benefit of others, as well as for themselves. With guidance and persistence, the work patiently unfolds, helping consumers to navigate their recovery. Cultivating hope and support is essential. Assistance is given in ways that respect the consumer's pace. An emphasis on interdependence in community is made meaningful through developing lasting connections with others.

Open Dialogue

Developed by Jaakko Seikkula and a team of Finnish academicians and clinicians, and affiliated with a larger network of similar services in Scandinavia described by Andersen (this volume), open dialogue has become a welcome alternative to traditional institutional and clinic-based care for the mentally ill. As Seikkula describes this community-based network model, professionals provide guidance in the use of dialogic process to transform and shape ways of making meaning of the experience and suffering of mental illness. Professional staff respond immediately to psychiatric crises by convening networks of involved participants to gain an understanding of the individual's current situation. This effectively reduces isolation and draws on multiple perspectives and new ways of understanding that shapes recovery. Open dialogue does not privilege professional knowledge but seeks to use this knowledge in a transparent way to create "openness" that makes it possible to join together the understanding of all involved to work together on an equal footing. Dialogue is conversation that depends on concerted attending to what others are saying. Based on the notion of dialogic process drawn from the work of the Russian linguist Bakhtin, the emphasis is on constructing meaningful communication so that connections with a supportive network are possible. Seikkula presents the evolution of open dialogue work in Finland, where an accumulated research base shows that this approach reduces the need for medication and the use of hospitalization and promotes integration into the community.

A Community-Based System of Care in Kosovo

Ellen Pulleyblank-Coffey, James Griffith, and their colleague in Kosovo, Jusuf Ulaj, describe a collaboration between the American Family Therapy Academy (AFTA) and the University of Prishtina that bridges two cultures to develop a community-based system of care for a people in a country ravaged by war. They focus on building capacity in the Kosovar professional community to work effectively, despite a scarcity of resources, but with unswerving commitment, to address the exceptional needs of the Kosovar people who are recovering from ethnic civil war. Working with family traditions, they provide outreach and home visiting and links to community and outpatient services as part of an evolving system of care. Multifamily work (McFarlane, 2002) is seen as complementary to the Kosovar cultural traditions that respect families as primary mediators for their members' care. Inviting families to come together becomes an effective way of crossing the barriers caused by shame and the stigma of mental illness. New ways of coping are shared that enhance mutual aid among families, and medical knowledge helps promote understanding of mental illness. Efforts are made to link families with needed services, scarce as they are, as a step toward integrating support that begins to work as a system of care. Training nurse-practitioners as outreach workers enabled them to work in families' homes, creating a solid bridge between the clinic and those who would not otherwise seek out needed services.

Critical Incident Stress Debriefing

Critical incident stress debriefing is introduced as an intervention used for vulnerable populations that have experienced disasters and trauma-inducing events. This approach was used after events like the high school shootings at Columbine, the bombing of the federal building in Oklahoma City, and the World Trade Center disaster of September 11, 2001, to bring people together as a means of support and mutual aid and to connect them to needed resources in their communities. The goal is to restore hope and enhance group survivorship and community recovery from devastating experiences where the social fabric that holds people together has been torn. Clinicians have teamed with national disaster organizations to provide critical incident stress debriefing to meet the unprecedented need of whole communities reeling from the disaster caused by terrorist acts.

In this volume Joshua Miller details the process involved in debriefings, describing how it helps individuals and members of a community understand and cope with their physical and emotional reactions and develop avenues for healing, self-care, mutual aid, and support so that they are able to reengage in their lives. Drawing from a diverse number of personal debriefings, he reflects on nuanced ways to shape the process to meet different participants' needs and preferred ways of relating. The use of strength-based and empowerment approaches, the creation of individual and group narratives, and the use of group process all contribute to the quality of the experience for participants and depend on the orientation and skill of the facilitators. Miller observes that benefits can be increased through training peers to work with clinicians, so that participants have the experience of gaining help from those who have worked beside them and are living with similar grief and trauma (e.g., fellow firefighters, construction workers, police, or volunteers from the community). He emphasizes that clinical judgment and skill are critical after events such as the attacks of September 11, 2001, because it is important to assess who might be at risk for depression and self-destructive behavior, thus requiring referrals for further treatment.

Miller acknowledges that there is limited evidence that debriefings prevent future post–traumatic stress disorder. He notes, however, that numerous reports indicate that those who receive debriefings find them helpful. Debriefings are acts of constructing and reconstructing a group narrative of tragedy and disaster. How this occurs is important for research and reveals how the community's culture of care can be facilitated by community-based clinicians.

Conclusion

In developing this geography of community-based services, we have conceptualized clinical practice in and with the community and introduced four practice arenas where community-based innovations are well established. We are optimistic that community-based clinicians will continue to facilitate a communal practice that integrates clinical knowledge and skill with community interventions, as there are robust examples of the transformative power of this work. Clinical approaches in systems of care and community-based programs depend on the special synergy of communal life to support mental health. Clinicians who work in communities have opportunities to be full citizens of those communities, committed to work together with shared concerns, in partnerships and collaborations with consumers as a catalyst for healing and change. Much has to be done to champion these advances. It is incumbent on practitioners to understand the paradigm shift that has occurred. These new and different assumptions about resilience, prevention, recovery, and clinical practice in community with consumers influence how we will continue to re-create this new culture of mental health care.

References

Adelman, H., & Taylor, L. (1997). Addressing barriers to learning: Beyond school-linked services and full service schools. *American Journal of Orthopsychiatry, 67,* 408–421.

Adelman, H., & Taylor, L. (2000). Shaping the future of mental health in schools. *Psychology in the Schools, 37,* 49–60.

Bix, P., Landergan, K., & Ford, R. (2000). The Ford School Village. *Collaborative for Integrated School Services Newsletter, Field Notes, 5:*4.

Burchard, J., Bruns, E., & Burchard, S. (2002). The wraparound approach. In B. Burns & K. Hoagwood (Eds.), *Community treatment for youth* (pp. 69–90). New York: Oxford University Press.

Burns, B., & Santos, A. (1995). Assertive community treatment: An update of randomized trials. *Psychiatric Services, 46,* 6669–6675.

Burns, B., Schoenwald, S., Burchard, J., Faw, L., & Santos, A. (2002). Comprehensive community-based interventions for youth with severe emotional disorders: Multi-systemic therapy and the wraparound process. *Journal of Child and Family Studies, 9,* 283–313.

Canavan, J., Dolan, P., & Pinkerton, J. (Eds.). (2000). *Family support: Direction from diversity.* London: Jessica Kingsley.

Catalano, R., & Hawkins, D. (1996) *The social development model: A theory of antisocial behavior.* In D. Hawkins (Ed.), *Delinquency and crime: Current theories* (pp. 149–197). New York: Cambridge University Press.

Chamberlin, R. (1996). Primary prevention and the family resource movement. In G. Singer, L. Powers, & A. Olson (Eds.), *Redefining family support: Innovation in public-private partnerships* (pp. 115–134). Baltimore: Brookes.

Comer, J. (1995). *School power: Implications of an intervention project.* New York: Free Press.

Committee for Children. (2004). www.committeefor children.org

Dryfoos, J. (1994). *Full service schools: A revolution in health and social services for children, youth, and families.* San Francisco: Jossey-Bass.

Hess, P., McGowan, B., & Bostko, M. (2000). A preventive services program model for preserving and supporting families over time. *Child Welfare, 79,* 227–265.

Joseph, R., Friedman, R., Gutierrez-Mayka, M., Sengova, J., Uzzell, J. D., Hernandez, M., & Contreras, R. (2001). *Final comprehensive report: Evaluation findings and lessons learned from the Annie E. Casey Mental Health Initiative for Urban Children.* Tampa: University of South Florida, Louis de la Parte Florida Mental Health Institute, Department of Child Studies.

Lightburn, A. (2003) Systems of care: Expanding the response to school violence. In J. Miller, G. Schamess, & I. Martin (Eds.), *School violence and children in crisis: School and community based strategies for social workers and counselors* (pp. 279–296). Denver, CO: Love Publications.

Lightburn, A., & Kemp, S. (1994). Family support programs: Opportunities for community-based practice. *Families in Society: The Journal of Contemporary Social Services, 75,* 16–26.

Lourie, I., Stroul, B., & Friedman, R. (1999). Community-based systems of care: From advocacy to outcomes. In M. Epstein, K. Kutash, & A. Duchinowski (Eds.), *Outcomes for children and youth and their families: Programs and evaluation best practices* (pp. 3–21). Austin, TX: Pro-Ed.

Lyman, R., Ayers, S., Siegel, R., Alvarez de Toledo, B., & Mikula, J. (2001). How to be little and still think big: Creating a grass roots, evidence based system of care. In C. Newman, C. Liberton, K. Kutash, & R. Friedman (Eds.), *A system of care for children's mental health: Expanding the research base* (pp. 49–58). Tampa: Research and Training Center for Children's Mental Health, University of South Florida.

McDonald, L., Billingham, S., Conrad, T., Morgan, A., Payton, O., & Payton, E. (1997). Families and schools together (FAST): Integrating community development with clinical strategies. *Families and Society: The Journal of Contemporary Social Services, March/April,* 140–155.

McFarlane, W. (2002). *Multifamily groups and treatment of severe psychiatric disorders.* New York: Guilford.

Pumariega, A., & Winters, N. (2003). *Handbook of child and adolescent systems of care.* San Francisco: Jossey-Bass.

Ronnau, J. (2001) Values and ethics for family centered practice. In E. Walton, P. Sandau-Beckler, & M. Mannes (Eds.), *Balancing family-centered services and child well-being* (pp. 34–54). New York: Columbia University Press.

SAMHSA. (1998–2001). *System of care: Promising practices in children's mental health* (Vols. 1 & 2). Washington, DC: Center for Effective Collaboration and Practice, American Institute of Research.

Santarcangelo, S., Bruns, E., & Yoe, J. (1998). New directions: Evaluating Vermont's statewide model of individualized care. In M. Epstein, K. Kutash, & A. Duchnowski (Eds.), *Outcomes for children and youth and their families: Programs and evaluation best practices* (pp. 117–140). Austin, TX: Pro-Ed.

Shore, L. (1997). *Common purpose.* New York: Doubleday.

Singer, F., Powers, L., & Olson, A. (1996) *Redefining family support.* Baltimore: Brookes.

Stroul, B. (1996). (Ed.). *Children's mental health.* Baltimore: Brookes.

Test, M. (1998). Community-based treatment models for adults with severe and persistent mental illness. In J. William & K. Ell (Eds.), *Advances in mental health research* (pp. 420–437). Washington, DC: NASW Press.

Warren-Adamson, C. (2001). *Family centres and their international role in social action.* Aldershot, UK: Ashgate.

Weiss, H., & Halpern, R. (1990), *Community-based family support and education programs: Something old or something new.* New York: National Center for Children in Poverty, Columbia University School of Public Health.

Weissbourd, B. (1987). A brief history of family support and programs. In S. Kagan, D. Powell, B. Weissbourd, & E. Zigler (Eds.), *America's family support programs* (pp. 38–56). New Haven, CT: Yale University Press.

Yoshikawa, H., & Knitzer, J. (1997). *Lesson from the field: Head Start mental health strategies to meet changing needs.* New York: National Center for Children in Poverty, Columbia University School of Public Health.

Paradigm Shift and Essentials in Community Practice

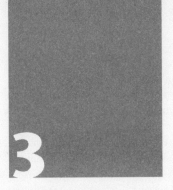

3

Ann Weick

In the Care of Strangers

The threads of caregiving are woven tightly into the fabric of human society. The reason for this is simple: human infants are among the most defenseless of any species. Without early, constant attention from others, they cannot survive. At the other end of the life spectrum, many elders require that same degree of intensive attention when their bodies and faculties begin to fail. Between these two life points, the vulnerability of the body and mind, in small ways and large, calls on the help of others. Both in growing and in declining, human beings are never more than one person away from the need for care.

As with most profound realities of human life, these intimations of our essential vulnerability are artfully disguised. Particularly in American society, we trumpet our individualism and fierce independence. We pride ourselves on "going it alone" and not needing anyone. Being dependent on someone is seen as a mark of weakness, something to be hidden and covered with apology. The more recent language of pop psychology has cast an even wider net of shame by naming the person who is helping as "codependent." The very idea of dependency shrivels our sense of agency, that thin but sturdy conviction that we are in charge of our lives, determiners of our fate, and free to choose how and when we need others.

At the same time, we are not without some collective awareness of the centrality of the caring function to personal and societal well-being. The pervasive needs of children, elders, those lacking financial means, and those with chronic illness or disability all serve as constant reminders of the demands of care. But within that awareness is a striking disconnection between what our experience undisputedly tells us and what our value-inspired myths lure us into believing. The notion that rugged individualism is a tenable social ideal flies in the face of the intricate interconnections required to sustain and support human survival. The challenges of caregiving, whether formal or informal, rest within the puzzling nexus of these contradictory values. Only by unraveling some of these contradictions can we create a more expansive context within which to consider the idea of social care.

The subtlety with which major cultural shifts occur within a society is often seen best in retrospect. When we take this long view, it is possible to discern patterns not always apparent in the kaleidoscope of current practices. What may seem in the moment to be an inevitable expression of "the way things are" becomes instead an opportunity to challenge and reformulate closely held beliefs and practices. With the benefit of this critical lens, we can stand back from our biases and culturally inspired distortions to examine how to create systems of care that respect people's self-determining, inner compasses and yet mitigate the risks of inherent vulnerability to which we are all subject.

The Meanings of Care

The idea of care is an ambiguous notion, freighted with the history and politics of human societies. Our strongest sense of it comes from the primeval interdependence that led our evolving species to cluster in groups for protection, sustenance, and survival. In ways that are still mirrored in some non-Western cultures, the concept of an independent identity apart from the group is incomprehensible. How one fares as a member of a group may involve complex obligations and rules of behavior, but it is through the group that individual needs are met. Thus, in its most essential form, care is tied to meeting, in some adequate fashion, our basic survival needs for food, shelter, and physical safety.

For those who have had the good fortune of consistent nurturing in childhood, the terms of care conjure memories of emotional sustenance: the attention and praise from family members; the watchfulness and cautions about childhood dangers, real or perceived; the expressions of affection in hugs, pats on the head, and playful teasing; and, inevitably, the setting of limits on behavior. These layers of emotion-based experiences provide the social narrative that shapes a widely held, if overly idealized, view of what it means to be cared for. Even if one's personal life did not contain these ingredients in sufficient quantities, there is a collective longing, often seen in media-inspired forms, to reconnect deeply with the real or imagined qualities of care that ensure our emotional and physical well-being.

Our language reveals the tension underlying our yearning for care and the act of providing care. The terms "caretaker" and "caregiver" are often used interchangeably, suggesting that taking and giving care are synonymous. However, the meaning of being "taken care of" seems unequivocal and is not easily confused with being a caregiver. Perhaps our language betrays an important element of caregiving: that in the act of giving care, both the receiver and the giver are being nourished by the care

given. The close relationship of these meanings may also help to begin deciphering the confusing layers of meaning attached to the notion of care. For example, what constitutes adequate care? Do we count it as adequate if physical needs are met but with hostility or chilly indifference? Are the observable measures of care—dry bottoms, filled stomachs, and basic hygiene—sufficient to satisfy our larger sense of care?

Blurred meanings further confound our judgments about what constitutes care. The individual and cultural memories of receiving care, so often tied to family, create a close association with caregivers as those familiar to us. Families are our "familiars." By dint of close, day-by-day connections, we learn what to expect from this cast of characters. Assuming some minimally adequate level of care provided by them and a continuity of relationship over time, family members may continue to serve as short- or long-term givers of care. As little as a generation ago, having children was seen as a protection against unattended need in old age. Now, it may be just as likely that a grandparent becomes the caregiver to grandchildren, or middle-aged parents provide a roof for once-emancipated adult children.

To recognize the strong link between families and caregiving does nothing to dim the myriad ways that family care is given or received. Even more important than the unassailable position of family within the network of care are the strong emotional beliefs, expectations, and assumptions surrounding this fact. To receive care from those who are familiar seems to epitomize the essence of care. It matters not that family care has many faces, some far from benign. The intimacy of the familiar may make the prospect of receiving care from a surly elder daughter more palatable than from an unknown aide in a nursing home.

The yearning for care that takes into account both body and spirit hides under the folds of the starchy costume of rugged independence worn by many. Because of this, the need for care suffers from both invisibility and stigma. Most of the threads of care that are wrapped around our human frailty are invisible to those but the most discerning. The commonplace sight of parents tending young children, neighbors helping an elder, and church members bringing food to someone who is sick inures us to the essential character of these informal, seemingly isolated acts. In the moment, they are unwitnessed. This invisibility leads us to carelessly underestimate the enormous human capital devoted to helping ensure that the species survives and flourishes. Absent this painstaking, intense, pervasive attention to the giving of care, it is impossible to imagine how the world of business, commerce, and government, dependent as they are on the secret service of caregivers, would continue to exist.

The invisibility of the care provided by "familiars," that is, those who have family or social ties to those in need of care, is plagued by an added burden when more formal structures in society step in to supplement or replace family care. In these situations, the caregiving enterprise is plagued by an added burden that trumps the taken-for-granted attitudes surrounding care by familiars. Those who must rely on society's ministrations in times of need feel the cold, unyielding signs of stigma, replete with deeply held cultural convictions about personal responsibility and the obligation to take care of one's own. The values that enshroud these societal expectations greatly diminish the sense of efficacy and well-being of those needing care and leave their judgmental residue on those who work valiantly to provide that care. The combined consequences of invisibility and social stigma surrounding the caregiving functions of our society add unnecessary barriers to the already challenging demands of nurturing, sustaining, and supporting members of our human family whose lives depend on our care.

At the same time, it would be a mistake to overly romanticize family care. Historically, the responsibility for care of young, ill, or otherwise frail individuals has fallen on those related by blood or marriage. To be more precise, this care has been lodged largely with women. Traditional social roles have placed women, more than men, in positions of caregiving. The fact that generations of women have risen to the challenges imbedded there has been a social asset beyond measure. At the same time, family care is not a singular phenomenon. Whereas scores of women in each age have moved into caregiving roles with determination and goodwill, others have faltered at the constant demands implicit in giving care. Family ties do not automatically translate into warm feelings. Even under the best of circumstances, which is to say, situations

where money, time, and motivation are present, there are many roadblocks in the path of consistent, skilled, and dedicated care by family members. Taking care of a crotchety grandmother or a chronically ill child or adult can stretch the limits of even the most devoted. The fact that millions of family members continue to meet these hard challenges is a resource to be counted.

Families and Strangers

It is interesting to note the shift that has required the ever-increasing development of non-family-based systems of care. While the presence of family care is a pervasive and essential ingredient of our society's social existence, the tremendous waves of social dislocation, occurring over several hundred years, have greatly attenuated the role of families, neighbors, and friends as caregivers. By the end of the nineteenth century, immigration, industrialization, and multiple forms of effective transportation had already rendered locality a less cogent magnet for permanency of place. The twentieth-century trends of major international wars, economic depression, chronic disease, and endemic poverty tested and eventually overcame the too-fragile abilities of families to predictably provide the care needed by their members over the life span. From county to state to federal and back to state auspices, the century saw a burgeoning of forms of care that extended and, increasingly, supplanted family care. Technological advances in medicine, with heightened abilities to diagnose and treat disease, began to create a divide between professional and family caregivers. Even if the treatment could not reverse or correct the illness or condition, the expertise associated with professional experience and credentials placed the frail, ill, or fragile person firmly in the hands of professionals.

Among other professions, social work came of age during the decades of that century. The desperate plight of immigrants served as a catalyst for launching an organized response to human need, but that response soon expanded to encompass other groups whose lives were challenged by poverty, abuse, addiction, chronic illness, and old age. The development of federal programs for public assistance and social security in the 1930s and the creation of the mental health movement in the

1950s placed social work within society's formal social welfare structures. It has largely been within these structures that the profession has carried out its helping mission and honed its helping skills.

As we begin the twenty-first century, formal systems of care are in the hands of strangers. In part, this arrangement matches a pragmatic analysis of reality. Many family members no longer live close to each other. This is true of elder parents and adult children, but it is also true of children whose biological parents are separated from them by divorce, geography, or the child welfare system. Even in situations where family members are available to provide direct care, the distance between family members and care providers can be significant. If an elder parent is in a care facility, the staff are those most knowledgeable about and most responsible for care. Family members can still provide social sustenance and direct help, but this is subject to negotiation within the larger system of care. Parents of children in organized child care face a similar situation. There is a role for family members to play, but it is circumscribed by the rules, practices, and policies of others.

It is tempting to use the term "systems of care" to describe the governmental, for-profit, and not-for-profit organizations that have taken responsibility for providing care. However, there is no system in evidence. The hodgepodge of agencies, programs, funding mechanisms, auspices, and categories of need lead to inevitable duplication, inadequacy of funding, competition for limited resources, and vast unmet need. Managed care is yet one more attempt to allocate services by cost, a last resort to test the theory that price is an appropriate mechanism for distributing needed resources.

Increasingly, the dominance of these formal structures of care has created divisions that obscure the development of other possibilities for meeting the needs for care endemic in human society. The overlay of managed care, a strategy of cost containment, skews even more the opportunity to examine creative responses to persistent human need. To break through the limitations of formal approaches and acknowledge the presence of vast assets within the arena of informal care, it is necessary to examine the fundamentals of care and, through this, begin to formulate a more expansive view that integrates the best of both formal and informal strategies. The challenge is to conceive a strategy that incorporates the strengths of both.

The Nature of Social Care

Use of the term "social care" is intentional. If we are to move beyond the limitations of current myths and divisions, it is necessary to begin with at least one basic assumption: that the notion of care is, in its essence, a social phenomenon. Human beings are a communal species. There is an implicit need for others, in terms of physical, as well as emotional, survival and well-being.

In spite of our societal reluctance to live gracefully with ideas that appear to be in opposition, forging a new notion of social care requires this mature perspective. Central to this maturity is a full-hearted acceptance of the equal measures of vulnerability and resilience that lie at the heart of the human condition. To be mortal poses the fearsome challenge of living with the ever-present fragility of human flesh. There is no moment during our lives that our essential vulnerability is not in play. At the same time, human bodies, as well as spirits, are immensely resilient. The research of recent years (Saleebey, 2002; Wolin & Wolin, 1993), as well as our own experiences, testifies to the body's and mind's sometimes astonishing recuperative and regenerative powers. Even in the face of extreme physical and emotional injury, the body's intricate systems, moment by moment, work valiantly and wisely to repair, protect, and sustain life. Walter Cannon's (1932) notion of body wisdom is a power to be reckoned with. Thus, the consideration of care must be deeply grounded in a profound appreciation for people's own capacities to survive and thrive, even in adverse circumstances.

While this caution may seem unnecessary, it is important to recognize that our essential vulnerability is always coupled with this innate capacity for self-righting. Because medically based approaches to care focus almost exclusively on the power of outside agents (drugs, surgery, chemotherapy), it is easy to lose sight of the body's own resources as a crucial partner in the healing process. Fortunately, the resurgence of complementary healing practices is gaining sufficient recognition to begin offsetting the exclusive lens associated with allopathic medical treatments, in which the suppression of symptoms is a primary goal.

The capacity of the body and spirit to heal and regenerate is a remarkable human resource. Any conception of care must be firmly anchored in an acknowledgment of and respect for this continuously surprising possibility. As the hospice movement has shown us, even in a person's final weeks of life, opportunities for emotional growth, for deepening relationships, and for receiving the devoted care of others can still be active ingredients in living that life and in preparing for its end.

The second layering of understanding needed to create a more generous conception of social care is the essential role of natural helpers. During the 1980s, social workers brought this term into the literature to highlight the informal connections that supported families and elders when there was need for care (Quam, 1984; Ballew, 1985; Patterson, 1987). As discussed earlier, family members, by virtue of proximity and relationship, may be central actors in the caregiving role. But it is increasingly probable that friends, neighbors, church members, and volunteers may assume some responsibility for meeting care needs of others. In these circumstances, the caregiving may be unnoticed by everyone but the person receiving the care. It is done quietly and connected by a common bond whether family ties, friendship, or shared group membership. In its most public form, this response can be seen in neighborhoods and towns across America when disaster or crisis occurs. People are touched by the suffering of others and reach out to help. Although the help may not be sustained beyond the crisis, the motivation and response reflect a capacity for care that deserves to be seen as a vital social resource.

While it is beyond the scope of this chapter to offer a specific design for a more integrated approach to care and caregiving, it is possible to tease out some of the principles that need to be present to spark creative development. The essential starting point is a radical acceptance of the realities of human vulnerability, couched within the equally radical possibilities of human transformation. Human beings can be crushed by life's challenges and still transcend them. Boldly embracing the tension implicit in this apparent contradiction helps move us away from the trap of individualism and the limitations it has imposed on the structure of social and health services. The nature of human society and human well-being is relational at its core. Beginning with a relational, rather than an individual, stance requires that the design of social care fully incorporate this principle.

Within this overarching principle rests a conception of care that is better seen as a web than a

system. It is already obvious to both providers and consumers that health and social services are not systems in any meaningful sense of the word. Their fragmented structures, shaped by history, political philosophy, and social ideology, are susceptible to tinkering but not to fundamental change. Usually these changes spring from strategies that try to systematize or rationalize services. Managed care is a case in point. The dilemma presented by these approaches is that they require the imposition of rationality or political will on the task of meeting human need. But the face of human need is far too various and interconnected to be satisfactorily salved by these efforts.

In contrast to the notion of a system of care, the image of a web of relationships seems a more apt conceptual anchor to use in thinking about framing the work of social care. The conception of a web of relations was popularized years ago by physicist Fritzof Capra (1975), who, along with other physicists, was struggling to articulate the unpredictable effects of subatomic particles. What they knew with assurance was that the explicit cause-and-effect theories developed by Isaac Newton and his successors were not sufficient explanations of what their research findings revealed. Instead, there needed to be a new language, not governed by linear, causal thinking. It may be useful to draw a lesson from this seemingly disparate field to reconceive the nature of health and social services. If the face of human need is as disparate and varied as we know it to be, then it seems more useful to imagine the responses to that need being accomplished through a complex yet interconnected web of formal and informal resources. The difference between this and current strategies is that all resources, both formal and informal, are equal partners in fashioning responses. Each is acknowledged and valued as a contributor in the overall task of supporting, protecting, and enhancing human well-being.

The most obvious context for envisioning this web is within community. Communities, whether formed by social ties, contiguity, or common purpose, function as webs of connection. The role of community, then, is critical in putting life and form into the idea of social care. However, it is important to not be limited by narrow definitions of community. The bonds creating webs of relationships may transcend geography and apparent commonalities. What must be searched for and included are those connections that arise serendipitously: the bonds that develop through a shared life crisis, a chance meeting in an unaccustomed place, or a shared interest or larger purpose. Both the subtle and the obvious connections form links in the web.

The image of a web is different in tone and substance from the image of a system. A system suggests the rational organization of disparate parts, with actions producing preidentified effects. If, however, we begin with the image of a web of connections as the frame for society's provision of social care, we find that many of the important pieces are already in place. Instead of a system-engineered approach, which tends to be based on a principle of exclusion, seeing social care as a web, nestled within community, embraces the principle of inclusion. Rather than concern about limiting, excluding, and rationing services, social care invites inclusion, redundancy, and creativity. It acknowledges that communities are already endowed with layers of connections that support human care. Parents and relatives are caring for children; neighbors are helping neighbors; church and social club members are reaching out within and beyond their own membership; strangers are responding to people who moments before were unknown to them. This caring impulse is evident in friendship and celebration, as well as in crisis, illness, and loss. Recognizing and harnessing these community strengths must be a cornerstone in expanding our notion of social care.

The challenge is to create a large enough frame for care so that these naturally occurring strengths can be integrated with the formal programs of care provided by governmental programs and not-for-profit organizations. This intentional partnership between informal and formal resources for care would bring together all strands of care into a new and seamless web, with the explicit goal of ensuring that no one in our society lacks the care they need.

Communities of Care

Given the long history and broad reach of formal programs of care, it seems daunting to imagine how the assets of naturally occurring care can be fully incorporated. To accomplish this, it is necessary to develop novel strategies that begin to create communities of care. Fortunately, a wide variety of community-based strategies are already beginning

to emerge. They vary significantly in terms of scope and focus, but they share some common characteristics. They begin with an understanding of people's need for social affiliation, sustenance, and care. They recognize the strengths and assets already evident in people's connections to one another and seek ways to broaden those circles of connections. They acknowledge the artificial separations caused by overly rigid and sometimes misguided notions of professional social work practice and work to form new, more equal partnerships between social workers and community members. And they see social service agencies not as bastions that isolate social work from their immediate community surroundings but instead as integral parts of the neighborhood within which they are located.

The work of John McKnight (1995) and Kretzmann and McKnight (1993) has been helpful in pinpointing the shape of this renewed sense of community. McKnight's (1995) caution is particularly apt: "Services provided in small towns or neighborhoods should not be called community services if they do not involve people in community relationships" (p. 116). This is particularly true for vulnerable groups who, by virtue of their being labeled as poor, mentally ill, or elderly, are segregated from community life rather than being more meaningfully incorporated into it. However, this exclusion occurs for many other community members as well. Many social services add to this exclusion by defining themselves and being defined by society as the primary agents in responding to human need. To right the balance, there is need for a renewed sense of shared social agency. The "agency" is no longer seen as a physical location but as a naturally occurring, human capacity that impels us toward association, caring relationships, and communal action.

The blurring of old lines of separation between worker and client and between agency and community requires the revaluing of essential professional skills and a new openness to the rich human resources present in the community. Because social work has a deep strand of its history tied to community work, where social workers settled into the neighborhoods of those they helped, the tradition is still accessible to us. We do not have to create this heritage but have only to dust it off and let it teach us how to support and strengthen naturally occurring processes of care. In that scenario, social workers can then take their well-established place as catalysts of change. In this role, they are not agents of change but, instead, help create a context in which individuals, groups, and neighborhoods can use personal and social assets and resources to meet their needs for care and for community enhancement.

What is of equal importance is the leadership role that social workers can play in helping the larger society fashion new responses to social care. To do so requires the very skills that social workers have in abundance. Social workers know how to deal with complexity and ambiguity, two of the elements that will be present in trying to forge a new path toward communities of care. Bringing to bear the skills of analysis, assessment, task planning, and strategic thinking, combined with the richly developed skills of interpersonal effectiveness, forms a necessary base for carrying these efforts forward. At the same time, social workers have a profound understanding of the need for social care and the many barriers to that care. What forms the energy for constructive action is the profession's commitment to fostering and strengthening the web of social connections that will help people achieve their full potential as members of a community.

Conclusion

As community-focused initiatives continue, it will be necessary to draw from social work's traditions and understandings a clearer evaluation of the profession's own assets and potential for growth. At what we might optimistically call the eve of a paradigm shift from systems of treatment to communities of care, it will be important to recognize the factors in current social work practice that limit our creativity and stunt our capacity for thinking outside the box. Central to this is a searching assessment of our beliefs about social work expertise. To the extent that the profession searches for and aligns itself with approaches that appear to make social workers experts on the lives and troubles of others, it will maintain its preoccupation with professional status and role-narrowing self-definitions.

However, if we can relinquish outmoded inclinations, social workers can fully contribute as web weavers. The skills of social work ideally suit social workers to be connectors, helping individuals, families, groups, and neighborhoods make connections with their own strengths and aspirations and with the informal and formal resources around them. When resources are limited or absent, social workers help create resources. When the problems and concerns of a few become the problems of many, they work as advocates to awaken the caring response of the larger community and help craft policy that redirects society's response into more constructive channels. These are the collective skills of good process. More than any other professionals, social workers know how to facilitate social processes. With such knowledge and skills, social workers can be the architects who help design and build a seamless web of social care. To accomplish this, they will create an alliance between the informal care by familiars and the formal care by strangers that can result in the reshaping of society's caring response and serve to remind us all of our interdependence and resilience.

References

Ballew, J. R. (1985). The role of natural helpers in preventing child abuse. *Social Work, 30*, 37–41.

Cannon, W. B. (1932). *The wisdom of the body*. New York: Norton.

Capra, F. (1975). *The tao of physics*. Boulder, CO: Shambala.

Kretzmann, J. P., & McKnight, J. L. (1993). *Building communities from the inside out*. Chicago: ACTA Publications.

McKnight, J. (1995). *The careless society*. New York: Basic Books.

Patterson, S. L. (1987). Older rural natural helpers: Gender and site differences in the helping process. *Gerontologist, 27*, 639–644.

Quam, J. K. (1984). Natural helpers: Tools for working with the chronically mentally ill elderly. *Gerontologist, 24*, 564–567.

Saleebey, D. (Ed.). (2002). *The strengths perspective in social work practice* (3rd ed.). Boston: Allyn and Bacon.

Wolin, S. J., & Wolin, S. (1993). *The resilient self*. New York: Villard Books.

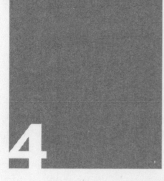

4

Dennis Saleebey

A Paradigm Shift in Developmental Perspectives?
The Self in Context

The idea that the development and socialization of children is a singular function of early life experience in the psychosocial interior of the family has been undergoing many challenges and revisions over the past three decades. In this chapter I will briefly describe the conventional views of child rearing, both professional and cultural, and present some challenges to those ideas. Gathering themes from those challenges, I would like to suggest a beginning of a different framework for understanding development and working with families and children. I understand all too well that anything that may present itself as new always has its fingers in the cookie jar of the past.

The Conventional and Time-Honored View of Human Development

It would be foolish, of course, to lump together the vast array of developmental and socialization theories that have influenced research, clinical practice, professional education, popular culture, and parental behavior. But perhaps we can distinguish some common features so that we may understand what the canonical view is about.

The most persuasive and shared doctrine of many influential developmental theories is that children move from some primitive state through a series of stages, phases, and challenges (some dictated by an epigenetic ground plan, others ordained by the nature of the child in relationship to the acts and orientations of parents and caretakers) to some state of maturity, full development, and self-actualization. This, of course, may not happen, depending on psychosocial constraints and barriers, traumatic events, toxic environments, abusive and difficult relationships, and the like. Nonetheless, prescriptions for achieving full maturity and depictions and characterizations of the normal paths of development have blossomed over the years. Major research enterprises have grown up around efforts to answer questions about the nature of maturity, the pathways to maturity, and the elements of life that thwart or forestall maturity. The socialization researcher asks the question, how does an untamed and uncivilized being become a citizen, a productive adult in specific sociocultural surroundings? In cases of both developmental and socialization inquiry and thinking, the parents are the prime movers of development. In the 1950s, the idea that parents are the molders of a child's personality became a firm part of the developmental psychology convention, even though the early research did not show much of a relationship between parental attitudes and behaviors (Maccoby, 1992). Before 1950 (the Freudians excepted here), there really was not much interest in parents as an influence on their children, but rather in how children were alike at certain ages and how one should approach their rearing (Harris, 1998). But the canon continued to maintain not only that parents help little children learn the conventions of a culture (language, dress, manners and morals, etc.) but that what they do is fateful for children's development into adults. That is, parental attitudes and behaviors produce personality traits, adaptive strategies, and, in some cases, psychopathologies that unfold during adolescence or adulthood. The parents are the sculptors of personality and character.

The Warrants of Psychoanalytic, Psychodynamic, and Ego Psychology Theories and Practices

The theories cast under this rubric have been most influential in claiming that parents are the critical factor in how children evolve—the kind of people they become, the accomplishments of their lives, and the torments they wrestle with. Children in interaction with, observation of, and fantasies about their parents develop the building blocks of their personalities: ego and superego, defense mechanisms (from healthy to neurotic to immature to psychotic), and ego ideals. These develop also as part of the civilizing of the id—the natural, untamed, avaricious self. The residue of conflicts that arise between parents and little children in the trials and struggles of development, and the urges of the id are usually unconscious, a place from which they work their exorbitant influence for good or ill. The ego, largely conscious, as it develops must master the greedy, atavistic urges from the unconscious, help mute the reverberations of early conflicts that have been buried in the unconscious, meet the demands of the "realities" of life, the increasingly insistent requisites of conscience, and resolve conflicts in the relationships that pertain in the child's life. The ego's management of these tensions over time appears as defense mechanisms. These are the adaptive strategies, largely unconsciously wrought, that are more or less successful in resolving these often competing demands. But it is within the nest of family that most of the groundwork for adaptation is laid, work that cannot be easily undone in

adulthood without special intervention like psychoanalytic therapy. It is the ghosts from our past (those unsettled conflicts, those dampened unacceptable urges, those primitive images of parents) that we cannot lay to rest. Janet Malcolm (1981) argues that

> the most original and radical discovery [of psychoanalysis] is that we invent each other according to early blueprints. . . . [Relationship] is at best an uneasy truce between powerful fantasy systems. . . . We have to grope for each other through a dense thicket of absent others. We cannot see each other plain. A horrible kind of predestination hovers over each new attachment we form. (p. 6)

Actually, Freud himself did not do much work on the defense mechanisms. That was left to the ego psychologists, starting with his daughter, Anna, and shortly thereafter Heinz Hartmann, Robert White, Erik Erikson, and others came along as well. These theorists and clinicians were much more devoted to understanding ego processes, the conscious mind, and how it fares in the larger sociocultural world. Nonetheless, the critical passages to adulthood passed through the geography of the parents. And development was thought to go through specific stages, each with an inherent crisis to be managed, universal to human nature, and obdurate to much change by culture and history.

By now there have been many variations on the original story, some definitely at odds with it. But the fact remains that many of these theorists, when they talk of the role of nature and nurture, do not give much room to nature (with the exception of suggesting that the stages of development are epigenetic—ground plans laid out by our species genetic inheritance) and define nurture primarily as what happens in the family as children grow. But the Harvard Study of Human Development of three different cohorts of 824 individuals, all selected as youth and followed throughout their lives, is now in its seventh decade. Although the theoretical perspective (applied later) seemed to be ego psychological, some of the general conclusions suggest that what we think of as toxic or difficult childhood experiences do not always differentiate very well between those individuals who had a favorable outcome (in late adulthood or old age) and those who did not fare so well. In fact, as a summary statement, the lead researcher and author, George Vaillant (2002), says this, *"What goes right in childhood predicts the future far better than what goes wrong"* (p. 95, italics in original). It would be unfair to say that every childhood trouble, like a bleak, loveless childhood environment, was not predictive of later outcomes, but there did seem to be a number of positive factors that affected the quality of aging, including loving well, maintaining healthy practices, having friendships, and an altruistic nature, among others. These clearly were not always or most significantly related to the quality of childhood relationships with parents.

Influences on Child Rearing and Family and Child Practice

As said, the conventional wisdom about development is not all of a piece, and is much more complex than I can possibly render here. But I think it may be fair to draw some conclusions.

While much of the argument over the years has been over the role of nature and nurture, it seems fair to say that, in most instances, nurture is defined as the influence of parents on their children. Other environmental factors appear as background to this center stage drama.

Parents are the single most important influence on a child's current behavior, as well as the shape and contours of the child's adult personality. The relationships between parents and children are a dense thicket of emotions, urges, folk knowledge, past experiences, and personality and must be navigated with great care on the part of parents and, even early in their development, children.

Parents can supplement their child-rearing techniques with knowledge usually wrought by a variety of experts—physicians, psychiatrists, psychologists, child development specialists, and even popular authorities. But for parents there will always be forces, some inner, maybe even unconscious, and others more obvious (as in overt responses) that imbue the parent-child relationship with a particular emotional and relational tinge.

The developmental canon has bred an astonishing and, for parents, occasionally bewildering array of popular and professional child-rearing experts whose advice can be found on bookshelves, on television, over the Internet, and in person. Much of the advice is contradictory at some points, and it has changed tenor over the years as new ideas

have emerged, cultural and social shifts in child-rearing practices have occurred. Data, as well as fads and fashions with respect to parenting, have changed. But the canon is usually preserved in its most rudimentary form.

Challenges to the Developmental Canon

In this section, I will examine some established and emerging views of the self and the development of the self.

The Resilience and Strengths of Families and Children in Improbable Places and Circumstances

Over the past 30 years, thanks initially to the work of people like Norman Garmezy (1993) and the groundbreaking research of Emmy Werner and Ruth Smith (1982, 1992), there is a rich and diverse literature on the resilience of children and families, especially those who have confronted daunting obstacles in their daily lives. Resilience is not a trait or an end point. Rather, it is the cumulative acquisition and expression of emotions, ideas, capacities, behaviors, motivations, understanding, and resources that lead a person to be more capable of overcoming or withstanding life's adversities and ordeals. Naturally, not all resilient souls can cope with everything that comes their way, but even in those situations where individuals are swarmed with pressure, there are things to be learned, and responses that may be transfigured into useful knowledge and behaviors in the future. The research and thinking on resilience is certainly not of a piece, but some ideas seem to characterize much of the literature. The cornerstone is the distinction between risk factors and protective factors in a person's life. The former are those elements of the intimate and distant environment or those life events that undermine adaptation or amplify the vulnerability of the individual. Protective factors, on the other hand, are those elements of relationships, environment, and contingency that augment the ability to adapt to stresses and challenges. I would add, as a parenthetical note, that another group of conditions may be involved here. Generative factors are those that are unexpected, hard to define in any given case, but that invigorate adaptation, growth, and understanding. Protective and generative factors, then, are "people, resources, institutions, and contingencies that enhance the likelihood of rebound and recovery, or that may exponentially accelerate learning, development, and capacity" (Saleebey, 2002, p. 278).

The resilience literature typically cites two clusters of resilience-enhancing factors: those that are related to personality, such as self-efficacy, realistic appraisals of the environment, empathy, humor, social problem-solving skills, and the like; and those related to interpersonal relationships, such as positive, caring relationships and "high enough" expectations of others (Norman, 2000).

The literature makes it clear that what we call development is shaped by the kinds of challenges and adversities that people, families, and communities face. It is not the case that individuals, at a given stage of development, face these threats with a particular personality (even if still forming) that dictates how they will respond. Rather, it is as much the nature of the ordeal itself and how a person (with help or not) responds fortuitously and/or unpredictably to that challenge. The Wolins (1996) remind us, through their research and clinical work, that many of the personality traits they saw in adults who had survived a childhood with parents struggling with alcohol and creating intimate havoc came from responding to the threats, uncertainties, and perils of their life.

Perhaps, as some researchers and clinicians think (Flach, 1997; Masten, Best, & Garmezy, 1990; Rutter, 1985), there are individuals who seem to be more resilient than others, who have some genetically endowed or early developmental disposition to be resilient. If that is so, it does not negate the fact that they also may strengthen some aspects of self because of their struggles, or even develop new capacities or qualities. It seems also true that, even in the case of genetically or developmentally endowed resilience, the role of social and interpersonal resources is critical (Benard, 2002).

Resilience, then, may be a nuclear potential for all human beings, enhanced or muted by external events, relationships, and internal factors. But at its roots it means, as the research has shown, that we would be hard put to predict how a child facing enormous stress will face it and how he or she will turn out because of it (Katz, 1997). The self is less predictable and more malleable than we might suppose. External factors (like relationships or institutions) are frequently the key to summoning up and extending the behaviors, attitudes, ideas, and emotions that may eventually become part of a resilient response to adversity.

Nature and Nurture: The Role of Genes, Temperament, and Experience

For centuries, people have been attracted to the idea that individuals are born with certain innate capacities and orientations, traits and virtues, personality and character. From the ancient Greeks to the Chinese, to the more modern conceptions of psychologists, anthropologists, and geneticists, the notion of certain inborn templates of emotion and cognition has held thrall. It is only more recently, as Kagan (1994) has observed, that the idea of intrinsic structures of personality or "types" has become much less popular, if not anathema, to our current sociopolitical scene. The impetus of democracy, egalitarianism, behaviorism (all behaviors are a result of environmental contingencies), and the idea that parental influence is the single most important force in a child's life all contrive to diminish or debase the idea of temperament as, in part, a genetic given. However, the notion of a temperament rooted in biology and shaped to an uncertain degree by experience is making a comeback (although it has always had supporters). The idea of temperament is related to but different from the concepts of character and personality. Robert Ornstein (1993) defines it as "more general, more basic than is the whole complex of personality; it concerns whether one does everything slowly or quickly, whether one seeks excitement or sits alone, whether one is highly expressive or inhibited, joyous or sullen" (p. 47). If temperament is inborn, it does not mean that you are stuck with being, say, shy and cautious or with being a thrill seeker and chance taker. There is a built-in flexibility here, and events in the environment may have a strong effect on temperament, either gradually over time or more immediately.

Jerome Kagan and his associates have studied inhibited and uninhibited infants and children since 1957 at the Fels Institute in Ohio. His findings are complex and very rich, so a summary is an injustice of sorts. By the time they are 2 years old, a certain percentage of the many children studied over these four decades plainly show one of the two extremes—either shy, inhibited, and anxious or bold, assertive, and relaxed. The inhibited children differ from the assertive children in terms of their behavior, emotions, and cognition, and in both groups a biological substrate underlies these differences. For example, more of the inhibited children have a number of physical characteristics that suggest high reactivity to external events. These include high levels of cortisol and the neurotransmitter norepinephrine, as well other markers that accompany a felt intense level of stress.

These findings raise questions that certainly a lot of parents would ask. Are these traits that my child is born with just the way it's going to be? Are they some sort of genetic fate? Can they change? Can my shy little poet become a floor trader at the New York Stock Exchange? Is my very inhibited child careening toward an adult life peppered with anxiety and depression? Is my assertive and extroverted son headed for trouble with the law? Actually, it may be hard to say. In the Fels study more than one third of the highly reactive, inhibited infants were not either exceptionally shy or fearful by the second year; a few were actually fearless. As Kagan (1994) observes, genes "necessarily share power with experience" (p. 262). Nonetheless, as they mature, a number of these children remain somewhat shy, inhibited, and cautious. The primary effect of these temperaments seems to be on the relative prominence of certain moods and feelings, the intensity and quality of relationships, and the choice of careers. But all of this is affected by early experience, too. Parents who are overly protective of a shy, inhibited, and reactive infant or toddler may inadvertently increase the social fears and fears of novelty or surprise of the child. In contrast, parents who have a sense of their own confidence and accept the child's behavior as it is but also gently prod him or her toward developmental milestone experiences may promote a greater sense of well-being and ease in the child. Experience with peers and with other adults, opportunities to participate in group activities, accomplishments at school, and many other factors can also influence basic temperament. Although Kagan and his researchers did not pursue other factors besides parental influences in any depth, his comments suggest that the experience that he speaks of extends beyond the family.

In the end, the relationship between nature and nurture, between temperament and environment is complex, dynamic, and in some ways yet to be revealed. But we must understand that our biology generally and our specific individual genetic inheritance do make a difference in how we approach and manage what life sets before us. Things do change, however, and we should honor the fact that the environment can influence change, often in a fairly dramatic way. It can even change the configuration of neural pathways in the brain (LeDoux, 2002). As time passes, thanks to a variety of complex influences, an extrovert may really become more reflective, and an introvert may become less preoccupied with certain fears and restraints, and neither of those outcomes is necessarily due to the behavior of parents.

The Power of Place: Contextual Influences on the Self Over the Life Cycle

A recent debate has arisen, occasioned in part by the controversial, summative work on development and personality by Judith Rich Harris. The debate concerns the relative influence of nature and nurture, more specifically, the influence of parents (or caretakers) on development and maturation versus the influence of genes, peers, the ambient environment of children, and other contextual factors. In our culture (the dominant culture, I should say), we confer enormous power (and pressure) on parents to shape and mold the personality and character of children. This can be a daunting prospect. On the one hand, the responsibility and possibility of contributing to the well-being of the family, community, and society by raising trustworthy, productive children is an intriguing, gratifying moral enterprise. On the other hand, being completely accountable for sculpting the malleable stuff of childhood into a virtuous, competent adult figure can be intimidating, to say the least. But the conceits of the developmental canon would have it so. There can be little doubt anymore that genes write many of the specifications for any number of physical, cognitive, emotional, and behavioral attributes. These are immanences, some of which may be fairly resistant to the influence of parents, and others that may even influence parental behavior. How relatively quiet and serene parents react to a child born with a strongly assertive temperament, for example, may require extensive behavioral and emotional adaptation on their part.

But the essence of this point of view is that while parents can do many things for their children, how the children turn out, leaving genetic factors aside for the moment, is mightily dependent on peers, the prevailing culture, and other elements of the environment, especially proximal ones. In his landmark array of research projects on behavioral ecology (behavior settings), as mentioned earlier, Roger Barker (1968) has given us a way of thinking about the proximal settings that effect our behavior. His claim is that the small nooks and crannies of life are critical to understanding behavior: *you cannot explain differences in the conduct and interactions of people in two different behavior settings (environments, usually small) on the basis of the individuals' cognitive patterns, characters, or personalities alone (or even at all)*. For example, in his comparison over time of two midwestern towns that he named Yoredale and Midwest, he examined those behavior settings for what he called "pressure" (he also examined them according to other criteria such as welfare). Pressure is the degree to which other forces act upon a person to enter or avoid or withdraw from a behavior setting (like a classroom, club, saloon, etc.). This was measured on a 7-point scale from required (children, for example, must enter the setting, if they are eligible) to prohibited (children are excluded). Seven percent of Midwest's habitats, for example, coerced and/or incorporated children into their ongoing programs; 14% of Yoredale's did. There also were settings that were childproof; 14% of Midwest's were; 19% of Yoredale's. According to Barker (1968),

> Forces for and against children are properties of a town's settings (its school classes, its pubs, its courts, its Golden Age club . . .). Transposing the children of Midwest to Yoredale, and vice versa, would immediately transform their behavior in respect to the parts of towns they would enter and avoid, despite their unchanged motives and cognitions. (p. 43)

And while people are an essential medium for these children, "their individuality is irrelevant to behavior settings" (p. 217).

Of course, people's psychology does play a part, and there are direct connections and feedback loops between people and their settings that, among other things, allow people to react and re-

form when there are changes in the setting—such as a sudden depopulation (workers are laid off from a factory, many children are home sick from school because of a flu epidemic, etc.). These require and elicit a number of processes, from perception to cognition, discrimination, judgment, motivation, and action in individuals and groups (Schoggen, 1989). The theory of behavior settings is rich and complex. It is important to note that these settings are often small or contained, are a part of the everyday life of everyone, and can have profound influence on the behavior of their inhabitants, especially if the normative clues and symbols are many and strong. It is also important to understand such settings in terms of the degree and quality of interaction and participation that they foster. Small behavioral settings and spaces, like classrooms, waiting rooms, or offices, that do not encourage much interaction or participation will probably have a different effect on those who enter and stay in them (Goodnow, 1995).

Related to Barker's thesis, some years ago Harold Proshansky and Abbe Fabian (1987) proposed the importance of "place identity" in the development of children. They argued that developmental theories of identity (e.g., those of Erik Erikson and Jean Piaget) almost completely neglected the role of the physical environment in the development of the identity of children. This long passage presents their argument:

> If a child acquires the knowledge and understanding of who it is by virtue of its dependent and continuing relationships to significant other people, then we must assume that such identity determinations are also rooted in the child's experience with rooms, clothes, playthings, and an entire range of objects and spaces that also support [I would add that some may challenge] its existence. . . . In effect, children learn to view themselves as distinct from the physical environment as well as from other people and do so by learning their relationships to various objects, spaces, and places including ownership, exclusion, limited access, and so on. (p. 22)

Think back on your childhood. How many memories and defining moments involve not only people but also nonhuman sentient beings, as well as places and spaces? Thus the issue here in some ways is the constancy of personality across social settings of various kinds. In discussing Cinderella and her two very different contexts, Judith Rich Harris (1998), in her engaging and wry fashion, puts it this way:

> Stability of personality across social contexts depends in part on how different or similar a person's various contexts have been. Cinderella's two social contexts [cottage and castle] were unusually divergent, so there was more than the usual amount of variation in her personality. But someone who met her after the prince carried her off to the castle wouldn't know that. They would see only her outside-the-cottage personality. (p. 73)

The basic assumption that we may take away from this is that all kinds of relationships, places, and spaces, in addition to genetic predispositions, have the power to mold character and personality, as well as the behaviors, feelings, motives, and cognitions that emanate from them. But even more important, it is to the small details of environment that we sometimes must turn our attention. These can be powerful and/or subtle but may have pronounced effects—over time or even in a short period of time—on how we behave. The fundamental attribution error (Nisbett & Ross, 1991) described by psychologists is to suggest that when we interpret other people's behavior we almost always go for a dispositional explanation (behavior is dependent on a person's personality and inner motivations) rather than a contextual one. Much research has shown that even when contextual changes are pointed out and quite dramatic, people still almost always reach for a dispositional or character interpretation (Gladwell, 2000); we are much more sensitive to personal than contextual cues. Walter Mischel (1996), in a new edition of his historic work, *Personality and Assessment*, underscores the importance of the context in understanding any given behavior: "It is evident [from the vast research] that behaviors which are often construed as stable personality trait indicators actually are highly specific and depend on the details of the evoking situations and the response mode employed to measure them" (p. 37). He does not deny the reality of stable, even genetically endowed traits but encourages us to understand the importance of the *immediate environment* in understanding any behavior. Later on, in discussing development, he touches upon resil-

ience, the contextual effects on self, and the idea of the relational self (although he uses none of these terms):

> Traditional trait-state conceptions of man have depicted him as victimized by his infantile history, as possessed by unchanging rigid trait attributes, and as driven inexorably by unconscious irrational forces. . . . [A different view] is that the dynamics of behavior involve intricate relations between what the individual does and the conditions that evoke, support, undermine or otherwise modify his behavior patterns. . . . A more adequate conceptualization . . . must also recognize that men can and do reconceptualize themselves and change, and that an understanding of how humans can constructively modify their behavior in systematic ways is at the core of a truly dynamic personality psychology. (pp. 300–301)

The Social Construction of Self: The Relational/Dialogic Self

A particular leitmotif of the Western world, at least since the Enlightenment, is that selves exist—selves that perceive, choose, analyze, observe, selves that are "inside." In this way, the self is the scaffolding of our consciousness. And the self stands in contrast, as an inner world, to the external world, that which exists out there, beyond our skin and sensibility. The self (subjective experience) has the power to discern and understand the external (objective) world. Thus, in the Western world anyway, we believe that a sane person has one central core self that is reasonably durable and knowable. But what exactly is the self? What is the stuff of the thought, the motive, the emotion, the act (Gergen, 1999)?

The idea of the "self-contained" individual is a peculiarity to many other cultures of the world. Clifford Geertz (1979), the anthropologist, observes:

> The western conception of the person as a bounded, unique, more or less integrated motivational and cognitive universe . . . organized into a distinctive whole and set contrastively both against other such wholes and against a social and natural background is, however incorrigible it may seem to us, a rather peculiar

idea within the context of the world's cultures. (p. 129)

Edward Sampson (1993) picks up on the idea of contrast by arguing that when we venerate the self-contained self, particularly if done in the context of domination and unequal power, we often celebrate it at the expense of a denigrated other; we not only honor the self but define it in terms of what it is not—the other. In the white, male Euro-American world, the other includes people of color, women, and gays and lesbians. They are constructed to be what the dominant group is not and in the service of that group's particular

> needs, values, interests, and points of view. . . .
> When I construct a you designed to meet my needs and desires, a you that is serviceable to me, I am clearly engaging in a monologue as distinct from a dialogue. . . . All such monologues are self-celebratory. They are one-way streets that return to their point of origin. (p. 4)

Clearly, if the self were considered from a dialogic point of view, it would be understood within the perimeters of relationships. "Dialogism" (Sampson, 1993) means that we understand people not in terms of what occurs inside them but on the basis of what occurs between them; all that is critical to understanding human nature and the human condition occurs as people interact with each other—usually with language and nonverbal communication. Meaning and conceptions of the self (even if felt as private) emerge in conversations and interactions with others over time.

This is a phenomenon of the postmodern world. It is a challenge to the view that there is an inner thing called a self and a world out there separate from the self but no less real or palpable. As Kenneth Gergen (1991) says,

> In a traditional community, where relationships were predictable, and repetitive and ongoing, and usually face-to-face, a stable and solid sense of self was preferred. There also was a strong sense of and agreement about what was right and what was wrong, so one could or had to be yourself, unselfconsciously. (p. 147)

But in this world of many voices, many values, overwhelming lines of communication, many possible identities, the requisite need for performances, sometimes style over substance, the many social

contexts in which one performs and operates, the concrete, immutable sense of self—that ego encased in a bag of skin, looking out at an external world through two peepholes, no longer holds up very well. Lewis Thomas (1974), the biologist, says "The whole dear notion of one's own Self—a marvelous old free-willed, free-enterprising, autonomous, independent, isolated island of the self—is a myth" (p. 142). It becomes clearer that we are selves only in relationship to others and to cultures. If finding meaning and meaning making is the crux of human nature, it is also born of interdependence. We share understandings of the world, but when we are in a state of flux, and context jumping, some of those understandings become precarious, challenged, or useless. Our self is subject to change in terms of changes in the relationships: shifts and alterations in the language, and the gestures that surround us; the medium of conversation; the material elements of the surrounding (it is one thing to profess love to one's partner in the subway as opposed to a secluded nook in Central Park). All those differences change the professing itself and the responding self. If there is no self outside a system of meaning, and that meaning is made and sustained over time in relationships, it may be understood that the self is a phenomenon of relationship. We do have a tendency for relationships and communications to become routinized and conventional—to seem like a kind of hard reality. The idea of the relational, constructed self is, that when the veneer of stability is taken away by circumstance or trauma or insight, that we are many selves, selves constructed out of our relationships with others and out of our historical and cultural experience.

For many Asians, for example, the idea of a self is a feeble one compared with the importance of a family. For many indigenous peoples the idea of a self shrinks in importance or substance when confronted with the web of relationships that are tribe and community. Although it means that the idea that our long-standing love affair with the autonomous freestanding self may be over, there are advantages to thinking about the self as a relational contextual epiphenomenon. Imagine that all our understandings, our manifestations of self are embedded in a social matrix, a matrix of relationships of one dimension or another, and that our self cannot be understood as standing alone. Would it be the case that our definitions of things like child development, parenting, socialization, mental health, and self-esteem, for example, would have to be recast in a different language, one that reflects context and relationship? For example, if a woman is seriously depressed, we know well that in some cases she would most probably be suffering from a serious dysregulation in certain pathways in her brain as a result of chronic stress. But she is not depressed by herself; to speak of her as a depressed person is a linguistic convenience and a modernist and medical preference. How she feels and thinks about herself depends mightily on how others (including those who treat her) think of her and respond to her, and how she responds to their responses. Weaning ourselves from a more individualistic, autonomous view of the monolithic self provides us with many possibilities for performance, for more playfulness and freedom in the articulation of selves as relational realities. This would apply, too, to the way we approach helping. Who helps whom? Where are the boundaries of the helping relationship? Maybe we cannot say with any certainty, except in response to this instance, this moment as it evolves. Helper, helpee, context are all part of the unfolding process driven by mutuality, pluralism, and uncertainty. We do not really know what this would look like, but the possibilities seem intriguing. A rethinking of that sort would require us to deconstruct (to probe the underlying assumptions and origins of) the language we currently use to see how it constrains our thinking—intervention, target population, assessment, client, helping relationship, professional, expertise. These are all individualistic notions for the most part. What new language would we construct together? How would we come to understand the complexities of child development?

The Matrix of Life: Community, Contingency, and Character

On the basis of the views just presented, we can see that there has been a gradual but pronounced move to understand the development of self (if we even can use that phrase) as occurring within a more refined filigree of relationships, institutions, and social contexts than ever before. Not all these views are commensurate, but there are some themes that we should quickly review before we pose possibilities.

1. The role of parents in producing certain kinds of children and being significantly culpable for later adult outcomes is very much in question. Clearly, parents or caretakers can provide, among other things, security, safety, a loving, caring environment, guidance, resources, and opportunities. But parents and their children are embedded in a larger communal, cultural, and relational environment. What goes on in those surroundings and how the parents and child affect it, as well as respond to it, is fateful for how they are (how they act, feel, think, are motivated) and how they relate at any given moment. And the surroundings that are most crucial in terms of immediate behaviors are close—the ambient, proximal environment. To say this is not to ignore the monumental and corrosive effects of poverty, oppression, and discrimination, but it is to say that the effects of these usually come down to and infuse the most immediate environment of adults and children.

2. Increasingly it is argued (at least by some psychologists, behavioral geneticists, and neuroscientists) that genes and environment form the superstructure of development. Joe LeDoux (2002), an eminent neuroscientist, puts it simply enough:

> Your brain was assembled during childhood by a combination of genetic and environmental influences. Genes dictated that your brain was a human one and that your synaptic connections, though more similar to members of your family than to those of members of other families, were nevertheless distinct. Then, through experiences with the world (whether selection, instruction, and construction), your synaptic connections were adjusted and altered further, distinguishing you from everyone else. (p. 307)

Two important things to take away from this disarmingly modest quotation are that when the environment has an effect on us, it may come from any source in the ambient or distal environment, not just parents and caretakers; and it may change, along certain pathways, the pattern of relationships or connections between neurons, which is critical for some aspects of cognition, emotion, and motivation.

3. The resilience literature particularly but not exclusively continues to show the importance of resources and generative factors in the environment in the life of children, youth, and adults. Two examples will serve to illustrate this. First, if there is one nearly constant finding in the resilience litera-

ture, it is that many children in dire circumstances, who cannot rely on their parents for support, protection, and guidance, often find a person in their environment (many times by dint of their own efforts) who will be steadfast (although not necessarily continually present), caring, reassuring, and understanding. Usually this person helps the young person connect with other resources in the community—a church, a boys' or girls' club, a family, an association of some kind. Second, professionals who work with families in dire trouble because of physical abuse or drug and alcohol abuse know that it is hard to inspirit resilience and to foster family strengths without support from the environment. Froma Walsh (1998) puts it this way: "Interventions aimed at enhancing positive interactions, supporting coping efforts, and *building extrafamilial resources* work in concert to reduce stress, to enhance pride and competence and to promote more effective functioning in these families" (p. 159, italics added).

4. From the ideas embodying the relational self come some convention-shattering notions. If the self is a phenomenon of and can only be understood in terms of relationships, and the medium of expression is performative (i.e., we are usually performing to one degree or another, responsive to the innuendo and expectations of the immediate social context) and dialogical (the construction of meaning—appreciative and affirming, directive and defining—with others), then we are immediately thrust into the social context as the hub of human understanding, knowing, and action. No act, no person, adult or child, can be understood apart from relational contexts (some may be historical, others may be culturally requisite; some may be intimate, others may be more extensive). Related to this idea is that what we think of as truth is a communal undertaking. Rather than being stultified by such a prospect, we might consider that such an assertion could mean understanding and action within a given interactional environment are to some extent context specific, giving us a luxuriant array of ways of being. Jerome Bruner (1986) sees this exciting possibility in relationship to education in this light:

If there is to be a new culture . . . its central technical concern will be how to create in the young an appreciation of the fact that many worlds are possible, that meaning and reality

are created and not discovered, that negotiation is the art of constructing new meanings by which individuals can regulate their relations with one another. (p. 149)

In his inquiry and writing on the education of children, school cultures, cognitive development, and the centrality of meaning making as a human activity, Bruner has increasingly come to believe that school cultures should foster mutual communities of learners who are jointly involved in developing projects that contribute to the collective good or that solve relevant problems. In this way everybody contributes to the education of the other. And education, to some degree, is always local.

Lois Holzman (2002), one of the developers of the East Side Institute for Short-Term Therapy in New York City, sees the therapeutic work that she and her colleagues do as essentially community building. She sees community not as a static or separate thing out there but as a process, "a collective, creative process of people bringing into existence a new social unit and sharing collective commitment to its sustainability" (p. 2). In their work, they are pushed by the idea that helping people, of any age, to grow and develop is best done in this process of creating a viable community. I suspect one reason for this is that, at some level, people understand that you best become who you are in the company of like-minded and interesting others.

In different ways, each of these perspectives contributes to the notion that development and growth, even if one chooses to define them from the modernist perspective as a phase-directed, linear process from conception to death, are to be understood in physical and social milieus. The "self," at any moment, is situated and distributed. The knowledge that one "has" and the actions that one engages in are nested in the confines of current, historical, social, and cultural relationships. Social "realities" are negotiated between people and distributed between them (Bruner, 1990). Additionally, the self can be understood in narrative terms. Donald Polkinghorne (1988) says this about narratives and the self:

We achieve our personal identities and self-concept through the use of narrative configuration, and make our existence into a whole by understanding it as an expression of a single unfolding and developing story. We are in the middle of our stories and cannot be sure how they will end; we are constantly having to revise the plot as new events are added to our lives. Self, then, is not a static thing or a substance, but a configuring of personal events into an historical unity which includes not only what one has been but also anticipations of what one will be. (p. 150)

Children, it seems, have a natural affinity for narrative and story, even before they are facile with language. Narratives and stories are an essential part of the fabric of all cultures and families. Narratives instruct, guide, reveal, suppose, rationalize, and imagine, but they usually have a point and usually, whether autobiographical or familial or cultural, point to a future possibility or state. It seems also the case, according to recent research, that narratives help shape neural connections and in turn are shaped, in part, by neurochemistry and anatomy. Daniel Siegel (cited in Wylie & Simon, 2002) argues that because storytelling is central to every culture, it must reflect a genetic predisposition and capacity. According to Siegel, "Coherent stories are an integration of the left hemisphere's drive to tell a logical story about events and the right brain's ability to grasp emotionally the mental processes of the people in those events" (p. 37). Extrapolating from this, it seems clear to a growing number of neuroscientists that the brain's development and articulation are very much a function of relationships with the environment, interpersonal relationships in particular (LeDoux, 2002). The plasticity of the brain, combined with rich interpersonal, institutional, physical, and natural environments, creates countless opportunities for learning, adaptation, growth, and resilience. Also, to the extent that our life is a narrative(s) unfolding, development is less a linear progression than a discursive tale and sometimes capricious plotline.

The Makings of a New Paradigm in Development?

In many traditional societies, in the past and the present, especially those that are agrarian or dependent on animal husbandry, many of our ideas about child rearing would seem irrelevant or at least curious. Each of these societies is unique, but they share some common practices. For our interest

here, one of these is that children at a young age, especially if another child is born into the family, are thrust out into the community, often in the company of an older sibling, and introduced into the world of peers, both younger and older. Elders and other community members sometimes look after them—at a distance—when they are away from home. At home, although they are cared for and made secure when they are infants, they are taught virtually nothing about the world outside that awaits their entry into a society of peers and the community (Harris, 1998).

From a very different angle, if one examines successful poverty-fighting, socialization, educational, child protection, and community-building programs, especially in those environments in economic distress, one thing stands out. These programs are deeply involved in the community, connecting families and individuals with one another (Schorr, 1997) and with both indigenous resources and more formal ones. They see the community as full of social capital to be mobilized and used in capacity enhancement, protection, and development in children and adults. The community is crucial, too, in strengthening developmental (socialization, education, participation) vitality in children; assuring the protection of vulnerable and dependent members of the community; and fostering involvement of residents as stakeholders in the well-being of the members of the community and the community itself.

It may be the sense and reality of community that makes us most humane and human. We were born to be together in small units of kinship, friendship, mutuality, and collaboration. That is how, as a species, we were able to defend ourselves against threatening elements in the natural and human world. It is also how we protected the very young, the frail, and the very old (Harris, 1998). Although community and neighborhood have taken a battering in recent decades thanks to the transience of families, highly mobile technologies, and the spread of the doctrines of individualism in the popular culture and the professions, for example, what the community provides is still a matter of urgency to individuals and families:

It is [in the community] where capacities of individuals and groups are summoned and deployed in the service of mutual aid. It is here where people may work to resolve common problems. It is here where the assets and resources of people are exchanges in terms of helping others or in securing a common goal. It is here where stories and narratives connect individuals and families to each other and the larger sense of their community. It is here where celebrations take place and tragedies are acknowledged and lamented. . . . And it is here where we can most clearly see the stunning effects of political, social, and economic oppression. (Saleebey, 2001, p. 213)

The message is unmistakable. Families are often a barometer of how things are going in the community or neighborhood. When there is disorganization, crime, violence, loss of resources, or a break in the ties to the outside and to institutions on the inside, families often reflect that with their own internal struggles (although many families do much better than one would expect under such conditions). But, even more pointedly, it is highly unlikely in this complex, rapidly changing world that any family can meet its commitments for the socialization, security, guidance, and protection of its children without support from the larger community.

To say this is not to discount the importance of parents, but it is to say that raising children effectively is a communal or collective endeavor or process. In recent decades we have overblown the role of parents and underplayed the role of the commons. At the very least,

The research makes clear . . . that the capacity of families to do their child-rearing job is powerfully dependent on the health of their communities. A few children, blessed with extraordinary resiliency or unflagging adult support will be able to beat the odds, but most children growing up in severely depleted neighborhoods face a daunting array of risks that greatly diminish their chances of escaping poor economic, educational, social, and health outcomes. Regardless of race, family composition, income or natural endowment, as Harvard's Robert Putnam of *Bowling Alone* fame pithily puts it, "of two identical youths, the one unfortunate enough to live in a neighborhood whose social capital has eroded is more likely to end up hooked, booked, or dead." (Schorr, 1997, p. 306)

Although the economic circumstances and the physical capital available may be clearly more propitious for children whose parents are relatively well-to-do, there still may be a paucity of human, resources, or connective capital for them. The group outcomes are nowhere near as dire, but the negative effect on the course of life is there (Coles, 1988).

The importance of the links between families and communities and the human, economic, social, cultural, and spiritual stock of a neighborhood cannot be overstated. Most families who struggle or whose children are not thriving usually do not lack decency or have "defective" value systems. Too many of our policies and practices with regard to these embattled families look only at the family's psychosocial interior without regard for the depleted community assets and capacities. Environments that are harsh because of poverty, diminished resources, isolated families, inadequate medical care, environmental toxins, neglect, poor nutrition, and violence are tough on a little person's brain. Chronic unrelenting stress can lead to brain cell death and can impede in a very direct way the ability of a small child's (or even older children's) cells to regenerate broken or disorganized connections. The miracle is that in such environments some children do make it and do better than anyone could have possibly expected. We know too little about them, but if they do make it, we have to at least consider the possibilities of strong, determined, and competent parenting or caretaking; extended family involvement; sources of support, guidance, and respite in the community, such as a child care or a tutoring program at a church, afterschool programs, the involvement of a caring, concerned nonfamilial adult; supportive peer relationships; or a sanctuary like a library or park—it is hard to say what it might be. In studying the assets of more than 250 communities, Peter Benson (1997) of the Search Institute suggests that there is a direct relationship between the assets and resources available to kids in a community, in their families, and in themselves and how they fare in school, on the street, in their families, and in the neighborhood.

Parents who have children with special problems or disabilities often find very quickly that they are alone in a vacuum of missing services and communal isolation. In writing of her experience as a mother to disabled children, Nancy Mairs (1996)

observes, "In a society where the rearing of even a healthy child is not viewed as a community undertaking, where much-touted 'family values' are always ascribed to the nuclear and not the human family, the parents of a disabled child will find themselves pretty much on their own" (p. 110). Again, connection and caring are essential community resources that families should be able to draw on and reciprocate.

For years, Jody Kretzmann and John McKnight (1993) have pointed out and demonstrated in their work that helping individuals, families, and associations bring their "gifts" to the community is a major factor in the revitalization of communities and the amplification of individual and familial well-being. Their approach to community building is assets based, internally driven (by residents of the community), and relationship focused (bringing people together in common activities and projects based on the sharing of their resources, capacities, knowledge, and skills). One of the most common focal points of "gift giving" in many communities is child care, child socialization, parental support, and knowledge about child rearing.

Finally, another word about meaning making. If the capacity to make meaning is the most distinguishing feature of human activity, the route to it is complex. Figuring out how children enter this world is in some ways difficult, but in any case, coming into the world is an incredible feat. A young human being, hardly formed, begins to recognize and express the interpretations and renditions of life typical of culture, class, context, gender, and kin. The coming of age of this kind of symbolic grounding is wrought through interactions with others and delivered usually through the medium of narratives and stories. The amazing human achievement of negotiating and renegotiating meanings is "enormously aided by a community's stored narrative resources and its equally precious tool kit of interpretive techniques: its myths, its typology of human plights, but also its traditions for locating and solving divergent narratives" (Bruner, 1990). This kind of symbolic opulence, and the aptitude for understanding and using it, cannot be brought and taught by parents alone.

Up to this point we have clues from many different sources that the development and growth of children are, at best, a communal undertaking, a partnership between families and communities. What might this mean for theory and practice?

Implications for Theory: A Modest Beginning

If the warrants of some of the views here are to be taken seriously, it may be time to move away from the idea that parents (usually a parent, the mother) or caretakers alone bear the most significant responsibility for meeting the basic needs of children (providing them with security, guidance, and comfort) and for how children ultimately turn out. Obviously, parents are strategic figures in the nurturing of children. But they do their work surrounded by a community—its residents and institutions— as members of a social class and a variety of peer groups (e.g., their own and their children's), imbued with culture or cultures, buffeted by ever-shifting ideas and interpretations of the nature of parenting and "good" parenting, and influenced heavily by a variety of media. To get to the point, as very few have pointed out, Judith Harris (1998) being the most recent, the effect of parental behaviors on children's personalities has not been demonstrated. If one defines nurture only as what parents do to and with their children, how they relate to them and educate them, there is no evidence that those are the most essential elements of forming character and personality:

> Experiences in childhood and adolescent peer groups modify children's personalities in ways they will carry with them to adulthood. Group socialization theory makes this prediction: that children would develop into the same sort of adults if we left their lives outside the home unchanged—left them in their schools and their neighborhoods—but switched the parents all around. (Harris, 1998, p. 359).

Recall from the earlier brief discussion of developmental psychology and socialization theories, the prevailing canon holds that the child's personality and performance in adulthood are related to early family experiences and trauma. Beyond the effect of genes (we will not discuss the genetic basis here, but in the case of personality traits, genes may account for, on the average, 50% of the variation of traits [IQ, personality traits, etc.] tested in population samples; obviously, then, the environment accounts for the other 50%), what do we have, then?

These ideas are tentative and beg for fuller expression. Let us agree that there are optimal times for the development of certain capacities in human infants and small children (e.g., language, recognition of strangers, crawling, and walking), but when it comes to other more psychosocial, emotional, motivational, and behavioral capacities, the variation within cultures and societies and between them is considerable. The variation in child-rearing fads and fashions and in the social and cultural surround of different historical epochs is as well (Germain & Bloom, 1999). Let us also agree that children, even in more traditional and physically confined or isolated societies, are a part of many environments and not just raised in the home. Many of these environments are discrete (they can be known and experienced as distinct places and spaces). They are composed of people (their behavior, interrelationships, cultural and ethnic tools and rituals); symbols; things (buildings, natural habitat); and sometimes a particular appearance or look, and a tempo, a rhythm of life. These are all mutable, of course, as people move in and out, and changes are wrought through larger natural and social forces—many of which fly on the wings of contingency and chance.

A Developmental Infrastructure

The development (driven to an extent by the relevant genetic dispositions) of any person, then, is guided, shaped, and influenced by many factors beyond parenting. Let us say that these factors make up, along with parents, a developmental infrastructure. We know about the physical infrastructure of cities (e.g., the condition of gas and electric mains and lines; the quality of bridges, road surfaces) and the resources that provide crucial services (e.g., sanitation, health, construction, firefighters, and police). But what if we began to conceive of and implement *a developmental infrastructure*? This might include peers, extended family, neighbors, media, physical environments (built and natural), key local associations (e.g., a parenting group, a genealogy study group, boys' clubs and girls' clubs) and institutions (a church, a school), as well as more formal services and resources. Each of them plays a role, even if not clearly understood or explicated, in the raising of children. Let us look briefly at one of these: the peer group.

Peer Groups

Children's and youth's peer groups wield influence in how the self unfolds. Since the famous robber's cave experiment by Muzafer Sherif and his colleagues (Sherif, Harvey, White, Hood, & Sherif, 1961) in the 1950s, which demonstrated the quickly developed and fanatic intergroup tensions between two groups of young males, the emphasis on peer groups has been not so much on socialization but on antagonisms, ganglike intergroup tensions, teasing and bullying, and leaders and followers. The following passage by Steven Pinker (1997), which seems pitched to males, primarily reflects this view:

> Children's cultural heritage—the rules of Ringolevio, the melody and lyrics of the nyah-nyah song, the belief that if you kill someone you have to legally pay for his gravestone—is passed from child to child, sometimes for thousands of years. As children grow up they graduate from group to group and eventually join adult groups. Prestige at one level gives one a leg up at the next. . . . [A]t all ages children are driven to figure out what it takes to succeed among their peers and to give these strategies precedence over anything their parents foist on them. (pp. 449–450)

In terms of females and peer groups, Mary Pipher (1994) also accentuates the negative:

> While peers can be satisfying and growth-producing, they can also be growth-destroying, especially in early adolescence. Many girls describe a universal American phenomenon—the scapegoating of girls by one another. Many girls become good haters of those who do not conform sufficiently to our culture's ideas about femininity. (p. 68)

But peer groups also afford the opportunity to learn about cooperation, leadership, playing by the rules, sharing, role-playing, being part of a collective or something bigger than the self, understanding how one can fit in, learning skills, figuring out the world of most insistent interest (like school or the street). It is here that children learn context-appropriate behavior—how people of their age, class, culture, and gender are supposed to act in a given situation. They identify with this group and are concerned about not being very different from its other members. This falls away as they grow into adults, although adults, while more likely to assert their distinctiveness, still hang out in groups of various kinds. Underlying the assertions about the socializing properties of the group are two dynamics. First, children's (and adult's) behavior, to an extent we do not appreciate, is context specific—sensitive and responsive to the people, norms, expectations, rites, rules, and physical attributes in that setting. What children learn at home about themselves and the world may not have much use or be transferable to their peer group or to the playground or classroom. Second, we still probably do not appreciate the sculpting power of genes. To put it as many behavioral geneticists do, the extent to which two siblings are alike is not because of their parents' behavior but because of their genetic heritage. But, in important ways, they are still different because of the role of experience and environment.

If we include peers as a part of the socialization infrastructure, we would give them more accountability for the socializing of each other into active and responsible citizens. This might occur through ensuring active participation in the moral and civic life of the community, group mentoring, high expectations for achievement and socialization, and affording the opportunity for them to be responsible for each other.

In my experience in a number of modest community-building programs, three things are apparent. First, there is a children's-eye-view of community. Children and youth are very aware of the community, the neighborhood, and they do not often see it the same way as adults do. Second, children and youth are often hungry for the experience of community and recognize it as important to their well-being. In our projects, programs that have been developed, at least in part, by youth have the development of the sense of community as an important goal—providing a sense of belonging, participation, and collaboration and giving and receiving the gifts of skills, work, and oneself. Third, activities that are positive in this way (youth developing a community sense and providing something to the larger community) have a valuable effect on that larger community.

Perhaps there are two ways to regard the developmental infrastructure. The most radical is that we organize to develop those elements of it beyond parents (peers, media, neighbors, etc.) that we think directly affect the socialization of children. As communities we develop programs and policies that organize and support this infrastructure so that, instead of always focusing on parents and their children, we focus on the web of relationships, the ambient environment in which children grow and change and thrive.

The more conservative view is the one that is alive and well but still weak-kneed because of lack of sufficient support from a variety of sources. This is the view that parents, in order to do their job, need more community support and resources. Lisbeth Schorr (1997) explains how this situation has changed: "In the past, extended family, neighbors, and teachers shared responsibility for children. The key was redundancy. Especially in minority neighborhoods, if a parent was unavailable, other adults were on hand to hurry a dawdling child to school, teach a new skill, or set another place at the table" (p. 120). But, in this view, it is the parents who are the singular and eminent socializers of children.

Conclusion

It is probably obvious to readers that the ideas and concerns here bear a relationship to ecological theory or person-environment frameworks, and to life course theories and ideas. (See Germain & Bloom, 1999, for an able accounting and detailing of these.) They do, to a degree. Environmental psychologists and developmental ecologists have taken on some of these ideas as well. As an example, let me quote from Urie Bronfenbrenner's (1995) latest propositions regarding his bioecological paradigm. In proposition 1, he claims that, in early life especially,

> human development takes place through processes of progressively more complex reciprocal interaction between an active, evolving biopsychological human organism and the persons, objects, and symbols in its immediate environment. . . . this interaction must occur on a fairly regular basis. . . . Such enduring forms of interaction in the immediate environment are referred to as *proximal processes*. (p. 620, italics added)

And, in proposition 2, he claims:

> The form, power, content, and direction of the proximal processes . . . vary systematically as a joint function of the biopsychological characteristics of the developing person; of the environment, both immediate and more remote, in which the processes are taking place; and the

nature of the developmental outcomes under consideration. (p. 621)

This is the kind of language that will yield useful hypotheses to be tested. But we want these ideas, too, to thrust us into the welter of forces, events, experiences, people, knowledge, and time that affect how people grow and change. Some of these ideas were evident in the past. This chapter is an attempt to take some of these ideas, new and old, and to add others about the nature of the self and socialization to see if we indeed might have the conceptual tools to create a view of human development nested in a web of relationships and environments; a view respectful of an individual's capacity to form the self, as well as culture and history's impact on the experience of growing and being and becoming. It probably is uncertain whether or not we have the beginnings of a new paradigm, but I think we have the conceptual tools to begin to assemble ideas about development that reflect our multiple realities and experiences. I think, too, that we need descriptions (or operational definitions) of these ideas that propel us in a dramatic way into the matrix of the daily life of people without beggaring its dimensions and variety. Perhaps the idea of a developmental infrastructure may give us a conceptual peg on which to begin hanging some new or different interpretations of the amazing experience of being and becoming human.

References

Barker, R. (1968). *Ecological psychology*. Palo Alto, CA: Stanford University Press.

Benard, B. (2002). Turnaround people and places: Moving from risk to resilience. In D. Saleebey (Ed.), *The strengths perspective in social work practice* (pp. 213–227). Boston: Allyn and Bacon.

Benson, P. (1997). *All kids are our kids: What communities must do to raise caring and responsible children and adolescents*. San Francisco: Jossey-Bass.

Bronfenbrenner, U. (1995). Developmental psychology through space and time. In P. Moen, G. Elder Jr., & K. Luscher (Eds.), *Examining lives in context* (pp. 619–647). Washington, DC: American Psychological Association Press.

Bruner. J. (1986). *Actual minds, possible worlds*. Cambridge, MA: Harvard University Press.

Bruner, J. (1990). *Acts of meaning*. Cambridge, MA: Harvard University Press.

Coles, R. (1988). *Children of crisis*. New York: Bookthrift.

Flach, F. (1997). *Resilience: The power to bounce back when the going gets tough*. New York: Hatherleigh.

Garmezy, N. (1993). Children in poverty: Resilience despite risk. *Psychiatry, 56*, 127–136.

Geertz, C. (1979). From the native's point of view: On the nature of anthropological understanding. In P. Rabinow & W. M. Sullivan (Eds.), *Interpretive social science* (pp. 120–132). Berkeley: University of California Press.

Gergen, K. (1991). *The saturated self: Dilemmas of identity in contemporary life*. New York: Basic Books.

Gergen, K. (1999). *An invitation to social construction*. London: Sage.

Germain, C., & Bloom, M. (1999). *Human behavior in the social environment: An ecological view* (2nd ed.). New York: Columbia University Press.

Gladwell, M. (2000). *The tipping point: How little things can make a big difference*. Boston: Little, Brown.

Goodnow, J. (1995). Differentiating among social contexts: By spatial features, forms of participation, and social contracts. In P. Moen, G. Elder Jr., & K. Luscher (Eds.), *Examining lives in context* (pp. 269–302). Washington, DC: American Psychological Association Press.

Harris, J. R. (1998). *The nurture assumption: Why children turn out the way they do*. New York: Simon and Schuster/Touchstone Books.

Holzman, L. (2002, December). *Practicing a psychology that builds community*. Keynote address, American Psychological Association Division 27, Society for Community Research and Action Conference, Boston.

Kagan, J. (1994). *Galen's prophecy: Temperament in human nature*. New York: Basic Books.

Katz, M. (1997). *On playing a poor hand well: Insights from the lives of those who have overcome childhood risks and adversities*. New York: Norton.

Kretzmann, J., & McKnight, J. (1993). *Building communities from the inside out: Toward finding and mobilizing a community's assets*. Evanston, IL: Northwestern University Center for Urban Affairs and Policy Research.

LeDoux, J. (2002). *The synaptic self: How our brains become who we are*. New York: Viking.

Maccoby, E. (1992). The role of parents in the socialization of children: An historical overview. *Developmental Psychology, 28*, 1006–1017.

Mairs, N. (1996). *Waist high in the world*. Boston: Beacon.

Malcolm, J. (1981). *Psychoanalysis: The impossible profession*. New York: Vintage Books.

Masten, A., Best, K., & Garmezy, N. (1990). Resilience and development: Contributions from the study of children who overcome adversity. *Development and Psychopathology, 2,* 425–441.

Mischel, W. (1996). *Personality and assessment.* Mahwah, NJ: Erlbaum.

Nisbett, R., & Ross, L. (1991). *The person and the situation.* Philadelphia: Temple University Press.

Norman, E. (2000). Introduction: The strengths perspective and resiliency enhancement—a natural partnership. In E. Norman (Ed.), *Resiliency enhancement: Putting the strengths perspective into social work practice* (pp. 1–16). New York: Columbia University Press.

Ornstein, R. (1993). *The roots of self: Unraveling the mystery of who we are.* San Francisco: HarperSanFrancisco.

Pinker, S. (1997). *How the mind works.* New York: Norton.

Pipher, M. (1994). *Reviving Ophelia: Saving the selves of adolescent girls.* New York: Ballantine.

Polkinghorne, D. (1988). *Narrative knowing and the human sciences.* Albany: State University of New York Press.

Proshansky, H., & Fabian, A. (1987). The development of place identity in the child. In C. Weinstein & T. David (Eds.), *Spaces for children: The built environment and child development* (pp. 21–40). New York: Plenum.

Rutter, M. (1985). Resilience in the face of adversities. *British Journal of Psychiatry, 147,* 598–611.

Saleebey, D. (2001). *Human behavior and social environments: A biopsychosocial approach.* New York: Columbia University Press.

Saleebey, D. (2002). The strengths perspective: Possibilities and problems. In D. Saleebey (Ed.), *The strengths perspective in social work practice* (pp. 264–286). Boston: Allyn and Bacon.

Sampson, E. (1993). *Celebrating the other: A dialogic account of human nature.* Boulder, CO: Westview.

Schoggen, P. (1989). *Behavior settings: A revision and extension of Roger G. Barker's ecological psychology.* Stanford, CA: Stanford University Press.

Schorr, L. (1997). *Common purpose: Strengthening families and neighborhoods to rebuild America.* New York: Anchor Books/Doubleday.

Sherif, M., Harvey, O. J., White, B. J., Hood, W. R., & Sherif, C. W. (1961). *Intergroup cooperation and competition: The robber's cave experiment.* Norman: University of Oklahoma Press.

Thomas, L. (1974). *The lives of a cell: Notes of a biology watcher.* New York: Penguin.

Vaillant, G. (2002). *Aging well.* Boston: Little, Brown.

Walsh, F. (1998). *Strengthening family resilience.* New York: Guilford.

Werner, E., & Smith, R. (1982). *Vulnerable but invincible.* New York: McGraw Hill.

Werner, E., & Smith, R. (1992). *Overcoming the odds: High-risk children from birth to adulthood.* Ithaca, NY: Cornell University Press.

Wolin, S., & Wolin, S. (1996). The challenge model: Working with strengths in children of substance-abusing parents. *Adolescent Substance Abuse and Dual Disorders, 5,* 243–256.

Wylie, M. S., & Simon, R. (2002). Discoveries from the black box. *Psychotherapy Networker, 26,* 26–37, 68.

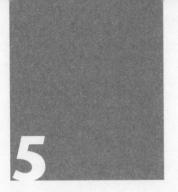

5 Carol R. Swenson

Ideas of Self and Community
Expanding Possibilities for Practice

Clinician 1: "The community is a source of referrals, but once clients are in the door, it makes no difference. . . ."

Clinician 2: "Community" has been extremely important in my personal life, but actually, . . . I guess I don't think about it in my work with clients."

Clinician 3: "I try to create 'community' in the session, by sharing my own 'broken places.' "

Clinician 4: "I am always trying to help my clients become more embedded in a community. They are so devalued and isolated, when actually they have so much to contribute."

These four clinicians express different ideas of community and, indirectly, different ideas of the self. The first clinician has a concrete and utilitarian idea of community—it consists of relationships with community representatives who facilitate referrals. The second clinician views community as personally meaningful but divorced from her professional life. The third clinician, by contrast, has an almost mystical sense of community—it is a deep connection at the level of personhood, which transcends but can be called upon in the clinical relationship, and which reduces the power differential between worker and client. And the fourth clinician has a

notion of community as a place of mutual respect and mutual help, which can be fostered by the clinician.

Conversely, these vignettes represent implicit, and differing, ideas of the self. The first and second clinicians appear to understand a client's self largely in individual or familial terms. (The second clinician is a puzzle, actually. She appears not to have questioned the discrepancy between her thinking about herself and her thinking about clients.) The third clinician imagines a self-in-relation and fosters it in the clinical dyad. And the fourth clinician has a vision of a self-in-community that guides her work.

These four quotations come from interviews with clinicians, in which they were asked about their ideas of community and its relation to their professional work (Swenson, 1995; Swenson et al., 1993). All the clinicians interviewed were considered by colleagues to be community oriented in their practice. And while it would be unjustified to draw major conclusions from just a few words, these phrases represent their speakers' views as expressed in extensive interviews.

As these vignettes illustrate, all clinical practice embodies, implicitly or explicitly, an idea of the self and an idea of community. If we do not work to make our professional understandings explicit, we are likely to adopt, uncritically, the concepts of the dominant culture (Sampson, 1985, 1988). In the United States, the dominant idea of the self is the "rugged individual," translated in much psychosocial theory into a bounded, masterful, autonomous self (Bellah, Madsen, Sullivan, Swidler, & Tipton, 1985, 1991; Cushman, 1990, 1995; Sampson, 1977, 1988).

However, social work values and traditions (Addams, 1910/1961; Council on Social Work Education, 2001; National Association of Social Workers, 1994; Reynolds, 1951/1973, 1963/1964; Schwartz, 1985; Specht & Courtney, 1994), as well as feminist, multicultural, and spiritual perspectives (Canda & Furman, 1999; Devore & Schlesinger, 1996; Swigonski, 1994), support an alternative conception of the self: a self-in-community. This expands the idea of "self-in-relation," which emphasizes both connection and individuation, beyond small and intimate units like the dyad or family (Miller, 1984). But how do we incorporate such ideas into our clinical practice? This chapter will suggest some possibilities.

Community clinical practice can be understood in concrete and utilitarian terms—traditional services delivered more accessibly to people who find it difficult to go to a hospital or agency. From another perspective, community clinical practice can represent a shift in our fundamental notions of self, of other, of community. Out of these ideas can come a more radical change, a different vision of what it means to be a human being, a vision in which participation in community, or communities, is at the heart.

In this chapter I will discuss some of the traditional ways that "selfhood" has been conceptualized and some of the critiques of those views. I will address various ideas about community. Drawing on expanded notions of the meanings of self and community, I suggest new possibilities for practice. The ideas and citations that follow are intended to be suggestive; they are not a comprehensive review.

Ideas of Self

One of the difficulties in discussing ideas of the self is that until recently "self" was taken for granted. We assumed that everyone's idea of the self was the same, over time (historically) and across place (cul-turally). This was true in social work, in other mental health professions, and in the wider culture. What attention anthropology paid did not seem to reach the professions. It is somewhat like the way "family" was understood by clinicians—as undifferentiated background—before family therapy made it a focus of inquiry.

Over the last few decades, however, scholars in various fields have begun exploring the idea of the self, and professions have begun to see the relevance of this exploration for their work. Christopher Lasch, Robert Bellah and his associates, and Michel Foucault began to consider historical and cultural variations of the self. Foucault (1980, 1981a, 1981b) was one of the early voices, describing the self as something that is formed and reformed in relation to various personal values, goals, and cultural standards. About the same time, Lasch (1979) was describing the contemporary American self as individualistic, self-absorbed, and living for the moment. Bellah, Madsen, Sullivan, Swidler, and Tipton (1985, 1987, 1991) have tried to reexamine America, following in the footsteps of the famous French cultural observer Alexis de Tocqueville. They were impressed by the overwhelming individualism (sometimes broadened to include the person's family) of contemporary Americans. This includes highly valuing personal expression, and a utilitarian framework for ethics. They conclude that America's dominant moral language moves little further than economic metaphors of costs and benefits, giving scant attention to commitment, values, traditions, or community.

Others, even within psychology, such as Edward Sampson (1985, 1988), have begun to compare Euro-American ideas of the self with those of other times and places. Michael White (1995), an Australian narrative therapist, says,

> There is a dominant story of what it means to be a person of moral worth in [Western] culture. This is a story that emphasizes self-possession, self-containment, self-actualization and so on. . . . The notions that accompany this dominant story . . . don't represent some *authentic way of living*, or some *real or genuine expression of human nature* but, rather, are really a specification or prescription of cultural preferences. (p. 16, italics added)

Philip Cushman (1990), summarizing, says "There is no universal, transhistorical self, only local selves; there is no universal theory about the self, only local theories" (p. 603).

Further, Cushman (1990, 1995) has tied the individualistic American self to the prevailing social order. He sees politico-economic powers in the United States as quite deliberately creating "empty" selves—consumers who will fill their emptiness by constant buying, thereby fueling capitalism. From this perspective, as helping professionals privilege individualism and encourage clients to become more separate and self-focused, they are supporting the dominant social order. In contrast, clinicians who withstand "the cult of the individual" and encourage self-in-community are challenging the dominant order and engaging in modestly radical practice.

Other, more subordinated, visions of the self can be found. Cushman (1990) and Bellah et al. (1985) describe an alternative self that is rooted in an experience of shared meanings and values, of common commitments, of rituals and traditions, of mutual appreciation and mutual aid. They particularly found expression of this subordinated view among people who were deeply religious, living a life of service to others, or strongly committed to an oppressed ethnic group.

In other cultures, however, elements of selves that are subordinate in our culture may be dominant. Thus Alan Roland (1988), for example, looked at ideas of the self in Indian and Japanese cultures. He identified, in addition to the Euro-American individualistic self, a familial self, an expanding self, and a spiritual self. The latter two are of particular interest here, since they suggest ideas that relate to self-in-community. The expanding self emerges from cross-cultural experiences and recognizes the differences between one's own culture and that of others, valuing both. The spiritual self includes a transcendent view of the connections between all living things, in which universal harmony is the goal. Similarly, in his later years, Erik Erikson added a spiritual self as a ninth stage of his famous typology (Erikson, Erikson, & Kivnick, 1986).

In social work, in addition to the "masterful, bounded, autonomous" self, there has always been a second, subordinated vision of the person. This vision has been important especially to social group workers and community workers. Jane Addams (1910/1961) was an early proponent of the view that living in relationship is central, and she espe-cially valued cross-class and cross-ethnic relationships. Bertha Reynolds (1951/1973; 1963/1964) had a vision of living in community and, indeed, saw a role for social work mediating "between client and community." This idea has been carried forward with the emphasis on mutual aid in social group work (Gitterman & Shulman, 1993). Judith Lee (2001) has been a strong contemporary social work voice expressing a vision of self-in-community.

Ideas of Community

Ideas of community have had quite a different history than ideas of the self. Perhaps because community is a less central commitment in Western thought than selfhood, it has been seen as needing definition. Hillery (1955) identified 94 definitions! He notes, however, that about three fourths of the definitions include the same three elements: geographic area, social interaction, and common ties.

Historically, sociology has considered two very different types of community: a small community with high degrees of interaction, commitment, and homogeneity, and low rates of change (gemein-schaft), and a large community that is more impersonal, specialized, quick changing, and diverse (ge-sellschaft; (Bell & Newby, 1972). Debate has addressed questions such as whether the first type of community is disappearing with urbanization, industrialization, and geographic mobility, and whether gemeinschaft is "better" than gesellschaft. Earlier beliefs that historical trends amplifying ge-sellschaft would destroy gemeinschaft have not been borne out. Close, personal ties appear to co-exist with more impersonal relationships.

Other distinctions are communities based on geography and communities based on shared interests or commitments. There have also been the contrasting perspectives of community as objective and measurable, on the one hand, and as subjective, a "psychological sense of community," on the other.

The "psychological sense of community" is especially important for considering self-in-community. Seymour Sarason (1974), one of the pioneers of the community mental health movement, stressed how much people's sense of well-being depends on their psychological sense of community. The psychological sense of community involves feelings of connectedness and mutual belonging, which arise out of shared goals, values, and actions. Lieberman (1988) used the concept of "internal representations of community" to point out that community is not only "out there" but also "within."

For our purposes, these various views can inform our thinking, and we do not need to choose one. Hutchinson (1995), writing for social work, says, "Community is people bound either by geography or network links (webs of communication), sharing common ties, and interacting with one another" (p. 8). Because of the varying perspectives, it is clear that we need to try to make our concept of community explicit. For example, Hutchinson suggests that the *territorial* community is often of considerable importance in the lives of society's more vulnerable members. She concludes that we need to pay particular attention to territorial community as we plan social services.

Currently, one important force in relation to community in the contemporary world is the Internet. But it is ambiguous, or perhaps multidimensional. On the one hand, the Internet has made it possible for huge numbers of people to be linked in very impersonal ways. On the other hand, it has broken geographic barriers, so people with unique bonds, such as sharing rare diseases or belonging to dispersed ethnic groups, can have relationships across vast distances. However, the enthusiasm with which many people absorb themselves in "chat rooms" and other Internet-mediated relationships does suggest an absence of community in their everyday lives. Social workers and other mental health professionals are experimenting with ways to use the Internet to enhance connections and to build community.

Intersections of Self and Community

As community clinicians, we can best direct our attention at the boundary or interface of self and community. Various intellectual traditions have strove to bring the ideas together. Frank and Keys (1987), community psychologists, observe that there can be no individuals without groups, and no groups without individuals. Object relations theorists Greenberg and Mitchell (1983) suggest, "The human community and culture transcend the individual life span; in some sense the community creates the individual life, giving it substance and

meaning" (p. 400). The social psychologists have always understood "self" as a social creation (Blumer, 1969; Gergen, 1985; Mead, 1934).

Community and Clinical Practice

As clinical practice has evolved, the early focus on individual development and pathology has been modified by more recent thinking that is more inclusive, first of family relationships and then of social relationships beyond the family (Adams & Nelson, 1995). In addition, the early emphasis on a single developmental path from dependence to autonomy (the "bounded, autonomous self" discussed earlier) has been questioned, especially by feminist developmentalists, who suggested that both interdependence and autonomy are developmental lines that mature (Gilligan, 1982; Miller, 1976, 1984). These ideas have resonated with practitioners who work with non-Western clients, where the "bounded, autonomous masterful self" may be less valued (Devore & Schlesinger, 1996; Roland, 1988).

Ecological, and general systems theories also have implications for ideas of self and community (Germain, 1991; Germain & Gitterman, 1996; Meyer, 1993). General systems theory, which emerged in the late 1960s and 1970s, provides a multidimensional framework for understanding human behavior. The theory focuses on the interdependence and interactions among people and emphasizes the many systems in which people interact. The theory is a means of conceptualizing the mutual interrelatedness of a series of nesting systems or networks: individuals, families, social groups, communities, and societies (Hartman & Laird, 1983). Hence, this theory appreciates community, but as a "general theory" it does not develop self-community in a substantive way.

The ecological perspective for understanding development was spurred by a recognition of environmental barriers that pose unavoidable challenges to growth (Bronfenbrenner, 1970, 1979). The focus of the ecological perspective is on identifying positive as well as negative influences in the environment with a goal of mobilizing and supporting natural resources of the client (Swenson, 1979, 1981). Natural helping networks also act as buffers against negative influences such as oppression and poverty. Self-sufficiency develops through social networks, which can be thought of as a "personal community."

More recently, social constructionist and narrative approaches have emerged. Constructionists emphasize the meanings that individuals and groups create about experience, rather than positing an objective "truth" to be found. They are interested in ways of intervening with clients that expand client experiences and create opportunities for clients to take the role of the acknowledged expert (Anderson & Goolishian, 1988). As an example of social constructionist thinking about self and community, Jo Ann Allen (1993) raised the concern that therapy may support the status quo through pathologizing explanations of client behavior that ignore external conditions such as oppression and poverty.

The strengths perspective has been developing out of concern with the pathologizing qualities of much clinical theory and interventions. It is both a critique and a new direction, as practitioners explore its implications for intervention (Saleebey, 1992, 1996). It is through building on strengths that positive change occurs, whether those are strengths of the individual or family, of naturally occurring or planned groups, or of the wider community. In fact, group or community resources can be mobilized to help address individual or family weaknesses; individuals and families can strengthen groups and communities as well.

Closely related to the strengths perspective is a collaborative helping stance. If clients are seen as experts in their own lives, the helper gives up the great power of the "expert role" (Madsen, 1999). This shift of power, especially in a group or community context, can have significant implications for people's lives (Freire, 1970/1973, 1992).

Mutual aid has been a key concept in the strand of social work that had its origins in the settlement house movement. As has been discussed, many writers from this tradition have eloquently expressed their vision of personhood. They see people, whom others might call "clients," as self-directed agents, reciprocally helping and being helped, living with others to whom the person feels ties of caring and belonging (Addams, 1910/1961; Reynolds, 1951/1973; Lee & Swenson, 1993). "Empowerment" is the outcome of a practice role that builds on and strengthens mutual aid, ultimately becoming political action on one's own behalf and on behalf of others (Lee, 2001).

A final related idea is social justice. Clinicians, especially clinical social workers, are "rediscovering" the significance of social justice (Swenson, 1998; Van Soest, 1995; Wakefield, 1988). Social justice concerns the ways in which society and its constituencies regard the needs, rights, and claims of individuals and subgroups. From a community perspective, injustice may be exclusion from full participation in the life of the community (Breton, 1989). A central function of communities is to be a location for mutual aid and reciprocal help.

All these ideas offer hints for new community-oriented interventions. Expanding these suggestions will be the focus of the remainder of this chapter.

Expanding Possibilities for Practice

The ideas that follow are derived from practice and research experiences, as well as from the literature discussed in the first part of this chapter. These ideas are particularly informed by the narrative therapists (e.g., Michael White & David Epston, 1990) and are rooted in four concepts discussed earlier: the strengths perspective, collaborative helping relationships, mutual aid/empowerment, and social justice. While all of these interventions are likely to be *accompanied* by direct action in the community, either with or on behalf of clients, the interventions discussed in this chapter will focus on *therapeutic conversations* with clients.

To back up for a moment, as a clinician in the community mental health field, I had struggled to articulate what "community" added to "clinician." I had a strong sense that community meant something important in my life and in many other people's lives. I saw that many clients of community mental health centers were isolated from meaningful communities, and that other people with few social relationships were apt to be lonely and unhappy. The resources I had for understanding community were largely theological and spiritual, however, rather than professional.

I was not clear what to do with these forms of knowledge about community. The practice theories of the day were still largely focused on individuals, with some attention to family work, group work, and prevention. Most professionals I knew were like the first and second clinicians in the opening to this chapter. Ideas about community led to some new practices in the community, such as consultation and education, but on the whole these ideas influenced clinical practice very little. As I became a scholar of practice as well as a practitioner, I developed my interest in community-related topics such as natural helping, social networks, and mutual aid (Swenson, 1979, 1981) and became more informed about the social group work tradition (Lee & Swenson, 1978, 1993). Over time, I became aware of the critiques of Lasch, Bellah et al., and Cushman, discussed earlier.

These various themes led me to become interested in what contemporary clinical social workers might think and say about community. I wondered if the ways of thinking that are part of social work's history would lead these clinicians to a more expansive and elaborated vision of the self than that of the people, including clinicians, that Lasch, Bellah, and Cushman describe. Different traditions of social group work, community organizing, and the settler's movement, as discussed earlier, seem to express a vision of self-in-community. Accordingly, with Dina Carbonell as a co-instructor and nine MSW students, I carried out a qualitative study of clinical social workers' ideas about community (Swenson et al., 1993; Swenson, 1995). We asked the participants to talk about the significance of community in their own lives and then asked them how ideas of community inform their work. This somewhat unusual initial focus on the clinicians' personal lives arose from our belief, and experience, that to start with questions about "community" in their clinical work was likely to lead to puzzled silence.

All the respondents could say something about community, at least that it signified a shared locality or a characteristic. Any deeper meaning of that which was "shared" was not emphasized. Even for those respondents who went a little deeper, recognizing community as a location of social support, the notion of community was relatively utilitarian—what it could provide to this individual or family.

There were two kinds of further elaborations, however. One of these was the idea of community identifications and participation being part of identity, part of the sense of self. Words like "embeddedness," "belonging," "relatedness," "affiliation," "meaning making," and "self in relation" were used or come to mind. Sometimes this identification was so expansive that it became an existential or spiritual sense of the interconnectedness of all human

beings, or even "the connectedness of all things in the universe." Only a few of the respondents used this kind of language, and it was still largely unidirectional: benefits *from* the community *to* the person.

A final cluster of responses, seen only fleetingly, and from no more than three respondents, was a deep sense of reciprocity, mutuality, and obligation with others who share a common history, symbols, ritual, and values. This included social participation, shared goals, and a commitment to create community for others. There was none of this final kind of talk in relation to clients, with one exception. "Deb" (this and any other names are psuedonyms) talked about how much her client community (disabled people) "have to give." Sadly, this opportunity was lost because people in the larger "community" shunned them.

But throughout the interviews, the participants' inarticulateness in describing community and their underdeveloped sense of community were most apparent. We concluded that there is a great need to develop a sense of self-in-community and to integrate it into our theories and practices.

To carry this work forward, I developed another qualitative study with the goal of explicating the idea of self-in-community, and elaborating clinical practices to realize it (Swenson et al., 1996). In this study the 12 participants (myself, Ruth Cope, PhD, co-instructor, and 10 MSW students) generated case vignettes that were enacted (role-played), audiotaped, and discussed. The focus was intensifying our attention to community, particularly self-in-community, and elaborating practice principles suggested by this scrutiny.

The ideas about community that follow are a synthesis of our reflections. They can be viewed as a very loose, nonlinear progression, but each element can also stand alone. They include (1) defining the presenting problem in a community-oriented way, (2) assessing from a community perspective, (3) examining and critiquing community/cultural stereotypes, (4) addressing pain and grief about difficult community relationships, (5) starting to dream of a community of choice, (6) identifying present or future potential communities, (7) acting in community, and (8) reflecting on acting in community.

1. Defining the presenting problem. The client may define his or her problem in a community-oriented way. More often, however, it will be seen

primarily as "individual failing" or "individual ill-ness." Community clinicians will wonder, however, "Is there any sense of the problem as 'loss of community/loss of connection,' or as 'community betrayal'?" These clinicians carry a sense of self-in-community that allows them to notice "absences" of community, as well as "presences." The presenting problem ultimately may be defined as a combination of these individual and community dimensions.

A man in his 50s, who is a member of a religious order, has been a very successful teacher within that community. He is experiencing an intensification of pain about his experiences as a child of sexual abuse within that community. He has never talked about the abuse within the community, nor about the neglect, if not abuse, in his family of origin. Now he is questioning whether he wants to remain in the order, where he feels bitterly betrayed, but he also sees it as the only community he has.

2. Assessing in a community-oriented way. Usual assessment questions may be asked, but with an additional, community focus. Clinician questions might include: What is your present support system like? Is there someone you call when you feel lonely? Tell me about important relationships you have had with other people or groups of people. Have you ever had a supportive community? What communities have you been a part of? How do you understand "community"? What have community connections been like for you? What are the "rules" in the communities in your life? Are certain emotions tolerated, and others not? Who had the power in the community? How were decisions usually made? Do you remember a time that you felt powerful in a community setting? Do you feel a part of any spiritual or faith community? What is this community like for you?

The client and the clinician construct a story of community and/or communities. What has community meant to this person? What is the history of community in this person's life? What are the legacies, both positive and negative, that this client carries? What values does this person hold?

A young woman sought help for her anxiety and sleeplessness. It transpired that her partner had been murdered just about a year ago. At the time, she had been prevented from seeing his body by well-meaning friends and neighbors who physically held her back, saying, "It's better for you not to see

him." The client felt quite strongly otherwise. She yearned to have seen him with her own eyes, to have touched him. No sight could be as terrible as this void she felt. Since then, when these people saw her, they would never talk about her boyfriend, "even though it's the primary thing on everyone's minds." When she tries to talk about him, everyone tells her, "It's time for closure, it's time to move on." She will be lying in bed, sleepless, missing him, and at the same time feeling that if she calls anyone, they will be impatient and judgmental. Thus the original loss has led to an interlocking series of "losses" of her family and friends, just when she needs them most. She feels betrayed by them but then feels guilty for her reaction.

3. Examining and critiquing community stereotypes. The clinician raises awareness of community stereotypes, for example, "the way men are" or "the way doctors are." These stereotypes may be held by the wider culture, by subgroups that are important to the client, or sometimes by both. When culture and community diverge, it may cause distress, but it can also be an avenue for coming to appreciate diversity. The clinician can call upon the history of a client's experiences to start to develop and use new categories. A new kind of rootedness and belonging can be created. Utilizing a strengths perspective is particularly important here.

Mrs. C., a Dominican immigrant who spoke little English, was anxious and worried about an official-looking letter that she had received. The community clinician was able to tell her that the letter simply said her children needed vaccinations, the ones she had already taken them for. Mrs. C., alternately laughing and crying, said, "You mean I did the right thing?" She was ready to see her own shortcomings everywhere, a situation that her adolescent daughters exploited. The clinician talked with Mrs. C. about the group she was starting for mothers who speak primarily Spanish, focusing on the special issues of bringing up teenagers in America.

The idea that problems are individually caused is, itself, a cultural assumption. It is a particularly important stereotype because it can lead to isolation, self-blame, and depression. While acknowledging the partial truth in this assumption, the clinician can ask questions in such a way that possible contributions of community, family, society, and culture may be seen. This may have a mobilizing effect for the client and lead to action. Possible questions to consider include the following: What is the community's role in the client's problem? What are maladaptive community responses, such as covering up pain or abuse? What responsibility does a community have to help a client heal?

A client who described his background as "working class" attended an elite college on scholarship. He survived and graduated, but the experience left him feeling diminished and self-doubting. He felt that students and faculty had constantly judged him because he was seen as "different," and this difference was judged "inferior." The client understood the class privilege being expressed, but he was still hurt. One consequence for him was having a hard time finding a personally meaningful career.

Clinicians need to be aware, as members of a clinical community, of our own cultural assumptions, rules, and values. One way that clinical communities vary is in terms of the stance of the clinician. For example, according to the social group work tradition, a social worker's stance is open and authentic. Other approaches call for a more reserved style. No matter the stance, self-awareness is essential. The clinician's own ideas and experiences of community are examined and understood. The clinician is ready to talk about community issues as it is appropriate to the clinical work. It is particularly important that clinicians do not assume that they know a client's experience, even if their own experience seems similar.

Marlene led a women's group, which gave much attention to the ways the women were burdened by their family responsibilities. One of the members, Suzanne, was discussing with pleasure her plans for a short vacation. The group rule of paying when unable to attend came up. "In spite of the fact that it was part of the original contract, and we understood it to symbolize respect for the group," the group members said, "it now looks ridiculous. Here is Suzanne, enacting one of the group's goals, and the leader wants to charge her!" Marlene wisely agreed that the members were absolutely right. Later she said, "I'll bet if I had insisted, they would have complied . . . and the group would never have worked well again. I'm going to have to think carefully about this before I start my next group."

4. Addressing pain and grief. This is the feeling part of dealing with community and cultural stereotypes and losses. The clinical work will go back

and forth between the cognitive (element 3), and the affective (element 4): acknowledging the pain that loss of connection and community cause; acknowledging the experience of feeling shamed over not conforming or not belonging; feeling betrayed and angry, lost, empty; acknowledging ambivalence; feeling torn between contradicting communities or warring values; needing community, but also being hurt by it at the same time.

Julie was a college freshman when she came to the counseling center. She was upset and grieving over a breakdown in the relationship between herself and her best friend from high school. She could not stop thinking about it, although she was sure she had made every attempt possible to reconcile, and that she had to "let it go." She was feeling alienated from her father, her only viable family relationship. Additionally, she had transferred from another college at the end of first semester because it seemed to be only a "party school." She was feeling completely alone. As she grieved the ruptured relationship in therapy, she began to take steps, tentatively at first, into some new relationships with other students. She began to find students who shared her interest in art and communications. As the term wound down, she decided she was ready to discontinue sessions at the counseling center.

5. Starting to dream of a community of choice. What kind of connections is a client looking for? With whom would a client like to establish connections? How will these connections be different from past connections? How will they be similar? What would one's ideal community look like? How would people interact? How would decisions be made? What values would members of the community share? What kinds of rituals would be shared? How would differences be addressed in this community?

The client is a young African American woman who persistently felt lonely and alienated in high school. She went to an intellectually challenging college, where she found others who were interested in ideas, the arts, progressive social action, and spirituality. She was thrilled to discover so many people like herself. She sought out a pastoral counselor to help her decide whether to pursue theological training or social work as a career. They agreed that neither was a "bad" choice, and that both directions offered the opportunity to be with many people who shared her values and commitments.

6. Identifying present or future preferred communities. Clients and clinicians might go back and forth between elements 5 and 6. They would be identifying possible supportive and collaborative relationships or groups for the client, given his or her preferences and values. These relationships may already be in the client's life, in which case an attempt to strengthen the ties might be helpful. If the client does not have a preexisting relationship with a group or a member of the group in which he or she is interested, strategies for connecting with this group would be discussed.

Questions about preferred communities might include the following: Where can we find support in a community that would "be there" for you? Are there places you could meet people, connect with people? What kinds of connections are meaningful or important for you? Perhaps we could think a bit about what kinds of relationships you might be looking for and in what kinds of places you might start looking?

A client whose marriage was failing because of his wife's alcoholism felt alone and unsure what to do. The clinician helped him to consider possibilities, such as joining Al-Anon, attending a men's group, or getting more involved in his church. They discussed the similarities and differences in what each choice would offer.

If joining an existing group is unappealing or insufficient for a particular client, another idea is to "recruit an audience" for the client's new story or newly discovered preferences. In this way the client, with the guidance of the therapist, starts to create his or her own community. A client might write a series of letters or have a series of conversations with more distant members of the community whom he or she perceives as likely to be receptive to a new story. As people respond or do not respond, a decision could be made (by client and therapist) about how to proceed. In some cases, a therapist and client might simply decide to discuss a community member's response. In other cases, the community member might be invited in to a session, alone or with other community members. They might be part of a reflecting team, or there might be a less structured conversation. There might be a ritual gathering planned, which includes symbols of significance to the client.

7. Acting in community. After possible strategies and resources are identified, the client makes a choice and takes some action in relation to her or his preferred community. Whether she attends Narcotics Anonymous for the first time, or again, or he writes letters to people in his community asking for a supportive response, the client has taken a step toward finding the self she or he wants to become within the context of a given community. Political action with others in the community might be a part of this stage as well.

8. Reflecting on acting in community, This might be reflecting in community, reflecting with the clinician, or reflecting alone. The client reflects on community actions taken and evaluates cognitively and emotionally what the community interaction felt like. Was it affirming? Was it confining? Is it something the client should try to continue in spite of discomfort? Is it something the client should stop, and instead try out another action in community?

At first, a client will probably reflect on these actions with the therapist, and eventually the client may involve the preferred community in these reflections. How does the community respond to reflections, new information, and critique? This reflection may result in further examination and critique of cultural stereotypes (element 3) and grief and loss (element 4) processes, or it may result in further identification of preferred communities (element 6). Ideally, if a client has found a community or communities that fits him or her well, the client may simply move back and forth between action and reflection (elements 7 and 8).

This reflection goes for the therapeutic relationship as well. As the client discovers aspects of the therapy culture that are not productive, he or she will discuss it with the therapist. Either a change will occur and the therapy will continue as a helpful activity for the client, or the therapy will appropriately end or recess.

In Marlene's women's group, mentioned earlier, the women used their newfound voices to question the group contract about payment. Marlene is probably correct that the group would have ceased being truly effective if there had not been a change.

I have discussed some of the ideas of self and community, both those from cultural commentators, such as Bellah, Cushman, and Lasch, and those within social work and other mental health professions. I have presented a study that examined the "languages of community" of a group of well-regarded community clinicians. The rather sobering outcome of this study is the realization that even people who value community in their lives and in their work have difficulty moving away from the individualism that is so dominant in our culture and reinforced in many professional theories.

This outcome led to a second study, which accomplished two purposes. It allowed the generation of an empirically based set of practice principles that weave ideas of community throughout the clinical process. It also demonstrated that its method is an effective means of teaching about significant clinical topics. Students commented that the course offered the most in-depth look at a clinical process of any of their courses. It offers a way to begin to develop best practices in a frontier area of practice, and a way to give students hands-on experience of knowledge building.

Conclusion

This chapter has considered community as an idea and its relationship to ideas of the self. Both of these concepts are elements of daily life and also of clinical practice, though they are seldom the focus of our attention. However, the idea of the "self" is the dominant one, and ideas of community are marginalized. Clinicians, especially community clinicians, need to become more sensitized to "community" and to expand its place in their clinical practice and thinking. This will take very deliberate effort because it opposes cultural and professional norms. Only when this occurs will the promise of community clinical practice be realized.

In the "Parable of the Long Spoons" (cited in *The Magic of Conflict*, by Thomas Crum, 1988), the protagonist, a man who was poor and still gave generously to others, was offered the granting of a wish by the archangel Gabriel. He wished, he said, to see heaven and hell. What he saw in hell was people with spoons bound to their arms, unable to feed themselves because the spoons were longer than their arms. They were starving and suffering. In heaven, to the man's surprise, at first things appeared to be the same. However, the people seemed happy and loving. Looking closely, he saw that they were using the long spoons to feed each other.

The community clinician sadly acknowledges that adversity will be with us always. However, we can bear that adversity best in the context of communities built on mutual aid and social justice.

References

Adams, P., & Nelson, K. (1995). *Reinventing human services: Community- and family-centered practice*. New York: Aldine de Gruyter.

Addams, J. (1910/1961). *Twenty years at Hull House*. New York: Macmillan.

Allen, J. (1993). The constructivist paradigm: Values and ethics. *Journal of Teaching in Social Work, 8*, 31–54.

Anderson, H., & Goolishian, H. (1988). Human systems as linguistic systems: Preliminary and evolving ideas about the implications for clinical theory. *Family Process, 27*, 371–394.

Bell, C., & Newby, H. (1972). *Community studies*. New York: Praeger.

Bellah, R., Madsen, R., Sullivan, W., Swidler, A., & Tipton, S. (1985). *Habits of the heart: Individualism and commitment in American life*. Berkeley: University of California Press.

Bellah, R., Madsen, R., Sullivan, W., Swidler, A., & Tipton, S. (Eds.). (1987). *Individualism and commitment in American life*. New York: Harper and Row.

Bellah, R., Madsen, R., Sullivan, W., Swidler, A., & Tipton, S. (1991). *The good society*. New York: Knopf.

Blumer, H. (1969). *Symbolic interactionism: Perspective and method*. Englewood Cliffs, NJ: Prentice Hall.

Breton, M. (1989). Liberation theology, group work, and the right of the poor and oppressed to participate in the life of the community. *Social Work with Groups, 12*(3), 5–18.

Bronfenbrenner, U. (1970). *Two worlds of childhood: U.S. and USSR*. New York: Russell Sage.

Bronfenbrenner, U. (1979). *The ecology of human development: Experiments by nature and design*. Cambridge MA: Harvard University Press.

Canda, E., & Furman, D.(1999). *Spiritual diversity in social work practice: The heart of helping*. New York: Free Press.

Council on Social Work Education. (2001). *Educational policy and standards*. Washington, DC: Author.

Crum, T. F. (1988). *The magic of conflict: Turning a life of work into a work of art*. New York: Simon and Schuster/Touchstone.

Cushman, P. (1990). Why the self is empty. *American Psychologist, 45*, 599–611.

Cushman, P. (1995). *Constructing the self, constructing America*. Reading, MA: Addison-Wesley.

Devore, W., & Schlesinger, E. (1996). *Ethnic-sensitive social work practice* (4th ed.). Boston: Allyn and Bacon.

Erikson, E., Erikson, J., & Kivnick, H. (1986). *Vital involvement in old age*. New York: Norton.

Foucault, M. (1980). *Power/knowledge*. New York: Pantheon.

Foucault, M. (1981a). The political technology of individuals. In L. Martin, H. Gutman, & P. Hutton (Eds.), *Technologies of the self* (pp. 145–162). Amherst: University of Massachusetts Press.

Foucault, M. (1981b). Technologies of the self. In L. Martin, H. Gutman, & P. Hutton (Eds.), *Technologies of the self* (pp. 16–49). Amherst: University of Massachusetts Press.

Frank, S., & Keys, C. (1987). Community psychology and the study of organizations: A reciprocal relationship. *American Journal of Community Psychology, 15,* 239–251.

Freire, P. (1970/1973). *Pedagogy of the oppressed*. New York: Seabury.

Freire, P. (1992). *Education for critical consciousness*. New York: Continuum.

Gergen, K. (1985). The social constructionist movement in American psychology. *American Psychologist, 40,* 266–275.

Germain, C. (1991). *Human behavior in the social environment: An ecological view*. New York: Columbia University Press.

Germain, G., & Gitterman, G. (1996). *The life model of social work practice* (2nd ed.). New York: Columbia University Press.

Gilligan, C. (1982). *In a different voice*. Cambridge, MA: Harvard University Press.

Gitterman, A., & Shulman, L. (Eds.). (1993). *Mutual aid groups, vulnerable populations, and the life cycle*. New York: Columbia University Press.

Greenberg, J., & Mitchell, S. (1983). *Object relations in psychoanalytic theory*. Cambridge, MA: Harvard University Press.

Hartman, A., & Laird, J. (1983). *Family-centered social work practice*. New York: Free Press.

Hillery, G. (1955). Definitions of community: Areas of agreement. *Rural Sociology, 20,* 779–791.

Hutchinson, E. D. (1995). *Toward a theory of community: Enhancing the HBSE curriculum*. Unpublished manuscript, Virginia Commonwealth University, Richmond.

Lasch, C. (1979). *The culture of narcissism*. New York: Norton.

Lee, J.A.B. (2001). *The empowerment approach to social work practice* (2nd ed.). New York: Columbia University Press.

Lee, J.A.B., & Swenson, C. (1978). Theory in action: A community social service agency. *Social Casework, 59,* 359–370.

Lee, J.A.B., & Swenson, C. (1993). The concept of mutual aid. In A. Gitterman & L. Shulman (Eds.), *Mutual aid, vulnerable populations, and the life cycle* (pp. 413–430). New York: Columbia University Press.

Lieberman, A. (1988). *Internal representations of community*. Unpublished master's thesis, Smith College School for Social Work, Northampton, MA.

Madsen, W. (1999). *Collaborative therapy with multistressed families*. New York: Guilford.

Mead, G. H. (1934). *Mind, self and society* (C. W. Morris, Ed.). Chicago: University of Chicago Press.

Meyer, C. (1993). *Assessment in social work practice*. New York: Columbia University Press.

Miller, J. B. (1976). *Toward a new psychology of women*. Boston: Beacon.

Miller, J. B. (1984). *Development of women's sense of self*. (Work in Progress, No. 12). Wellesley, MA: Stone Center Working Papers Series.

National Association of Social Workers. (1994). *Code of ethics*. Washington, DC: Author.

Reynolds, B. (1951/1973). *Social work and social living* (2nd ed.). Washington, DC: National Association of Social Workers.

Reynolds, B. (1963/1964). *An uncharted journey* (2nd ed.). Hebron, CT: Practitioners Press.

Roland, A. (1988). *In search of self in India and Japan*. Princeton, NJ: Princeton University Press.

Saleebey, D. (Ed.). (1992). *The strengths perspective*. New York: Longman.

Saleebey, D. (1996). The strengths perspective in social work: Extensions and cautions. *Social Work, 41,* 296–305.

Sampson, E. E. (1977). Psychology and the American ideal. *Journal of Personality and Social Psychology, 35,* 767–782.

Sampson, E. E. (1985). The decentralization of identity: Toward a revised conception of personal and social order. *American Psychologist, 40,* 1203–1211.

Sampson, E. E. (1988). The debate on individualism: Indigenous psychologies of the individual and their role in personal and societal functioning. *American Psychologist, 43,* 15–22.

Sarason, S. (1974). *The psychological sense of community: Prospects for a community psychology*. San Francisco: Jossey-Bass.

Schwartz, W. (1985). The group work tradition and social work practice. *Social Work with Groups, 8*(4), 7–27.

Specht, H., & Courtney, M. (1994). *Unfaithful angels: How social work has abandoned its mission*. New York: Free Press.

Swenson, C. (1979). Social networks, mutual aid, and the life model of practice. In C. B. Germain (Ed.), *Social work practice: People and environments* (pp. 213–238). New York: Columbia University Press.

Swenson, C. (1981). Using social networks to promote competence. In A. Maluccio (Ed.), *Promoting competence in clients* (pp. 125–151). New York: Free Press.

Swenson, C. (1995). Professional understandings of community: At a loss for words? In P. Adams & K. Nelson, (Eds.), *Reinventing human services: Community- and family-centered practice* (pp. 223–243). New York: Aldine de Gruyter.

Swenson, C. (1998). Clinical social work's contribution to a social justice perspective. *Social Work 43*, 527–537.

Swenson, C., Carbonell, D., Bayer, T., Carleton, E., Costikyan, N., Curtis, R., Gallagher, M., Lippolis, G., Nada, M., Shapiro, I., & Weingast, L. (1993). *Clinical constructions of community*. Unpublished manuscript, Simmons College School of Social Work, Boston.

Swenson, C., Cope, R., Buckley, E., Clifton, R., Cohen, S., Decter, P., Gillis, J., Madsen, M., Norton, W. Taylor, M., Telega., & Wisler, M. (1996). *Toward a conception of self-in-community*. Unpublished manuscript, Simmons College School of Social Work, Boston.

Swigonski, M. (1994). The logic of feminist standpoint theory for social work research. *Social Work, 39*, 387–393.

Van Soest, D. (1995). Peace and social justice. In R. Edwards (Ed), *Encyclopedia of social work* (pp. 1810–1817). Washington, DC: NASW Press.

Wakefield, J. (1988). Psychotherapy, distributive justice, and social work, Parts I & II. *Social Service Review, 62*, 187–210, 353–382.

White, M. (1995). *Reauthoring lives: Interviews and essays*. Adelaide, Australia: Dulwich Centre Publications.

White, M., & Epston, D. (1990). *Narrative means to therapeutic ends*. New York: Norton.

6

Lynn Hoffman

A Communal Perspective for the Relational Therapies

This chapter proposes a framework for the relational therapies that focus on the communal creation of meaning. The therapist is both the knitter and the yarns, singular, yet one of many. Just as family therapists took advantage of a newly seen unit, the family, to enlarge their range of choices, so can postmodern therapists take advantage of the shift to the nonessentialist position of social construction theory. However, even that theory takes a backseat to a heightened interest in practice. Instead of asking, "What are the philosophical underpinnings of our work?" we now ask, "What is the knit one, purl two, of the kind of social knitting preferred by effective therapists of any school?" The nature of these more communal practices is considered within the historical context of the family therapy field.

Systemic therapy as a genre and constructivism as its philosophy have been the bridge that connects the modern, essentialist framework of traditional family therapy to the postmodern constructionist one. The difference between these positions is neatly summed up in the story of the Three Umpires:

First umpire: I calls 'em as they are. (essentialism)

Second umpire: I calls 'em as I sees 'em. (constructivism)
Third umpire: They ain't nothing till I calls 'em. (constructionism)

Translated for the purposes of therapy, the essentialist looks for the cause of the problem and tries to fix it. The problem exists in the real world "out there." Constructivist therapists say we cannot know what is out there, even though it may exist, because what we perceive is always filtered through the screens of the nervous system. That is why biologist Humberto Maturana (Maturana & Varela, 1980) always started a lecture by drawing an observing eye in the upper right-hand corner of the blackboard. The constructionist moves to the social web. Feeling him- or herself to be part of a tapestry woven from elements like language, customs, and culture, he or she is at the same time one of the weavers and one of the threads. Kenneth Gergen (1994), the chief proponent of social construction theory, speaks of conversation as the communal creation of meaning. Having taken up a constructionist position myself, I have been exploring the dimensions of this communal perspective and the practices that fall naturally out of it.

But let me start with where family therapy in

the United States is now. Managed care, with its demands for accountability, has pushed the field of family therapy up against the wall. Many of us are asking what, if anything, backs up our claims. Research results are not outstanding, in part because many of our approaches do not emphasize outcomes, but also because studies of family therapy results are not compelling (Shadish, 1995).

Worse yet, we do not even agree on what kind of issues family therapy should deal with. Starting modestly with schizophrenia, we moved on to parent-child problems, marital woes, developmental traumas, life stage stuckness, gender discrimination, sexual abuse, violence, addiction, poverty, and all the injustices of class, ethnicity, and race. At the same time, the competition among the "helping professions" for the right to treat these woes has intensified.

This seemed like a good time to assess the field. Even though I am not in the same place as where I started, I did not want to abandon all the good ideas I learned on the way. So I tried to think of family therapy as a braided Easter bread or (in the Jewish tradition) a challah, with strands from early on disappearing and then reappearing in a changed position or on another side. Each new strand suggested an answer to a question that had been brought to the fore by a previous one. However, it was the continuing conversation between the strands that made the entire braid so special.

The Early Strands

In a former article (Hoffman, 1998), I described the influence of psychodynamic ideas on early family therapy, citing psychologist Margaret Singer's (1996) view that the ascendance of psychoanalytic and developmental theories after World War II rested on an etiological framework. Singer and others have called this view the "blame and change game." If you can find someone or something to blame, you can change. Instead of the finger being pointed at the character of the individual, it was pointed at some influence, person, or event in the past.

Early family therapy developed a blame and change game of its own. Family researchers ascribed the cause of emotional distress to underlying factors like unacknowledged conflict or family se-

crets. These conditions, like festering sores, needed to be exposed to light and air. From early on, the key example was the idea that the symptoms of the child hid the parents' pain. Once the therapist focused on the marital conflict, it was thought that the child's symptoms would disappear. This paralleled the psychoanalytic belief that symptoms were surface manifestations of a deeper wound.

This position was usually benign in individual therapy, because the people who were implicitly most at fault remained outside, but it had a chilling effect on family therapy because these guilty ones were present. At first, mothers were to blame. Then therapists zeroed in on the parents, who were seen as "triangling" the child into their own conflicts. The kin group was the next focus, then the other helpers who might be connected to a case. As time went by, the lens widened steadily, but the blame remained.

It was a relief when, in 1968, I stumbled upon E. H. Auerswald's ecosystemic point of view. I had been thinking of family therapy as an "indoor therapy" that sometimes degraded its customers. When I met Auerswald and began to work with him as the historian for his Applied Behavioral Sciences Program at Gouverneur Health Services on the Lower East Side of Manhattan, I finally found the "outdoor therapy" I was looking for (Hoffman, 2002). Auerswald had come up with a systemic version of community mental health that took ecology as its guiding metaphor and seems like a precursor to the "wraparound" concept being used by the community care movement today. Taking this wide-angle view, Auerswald set up a pilot project: a family health team that would serve all family members from a given catchment area. In this way he hoped to make a transdisciplinary dialogue a fait accompli. The team was composed of an internist, a pediatrician, a gynecologist, a public health nurse, a social worker, and a psychiatrist.

Another innovation was the mobile crisis unit, a roving bus that responded to crises wherever they might be found, at any time of day or night. This unit included a psychiatrist, a social worker, and a Puerto Rican health technician. Implicit in all of Auerswald's work was the recognition that both the providers and those they treated are embedded in social networks. Rather than seeking diagnoses, Auerswald relied on the strength to be found in people's natural connections. Often, in that neighborhood, a woman who was fresh from Puerto Rico and was afraid of the "junkies" outside her door would be brought to him with a diagnosis of agoraphobia. In one such case, after hearing the woman's story, Auerswald called the department of welfare and had a telephone installed in her apartment. Somewhere in the city, he told us, there must be other people from her village who could relieve her fears.

Another exception to a blaming perspective was the interactional view of the Mental Research Institute (MRI; Watzlawick, Weakland, & Fisch, 1974). Drawing on Milton Erickson's hypnotherapy (Haley, 1973), the MRI group ignored causes and took a rhetorical approach instead. Being constructivists, they held that reality is constructed, and that it was the therapist's job to shape it differently. Strikingly, the MRI never targeted any treatment unit except the complaint and never insisted the whole family be called in. The downside of this approach was its condescending view of the customer. Family therapy was likened to a game of chess. The therapist, who knew the rules of the game, was the master player, while the family members were the pieces on the board. An approach like this would naturally tend to hide the thinking behind its moves. If the customer knew the reason for maneuvers like paradoxical interventions, this could undermine their success. One had an extraordinary sense of a band of therapists conducting guerrilla warfare against customers determined to outwit them.

Fascinated by the interactionists' use of paradox, the Milan systemic team of Mara Selvini-Palazzoli, Luigi Boscolo, Giuiana Prata, and Gianfranco Cecchin (1978) began to use similar tactics to treat the problem in context. They came up with a systemic amalgam that involved not only the kin group, always important in Italy, but also the other professionals attached to a case. Their chief intervention was a "counterparadox" that prescribed the problem within the net of relationships in which the symptom had its being. True to the group's research orientation, all interviews were watched by a team behind a screen and videotaped, to be studied later. The team idea, which had not been used so formally before, fascinated therapists and was widely imitated, but over time it put a gulf between clinicians and clients and turned the one-way mirror into a one-way street.

In 1981, however, Boscolo and Cecchin broke away to start their own training center. The invention of "circular questioning" (Selvini-Palazzoli, Boscolo, Cecchin, & Prata, 1980) gave Milan-style therapists a tool for placing family members in a position to reflect on the machinery they were caught in. Cecchin (1987) added concepts like "curiosity" and "irreverence" to the description of the therapeutic dialogue. As a result, the often pejorative "systemic hypothesis" began to be replaced by reflexive conversations that did not necessarily imply innocence or guilt.

The interactional approach of the MRI mutated, too. Steve de Shazer (1985) and Insoo Berg (1994), along with colleagues like Eve Lipchik (1993) and William O'Hanlon (1999), moved from an emphasis on problems to an emphasis on solutions. Berg and de Shazer refined their approach, calling it solution focused, and creating a model that had immense influence in the family field. Solution talk, taking the "emphasis on the positive" that Milton Erickson brought into therapy, looked at possibility rather than pathology and had an extremely sympathetic feel (Haley, 1973).

These developments were all shifts in a less essentialist, less blaming direction. However, a seismic movement called postmodernism now began to threaten the underpinnings of the entire craft. It was not a question of just a new model but a new way of thinking. Instead of asking, "What is the thing in the bushes?" (Hoffman, 1981), we asked, "How do our ways of knowing create the thing in the bushes? How do intellectual frameworks like normative psychology constrain what we can know?" For me, this was a watershed. Never before had I stepped outside the assumptions of my education on so large a scale.

The Influence of Postmodernism

I think it is correct to call postmodernism a true paradigm shift. Paradigms are explanatory systems that shape the sensibility of large communities of "knowers," in our case the Anglo-European "knowers" of the Western world. Every once in a while these frameworks wear out, and then all the little subfields that dangle from them need to change, too. Instead of believing in stable unities such as the "self," the "family," "nature," we began to question them. As philosopher Richard Rorty (1979) says:

> The picture which holds traditional philosophy captive is that of the mind as a great mirror containing various representations—some accurate, some not, and capable of being studied by pure nonempirical methods. Without the notion of mind as mirror, the notion of knowledge as accuracy of presentation would not have suggested itself. (p. 12)

In the course of this revolution, academic, scientific, and professional certitudes were placed, as the French philosopher Jacques Derrida (1978) would say, "under erasure." Also under erasure was the "Western canon" that was founded on the "great books" and the "dead white men" who wrote them. Critical feminists like Rachel Hare-Mustin (1994) began to prod family therapists about their blindness to gender and race and asked a pointed question: Must all our therapy discourses be kept within the "mirrored rooms"?

Particular scorn was heaped upon the not-yet-dead white males of family therapy. In *The Family Interpreted* (1988), Deborah Luepnitz took issue with the psychiatrists who were family therapy's pioneers and questioned the teaching of philosopher-kings like Gregory Bateson. Systemic therapists were particularly attacked for blaming women, for downplaying questions of power, and for ignoring issues of social justice (Erickson, 1988). It became clear that the ecosystems metaphor threatened to make the rights of individuals subservient to the balance of the whole.

But I was struggling with other concerns. In my article "Beyond Power and Control" (Hoffman, 1985), I tried to offer an alternative to what felt to me like a masculinist takeover of family therapy. I wanted to use the power of what psychologist Carol Gilligan (1982) had called a "different voice." I did not think that this different voice belonged to women, only that the authoritative stance of the male hierarchy should not be the only one. But the prevailing wisdom framed what was then called "difference feminism" in a very negative light. For the next few years, the academic playing field became increasingly concerned with the contests that took place around identity politics, and my idea of a different voice seemed not to fit.

For a long time I felt stuck. Then philosopher Lois Shawver (1983) introduced me to French postmodernism, and I discovered an ally in French philosopher Jean-François Lyotard. In *Just Gaming* (Lyotard & Thebaud, 1996), he compares the "game of speculation" of the Western philosophical tradition, in which the speaker competes, to the "game of audition," in which the purpose is to listen and understand. He says this amazing thing:

> For us, a language is first and foremost someone talking. But there are language games in which the important thing is to listen, in which the rule deals with audition. Such a game is the game of the just. And in this game, one speaks as a listener, and not as an author. It is a game without an author, in the same way as the speculative game of the West is a game without a listener, because the only listener tolerated by the speculative philosopher is the disciple. (p. 71)

Certain phrases resonated in my head: "the game of audition." "the game of the just." I was electrified, because I had long felt that all therapy approaches were too mandarin, too remote from the experience of the people who came to us, and that they were anything but just. The fact that there is a school of community work in New Zealand (Waldegrave, 1990) that chose the name "just therapy" is by itself a comment on the usual state of affairs.

Lyotard's ideas supported another approach that broke sharply with traditional family therapy that called itself narrative. The originators, Michael White and David Epston (White, 1995), were influenced by the ideas of social philosopher Michel Foucault (1972), who had brilliantly "outed" the oppressive cultural discourses of everyday life. White and Epston (1990) applied these ideas to the discourses of psychotherapy and psychiatry. Using a technique they called "externalizing," they replaced diagnostic terms with phrases from ordinary language. Thus "schizophrenia" became an "in the corner life-style," and "encopresis" became "sneaky poo." This device gave them a way to align themselves with the person against the problem and allowed them to put moral agency back into family therapy, a great relief to many after the neutral stance of the systemic years.

In keeping with his Foucauldian stance, White (1995) does not talk about postmodernism but prefers the term "poststructuralism." "Structuralism" seems to be similar to "essentialism" in that both concepts assume that there is a hidden essence or structure within the unit or event being described. Proponents of both views are eager to point out the error of the antediluvian ways. There is an us-versus-them implication in both views, which we would do well not to ignore.

One limitation of the Foucauldian vision for therapy is that its defining parameters are imprisonment, surveillance, and resistance, though not overt revolution. In the wrong hands, this polarizing language could easily become another "blame and change" game. However, White has moved in the opposite direction. His interviewing style has become much less hard-edged. Early on, the externalizing questions gave the impression of sheepdogs herding their charges into the little corral. Now he takes seriously his own advice to "stay one step behind," and as a result, an unprecedented tenderness pervades his work.

A second postmodern strand, called a collaborative language systems approach, came out of the teamwork of the late Harry Goolishian and Harlene Anderson (Anderson & Goolishian, 1988). This view looks for support to linguistic philosophers like Ludwig Wittgenstein (1953) and Mikhail Bakhtin (1981), and to social constructionists like Kenneth Gergen (1994) and John Shotter (1993). In applying postmodern theory to therapy, Anderson (1996) believes that the critical piece is that the therapist shed the mantle of expertise. As a result, she goes directly to the persons who consult her, asking what their own opinions are and what they feel would be useful. For her, solutions can only be arrived at from within the therapeutic conversation, through a process of what she calls "mutual puzzling."

Extending this position, John Shotter (Bayer & Shotter, 1998) moves away from a linguistic metaphor to one derived from physical embodiment and touch. I am extremely sympathetic to this view. The notion of sublingual communication, which I see as the underground rivers of sensed feelings that flow between people when they connect, describes the process of our work much better than the more remote analogies of narrative and text. In a previous article, I compare therapy to the process of kneading yeast bread. The reason I like this metaphor is that it fits with Wittgenstein's (1953) idea that language is not just the speaking of words but part of an activity or "form of life."

Don Schoen supports this view in his book *The Reflective Practitioner* (1984). He says that the actual practice of therapy should be the source of one's knowledge about it, and this is why it is so important to watch at first hand what self-styled postmodern therapists actually do. Their interviews contrast sharply with those of family therapists who take a more modernist position. There are no lists of questions, no interviewing guidelines, no interventions, no goals. Constructionist therapists refrain from going into therapy with a blueprint of any kind. But they do attempt to influence the atmosphere in which therapy takes place by presiding over the equivalent of a virtual quilting bee. Looking for a descriptive phrase, I turned to the idea of "communal practices."

Communal Practices

In *Realities and Relationships* (1994), Gergen links the word "communality" with social interaction. Observing that the traditional view that meaning originates within the individual mind is deeply problematic, he goes on to say:

> Words (or texts) within themselves bear no meaning; they fail to communicate. They only appear to generate meaning by virtue of their place within the realm of human interaction. It is human interchange that gives language its capacity to mean, and it must stand as the critical locus of concern. I wish then to replace *textuality* with *communality*. This shift allows us to restructure much that has been said about meaning within texts as a commentary on *forms of relatedness*. (pp. 263–264)

It was Tom Andersen (1991), however, who first used the phrase "communal perspective" to describe a stance toward therapy. He had asked me to do a workshop on that subject in Norway in 1999. I had long been brooding on the subtle communicational weaving that I saw in Andersen's reflecting teams. It was not the reflections themselves that so impressed me but the fact that one group would comment on what another group said, and then another group would comment in turn, creating a juxtaposition out of which surprising meanings could arise. My phrase for this process was "knit one, purl two." Michael White calls it "telling and re-telling." Now I think of it more generally as "communal practice."

As a result, the work of postmodern therapists

goes in the direction of what I call "world building." In his classic text, *The Timeless Way of Building* (1979), architect Christopher Alexander invokes a time before blueprints existed. Then he asks the important question: If we refuse to follow formal guidelines, what is the central quality we look for when we build? After much discussion with himself, he finally comes up with "aliveness." We instinctively know when a house, a garden, a town, is "dead" because we do not want to go there. If it feels alive, we do. He talks about the patterns used before there were architects, patterns that have a folk feel and are intuitive rather than mechanical. Among these he lists such elements as "farmhouse kitchen," "child caves," and, for the garden, "sunny corner."

Some of the early family therapists were folk builders in that sense. The person who comes most to mind is Virginia Satir. She was in one sense a constructivist, in that she specialized in pointing out conflicting perceptions of reality. She had a hundred ways to call attention to the "discrepancies," as she called them, that created so many family divides. But Satir was also an early constructionist. Her "reframing" techniques were not so much a way to disarm resistance as a method for softening the way people heard each other. My favorite example (1967) is an interview with the family of a minister and his wife. Their teenage son had impregnated two of his classmates and was sitting in a corner with his head down. The first thing Satir did on coming into the room was to say to him, "Well, we know one thing. God gave you good seed."

Instead of calling this move "reframing," Lois Shawver (1983) prefers "transvaluation." This term describes a way of changing the significance of a situation, usually from pessimistic to hopeful, but always from an expected to an unexpected point of view. I like Shawver's term because it embraces a shift that, even if suggested by the therapist, does not exempt her from the experience of change. And the source of the transvaluation may be any person present. Unlike "reframing," which is a strategy that can be learned by rote and is imposed by the therapist, it arises spontaneously from the conversation.

Looking back at Satir's work gave me a new perception of Tom Andersen's (1991) invention of the reflecting team. The "reflecting process," as Andersen later called it, gave concrete form to the "overhearing" position, as opposed to the "observ-ing" position of every other approach to therapy I had known. It turned out that a reflecting conversation could be applied to many settings: teaching, supervision, mediation, workshops, even conferences. Like the legendary little black dress, it could be dressed up or down; it could go anywhere. In fact, the reflecting team changed therapy as I knew it. Wherever it went, it brought connection. As soon as I began to use it, a more horizontal relationship sprang up between me and the people who came to see me. It turned opposing voices into parallel voices. The "therapeutic boundary" began to melt, and interventions became a thing of the past. Most amazing of all, the atmosphere of the session became intent and focused, as if we were all experiencing the pull of a good mystery story. In fact, we were often rewarded by a denouement of unexpected beauty and force.

I call this the Lake Titicaca effect. High up in the Andes Mountains of Peru is a lake surrounded by reeds. My mother was the first person I ever knew who had seen this lake, because she had gone to South America in 1942 to study the woven fabrics of the Mayan people. When the people there build a house, they lay reeds on top of reeds until there is a floating platform 6 feet thick. They use the same reeds for their houses. The reflecting team or, as Andersen now calls it, the "reflecting process," works the same way, by creating a deeply layered platform on which a house or village can be built.

White, too, has gone in an increasingly communal direction (Hoffman, 1998). Citing Myerhoff's (1986) idea of definitional ceremonies, he started using the format of the reflecting team as a source of "outsider witnesses," people whose words could enrich the stories of the persons who consulted him. As part of this enterprise, he conscripts workshop participants or brings in individuals from a person's natural environment, in spirit or in life. Through these ceremonies of "telling and retelling," White tries to create "thicker descriptions" for the people who are present to overhear.

Two less well-known communal approaches are worthy of mention. One, a social network–based approach to psychosis in Finland, is called Open Dialogue. The persons who are most identified with this idea and have written extensively about it are psychologist Jukka Aaltonen (Seikkula, Alakare, & Aaltonen, 2001), who pioneered "need-adapted" social interventions in Finland, and psychologist Jaakko Seikkula (Seikkula & Olson, 2003), who worked at Keropudas Hospital in northern Finland, and who believes that the chief architect of therapy is a dialogue with a community. This is another method that falls consciously into the postmodern category, influenced, I think, by the fact that Harry Goolishian often visited Norway and Finland in the years before his death. His interest in postmodern ideas was contagious, as was the personal democracy of his style of work.

The heart of Keropudas's team-style organization is its insistence on working with the social network, as well as a policy of meeting the afflicted family within 24 hours of getting a call. The team continues meeting daily for however long it takes, although individual or family therapy is sometimes added to the mix. To me, this was E. H. Auerswald's family health team and mobile crisis unit rolled into one. One key change was Keropudas Hospital's insistence on breaking down interdisciplinary barriers. It instituted a policy that required all hospital personnel, from the chief psychiatrist to the nursing interns, to take the same 3-year course in family therapy.

An article on Open Dialogue by Seikkula and family therapist and writer Mary Olson (2003) is available in *Family Process*, and I hope it will be widely read. Written by Olson but based on an illustration of the dialogic method taken from an interview that Seikkula and the Keropudas team had with a psychotic husband and his wife, the piece should be of particular interest to family therapists. Olson traces the lineage of the approach back to earlier systemic approaches, but she includes three precepts for the work as its practitioners now describe it, the last two taken from the thinking of Russian philologist Mikhail Bakhtin (1981): tolerance of uncertainty, polyphony, and dialogism. In working with first-time psychotic breakdowns, the Keropudas team stresses the importance of listening to the distressed person's language and will even adopt it. The eventual hope is that a new language for the disturbing event will evolve from the conversations between the team, the person, and the social network, preventing the isolation that so often feeds into chronicity.

The importance of Open Dialogue has been demonstrated by its remarkable success rate compared with "treatment as usual" of first-episode psychotics in other hospitals in Finland. Results of a 5-year study show that only half of the patients treated were hospitalized, for an average of 19 days, only 35% were given neuroleptics, and at the 5-year mark, 80% were working, studying, or looking for a job. In treatment as usual, average hospitalization was 110 days, 93% were given neuroleptic medication, and 62% ended up living on disability allowance. The most striking finding was that in the 5 years since Keropudas Hospital has been using Open Dialogue, there have been no new cases in the area covered of chronic psychosis.

Chris Kinman (1996) is another communal practitioner whose work I described in my last book (Hoffman, 2002). Kinman started out by working with young people from First Nations communities in Vancouver, British Columbia. Using a "language of gifts," Kinman set out to replace the traditional problem framework of community mental health with a gift framework. Instead of the usual problem-focused intake form, Kinman has devised what he calls a "collaborative action plan," which starts out by asking about a person's "gifts and potentials." Only when there is a long list of gifts will the conversation move on to the "roadblocks" that might get in the way of the person's potential. Kinman always includes the meaningful network in his meeting: parents, school people, other kids, helpers, and sometimes the spirit animal that belongs to the child.

Over the course of 10 years, Kinman and I came up with a type of event we called "honoring community." Partly this was because I could not come out from the East Coast very often, so I would take advantage of these visits to meet the people Kinman was currently working with. I would sit and talk with various groups of helpers or families while the others listened, going from group to group, and looking for the special ways in which each group had made a difference. Central to this process were the reflecting practices I had learned from Tom Andersen and from Lyotard's idea of the "game of audition." In traditional professional meetings, the presenters listen in order to speak. In these meetings, we spoke in order to listen. The effect was that everybody ended up hearing new things, both from each other and from themselves reflected back.

To me, the most remarkable of these events was when I was invited in 2002 to a meeting of the public health nurses in the Frasier Valley area outside Vancouver. The nurses had been looking for a more positive alternative to their problem-focused record, and when they met Kinman they adopted his collaborative action plan right away. In two years, the idea of a language of gifts had had an enormous impact. Present at our conference were representatives of the administrative staff who had backed these changes, faculty from the public health nursing program at the University of Vancouver who were now teaching these ideas, and the pioneering frontline staff who were putting them into practice. The star of the event was a couple: a young woman recovering from a postpartum depression and the young nurse who was working with her. In speaking with all these groups and persons over the course of the day, while everyone else listened in, I experienced something I had never seen before: a change at every level of a complex community agency.

Communal practices like these make up a category that defies borders. As I said, many so-called modern therapists use them; postmodern therapists do, too, but with more self-consciousness. But there is one irreversible advance that comes with postmodernism: an awareness of the limitations of knowing. In a recent paper (1999), Fred Newman describes postmodern therapy as a study of the unknowable, meaning the domain of things that cannot be discovered in the same way that things in the physical universe can. For this reason, he states that storytelling should not be turned into a kind of explanation but should be seen instead as a nonexplanatory mode of understanding the activity of human life.

I like that idea. I want to continue to be "not knowing" at the level of the road map while still exploring the road. If you are like me, you will remember the sand tunnels we used to dig as children at the beach, and that delicious final moment when our fingers touched.

References

Alexander, C. (1979). *The timeless way of building*. New York: Oxford University Press.

Andersen, T. (1991). *The reflecting team: Dialogues and dialogues about the dialogues*. New York: Norton.

Anderson, H. (1996). *Language, conversation and possibilities*. New York: Basic Books.

Anderson, H., & Goolishian, H. (1988). Human systems as linguistic systems. *Family Process, 27*, 371–393.

Bakhtin, M. (1981). *The dialogical imagination* (M. Hol-

quist, Ed., & C. Emerson, Trans.). Minneapolis: University of Minnesota Press.

Bayer, B., & Shotter, J. (1998). *Reconstructing the psychological subject: Bodies, practices and technologies*. Thousand Oaks, CA: Sage.

Berg, I. K. (1994). *Family based services: A solution-focused approach*. New York: Norton.

Cecchin, G. (1987). Hypothesizing, circularity and neutrality revisited: An invitation to curiosity. *Family Process, 25*, 405–413.

Derrida, J. (1978). *Writing and difference* (A. Bass, Trans.). Chicago: University of Chicago Press.

de Shazer, S. (1985). *Keys to solution in brief therapy*. New York: Norton.

Erickson, G. (1988). Against the grain: Decentering family therapy. *Journal of Marital and Family Therapy, 14*, 225–236.

Foucault, M. (1972). *The archeology of knowledge*. New York: Pantheon.

Gergen, K. (1994). *Realities and relationships*. Cambridge, MA: Harvard University Press.

Gilligan, C. (1982). *In a different voice*. Cambridge, MA: Harvard University Press.

Haley, J. (1973). *Uncommon therapy: The psychiatric techniques of Milton H. Erickson*. New York: Ballantine.

Hare-Mustin, R. (1994). Discourses in the mirrored room. *Family Process, 33*, 19–35.

Hoffman, L. (1981). *Foundations of family therapy*. New York: Basic Books.

Hoffman, L. (1985). Beyond power and control. *Family Systems Medicine, 3*, 381–396.

Hoffman, L. (1998). Setting aside the model in family therapy. *Journal of Marital and Family Therapy, 24*, 145–156.

Hoffman, L. (2002). *Family therapy: An intimate history*. New York: Norton.

Kinman, C. (1996). *Honouring community*. Abbotsford, British Columbia, Canada: Fraser Valley Education and Therapy Services.

Lipchik, E. (1993). Both/and solutions. In S. Friedman (Ed.), *The new language of change* (pp. 25–49). New York: Guilford.

Luepnitz, D. (1988). *The family interpreted*. New York: Basic Books.

Lyotard, J-F., & Thebaud, J-L. (1996). *Just gaming* (W. Godzich, Trans.). Minneapolis: University of Minnesota Press.

Maturana, H., & Varela, F. (1980). *Autopoiesis and cognition*. Dordrecht, Netherlands: D. Reidel.

Myerhoff, B. (1986). Life not death in Venice. In V. Turner & E. Bruner (Eds.), *The anthropology of experience* (pp. 261–285). Chicago: University of Illinois Press.

Newman, F. (1999). Does a story need a theory? In D. Fee (Ed.), *Pathology and the postmodern: Mental ill-*

ness as discourse and experience (pp. 271–286). London: Sage.

O'Hanlon, W. (1999). *Guide to possibility land.* New York: Norton.

Rorty, R. (1979). *Philosophy and the mirror of nature.* Princeton, NJ: Princeton University Press.

Satir, V. (1967). A family of angels. In J. Haley & L. Hoffman (Eds.), *Techniques of family therapy* (pp. 97–173). New York: Basic Books.

Schoen, D. (1984). *The reflective practitioner.* New York: Basic Books.

Seikkula, J., Alakare, B., & Aaltonen, J. (2001). Open Dialogue in psychosis: An introduction and case illustration. *Journal of Constructivist Psychology, 14,* 267–284.

Seikkula, J., & Olson, M. E. (2003). The Open Dialogue approach to acute psychosis. *Family Process, 42,* 403–418.

Selvini-Palazzoli, M., Boscolo, L., Cecchin, G., & Prata, G. (1980). Hypothesizing-circularity-neutrality. *Family Process, 19,* 3–12.

Selvini-Palazzoli, M., Boscolo, L., Prata, G., & Cecchin, G. (1978). *Paradox and counterparadox.* New York: Jason Aronson.

Shadish, W. (1995). The efficacy and effectiveness of marital and family therapy. *Journal of Marital and Family Therapy, 21,* 345–360.

Shawver, L. (1983). Harnessing the power of interpretive language. *Psychotherapy: Theory, Research and Practice, 20,* 3–11.

Shotter, J. (1993). *The cultural politics of everyday life.* Toronto: University of Toronto Press.

Singer, M. (1996). From rehabilitation to etiology: Progress and pitfalls. In J. Zeig (Ed.), *The evolution of psychotherapy: The third conference* (pp. 349–358). New York: Brunner/Mazel.

Waldegrave, C. (1990). Just therapy. *Dulwich Centre Newsletter, 1,* 6–47.

Watzlawick, P., Weakland, J., & Fisch, R. (1974). *Change: Principles of problem formation and problem resolution.* New York: Norton.

White, M. (1995). *Reauthoring lives: Interviews and essays.* Adelaide, Australia: Dulwich Centre Publications.

White, M., & Epston, D. (1990). *Narrative means to therapeutic ends.* New York: Norton.

Wittgenstein, L. (1953). *Philosophical investigations.* Oxford: Blackwell.

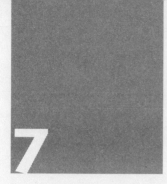

7

Marcelo Pakman

Toward Critical Social Practices

Hermeneutics, Poetics, and Micropolitics
in Community Mental Health

Machiavellian intelligence . . . instead of contemplating unchanging essences, is directly involved
in the difficulties of practical life with all its risks, confronted with a world of hostile forces
which are disturbing because they are always changing and ambiguous.
(Detienne & Vernant, as quoted in Campbell, 2001, p. 53)

There is dissatisfaction among community mental
health professionals. Loss of professional privileges,
including a decline in reimbursement and benefits,
and increasing limitation of their independence to
choose adequate treatments or preferred methodologies have accompanied the frequently overwhelming need to treat large volumes of people.
During the last decade many clinicians, administrators, academics, and policymakers in the field,
committed to fostering egalitarian care, welcomed
that patients were relabeled as "consumers," seeing
the new name as a sign of people becoming agents
in their interaction with professionals. They overlooked, however, that this change was also a sign
of the pervasive advance of market theory language,
an aspect of the onslaught of neoliberal policies that
followed the end of the cold war. Thus, an "in principle" legitimate aspiration to promote the rights of
the patients inadvertently added to the progressive
loss of a social stance of relative autonomy for professionals, who became a link in the assembly line
of mental health care. Large insurance companies
implemented the "managed care" concept, driven
mostly by financial goals, and unanimously recognized as the necessary solution for the health care
crisis (Pakman, 2003). Patients became consumers,
professionals became intermediaries between the

large companies funding community care and the
consumers, and care itself became a commodity.

These changes beyond the consulting room inevitably affected what happened inside the consulting room, the traditional arena of mental health
professional practice. With their practice manda-
torily channeled and restricted by procedures dictated by insurance companies and institutional administrators who adopted their goals, professionals
view their own attempts at applying sound theories
to the treatment of their patients as increasingly
compromised. But there is a prior history to the
attempts of mental health professionals to adjust to
the community context in order to practice psychotherapy in a way that is congruent with the theories of academic standing they prefer. This chapter
will examine the sources of strain for community-
based practitioners historically and how an understanding of the "poetics" and "micropolitics" of
practice currently can help in the actual conditions
of public mental health practice.

Hermeneutics

Confronted with irrational behavior that did not
appear at first view to make sense, the psychoana-

lyst, the common ancestor of psychotherapists, became an interpreter looking for the hidden meaning of apparent, manifest riddles. Thus psychotherapy has been, since its beginning about a hundred years ago, a practice of interpretation of human behavior, frequently focused on those aspects of behavior that appear in principle not to make sense, to escape being captured by reason.

Many psychotherapeutic practices still reveal that they fall within the scope of that interpretive, hermeneutic tradition. Hermeneutics, the twentieth-century discipline of interpretation, was named after the Greek god Hermes. Incarnating Prologus in the theater, Hermes would present to the audience things that the actors themselves did not know. Hermes, anticipating the performance of the actors, represented it as one among many possible ways. Representing what was absent in the presentation of the actors, Hermes was making what in French is called an "explicitation," and in English an "interpretation." Hermes, as Prologus in his own acting performance, not only made present, but also represented what was not present: he interpreted.

But we see what is present through what is represented. Ultimately, human behavior is always presence and representation. It is always not only interpretable but interpreted. And presentations ultimately regress to infinity; as Jacques Derrida has pointed out, every presentation, when deconstructed, leaves us only with further representations (Derrida, 1978). Representations frame what is present and make it available to perception and reason, to emotion and action, to meaning and further representing.

From its origins in religious practice (as in Talmudic, "midrashic" Torah commentaries among Jewish scholars) and the law (as in debates of how to interpret law), hermeneutics would more recently undergo the postmodern turn. Postmodern hermeneutics led to the questioning of all metanarratives, and more specifically of Cartesian reason, which would undermine the authority of the true interpretation, leaving us, instead, in a multiverse of competing ones. However, psychotherapists who fall within a hermeneutic tradition are capable of interpreting because they can map individual, family, couple, group, or organizational manifest behavior on grids provided by different psychological, biological, and social theories as underlying metanarratives. Although escaping the actor's awareness, those metanarratives are still frequently assumed to be at work as efficient underlying causes. Whether psychotherapists follow psychodynamic, psychoanalytic, neuroscientific, or developmental psychology schools, or certain more or less vaguely defined systemic models, they invoke, explicitly or implicitly, these typically modern metanarratives that the adoption of more postmodern language could not totally erase (Pakman, 2003).

Psychotherapists in a hermeneutic tradition look for meanings in behaviors otherwise viewed as irrational, abnormal, or enigmatic, as well as in behaviors that, although meaningful in a common sense, are conflictual and thus in need of further interpretation. Hermeneutics, interpretive practice, is not just a professional prerogative but is everybody's permanent exercise; it is not an a posteriori add-on to behavior but is instead constitutive of it. What professionals add are supposedly scientific interpretive frames as academically approved sources for their interpretations.

At the beginning, the practice of interpretation required certain ideal conditions of "isolation" for its practice to be considered legitimate. Modeled on the research practices of "hard science," the psychotherapists attempted to fix certain variables and, like surgeons, tried to isolate a field for intervention, thus creating the conditions for valid interpretation. This methodology created in itself a "world out there" that was not supposed to contaminate the psychotherapeutic field, seen as an experimental one. Once certain variables were eliminated, we could operate on a clean field in which an equally aseptic "mind" would show its constitutive phenomena, "transference" being one of those that would constitute the arena for therapeutic intervention. The "reality out there," actually created by the methodological attempts at controlling the environment for psychotherapy and a rather disembodied view of the mind, erupted uncontrollably in the therapy, seriously challenging the professional attempts at being "scientific" following the tenets of their "espoused" theories (Schön, 1983).

If a controlled environment for psychoanalytic practice was already difficult to maintain, the democratization of mental health care, with its concomitant attempt at treating large volumes of patients in the settings in which they were encountered (general and mental health hospitals, correctional facilities, schools of different types, etc.) by professionals with a wide array of credentials and levels of training, made the creation and maintenance of that ideal setting practically illusory. Psychodynamic psychotherapy was born from this negotiation between the aspiration to maintain allegiance to a purely psychoanalytic frame and the constraints that prevented the therapist from controlling the environment and creating a setting adequate for that endeavor. Many psychotherapeutic schools and models followed the footprints of psychoanalysis and psychodynamic psychotherapy, without changing substantially their theoretical frame and their allegiance to be interpreters of human behavior, and relegating interventions difficult to justify under the interpretive frame to be inevitable, contextually needed add-ons without actual therapeutic value. In other cases, when they surrendered their allegiance to the interpretive frame, without any other comparably prestigious frame to justify what they were doing professionally, they saw their professional identity demoted as lacking an academic stance. Others, such as some social workers and nurses, chose to accept that their effective interventions should not be called psychotherapy.

The interpretive frame of the hermeneutic tradition has maintained its prestige, and psychotherapists have tried to identify with it, in order to protect their challenged professional identity. Thus, many mental health professionals have maintained a vacillating allegiance to working, as much as possible, in an ideally interpretive tradition that always treats the eruptions of "reality" as a contextual constraint. This allegiance to the ideal of a purely hermeneutic model is an important and rather overlooked aspect of current dissatisfaction among professionals in the field. It condemns them to an "I know how to do it, but the context in which I work does not let me" frame of mind. They find themselves like dentists trying to fix the teeth of patients running across a park in the middle of a storm. And even though "reality" increasingly bothers mental health professionals, they have contributed to the construction of that reality by trying to maintain a practice born in the ideally controlled environment of a middle-class intellectual context. This practice is based on a modernist view of science and a longing for a status similar to that of a hard science. The "reality" being excluded is one created by a privileged frame in the powerful tradition of disciplinary psychology, which invented the "mind" as an internal, individual phenomenon, putting forward a disembodied, asystemic, and nonreflective view (Pakman, 1999).

Knowledge-in-Action

Even in conditions more ideal than the ones we confront day in and day out in community mental health, a close view of the actual therapeutic conversations and interventions shows that maintaining a purely hermeneutic, interpretive practice tends to be a rather chimeric project. These observations show that psychotherapy is not a coherent practice and that in any given session multiple sources can be traced for the therapeutic interventions. As Donald Schön conceptualized (1983), the "knowledge-in-action" that therapists display when they are practicing their professional trades is a mosaic of "theories-in-use," born from the practice-based intertwining of multiple sources, both academic and nonacademic. These "espoused theories" are, typically, the overarching principles professionals claim to be the foundation of their interventions when asked about their theoretical persuasions (psychoanalytic, psychodynamic, structural, bio-psycho-social, strategic, feminist, narrative, etc.). As more or less well-defined schools with academic standing, they are, however, only one among many sources of learning informing their practice, all of them structured as "theories of action," tacit, rather personal and idiosyncratic at times, and are able to be reconstructed in reflective dialogues that examine examples of therapeutic conversation and aim to extricate the patterns of actual intervention practices.

Among the nonacademic sources of learning, everything counts: "commonsense" truths pervading the culture at large; family and cultural traditions of the practitioner; life experiences and tacitly incorporated "know-how" about how to get out of difficult social situations; the so-called school of pain by which practitioners have learned how to overcome different types of painful experiences; and social prejudices, including gender, ethnicity, language, and social class determinants.

Not infrequently in psychotherapeutic practice there seems to be no congruence between the espoused theories and the theories-in-use. Therapists use interpretive frames from different traditions. Some of their interventions cannot be understood as interpretations within the frame the therapists intend to pay allegiance to and identify as foundations for their work, although they may be connected with other traditions. And all traditions, academic and nonacademic ones, are ultimately interpretive because they provide frames for interpretations of behaviors to happen. During the last decade, insurance companies have tried to implement, through many different procedures, evidence-based practices, modeled on medicine that fit with their financially driven agendas for cost containment. These procedures, the embodiment of the current structure of the mental health field, gained rapid dominance in informing the theories-in-action professionals put to work in their actual practice. Although the argument is that people are free to apply any evidence-based theory as long as they follow the prescribed procedures of that theory, those procedures add to nonacademic sources of learning and end up constituting theories-in-use of which practitioners are, by definition, unaware. Only those aspects of the espoused theories able to be channeled within those procedures survive. Thus, in the natural selection of sources of learning, academic ones do not tend to fare well under the adaptive advantage of procedural and nonacademic ones. Lying, distorting, and manipulating information to fit the requirements are commonsense adaptive strategies practitioners use to maintain their shaken professional identity. Dissatisfaction grows for the professional honestly trying to practice a kind of therapy that would make him an interpreter of behavior, and to defend the affiliation to a hermeneutic tradition that still signals a link with academic legitimacy.

I have progressively come to believe that a new language is necessary not only to describe professional practice but also to legitimate its complexity and to make room for the elements that do not fall within a hermeneutic, interpretive tradition. If therapeutic practice is, as we said, not congruent with a purely interpretive tradition, we need an approach that does not take that incongruence as a weakness to be ashamed of because it spoils the ideal practice we aspire to. The multiple sources of interventions and interpreting frames, including those procedural ones so relevant in today's managed care–funded institutions, and recognizable in clinical practice, can be taken as a source of creativity and as therapeutic tools in themselves. But we are not calling for eclecticism, as has been re-

peatedly done, to cover up the growing discomfort and dissatisfaction in the field. No well-argued and sound approaches have systematically been based on this vaguely claimed eclecticism, which seems to be a name for the obscure awareness that clinical practice is far from being the pure application of abstract theories, but does not help to find a way out from the trap. We are calling instead for a reflective frame that would allow us to start with actual therapeutic conversations instead of seeing them as the outcome of the application of abstract theories. We call also for a concept that would legitimize many noninterpretive interventions in psychotherapy, while allowing us to move among frames and generate new ones.

Poetics

To view professional practice from this perspective, it is necessary to make a reflective turn in the technical-rational traditional epistemology of practice, as it was postulated by Donald Schön in the field of organizational consultation (Argyris & Schön, 1996), and as I have both promoted and made preliminary steps to implement, over the last decade, in the practice and teaching of community mental health and systemic therapy.

As I have time and again seen in consultations structured in a setting taken from the design studio (Schön, 1987), this mosaic of sources of learning, traced and reconstructed as the theories-in-use therapists bring to their actual practice when they are in the mode of doing their professional work, is the rule and not the exception. Therapists operate as *bricoleurs* and build ways of dealing in action with the situations they encounter professionally, using all the materials they find at hand and all their sources of learning. To maintain, under these circumstances, an allegiance to an interpretive, hermeneutic frame obscures the multilayered quality of their practice and obliterates their ability to critically reflect on their own practice, in order to tap into their expertise at the fingertips (Hoffman, 2002).

The concept of poetics (Culler, 1990, 1997; Rimmon-Kenan, 1983) seems to be quite fertile when used in the context of a reflective stance as the one I have initiated, bringing Donald Schön's (1991) reflective turn to the mental health arena. Poetics captures well and allows us to locate in an alternative tradition many interventions that have flourished over the years, mainly in the systemic/family therapy field, as well as in some social work and communal practices that are separate from the dominant hermeneutic tradition in psychotherapy.

A "poetics" is a constructive practice that, instead of looking for meanings in behaviors that otherwise seem irrational, abnormal, or enigmatic, assumes that all behaviors are socially viable and effective, to the extent that they cause effects and that they affect others, and creates an opening for meaningful interpretations that focus on making explicit the mechanisms that allow them to be so. Thus, a poetics necessarily reflects on the social and contextual architecture that allows meaningful behavior to happen, on the competence human beings display in their social interactions, and on the techniques that are at work in the human drama in which we are constantly involved (Pakman, in press). However, as mentioned earlier, human behavior always shows its presence through representation; it is not only interpretable but interpreted. Poetics, then, asks for the context that allows for interpretations to happen, and for the ways in which interpretations become more or less successful, dominant, or useful. Poetics deals not with interpretations of what is given but with generation of possibilities. This generative, as opposed to interpretive, quality of poetics includes at its core the possibility of finding new or unexplored interpretive frames. Poetics is also generative in another sense: it tries to explore how it is that the interpretive frames for a given situation are themselves able to generate different realities.

This poetic approach allows us, then, to move among different interpretive frames, adopting a metaposition from which they are explored, without paying total and unreflective allegiance to any of them. Psychotherapies can be, then, not only hermeneutics, an interpretive practice in search of meaning, but poetics, the competence to act socially and to review reflectively the context in which interpretive practices happen and are born, promoted, or maintained. Poetics embodies the proposed reflective turn, which we use both in consultations with colleagues and in therapeutic work with clients.

The reflective observation of a piece of interaction during a therapeutic session can identify some of the sources of what a therapist says. I will briefly present a clinical case in which I operated as a consultant for the therapist, as I could construct it for myself listening to her initial presentation.

Case Study

Elvira is a 42-year-old Caribbean, Spanish-speaking woman, living with her 48-year-old companion, Pedro, recently immigrated from another Caribbean country. They are both unemployed, and they speak poor English. Elvira is illiterate and poor, and she completed high school with difficulties. An overweight woman, Elvira has been diagnosed with type 2 diabetes mellitus and suffers also from hypertension, hypothyroidism, and glaucoma. She is harsh in her interactions, uses foul language, and frequently alienates people, particularly workers of state agencies with whom she has occasionally had interactions related to family matters. Pedro has a history of being a temporary worker in tobacco fields during previous stays in the United States, has chronic pain from a herniated disk, the result of an accident, and has been incarcerated many times for drug-related offenses. He has two sons and a daughter from three different women. He has had no contact with any of those children over many years. He was married to one of these women, and all of them refuse to see him, accusing him of domestic violence. He also may have served time on charges related to those episodes. He currently smokes two packs of cigarettes a day. Elvira has been a pot smoker for many years, which she explains by saying, "Weed relaxes me." Although Pedro has never been abusive toward her, she had previous relationships with physically abusive men. Soon after arriving in the United States, she took charge of two granddaughters from her daughter Mary, who was deeply involved in drug use and deprived of custody of her children by the Department of Social Services. Another daughter, Ema, has not been in touch with her for several years, but Elvira has received news that she is married and doing well in another state. Her son, Angel, was in jail and is about to be released. Elvira and Pedro were planning to have him live with them temporarily, although Pedro and Mary were somewhat reluctant about this plan because Angel was incarcerated due to a sexual offense against a minor. His stay with them could jeopardize their housing because it would violate housing authority regulations. Elvira had been showing signs of depression prior to coming to the United States. These symptoms worsened shortly after her arrival, and panic attacks ensued. She applied for disability and was rejected. Pedro was planning to apply as well, and Elvira was planning to appeal saying, "I'm fighting for it." Both were living on welfare payments. Their social network was limited to a cousin of Elvira, Francisco, who had encouraged her to emigrate to get better medical services, and a few neighbors, Juana and Ricardo, with whom they were building a friendship. The other neighbors were a source of conflict in their view; the neighborhood was quite dangerous, shoot-outs occurred frequently, and the building in which they lived was a well-known spot for drug-related transactions. There were escalating family arguments, and Elvira was accusing Pedro of having an affair and misusing the little money they counted on. This escalation has prompted their referral to this agency by Elvira's primary care physician after he had ineffectively tried to treat her depression with antidepressants, which she did not take regularly.

The therapist was a woman in her 40s, an experienced practitioner, well credentialed and trained, ethically sound, well motivated, and committed to working in community mental health. She identified a psychoanalytic frame as the most basic overarching theoretical foundation of her practice, acquired during her early training in a midwestern institute in which she had little contact with minorities, as opposed to the many intercultural connections she had had in college. We worked with the format of a design studio, in which we typically use a poetic frame aimed at making explicit the theories-in-use the therapist puts to work to be able to gain a critical perspective on them, to overcome difficulties, and to expand the repertoire of interventions. Working with her in this way, we were able to trace some of the sources of things she said during an hour-long fragment of a family psychotherapeutic session, plus two other minor fragments from other sessions whose video recordings we observed together with other practitioners. She also commented about other interactions we did not observe.

After some initial conversation about the case being a typical one among the many multiproblem families she and I deal with regularly in clinical practice, we started reviewing the therapist's interventions. We agreed initially that the therapist used some loosely defined "psychodynamic" concepts to assess Elvira's depressive symptoms and the couple's issues related to substance abuse, which appeared to be pervasive in the family. The family had had some consultations in the past in which they had picked up some "psychological" talk, making for an easy start in navigating a territory of common language.

Some elements coming from readings of "structural therapy" were then traced to attempts at rebuilding a closer connection in the couple to legitimize Pedro's "authority." Structural therapy also came to mind for the therapist when she tried to disrupt a coalition of Mary with Pedro, which in the therapist's view was detrimental to Elvira and ineffective in raising Elvira's granddaughters, who were showing some evidence of initial learning difficulties and "out-of-control" behavior at school.

Some things never studied academically but assumed to be part of "psychoanalytic" understandings were identified in the therapist's comments about the effects of traumatic experiences in their lives on the family. Interestingly, the therapist would make continuous efforts to try to go back to the "psychoanalytic" and "psychodynamic" types of intervention and tended to see those moments as the only therapeutic ones. All the other interventions were seen as mere "talk" or were downplayed as irrelevant, although in many cases the family members would be clearly motivated or engaged in those moments. Some advice given by the therapist regarding the need to "put emotions in words" seemed to come from not clearly identifiable sources studied in "psychosomatic medicine."

A whole discussion about how to solve role conflicts for women who work, during a session with Mary and Elvira around Mary's attempts at staying clean and getting a job, was traced back to some commonsense ideas linked also to human rights promoted by a poorly defined "feminist movement." The therapist was sympathetic toward this movement, and had a few friends who were deeply involved with it.

A piece of advice from the therapist's grandmother popped up in some recommendations for how to deal with Elvira's suspicion of Pedro's infidelity. The therapist viewed other discussion regarding how to deal with violent men as linked to notions coming from some personal experiences with a minority roommate in college. Multiple mini-interventions had to do with forms the therapist had to fill out to be reimbursed by an insurance company.

Finally, we identified some hesitations and emotional upset of the therapist that appeared to be connected to an internal dialogue she was having with her usual supervisor, strongly identified with a school of thought the therapist liked but was not knowledgeable about, except through reading. A discussion followed about how this reflective process could be used in a consultation with the family as well as in therapy, helping them to trace the different sources of their understanding of their difficulties and of the family life situation, in order to widen the repertoire of possible actions toward the future.

When poetics is added to a purely hermeneutic frame, the main task of psychotherapy becomes not only to interpret behavior but also to contextualize, analyze, and ponder alternative actions, perceptions, and emotions, and the multiple mutual interpretations of them that are always part of what they become in actual relationships. The psychotherapist is not, then, a privileged interpreter but a provider of expertise, designing reflective strategies to navigate multiple and competing interpretations embedded in the actions, perceptions, emotions, and judgments that build the tapestry of social, psychological, and biological human life.

In a psychotherapy based mostly on hermeneutics, behavior calls for interpretations in terms of underlying truths beyond what is manifest. But when poetics plays an essential role in psychotherapy, significant effort goes into a reflective construction of the embedded patterns or architecture of the techniques and contextual factors at work in viable and effective behavior. This reflective construction is not detached and analytical but participatory, and new alternative viable behaviors are always born during the process. While interpretation privileges the past as a source of mostly causal explanations, poetics understands that the present opens it up into the future.

In my preliminary discussion with the therapist and the other practitioners present for the consultation, I kept asking what the therapist's "intentions" were in saying the different things she said in her interventions. Tracing the concepts back to possible learning sources was an aside, but it provided a step in exploring what she was trying to do. Asking about intentions allowed us to become future oriented, moving away from looking for bet-

ter causal explanations. When the different sources of interventions were discussed, we became progressively imbued with a spirit of research among equally valid explanations, and we became ready to start a similar exploration with the family. A metastance from which to look at our different interpretive frames launched us toward interventions that the therapist confided have not traditionally been considered part of the therapeutic endeavor with which she was having conflict. We share some extended prejudices in the professional world related to seeing interpretive interventions as more "profound" and showing better theoretical foundation than others having to do with more future-oriented, hands-on approaches, often seen as second-class communal interventions. This was a heated issue that had prompted tensions in the agency the therapist worked for. This whole approach worked as a microsocialization into seeing supposedly lateral aspects of the therapeutic intervention as full-fledged interventions, with the potential to sometimes open therapeutic avenues. Given that this consultation had an educational goal, I then introduced the idea of a table of "bricolage," in which we find elements for building something acceptable for everybody. We can add our own elements at times, but we cannot totally control them or eliminate the ones we find to be more obstacles than helpers. We naturally tend to amplify the ones we have in action to do something helpful with, and to tone down the ones we find more difficult to work with (Schön, 1991). This also prepared the terrain for further exploration of untapped areas and methods of intervention.

The relationship between hermeneutics and poetics is not only one of side-by-side addition but also one of circularity. In the poetic exploration of the contexts that allow interpretations to happen, we also can use different frames, themselves heirs of and open to different interpretive traditions. Thus, in a poetic activity, meaningful behavior is reconstructed to understand the biological, psychological, and social mechanisms that make it possible, the context of the interpretations at work in its construction, and the possible interpretations of multiple social actors that would influence its future meanings.

A psychotherapist within a hermeneutic tradition tends to focus, when confronting any human behavior, on the meaning of such behavior and tries to make interpretations based on the specific frame he or she pays allegiance to. However, as was apparent in the previous example, the psychotherapist is not able to avoid making interpretations and other noninterpretive interventions, whose roots are embedded in procedures dictated mostly by the context in which he or she works, the culture at large, or the sources of learning he or she has incorporated over time. Although clinical work based on a hermeneutic tradition tends to seek coherence, it cannot ever achieve it.

As a consultant positioned within a poetic tradition, I invited the therapist to instead assume that Elvira's, Pedro's, Mary's, Angel's, and the granddaughter's specific problematic behaviors were already meaningful for them in their circumstances, that they did not need explanation, and to explore what made those behaviors preferable to others. What were their intentions when acting that way, and what were the perceived consequences? What were their justifications and interpretations from different perspectives, and what were the opinions and interpretations of people around them, including professional people? What were the circumstances that made possible their acting that way? What made the behavior viable? What was their evaluation of how effective or ineffective, according to different goals, those behaviors were? I invited them to explore these issues over time around concrete problematic behaviors like Elvira's difficulties in treating her physical condition, her search for disability, smoking pot, her suspiciousness of Pedro, Pedro's substance abuse, his history of abusing women, his experience in jail, the upbringing of the granddaughters, their conflictual behavior at school, their arguments, Angel's return home, and their immigration to the United States, among others, and we decided to discuss with them how to choose the issues to be discussed. I also asked, What are the already existing and other possible effects of these behaviors and their attributed meanings for different family members and for others? How is that already affecting them and others? What type of configurations described by multiple academic (psychological, biological, social, economic, communicational, linguistic, political, etc.) and popular views of these types of phenomena can be considered to be at work in their behaviors and their effects? What alternative developments can we imagine as a consequence of the multiple meanings of these behaviors in their own social situations, as well as in others? Of course I did not intend to get an exhaustive answer to these questions. I was looking not for information but for a certain frame to be incorporated, thus switching to a generative poetic frame.

The addition of a poetic frame complements and interacts with a hermeneutic frame and seems to be particularly helpful when we recognize that actual work in context is never totally coherent or congruent with abstract allegiances. It allows the psychotherapist to increase her degrees of freedom regarding any specific interpretive frame, but not in a random, eclectic way. Although fluctuation between frames happens always as a matter of fact, this poetic tradition seems to allow for a reflective consideration of the alternative frames and for the creative use of the alternation itself.

Creating an opportunity to look at the many sources of frames for exploring the problems at hand positioned the therapist and the consultant to introduce a similar critical stance in her interaction with the family. In this case, I asked the therapist, prior to meeting with the family, what significant things she had in mind that she was, for whatever reason, unable to bring to the actual conversation with the family. At that time, I had started to be interested in revisiting secrets in psychotherapy and had focused on "secrets" of the therapist. She mentioned two things: one was that she was overwhelmed at times by the actual arguments during the sessions, during which she started to feel useless and ineffective, as if "talking to deaf people." She also mentioned that she doubted at times the authenticity of some of the statements Pedro and Mary were making, that they sounded like "preaching." In both cases the therapist did not talk about this with the family because she was afraid that, getting somewhat upset about it herself, she would offend them. Further exploring this fear, and in a climate of more open transparency, she also said she could not get herself to like Elvira, whom she saw as subtly encouraging some of Pedro's, and even Mary's, behavior. She acknowledged that this inability to empathize went against her beliefs and ideas about domestic violence and was, in a way, influencing her interventions. This had not been brought to the conversation explicitly either. We were now increasing our understanding of the different sources of interventions. I proposed to use these "secrets" to expand the repertoire of possible avenues of change for the family, adding again more elements to the "bricolage" table. We agreed that, as the person consulting me, she was my primary "client." I would try to help her in her difficulties with the family around these issues, which were probably significant for unlocking the therapeutic impasse she now complained about more overtly. I said I would try to make room for a more likable Elvira to appear in the session, given that it is very difficult to ask people we do not like to change, something I have probably learned more from some people I have worked with than from any therapeutic model.

I started the consultation by telling Pedro, Elvira, and Mary that I was there primarily to help the therapist help them, saying I understood they were very talented in getting at each other's throats. They laughed in agreement, and I asked them generically, but looking at each of them individually until they answered the question, What are you better at, listening or talking? They all agreed they were better at talking. I looked then at the therapist, saying, "You have a very difficult task here. When working with people who are better at talking than at listening, it is very easy to feel useless, as if you were talking to deaf people who did not learn alternative ways of communicating. Have you ever felt like this with this family?" She immediately answered she had. We have rapidly brought to the foreground one of the secrets of the therapist, an element that is not part of any formal model of psychotherapy but one that I was getting good at using within my poetic generative frame as an element with which to build therapeutic conversations. I proceeded to tell them, jokingly, and also using my "one up" position as a consultant, that I did not like to feel useless, nor did the therapist, and that I tended to think that whenever we felt useless, they were not learning anything new either, which was the purpose of the sessions. So, to prevent such a poor use of time whenever they started arguing, something they could well do without us at home, we were going to interrupt them, and if that proved to be continuous, we would invite them to come back at a better time, after they argued among themselves at home. We knew that no violence had transpired and that the arguments were verbal ones, but we warned them also that if they were in need of being controlled, that had to be done by other social agencies, apart from the therapy. This intervention worked during the consultation, and we did not have to interrupt them more than once. We stressed the fact that they were

doing something new a couple of times during the session. I took a very active role, building on my position as a consultant, and I told Elvira I was curious to know what circumstances of her life made her be involved with abusive men and surrounded by people with drug abuse problems. A view of how she learned to adapt to very bad circumstances emerged progressively, and at some point I was able to tell Pedro that a woman with those experiences was prone to adjust to bad things and could be inviting everybody to take advantage of her. I then asked Mary and Pedro how they were going to avoid taking advantage of Elvira, and who was going to make sure that that would not happen. I proposed that they should temporarily tolerate the family therapist being biased for Elvira. The therapist, now better connected with this more likable woman who had emerged during the session, agreed she could do it, and I reassured her I would be backing her from the outside in this regard.

We add a poetic stance not to try to build coherence but to question coherence altogether as an unnecessary illusion. We do expect, however, that bringing forth a different theoretical tradition may serve as an umbrella to encompass many already introduced creative interventions in community mental health, to help generate new ones, and to allow their critical transmission in a frame of theoretical legitimacy.

Although a postmodern turn has brought recognition of uncertainty, the inability to reach the ideal interpretation, and the impossibility of closure to the hermeneutic field, the stress in a hermeneutic tradition is always on optimizing interpretations. The context of the totality is incorporated mostly to make the interpretation of the parts or elements more accurate, and vice versa. The main question is, What is the meaning of the event? The present is studied in the light of the past. In a poetic approach, instead, there is a process of interpretive frame reflection (Schön & Rein, 1994) that allows for even contradictory or confronting frames to be explored or transcended in cases of conflict. There is, then, movement among both congruent and competitive frames, and the emphasis is on generating alternatives. Poetics is mostly generative, not interpretive in itself. Although there is in hermeneutic practice a certain amount of reflection on the interpretive frame (as described in the hermeneutic circle), the process always goes back to interpreting more accurately, not toward generating alternative frames for the material (clinical in our case) we are working with. Poetics asks, How is a given meaning possible as determined by its context, and how can it be different or changed? In doing so, it looks at the present from the standpoint of the future, exploring expectations.

Poetic Elements and Micropolitics

The psychotherapist takes, during his professional work, alternative generative positions, constitutive of its poetics, which are put to work through certain favorite technical tools: a certain use of temporality, language, reflexivity (Pakman, in press), in a personal and idiosyncratic style that can be explored and reflectively reconstructed. The elements of the therapist's poetics are not abstract theories to be applied to concrete cases. They are not consciously adopted as an a priori decision followed by the application of techniques. They are born from action in specific circumstances, in which the therapist puts to work his talents and idiosyncrasies, his personal style, preferred metaphors, rhetorical means, sense of humor, physical presence, and favorite rhythms in which to conduct the session, as well as a sense of timing. They become constantly intertwined with the therapist's academic and nonacademic sources of learning, including the procedures driven by the social-economic-cultural context in which professional practice occurs. They can, a posteriori, be reconstructed, and when and if that happens, they become more conscious elements in guiding therapeutic interventions. These elements organize the conversation from a certain perspective, as overarching preoccupations orienting the therapeutic process at any given moment. They are not only implicit elements of constructing therapeutic conversations but also parameters to judge the ongoing construction during its making.

I like to characterize the elements of the poetics I am reconstructing as an ethics, an aesthetics, a pragmatics, and a micropolitics. The first three elements are put to work in the consulting room and exist only as embodied technologies for dealing with the concrete situations a therapist faces. Ethics is mainly generative of alternatives; aesthetics has to do with a thorough evaluation of these alternatives, in order to choose the more desirable ones; pragmatics deals with the generation of concrete strategies to make the chosen alternatives come

about. I have taken and put to work, and explored in-depth elsewhere, two concepts of cybernetician Heinz von Foerster, who defined two constructivist imperatives—an ethical one: "Act always so as to increase the number of choices"; and an aesthetic one: "If you want to see learn how to act" (Pakman, in press).

From an ethical position, we ask these types of generative questions: What are the other interpretations we could make of this concrete situation? How can we describe the situation, and the other possible alternatives and interpretations, from now on? What other alternatives and interpretations were present at some other point but, for whatever reason, were not followed? Is there any way to reinstate any of those alternatives as current ones? How can we explore the options at hand and make them as explicit as possible, multiplying the details while describing them, portraying them as possible scenarios, including how they would change the position of different people should they occur? Are there other people involved who see, would see, or would recommend any other alternative or interpretations? What are, in each case, the sources and the consequences of alternative interpretations for all those involved in the situation?

After Pedro agreed to avoid taking advantage of Elvira's weaknesses and to allow the therapist to be her "defense lawyer," we said we needed to take concrete steps in this regard. We started discussing the financial situation of the family and pointed out how his evasiveness in this area was fueling Elvira's suspiciousness. He insisted on attending church as a possible solution for different problems, while Mary made some sarcastic comments about it. Pedro then insinuated that he did not believe Elvira's aggressive behavior would change unless she had total control of him. After a while it became clear that there was a feeling of mistrust, and I was able to say that many good intentions needed further exploration if we were serious about introducing positive changes. This addressed the remaining issue the therapist had brought up as a difficulty, namely, the lack of credibility of many stated plans to improve the situation. I mentioned "preaching" possible good deeds as something that could stay only as a good intention without helping much to be pragmatic. Pedro talked briefly about being raised by an uncle who was a "preacher" with a double life.

Instead of looking for psychological reasons for

the extended mistrust, I proposed being very clear and detailed in discussing alternatives for their actual problems. Thus, mistrust was considered a "sociological" problem that could be overcome through a change in their interactive practices. We started discussing what were their everyday problems, asking them to enlarge the list of problematic situations without intensely focusing on any of them. We were then able to identify as problems substance abuse, depression and other symptoms, physical illness, poor housing conditions, living on welfare, the contested disability of some of them, poor education, illiteracy and lack of opportunities, unemployment and poor employment history, recent immigration, poor English skills and the difficulties ensuing from dealing with the school, the legal, the health, and the mental health systems under those circumstances, and the poverty of their social network further weakened by the climate of mistrust we had talked about. We discussed briefly some of the circulating family and professional theories and interpretations regarding some of these issues, as well as how to prioritize them. We agreed that some interpretations of problems in one area were triggering, increasing, or maintaining problems in other areas, and we came up with some examples of this. We presented possible avenues of action regarding some of these many problems, making explicit the assumption that improvement in one area may slowly bring improvement, or at least movement in a positive direction, in other areas.

We focused on one problematic situation they all chose as a priority: there was a good chance that Angel would be released from jail in 2 weeks, provided a plan for him to be on probation for a few years was approved. The alternatives, discussed in some detail and written on a blackboard, were, first, that he might not be finally released, which would postpone the problem for about a year. They could hope for that and avoid discussing the issue. Second, Angel could be released, and in that case it remained to be seen if there were requirements of the court regarding where he could stay. If Angel stayed with Elvira and Pedro, there could be a problem regarding the housing authority, and the family would have to decide whether or not to hide this from it. If this were discovered, they would be given a warning and would lose that benefit and look for another place with or without Angel. The care of the granddaughters would need to be de-

cided. Angel had a history of abusing minors, and it was not clear whether he had received any treatment. We informed them also that there were many different professional and legal opinions about the follow-up and rates of reoccurrence of sexual abuse among perpetrators. The state mandated that the location of sexual abusers be public information, and trying to avoid that could bring further problems to Elvira and Pedro. Mary could soon be graduating from a substance abuse program herself, and the chance for her to recover custody of her daughters was a related issue. Should that happen, she could take the girls with her, and Angel could stay with Mary's mother and Pedro. Contact of these children with Angel was going to be an issue. Chances of substance abuse for both Elvira and Pedro could probably increase with Angel in the house, especially if the granddaughters left, because they were a factor in motivating Elvira to reduce her marijuana smoking to a minimum. Angel also had his own history of drug abuse. The prospect of arguments between Angel and Pedro was also a consideration, given that Angel had traditionally not gotten along with his mother's partners. Mary herself was rebuilding a relationship with Elvira, already strained because of Mary's mistrust of Pedro, and the addition of Angel to the picture could make this process even more difficult. Tensions could also arise if Angel's history became known in the neighborhood, jeopardizing Pedro and Elvira's attempt to establish a sounder social network. Substance abuse issues, if reoccurring in the house, could also put their welfare help at risk. Angel's fluency in English could help Elvira and Pedro negotiate with some agencies, but it could also make it more difficult for them to know what type of acquaintances he was with. Prospects for Angel to work were not very good, and that would further burden Elvira and Pedro financially, also bringing further themes for confrontations to happen. Financial issues could make it more difficult for Elvira to take care of her physical condition, as well as to follow through on her plans to enroll in a literacy program.

From an aesthetic position, we orient our interventions, asking these types of generative questions: From the options and interpretations, and their consequences, that we have discussed and that seem to be available, which ones does our client prefer to see happening? Which ones does he believe those around him would prefer to see happening? What are the criteria that make these choices preferred ones? What are the parameters used to judge them as more desirable? What are the parameters that different people involved in the situation are using? What are the conflicts that arise when the client sees that some options are more desirable according to one set of values or parameters, but not according to others? Which are the values used as parameters? Pleasure? Well-being? A sense of loyalty? Financial gains? Moral principles? Religious mandates? Fashion? Convenience? Avoiding blame or shame? Patriotism? Others? And what does each of these values mean for different people trying to decide what makes a choice more desirable?

In the situation we were discussing, there were, as is usually the case, contradictory needs and values. At this point it became clear this was not a problem to be solved easily but a dilemma that called for taking overt positions. They agreed finally that they would all like to protect the granddaughters; to give Mary a chance to continue reconnecting with Elvira and Pedro, and try to regain custody of her children; to make sure that plans for abstinence were maintained and reaffirmed; to maintain Elvira's treatment of physical ailments; to continue open discussions about the family finances; to help Angel, if possible, readjust to living in the community; and that these issues would take priority. Any concrete step would respect the stated goals. They would be discussed during the follow-up sessions, touching as many interactions among events as possible and including any needs to change them according to new information, events, or possibilities. We made a document with their choices for them to keep on the door of the refrigerator (the place they agreed to go to every day), with a copy held by the therapist. We agreed to have two of the practitioners present in the consulting session (both workers at the same agency as the therapist) to be available for further consultation in crises.

From a pragmatic position, we orient our interventions, asking these types of generative questions: Does the client know what to do to move toward the realization of his or her preferred options? How would the client go about starting to move in the desired direction? What are the missing pieces he or she would need to count on to facilitate moving toward that chosen future? Is starting to move in this direction something that will further increase the client's options? Or would

it lead, instead, to dead ends? Which ways of acting might change the choices, either for the client or for others? And how could it make them more or less desirable, either for the client or for others?

These three elements—ethics, aesthetics, and pragmatics—operate as positions alternatively taken by the therapists along the course of the sessions and constitute the task-specific skills, structured as theories-in-use, that we develop over time to deal with the specific situations our clients bring to us regularly.

We then discussed how to start moving toward realizing the stated options among the possible alternatives. Mary, who speaks English, was going to help Elvira and Pedro to prepare an expanded follow-up meeting in which their neighbors would be involved. She would also contact an agency for public representation that would tell them the legal situation regarding Angel and the possible probation. Elvira and Pedro were going to accompany Mary to a planned meeting at the facility where she was soon to be discharged to discuss the prospective plans of regaining custody of her daughters. This would also enlarge the circle of people working on the many problems of the family. We made contact during the session with this agency and left a message for Mary's main counselor to contact the family therapist and be incorporated into the loop of working toward the overall goals of the family. Elvira mentioned she was relying on her neighbor Juana, a nurse's aide, to help her with some of her physical issues. Pedro, in turn, knew that Juana's partner, Ricardo, had a brother who was a probation officer. We discussed calling Ricardo and Juana from our office to explain what we were doing, to request information about options for people being released from jail, and to locate a better medical institution with services for Latinos. Ricardo and Juana immediately agreed to come for a meeting with the therapist. Later on, Pedro offered to bring the pastor of the church he had been attending. Plans were made to reconnect Elvira with the literacy program and to follow up with Juana, the neighbor, regarding a more user-friendly health care system in the next session.

Micropolitics

Micropolitics has to do with the regulation and negotiation of spaces of power, when power is understood as the context that allows us to define what kind of reality is going to be considered for us and/or for others. Although micropolitics is another poetic element, I choose to elevate it to a category in itself, at the same level of relevance as that of hermeneutics and poetics, to stress that the locus of interventions is the social/institutional/policy-making instances that are part of the context in which we work. We try to operate on them to generate situations in which our ethics, aesthetics, and pragmatics could be more effective. In doing so, micropolitics operates with the other poetic elements, more intrinsic to the consulting room, to generate agency, potentiating the forces at work for desired change.

From a micropolitical position, we orient our interventions, asking these types of generative questions: What actions should be initiated, maintained, or amplified to increase the chances that our clients and our own movements will make desirable options happen? At what level should both our clients and ourselves be acting in this regard? Who should be involved in this process? With whom should we and our clients be interacting? Whose forces should be activated to better position us so as to make our psychotherapy more effective, thus enhancing our clients' options to change in the desired direction?

I learned later on that the follow-up session started a series of events that led to Angel being assigned to a prerelease program, which in turn allowed Mary to complete her substance abuse program and regain custody of the children, who maintained frequent contact with Elvira and Pedro. The conflicts among them diminished when Pedro became more involved in helping Elvira to take care of her health, and his relationship with Mary became progressively closer, to the point that Mary was designated to be in charge of Elvira and Pedro's finances. Elvira found the literacy course too taxing, but she started volunteering in the kitchen of a neighborhood center. She gave credit to her neighbor Juana for helping her abandon the marijuana after seeing that conflicts with Pedro followed days of heavy smoking. The therapist continued working with the family in close contact with a new primary care physician who started working with the whole family. Four months later, Angel got a place to live on his own, on the advice of a jail counselor and the probation officer connected with Ricardo's brother, with whom he became very close. He was attending a group for sexual perpetrators mandated by the court after his release from jail. The updated plans became a feature on the door of Elvira and Pedro's refrigerator, copied from the therapist's record.

The therapist and the other practitioners involved in this case became active in their agency, discussing ways to facilitate networking mechanisms with other agencies connected with the legal system, the school system, disability and welfare institutions, the police, the child and geriatric protection systems, the health care neighborhoods in the area, other mental health and substance abuse agencies, and so forth. Discussion ensued about how to respect new confidentiality policies without losing flexibility for creative interventions. Human rights concerns and ways to mobilize political contacts became part of the regular work of this agency, as usually happens when repeated instances of work like the one with this multiproblem family reach a critical mass in a given agency.

We operate micropolitically when we try to negotiate "procedures" to be followed, coming both from our own institutions and from those whose regulations we are mandated to follow; when we negotiate reimbursement fees with the insurance companies paying for them, and preferred treatments with agencies dictating general guidelines for health care; when we take political action to avoid the elimination of programs; when we try to influence policymakers and support "consumer" associations; when we explore technologies to prevent information systems from being restrictive, instead of empowering; when we lobby to make credentialing processes instruments to maintain, hire, and promote resourceful and experienced clinicians; when we ask that documentation guidelines be adequate supporters of our specific tasks instead of sources of alienation; when we network and cooperate extensively with other medical, social, mental health, and substance abuse services to integrate care with clients, not "about" them; when we try to involve academic resources to bring reflection to practice, and action to detached contemplation.

Micropolitics leads to interventions in larger systems and legitimizes the learning of these interventions as intrinsic to the duties of a psychotherapist, validating what is generally seen as part of a devalued role. A poetic stance generates openings within and beyond the consulting room, leading the psychotherapist to take a critical social role together with the patient, not only in optimizing the applicability of our more specific technologies but also in increasing awareness of the role of the social as a text of the mental, and not as a mere context for it. During this conjoint micropolitical operation on larger systems, and the poetic generative stance inside the consulting room, we explore together with our clients the background of "normalcy" against which abnormal and problematic behavior is defined as such. Therapy becomes, then, a critical social practice.

To bring poetics and micropolitics to the therapeutic field is part of a general movement, in the last decade, from contemplative to action approaches. This movement entails revisiting and transforming classical concepts, as John Rawls (1971) did by reframing justice as "fairness" and Stephen Toulmin (2001) did by moving from rationality to "reasonableness." In all cases the reorientation of the theoretical concepts is the outcome of a revived interest in, and of an attempt to legitimize, the type of intelligence put to work when we try to operate and reflect from within the situations we deal with. This participatory approach, at the heart of a conception of psychotherapy as a design profession (Schön, 1983), implies moving away from a sole allegiance to a hermeneutical, interpretive approach that, although admittedly postmodern in many of its forms, still slides frequently toward a rather detached and contemplative type of position, when monopolizing the making of therapeutic conversations.

Poetics and micropolitics, as generative frames, legitimize the local social arena as a locus of a necessary expertise for psychotherapists. They are action-oriented frames that bring to the field the power of the mythical, generative, metaphoric word, opposed to the logos, the illusory literal word at the center of the Western metaphysical tradition that Jacques Derrida has relentlessly deconstructed. They bring poiesis, generation, to its place in a well-developed, theoretically sound community mental health, as an area of participatory action-oriented science (Argyris, 1985).

The addition of poetics and micropolitics, both generative, action-oriented approaches, requires putting to work the type of intelligence that Detienne and Vernant call, in the epigraph to this chapter, "Machiavellian." They say that "its suppleness and malleability give it the victory in domains where . . . each new trial demands the invention of new ploys, the discovery of a way out (*poros*) that is hidden" (Detienne & Vernant, quoted in Campbell, 2001, p. 54). Jeremy Campbell (2001) adds that such an intelligence opposes "the philosophical brand that emerges from the work of Parmenides and others who look for unalterable core truths behind the surface ephemera of the world" (p. 53).

A new generation of psychotherapists can be socialized to tap into and develop this intelligence to facilitate their being at home in a world in which a rationality-in-action (Searle, 2001) is adaptive. For these community professionals, engagement in the social arena could be promoted as the legitimate territory of both the systemic structure we call a brain and the mind that, as Foucault (1965) claimed, disciplinary psychology has built and tried to capture, although it still remains at large.

References

Argyris, C. (1985). *Action science: Concepts, methods, and skills for research and intervention.* San Francisco: Jossey-Bass.

Argyris, C., & Schön, D. A. (1996). *Organizational learning II: Theory, method, and practice.* New York: Addison-Wesley.

Campbell, J. (2001). *The liar's tale: A history of falsehood.* New York: Norton.

Culler, J. (1990). *Structuralist poetics: Structuralism, linguistics and the study of literature.* Ithaca, NY: Cornell University Press.

Culler, J. (1997). *Literary theory: A very short introduction.* Oxford: Oxford University Press.

Derrida, J. (1978). *Writing and difference.* London: Routledge & Kegan Paul.

Foucault, M. (1965). *Madness and civilization.* New York: Pantheon.

Hoffman, L. (2002). *Family therapy: An intimate history.* New York: Norton.

Pakman, M. (1999). Designing constructive therapies in community mental health: Poetics and micropolitics in and beyond the consulting room. *Journal of Marital and Family Therapy, 25,* 83–98.

Pakman, M. (2003). A systemic frame for mental health practices. In P. S. Prosky & D. V. Keith (Eds.), *Family therapy as an alternative to medication: An appraisal of pharmland* (pp. 93–110). New York: Brunner-Routledge.

Pakman, M. (in press). Elements for a Foersterian poetics in psychotherapeutic practice. In *Cybernetics and Human Knowing.*

Rawls, J. (1971). *A theory of justice*. Cambridge, MA: Belknap Press of Harvard University Press.

Rimmon-Kenan, S. (1983). *Narrative fiction: Contemporary poetics*. London: Methuen.

Schön, D. A. (1983). *The reflective practitioner*. New York: Basic Books.

Schön, D. A. (1987). *Educating the reflective practitioner*. San Francisco: Jossey-Bass.

Schön, D. A. (1991). Introduction. In D. A. Schön (Ed.), *The reflective turn: Case studies in and on edu-cational practice* (pp. 1–12). New York: Teachers College, Columbia University.

Schön, D. A., & Rein, M. (1994). *Frame reflection: Toward the resolution of intractable policy controversies*. New York: Basic Books.

Searle, J. R. (2001). *Rationality in action*. Cambridge, MA: MIT Press.

Toulmin, S. (2001). *Return to reason*. Cambridge, MA: Harvard University Press.

8

Maria D. Corwin

Culturally Competent Community-Based Clinical Practice

A Critical Review

The community-based systems of care model and the cultural competence model have been in development for two decades. The systems of care model has always included culturally responsive services as part of its "comprehensive spectrum of mental health and other necessary services which are organized into a coordinated network to meet multiple and changing needs" and which are delivered in the client's natural environment (Lourie, Stroul, & Friedman, 1998, p. 6). However, apart from a commitment to recruiting bilingual, bicultural clinicians and the offering of diversity training sessions, the integration of organizational and individual multicultural competence concepts into the systems of care model has progressed slowly during this period (Bernard, 1998). The reasons cited for the lack of progress toward full integration have included (1) the lack of adequate organizational and practice theories to guide implementation of strategies to increase cultural competence of agencies and staff; (2) difficulty in operationalizing abstract concepts of cultural competence; and (3) lack of understanding of the need for a planned approach and long-term commitment to the developmental process of becoming a culturally competent organization or clinician (Jordan, 1998; Sue et al., 1998). This chapter will examine the mandate for cultural competence and the advances in theory, organizational strategies, and practice techniques that are now available to guide agencies and clinicians in making progress toward making culturally competent services in community-based systems of care a reality (Hernandez, Isaacs, Nesman, & Burns, 1998).

The constructs of culturally competent practice and community-based clinical practice are coterminous. Practice cannot be considered to be culturally competent unless service delivery and practice methods are based on knowledge of the contextual forces affecting people's lives, and unless interventions are targeted toward helping people to be successful in their ecological niches or contexts (Roosa, Dumka, Gonzales, & Knight, 2002). Likewise, implementation of community-based practice principles of comprehensive, coordinated, capacity-enhancing, client-centered services requires knowledge of how culturally diverse clients conceptualize health and illness, define help, and utilize and experience mental health services, as well as the ability to recognize intercultural misunderstandings that can render services ineffective or underutilized.

Since the inception of the community mental health center (CMHC) system in the 1960s, there has been a growing awareness that ethnic minorities and poor and working-class individuals were underserved or poorly served by programs and clinicians that were insensitive to or ignorant of their needs, expectations, and competencies. Following the civil rights movement and the War on Poverty program in the late 1960s, the mental health field recognized that contextual factors such as poverty, marginalization, inequality, and political underrepresentation strongly contributed to the mental health problems of these groups. There were sporadic attempts to better serve these populations through the use of branch offices and paraprofessionals and the adoption of a public health/primary prevention model. However, without a conceptualization of the role that cultural differences play in the quality of services offered or in their utilization, and lacking organizational and practice theories to guide reforms in service delivery and community organization, these efforts were often ineffective. According to Sue and colleagues (1998),

> Mental health professionals, who had never received the training appropriate for their new obligations, were now being asked to set up shop in unfamiliar social and cultural settings and to develop a delivery system from an array of disparate services. These same well intentioned professionals, mostly White, were also sometimes perceived as being agents of the repressive system they hoped to reform and were rejected by minority communities. (p. 97)

In 1977, under President Jimmy Carter, the President's Commission on Mental Health detailed the mental health needs of groups that were continuing to be underserved by the community mental health system. The commission made recommendations for a federal grant program that would give priority to underserved and unserved vulnerable populations and to mental health programs developing outreach and prevention programs. However, the Reagan administration immediately cut CMHC funding and converted federal funds to block grants to states to use as they saw fit (Cutler, 1992). With the funding cuts, states tended to ignore outreach and prevention programs for minority groups and to focus on services for the most acutely and chronically mentally ill. However, demographic shifts due to large-scale migrations from

non-Western countries in this period resulted in the need for states to attend to language and cross-cultural issues. States such as California, for example, found by 1988 that the majority of the clients in public mental health programs were ethnic minorities. By the year 2000, ethnic minorities constituted 30% of the total population and 40% of the child population and were the fastest-growing segments of the population (Raajpoot, 2000). This means that, at least in the public mental health sector, which includes schools, child welfare, and criminal justice agencies that provide counseling services, all mental health workers are working with culturally diverse clients (Sue et al., 1998).

Among the first policy responses to the changing demographics was the National Institute of Mental Health child mental health initiative, the Child and Adolescent Service System Program (CASSP) of 1984, which stipulated that the health care delivery system being advocated for children and adolescents should incorporate the special needs of cultural and ethnic minorities (Lourie et al., 1998). As described by Hernandez and colleagues (1998),

> In 1989, cultural competence was incorporated as a major system of care component, along with the core components of interagency collaboration, meaningful family involvement, community-based service and individualization of service. After 1989, each existing and future CASSP grantee was required to develop specific strategies for ensuring that cultural competence had been addressed by the state in which it was located. (p. 12)

Since 1989, the federal CASSP mandate for culturally competent systems of care has been matched by states and localities and by managed behavioral health organizations that manage state Medicaid programs (Stork, Scheolle, Greeno, Copeland, & Kelleher, 2001). In addition, a plethora of books and journal articles have been published on cultural diversity and culturally competent mental health practice in the past decade. Yet despite good intentions and adoption of policy statements, operationalizing of multicultural concepts in practice and administrative procedures and implementing service modifications have been slow and difficult (Hernandez et al., 1998). In fact, in 2001 the

United States Surgeon General's office issued a report, *Mental Health: Culture, Race, and Ethnicity*, that documented the disparities in availability and access to adequate mental health services for racially and culturally diverse groups, women, and the elderly. The report surveyed the needs of cultural and ethnic groups and the availability, utilization, and effectiveness of mental health services for them, concluding that there was a "constellation of barriers" to these groups receiving adequate care. In addition to the "cost of care, service fragmentation, lack of available services and stigma" that all Americans must deal with in getting mental health services, minority groups also "must deal with racism and discrimination; mistrust and fear of treatment; and differences in language and communication" (Manisses Communication Group, 2001, p. 34).

The Surgeon General's report also stressed the need to take cultural differences into account when designing and delivering mental health services (Criminal Justice/Mental Health Consensus Project, 2002, p. 1). The report noted that culture influences whether or when a person will seek help, what kind of help is sought, and from whom. It further noted that cultural differences might affect the presentation of illness or distress and that the beliefs and biases of Western mental health professionals could lead to inaccurate clinical assessments and ineffective or harmful treatment. The report called for culturally competent mental health services, which were defined as those with a respect for, and understanding of, diverse ethnic and cultural groups, an appreciation for the variable responses people have to their life circumstances, and ways of delivery of services to ethnic minority communities that reflected their different needs and styles of utilization (Bush, 2000). Among the recommendations for reorganizing service delivery were improving geographic availability, integrating mental health with primary care, improving language access, and increasing early intervention programs to high-risk populations (Manisses Communication Group, 2001). The development of culturally competent mental health services and specialists was deemed necessary to address the problems of high rates of attrition, late entry into the mental health system at a more severe stage of illness, underconsumption of community-based care, and overconsumption of inpatient psychiatric care (Bush, 2000).

Evolution of the Concepts of Culture and Cultural Competence

The definition of cultural competence used in the Surgeon General's report goes beyond an understanding of how culture mediates behavior, a valuing of cultural differences, and an ability to work effectively in cross-cultural situations to include broader system changes such as fundamental shifts in organizational structures, modes of service delivery, and funding policies (Hernandez et al., 1998). This more expansive definition of cultural competence represents the culmination of several decades of theory development and research on the nature of culture and the delivery of mental health services to culturally diverse groups. At the inception of the community mental health movement in the early sixties, culture was seen primarily in essentialist terms, as a "montage of specific ways of thinking, feeling, acting which is peculiar to the members of a particular group" (Webb-Watson, 1989, p. 466), a set of traditional ideas, values, and beliefs that organize and interpret and give meaning to existence. Cultural differences tended to be evaluated against the dominant, white middle-class standards of "thinking, feeling, and acting" and were determined to be deficient or deviant, the result of cultural deprivation. The emphases in mental health services and social services were on personal change through the remediation of personal deficiencies (e.g., ego deficits) and programs designed to compensate for familial and community inadequacies. The assessment of dysfunction was based on behavioral theories of personality development and functioning that were presumed to contain "culture-free constructs" or universal standards of healthy development (Webb-Watson, 1989).

The civil rights movements, affirmative action, and the entrance of more ethnic minorities and women into the mental health field led to a reframing of the culture of minorities as differences rather than as deficiencies, and to the beginning of attempts to develop ethnic-sensitive practice models. Operating with an essentialist notion of culture, these early attempts at culturally competent practice centered on increasing awareness of cultural differences through providing information about the cultural traits presumed to be characteristic of specific ethnic minority groups. Recommendations for cross-cultural practice centered on ethnic matching between client and clinician or the modification of treatment style to be congruent with the expectations of minority clients. This approach was problematic because it too often veered into stereotyping, while the contributions of stressors such as acculturation or membership in a devalued group were overlooked (Dean, 2001).

The adoption of systems theories, ecological models of human functioning, as a central organizing principle in social work in the 1980s refocused attention on the environmental context in which people function. The ecosystemic perspective on culture and mental health made clear the inextricable linkages between individual and societal mental health and broadened the definition of cultural competence to include a commitment to social justice, empowerment, and activism. Marsella and Yamada (2000) state:

> Thus, mental health is not only about biology and psychology, but also about education, economics, social structure, religion, and politics. There can be no mental health where there is powerlessness, because powerlessness breeds despair. There can be no mental health where there is inequality, because inequality breeds anger and resentment. There can be no mental health where there is racism, because racism breeds low self-esteem and self-denigration; and lastly, there can be no mental health where there is cultural disintegration and destruction, because cultural disintegration and destruction breed confusion and conflict. (p. 10)

The ecosystemic perspective also provided a framework for understanding how cultural factors influence the incidence and expression of health and illness and the giving and seeking of care. The idea of "cultural competency" came to encompass being knowledgeable about the role of culture in the onset, expression, course, and outcome of psychological distress, and the role of culture in shaping how individuals define, categorize, and explain illness and make their choices in methods for seeking relief from distress (Green, 1999). Transcultural psychiatry researchers such as Kleinman (1988), in addition to delineating the elements of help-seeking behavior, made clear that cultural orientations toward health and illness are not limited to culturally diverse clients but are shared by health care professionals as well. Kleinman noted that the etiological frameworks used to diagnose and treat

mental disorders reflect both broader cultural conventions and professional ideology, and that mental health professionals could not effectively work in cross-cultural situations unless they acknowledged the biases, vested interests, and deep feelings embedded in their theories (Fadiman, 1997). The fourth edition of the *Diagnostic and Statistical Manual of Mental Disorders DSM-IV;* American Psychiatric Association, 1994) included a section on culture-bound disorders but did not include in that section disorders such as anorexia nervosa that are found largely in Western cultures, reflecting the ethnocentrism inherent in any classification system.

Kleinman's admonition that mental health professionals need to recognize that the theories that guide mental health care are social constructions reflecting the biases and assumptions of Western society is a postmodernist view. Postmodern thought, a collection of phenomenological, interpretive, and social constructionist theories that posit the existence of multiple realities and belief systems rather than universal truths, has influenced how culture and cultural competence are currently conceptualized. In postmodern thought the notion of culture has changed from an essentialist, static listing of traits to a conception of culture as an emergent, constantly changing phenomenon shaped by historical and contextual forces:

> Today culture is increasingly seen to be more than a fixed set of guiding principles or latent structures that mechanically guide aggregate or individual behavior. Rather culture is recognized as a set of malleable and changing cognitive options, "a tool kit" . . . from which individuals and groups choose in order to accomplish specific goals. (Angel & Williams, 2000, p. 27)

Other postmodern philosophical tenets, such as the importance of subjective experience, the cultural relativity of knowledge, inquiry as being value-bound, reality as socially constructed, and the role of power and privilege in the construction of canon (Robbins, Chatterjee, & Canda, 1998), have contributed to a shift in emphasis in culturally competent practice away from learning about the content of culture to focusing on cultural self-knowledge and meaning systems or worldviews. Cultural differences are seen as situated within oneself and intercultural interactions as shaped by the cultural lens that each party brings to the interaction. From this perspective, awareness of one's personal and professional "biases, vested interests, and deep feelings" becomes the first step in developing an understanding of how an individual perceives and interprets life experiences and accommodates to his or her life situation. Green (1999), in *Cultural Awareness in the Human Services*, defined cultural competence as consisting of five essential components, with the first component the awareness of one's own cultural encapsulation and the limits it places on one's ability to understand and accurately assess a client from a different cultural background. The other components are (1) openness to and valuing of cultural differences; (2) a client-oriented, systematic learning style in which it is necessary to see the other as an expert in his or her culture and oneself as the student; (3) appropriate utilization of cultural resources in the client's naturally occurring social support systems; and (4) engaging with diversity by "learning about clients through direct observation and participation in their everyday routines in naturalistic settings" (p. 93).

Other current definitions of cultural competence include additional dimensions: awareness of how the history of minority-majority relations shapes current intercultural encounters; understanding of how organizations and institutions can enhance or obstruct culturally competent practice (Sue et al., 1998); recognition of cross-cultural dynamics such as differences in communication and problem-solving styles; development of policies and interventions that are congruent with clients' cultural perspectives; need to institutionalize cultural knowledge at organizational, policy, program development, and research levels; and understanding that cultural competence is a long-term, complex developmental process (Cross, Bazron, Dennis, & Isaacs, 1989).

At the same time that advances were being made in the conceptualization of culture and culturally competent practice, research on diversity in the workplace was leading to advances in multicultural organizational theory. The research examined the components of culturally attuned organizations and the processes involved in developing workplace environments that were sensitive to, and supportive of, the needs of a multicultural workforce and maximized the benefits of having a diverse workforce. Three stages were identified as characteristic of organizations as they moved from monocultural norms of behavior and standards of

performance to nondiscriminatory behaviors to cultural pluralism (Sue et al., 1998). Cross et al. (1989), building on this research, developed a six-stage Cultural Competence Continuum for evaluating organizations. At one end the continuum described organizations that were inadequate in meeting the needs of culturally diverse clients, in terms such as cultural destructiveness, cultural incapacity, and cultural blindness. At the other end of the continuum were organizations characterized by cultural precompetence, basic cultural competence, and cultural proficiency.

The inclusion of criteria for measuring the adequacy of organizations in providing culturally appropriate services adds another important dimension to the construct of cultural competence. The expansion of the conceptual framework guiding cross-cultural human services has increased the likelihood of achieving the long-standing but incompletely realized goal of culturally responsive systems of care. The following sections will examine how the organizational and practices theories of cultural competence that have evolved over the past two decades can be integrated into community-based clinical practice to achieve the mutual goals of improved access and utilization of services, equitable services, and equitable outcomes (Bernard, 1998).

Organizational Cultural Competence and Community-Based Clinical Practice

Several steps have been identified as necessary for organizations to achieve basic cultural competence and cultural proficiency. At this positive end of the continuum, organizations are characterized as valuing diversity, having a diversified staff at all levels, providing ongoing training in cultural diversity and culturally competent practice, having workers skilled in culturally competent practice, promoting social justice, and advocating "more broadly for multiculturalism within the general health care system and [engaging] in original research on how to better serve culturally different clients" (Diller, 1999, p. 13). Multicultural organization development models stress the importance of strong leadership: a commitment from the top down to make the changes necessary to provide effective services to culturally diverse groups. Other important elements in developing organizational cultural competency are (1) a mission statement articulating long-range goals and an action plan for achieving those goals; (2) a committee or superordinate group assigned to perform cultural auditing of an organization (systematic analysis of an agency's culture) and to implement policies and monitor progress; (3) methods for recruiting and retaining a diverse workforce; (4) institutionalization of diversity training; (5) outreach to and involvement of community members in program planning, diversity training, and policy development; (6) recognition of and building on family and community resources; and (7) planning to remain responsive to changing community needs (Adams & Krauth, 1995; Sue et al., 1998).

The last two elements, linkage to communities served and responsiveness to changing demographics and community needs, are particularly relevant to a systems of care approach to mental health services. Cross et al. (1989) noted that conducting culturally based needs assessments and incorporating the findings of the assessments into policy, program development, and direct practice are important steps in building culturally competent systems of care. To ensure that programs are culturally appropriate and truly community based, Delgado (1998b) and Green (1999) advocate for a high level of community involvement, a sharing of the decision making, and power in developing and administering programs. Methods such as using minority community members as interviewers or as participants in focus groups are likely to lead to more culturally valid needs assessments and program designs. Delgado (1998b) described such a community-based research project in which Puerto Rican teenagers in Mount Holyoke, Massachusetts, were trained to conduct asset assessments of their community preparatory to developing an adolescent substance abuse prevention program. The use of community youth not only increased the validity of the findings but also was an empowering experience for the teenagers, who gained a greater sense of control over their own lives and those of their families and community, as well as gaining skills and knowledge that might lead to a more positive life trajectory for them.

The Mount Holyoke project, in its approach to planning a prevention program, also employed a strengths perspective rather than a deficiency perspective; that is, it focused on mapping of community capacity through the identification of assets

and natural support systems rather than just on assessment of unmet needs. Once natural support systems were identified, efforts were directed toward engaging the members of these support systems in collaborative activities such as resource sharing, knowledge building, and outreach to the broader community. In a longitudinal study of Puerto Rican families with children in bilingual classes in an elementary school that examined how to improve collaboration between natural support systems, schools, and human service agencies, Delgado (1998a) again stressed the importance in community-based practice of including minority community members in the planning and delivery of services. The interviews of the Latino parents yielded many important insights into how this particular community viewed and utilized human service agencies, perceived the role of the school in their community, and wanted services to be delivered (e.g., in the schools with better integration of home, school, and human service organizations).

The model for school-linked services that has emerged is one that places equal emphasis on establishing linkages between schools, parents, and communities and linkages between schools and human service organizations (Cahill, Perry, Wright, & Rice, 1993; Clancy, 1995; Delgado, 1998a). The full-service school model "transforms schools into community hubs for services, activities, and support" (Dupper, 2003, p. 198). To achieve this community hub model, it is recommended that parents, school personnel, and representatives of service organizations participate in advisory committees; school social workers participate in community-based social service agency boards; community resources be identified and cataloged into a resource directory; and community members be utilized for educating school and social service agency personnel about relevant cultural dimensions of children's development and family functioning.

Green's (1999) "systematic learning style," one of the elements of cultural competence in his definition, is another approach for ensuring that members of a community are involved in the planning and implementation of programs intended for their benefit. In this approach, cultural guides are employed to plan for making community contacts. Interviews are then planned with key respondents, and participant observation studies are undertaken at religious, social, political, or community events to map the community resources and gain a fuller understanding of the community ecology, cultural milieu, and stresses of daily life. To design intervention programs, particularly preventive ones attractive to, and effective with, ethnic minority groups, it is necessary to develop a deep understanding of the cultural values that influence how individuals adapt to their local ecological niche, seek help, and deal with acculturation challenges (Roosa et al., 2002). Community outreach, participation in the life of the community, and involvement of community members on advisory boards and in the needs assessment, program planning, and implementation process are ways of achieving that deeper understanding.

Although it is now generally accepted that "a culturally competent system of care reflects and responds to the communities it serves through its administrative policies and procedures, hiring practices, training and professional development, and the active participation of community members and consumers" (Center for the Enhancement of Healthcare Training and Outcomes, 2003, p. 1), issues of implementation and evaluation of effectiveness have only recently begun to be addressed (Bernard, 1998; Jordan, 1998; Stork et al., 2001).

Bernard (1998) stresses the importance of effective leadership and a planned approach to creating a culturally competent system of care. The planned approach begins with the development of a shared definition of cultural competence and the presentation of a rationale for embarking on a long-term developmental process, such as an articulation of the benefits of culturally responsive services for all consumers and for providers. The next step is to conduct a thorough review of policies, administrative practices, staff resources, services offered, and evaluation procedures. This is followed by an assessment of organizational culture and an evaluation of the assumptions, values, and beliefs that organize and drive agency services and that present as resources or as obstacles to change. Diversity training then should be thoughtfully planned and implemented and a plan of action developed. The plan of action should contain short- and long-term objectives for jointly achieving the system of care and cultural competence goals, for example, "clients actually experience equal access, receive equitable services, and achieve equitable outcomes" or "the agency makes a complete paradigm shift, making cultural factors an integral part of its day-to-day business" (Bernard, 1998, p. 43).

Cultural Competence and the Systems of Care Integrated Planning Model

Jordan (1998) devised a model that merges the cultural competence and systems of care models into a single planning framework that allows for an assessment of how effectively principles of cultural competence have been incorporated into a comprehensive network of human services. In this integrated model, the categories that make up the systems of care delivery model (risk pools/targeted populations, system goals, partnerships, collaborative services, and evaluation methods) are evaluated along the cultural competence continuum (Cross et al., 1989) from destructiveness to advanced cultural competence. Advanced cultural competence is defined here in systems of care terms; that is, systems of care that are culturally proficient are characterized by equal access, appropriate services, and equitable outcomes. Equal access to services implies that outreach efforts have been made to make services known and acceptable; services are offered or denied at similar rates for all ethnic and cultural groups; and once clients are admitted into the system of care, they have equal access to the same quality of services. Appropriate services are defined for the systems of care model as services individualized to meet individual or family needs, including the need for culturally congruent services. Equitable outcomes refer to outcomes where there is a similar level of satisfaction and improvement in client functioning and living situation across cultural groups (Jordan, 1998).

At the advanced cultural competence end of the continuum, community-based service systems would be characterized as demonstrating that each dimension of service delivery has demonstrable characteristics of equal access to services, appropriate services, and equitable outcomes. Thus, with regard to the category of risk pool/targeted population, examples of a culturally proficient service system would be responsiveness to new ethnic groups in the client pool, outreach efforts to all ethnic groups, and proportional representation of all ethnic groups among clients served. Examples of advanced culturally competent system goals would include not only provision of culturally relevant services but also a proactive stance with regard to learning about the cultures of new ethnic groups in the community and continual mutual education between the agency and ethnic minority groups.

Partnerships in a culturally competent system of care would be proactive in seeking out and involving organizations serving new ethnic groups, advocate for diversity training in partnering agencies, and coordinate public and private service delivery to ensure equal access and culturally responsive services. Services would be characterized by an adequate number of multicultural and multilingual staff members, an inclusion of the strengths of ethnic groups in program planning and service delivery, and the employment of culturally sensitive assessment tools and treatment plans.

The final category, evaluation, would also involve the use of culturally sensitive instruments in the evaluation of programs and practice, and input from community members about the design of the evaluation studies. Evaluation studies at the advanced level of cultural competence would examine differences in outcomes across cultural groups, distribution of clients in comparison to distribution of ethnic groups in the targeted population, and evaluation of collaborative efforts with other agencies with regard to diversity training and distribution of clients served in these agencies (Jordan, 1998).

The remaining five levels in the combined cultural competence and systems of care planning model describe decreasing adequacy in providing equal access, appropriate services, and equitable outcomes to diverse populations served by a network of providers in a system of care. This combined planning model should prove to be as useful for assessing progress toward cultural proficiency for systems of care as the cultural competence continuum has been for individual organizations. A planned approach to achieving organizational cultural competence can reduce some of the anxiety, tension, and resistance that can accompany changes in organizational structure and service delivery procedures. A framework for evaluating the effectiveness of the integration of cultural diversity principles into a system of care makes it possible for interagency partners to locate problem areas and problem solve, as the following case example illustrates.

Case Example

This midsize community mental health center located in a small city participated in the wraparound system of care, providing mental health, case management, and family support services to children and adolescents identified by the schools or child welfare as exhibiting behaviors that placed them at risk for removal from their families and communities. The agency had made attempts to deliver more culturally appropriate services by diversifying its staff, occasionally offering training in diversity, printing literature and intake forms in Spanish, and assigning a Latina social worker to do outreach work in addition to her regular clinical duties. However, even though there was a significant black and Latino population in the city, and a majority of the students in the public school system were students of color, the clients served by the center were still disproportionately white. At the annual diversity training in-service session, staff of color raised their concern about this issue, as well as concern about the minimal outreach efforts and insufficient efforts to make ethnically or culturally diverse clients feel welcome. After a very tense meeting, the decision was made to bring in a consultant.

The consultant determined that there was solid general agreement about the goals of all clients having equal access to services and a right to culturally appropriate services, and that there should be equitable outcomes in treatment. However, polarization of the staff had developed over what, if anything, needed to be done to achieve these goals. White staff members were puzzled about why their efforts at hiring culturally and linguistically diverse staff and providing diversity training were considered insufficient, and they feared losing programs and changing practice methods that they perceived as constituting good clinical work. The staff members of color were angry about "token efforts" and demoralized by what they perceived as lack of concern and commitment to cultural competence by the agency administrators and staff. The consultant then outlined Bernard's (1998) commonsense approach to developing a plan of action for moving the agency forward in meeting its cultural diversity goals, emphasizing the importance of leadership and commitment from the top down to meeting these goals.

The introduction of an organizational plan with action steps, such as assessing organizational culture and working to establish a common understanding of cultural competence, was reported to have defused tension and anxiety and to have generated enthusiasm for participating in the change process. Each side felt heard and believed that such a planned approach could address its concerns. The director and assistant director clearly heard that strong leadership was essential and quickly took steps to form a standing committee on cultural diversity, whose first tasks were to evaluate the agency level of cultural competence using criteria derived from Cross et al. (1989) and Sue et al. (1998) and to assess the agency's cultural beliefs and expectations and definitions of culturally competence as steps towards developing a mission statement.

As the mission statement began to coalesce, following several reports from the committee to the clinical staff, the committee began to examine ways to work with its referral sources, as well as other members in the system of care, to evaluate obstacles to accessing services and receiving culturally appropriate services. Given the limitations in terms of staff time and expertise, the current plan was to partner with a school of social work to conduct research on access and outcomes problems and to assist staff in conducting consumer satisfaction focus groups. Plans were also under way to have regular rather than episodic training in diversity, which would include inviting ethnic community leaders in to educate staff about their communities. A longer-range goal was to offer in-service diversity and mental health training for teachers and school administrators, as the schools were seen as the partners that could benefit most from such training, and this training would have a positive impact on the types of referrals made.

Individual Cultural Competence and Community-Based Clinical Practice

The cultural competence continuum has also been used to measure progress in the achievement of cultural competence skills for individuals. The cultural competence continuum and the domains of multicultural competence model (Pedersen's Model of Training) are currently the central conceptual frameworks for organizing curricular and training programs for individual multicultural competence (Hong, Garcia, & Soriano, 2000). The next section will examine the developments in cross-cultural practice theory that are of particular relevance and utility for clinicians practicing in community-based systems of care.

The multicultural competence model identifies three dimensions of knowledge and skills that mental health practitioners have, over the past 20 years, found to be important for working effectively with individuals from diverse ethnic, cultural, political, economic, and religious backgrounds. The three domains are (1) awareness of how one's own beliefs, values, and attitudes influence perceptions of others; (2) knowledge of a client's culture and life experiences; the impact of racism and oppression on development and functioning; and cross-cultural communication, assessment, and intervention; and (3) skills in cross-cultural therapeutic techniques for improving clients' life situations and well-being (Hong et al., 2000).

Examination of one's own cultural values and attitudes and uncovering unconscious biases, stereotypes, and negative emotional reactions toward other ethnic groups are considered important first steps in becoming aware that there may be major differences in worldviews between clinicians and clients, and in developing respect for alternative views and lifestyles. In addition to developing self-awareness, clinicians working in a systems of care service delivery model must also become aware of the core values, beliefs, assumptions, and biases of the dominant American culture and of the mental health profession, as these biases may be at variance with the stated principles of the systems of care model, as well as conflicting with clients' conceptualizations of health and illness. The American mental health profession is still dominated by core values of individualism and scientism that conflict with stated beliefs in an ecosystemic perspective, a belief that mental health problems need to be understood within the context of people's lives. Individualism and scientism

> address two basic cultural assumptions of Western mental health professionals and scientists: (a) problems reside in individual brains and minds, and thus, individual brains and minds should be the locus of treatment and prevention; (b) the world in which we live can be understood objectively through the use of quantitative and empirical data. (Marsella & Yamada, 2000, p. 8)

The ecosystemic perspective is not culturally syntonic for clinicians because it conflicts with the central ideology of individualism and personal responsibility in American culture, which may be one reason that multisystemic intervention plans are less common than micro-level intervention plans and parent blaming is still prevalent (Markus & Kiyama, 1994; Webb-Watson, 1989).

Legault (1996), in a study of public social service agencies serving immigrant and minority populations, found that certain cross-cultural encounters frequently resulted in misunderstanding and failure in establishing a working alliance. She identified five common situations of intercultural misunderstanding: (1) differing notions of help and the role of social services; (2) differing views on child rearing; (3) unequal relationships between men and women; (4) differing concepts on family roles, relationships, and obligations; and (5) different concepts of physical and mental health. Legault suggests that awareness of one's cultural framework enables workers to decenter from their own worldview and center on the client's perspective. Knowing that clashes in perspective are inevitable especially around core beliefs about interpersonal relationships enables the clinician to be proactive rather than reactive in these encounters, being prepared to find a common language for negotiating differences when necessary.

One of the key areas for mastery for community-based practitioners with regard to the second dimension of becoming knowledgeable about the worldviews of culturally different clients is the culturally valid assessment (Glover & Pumariega, 1998). Practitioners need to recognize the inherent bias toward the dominant culture's norms of behaviors in the prevailing assessment paradigms and the distortions of the client's reality that occur when that reality is assessed only through Western psychological constructs. Culturally valid assessments will include information about cultural variations in expectations about behavior and standards of normality and abnormality relevant to the client's difficulties in functioning. Particular attention will need to be paid to identifying individual, family, and community strengths and resources because the tendency to see cultural differences as deficits or pathology still persists, and/or there may be differences in defining strengths or healthy functioning. Cultural influences on the nature, origin, and course of problems in functioning and on coping responses also need to be understood and factored into the intervention plan (Marsella & Yamada, 2000). To learn about the client's experience of a problem or illness from within his or her cul-

tural framework, Kleinman, as reported in Fadiman (1997), proposes a set of questions to be asked in the assessment interview. The questions are designed to elicit the client's definition of a problem or illness, his or her explanation of what caused it, why it occurred when it did, how the dysfunction or illness affects the client and his or her family, and the client's views of how severe and lengthy he or she expects it to be, and what should be done to resolve the problem. From this exchange, one can learn cultural attitudes, values, and behaviors related to illness categories, help-seeking patterns, attitudes toward help, and idioms of distress that are likely to influence the course of an illness or problem in functioning. Other significant contextual factors to be assessed for their stress potential are the client's degree of acculturation, cultural or ethnic identity, and migration experiences (Arroyo, 1998).

Culturally Valid Assessment Models

Amodeo and Jones (1997) developed a cultural framework for evaluating the use of alcohol and other drugs (AOD), which illustrates how cultural influences can be integrated into the assessment of problem behaviors for developing culturally competent strategies of intervention. On one axis are the "personal characteristics and experiences affecting an individual's relation to AOD" (subgroup membership, context of migration, degree of acculturation, and personal risk factors for alcohol and drug problems); on the other axis are "culture-specific dynamics: the culture's belief system (e.g., values, attitudes) and behavior patterns (e.g., communication styles, help-seeking) related to AOD" (Amodeo & Jones, 1997, p. 247). The consideration of both personal and cultural dimensions provides a more accurate assessment of how a problem behavior came into being and the forces present for maintaining or resolving it.

The final dimension in the domains of multicultural competence model is the skill dimension, the ability to develop culturally competent intervention strategies and techniques. For the community-based clinician, a key skill would be the ability to devise intervention plans that access and enhance family strengths and community support networks so that the client can remain in his or her community or be rapidly reintegrated when an out-of-community placement is required. The community-based clinician also should be skillful in devising ecological interventions that address the stresses associated with a devalued minority status and acculturation (Cuellar, 2000). Culturally skilled clinicians are "able to engage in psychoeducational or system intervention roles, in addition to their clinical ones. . . . [O]ther roles such as the consultant, advocate, adviser, teacher, facilitator of indigenous healing, and so on may prove more culturally appropriate" (Sue et al., 1998, p. 42). Skill in collaborating with indigenous healers, spiritual leaders, and community leaders is also indicated, given the important roles such leaders can play in supporting individuals and families in getting help and sustaining them through the helping process.

Future Directions for Culturally Informed Community-Based Clinical Practice

As this review indicates, several advances in culturally informed organizational and practice theories have moved the mental health field closer to its professed goal of serving appropriately, and effectively, individuals from diverse cultural backgrounds (Wright & Leonhardt, 1998). However, there has been insufficient research that tests the effectiveness of culturally informed intervention strategies and techniques. There is also a need for epidemiological studies of the risk factors associated with minority status, differences in clinical presentation, cross-ethnicity prevalence rates, and differences in the use of mental health services in order to develop more effective prevention and early intervention programs. In general, there is a need to identify the "critical psychological, biological, and social aspects of serving culturally diverse populations" if systems of care are going to be able to effectively serve a significant proportion of their client population (Glover & Pumariega, 1998, p. 289).

References

Adams, P., & Krauth, K. (1995). Working with families and communities: The Patch approach. In P. Adams & K. Nelson (Eds.), *Reinventing human services: Community and family-centered practice* (pp. 87–109). Hawthorne, NY: Aldine de Gruyter.

American Psychiatric Association. (1994). *Diagnostic and statistical manual of mental disorders* (4th ed.). Washington, DC: Author.

Amodeo, M., & Jones, L. K. (1997). Viewing alcohol and other drug use cross-culturally: A cultural framework for clinical practice. *Families in Society, 78,* 240–254.

Angel, R. J., & Williams, K. (2000). *Cultural models of health and illness.* In I. Cuellar & F. A. Paniagua (Eds.), *Handbook of multicultural mental health* (pp. 27–44). San Diego, CA: Academic Press.

Arroyo, W. (1998). Immigrant children and families. In M. Hernandez & M. R. Isaacs (Eds.), *Promoting cultural competence in children's mental health services* (pp. 251–270). Baltimore: Brookes.

Bernard, J. A. (1998). Cultural competence plans: A strategy for the creation of a culturally competent system of care. In M. Hernandez & M. R. Isaacs (Ed.), *Promoting cultural competence in children's mental health services* (pp. 29–46). Baltimore: Brookes.

Bush, C. (2000). Cultural competence: Implications of the Surgeon General's report on mental health. *Journal of Child and Adolescent Psychiatric Nursing, 13,* 177–179.

Cahill, M., Perry, J., Wright, M., & Rice, A. (1993). *A documentation report on the New York City Beacons initiative.* New York: Youth Development Institute.

Center for the Enhancement of Healthcare Training and Outcomes. (2003). http://www.usuhs.mil/cehto/learning-material.htm.

Clancy, J. (1995). Ecological school social work: The reality and the vision. *Social Work in Education, 17,* 40–47.

Criminal Justice/Mental Health Consensus Project. (2002). http://consensusproject.org/the_report/toc/ch-VII/ps40-cultural-competency

Cross, T. L., Bazron, B. J., Dennis, K. W., & Isaacs, M. R. (1989). *Towards a culturally competent system of care: A monograph on effective services for minority children who are severely emotionally disturbed.* Washington, DC: CASSP Technical Assistance Center, Georgetown University Child Development Center.

Cuellar, I. (2000). Acculturation and mental health: Ecological transactional relations of adjustment. In I. Cuellar & F. A. Paniagua (Eds.), *Handbook of multicultural mental health* (pp. 45–63). San Diego, CA: Academic Press.

Cutler, D. L. (1992). A historical overview of community mental health centers in the United States. In S. Cooper & T. H. Lentner (Eds.), *Innovations in community mental health* (pp. 1–22). Sarasota, FL: Professional Resources Press.

Dean, R. (2001). The myth of cross-cultural competence. *Families in Society, 82,* 623–631.

Delgado, M. (1998a). Linking schools, human services, and community: A Puerto Rican perspective. *Social Work in Education, 20,* 121–129.

Delgado, M. (1998b). *Social services in Latino communities: Research and strategies.* Binghamton, NY: Haworth.

Diller, J. V. (1999). *Cultural diversity: A primer for the human services.* Belmont, CA: Brooks/Cole Wadsworth.

Dupper, D. (2003). *School social work: Skills and intervention for effective practice.* New York: Wiley/Jossey-Bass.

Fadiman, A. (1997). *The spirit catches you and you fall down: A Hmong child, her American doctors, and the collision of two cultures.* New York: Farrar, Straus and Giroux.

Glover, S. H., & Pumariega, A. J. (1998). The importance of children's mental health epidemiological research with culturally diverse populations. In M. Hernandez & M. R. Isaacs (Eds.), *Promoting cultural competence in children's mental health services* (pp. 271–304). Baltimore: Brookes.

Green, J. W. (1999). *Cultural awareness in the human services: A multi-ethnic approach* (3rd ed.). Needham Heights, MA: Allyn and Bacon.

Hernandez, M., Isaacs, M. R., Nesman, T., & Burns, D. (1998). Perspectives on culturally competent system of care. In M. Hernandez & M. R. Isaacs (Eds.), *Promoting cultural competence in children's mental health services* (pp. 1–28). Baltimore: Brookes.

Hong, G. K., Garcia, M., & Soriano, M. (2000). Responding to the challenge: Preparing mental health professionals for the new millennium. In I. Cuellar & F. A. Paniagua (Eds.), *Handbook of multicultural mental health* (pp. 455–476). San Diego, CA: Academic Press.

Jordan, D. J. (1998). Cultural competence and the systems of care planning model: Consolidation of two planning strategies. In M. Hernandez & M. R. Isaacs (Eds.), *Promoting cultural competence in children's mental health services* (pp. 47–66). Baltimore: Brookes.

Kleinman, A. (1988). *Rethinking psychiatry: From cultural category to personal experience.* New York: Free Press.

Legault, G. (1996). Social work practice in situations of intercultural misunderstandings. In Y. Asamoah (Ed.), *Innovations in delivering culturally sensitive social work services* (pp. 49–66). Binghamton, NY: Haworth.

Lourie, I. S., Stroul, B. A., & Friedman, R. (1998). Community-based systems of care: From advocacy to outcome. In M. K. Epstein, K. Kutash, & A.

Duchnowski (Eds.), *Outcomes for children and youth with behavioral and emotional disorders and their families: Programs and evaluation best practices* (pp. 3–20). Austin, TX: Pro-Ed.

Manisses Communication Group. (2001, September 3). Culture counts in MH treatment, says Surgeon General's report. *Mental Health Weekly, 11,* 33–36.

Markus, R. M., & Kitayama, S. (1994). The cultural construction of the self and emotion: Implications for social behavior. In S. Kiyama & H. R. Rose (Eds.), *Emotion and culture: Empirical studies of mutual influence* (pp. 89–132). Washington, DC: American Psychological Association.

Marsella, A. J., & Yamada, A. M. (2000). Culture and mental health: An introduction, and overview of foundations, concepts, and issues. In I. Cuellar & F. A. Paniagua (Eds.), *Handbook of multicultural mental health* (pp. 3–26). San Diego, CA: Academic Press.

Raajpoot, U. A. (2000). Multicultural demographic developments: Current and future trends. In I. Cuellar & F. A. Paniagua (Eds.), *Handbook of multicultural mental health* (pp. 79–94). San Diego, CA: Academic Press.

Robbins, S. P., Chatterjee, P., & Canda, E. R. (1998). *Contemporary human behavior theory: A critical perspective for social work.* Needham Heights, MA: Allyn and Bacon.

Roosa, M. W., Dumka, L. E., Gonzales, N. A., & Knight, G. P. (2002). Cultural/ethnic issues and the prevention scientist in the 21st century. *Prevention and Treatment, 5,* 1–12.

Stork, E., Schoelle, S., Greeno, C., Copeland, V. C., & Kelleher, K. (2001). Monitoring and enforcing cultural competence in Medicaid managed behavioral health care. *Mental Health Services Research, 3,* 169–177.

Sue, D. W., Carter, R. T., Casas, J. Manuel, Fouad, N. A., Ivey, A. E., Jensen, J., LaFromboise, T., Manese, J. E., Ponterotto, J. G., & Vazquez-Nutall, E. (1998). *Multicultural counseling competencies: Individual and organizational development.* Thousand Oaks, CA: Sage.

Webb-Watson, L. (1989). Ethnology: An epistemology of child rearing. In L. Combrinck-Graham (Ed.), *Children in family contexts* (pp. 463–481). New York: Guilford.

Wright, H. H., & Leonhardt, T. V. (1998). Service approaches for infants, toddlers, and preschoolers: Implications for systems of care. In M. Hernandez & M. R. Isaacs (Eds.), *Promoting cultural competence in children's mental health services* (pp. 229–250). Baltimore: Brookes.

9

Catherine Nye

Similarity and Difference in Cross-Cultural Practice
An Anthropological Perspective

As citizens in increasingly diverse societies, we are interacting more and more frequently with individuals from different cultures. Our workplaces, schools, shops, and recreational activities provide us with opportunities for contact with people who are culturally different. As we begin to develop relationships across lines of culture, questions about similarity and difference emerge. How are people from different cultures alike and different? What do we share as a result of our common humanity, and what varies as a result of culture? Are there human qualities and characteristics that are shared across cultures, or is variability the rule? Where does difference begin and end?

These questions are relevant to everyone in our increasingly multicultural society, but they are particularly urgent for us, as human service professionals. As we more and more frequently find ourselves sitting with clients whose cultural backgrounds differ from our own, we must ask how our subjective experience and cultural knowledge are relevant to their treatment. Is what we "know" as human beings and members of a particular culture relevant to work with clients from different cultures? How much can we rely on the taken-for-granteds of our clinical practice skills, our use of self, our intuitions and empathy? Are these skills

cross-culturally valid? Are, for example, our culturally shaped intuitions relevant to the affective world of a client from another culture? At a more abstract level, are our theoretical models, our social work values and ethics, relevant to the experience of individuals from other cultures? At base these are questions about how individuals from different cultures are alike and different and what consequences these similarities and differences have for clinical practice. Understanding how—and how much—individuals vary from culture to culture, and how much, if at all, they share a common substrate across cultures, is essential for responsible clinical practice.

In the past, for example, the profession of social work focused on similarity. Social work is a value-based profession, and social work values and ethics were understood to be valid for all. In the service of ideals of equality and social justice, fearful that recognition of difference would contribute to discrimination and inequality, social work ignored and minimized difference. The "color-blind" stance of the 1940s and 1950s, for example, represented a denial of consequential racial and cultural difference. The "we are alike" implicit in this stance too easily devolved to "you are (or should be) like me." As a result, important cultural differences, which should have been acknowledged and respected, were denied and subjugated.

At present, social work is correcting for this historical denial. As a discipline it is focusing on diversity, recognizing and valuing cultural difference. The current emphasis in social work practice on "cultural competence" involves awareness of and knowledge about these differences. But questions about the extent and depth of similarities and differences remain. Are there underlying similarities—shared species-wide characteristics—across cultures that we can rely and build on in clinical practice? How does cultural difference circumscribe similarity? What are the limits of our shared humanness across cultures? To function effectively as clinicians, to recognize important differences and build on similarities, we need to know more about what is alike and what is different.

Differences in cultural practices at the behavioral level are obvious. How families are constituted, who sleeps by whom, what people eat, what work they do, their child-rearing practices, all vary from culture to culture. Much of the early literature on diversity focused on difference at this behavioral level. Differences in meanings, ideals, and values, which are enacted in cultural practices, are more subtle and complex. For clinicians, questions about the impact of difference at both the behavioral and the symbolic level on the intrapsychic world of the individual are most complex and most relevant. How do differences in cultural practices and meanings shape the intrapsychic world of the individual? How are the individual's affects, cognition, and experience of self and other shaped by culture? How profound are the differences? Are there areas where cultural differences do not make a difference?

Though these questions are relatively new to the human services, they have been central to the discipline of anthropology since the 1920s. Within anthropology, the conversation about similarity and difference across cultures is framed in terms of "universalism" and "cultural relativism." For more than 80 years proponents of "universalist" and "relativist" perspectives in anthropology have been engaged in a lively debate about their relative merits. In the hope that we, as clinicians, can build on the knowledge generated by this ongoing debate, this chapter will briefly review the history of these ideas in anthropology, explore the current state of this debate, and then discuss the implications for clinical practice.

Universalism and Cultural Relativism: Similarity and Difference in Anthropology

Universalists in anthropology focus on similarity. They seek to identify universal, shared attributes of humankind and culture. They are looking for ways in which all cultures, and individuals in all cultures, are alike. The universalist perspective was originally linked with biology. It was an essentialist, "biological determinist," view of human beings, based in the idea that as a species, humans share certain basic qualities and needs and that these shared, species-wide characteristics shape culture. In our postmodern world this essentialist argument is no longer popular. New rationales, which will be explored later, are currently used to justify universalist claims.

Cultural relativists, in contrast, focus on difference. They are interested in the variability of culture and ways of being human. They have traditionally minimized the importance of biology and see man as a "tabula rasa," a blank slate. From a relativist perspective, the environment—culture—determines what humans are. Human beings are therefore understood to vary widely from culture to culture. This "cultural determinist" view is congruent with a postmodern, social constructivist stance.

Recently a new synthesis of these two positions has emerged within anthropology. Cultural pluralists are proposing a creative both/and resolution of the tensions between universalist and relativist perspectives.

Context and History

The conversation between universalists and relativists has been going on within anthropology since it emerged as an academic discipline in the United States in the early decades of the twentieth century. The history of this debate is closely tied to its historical context. Anthropology emerged during a period of high immigration and rapid industrialization. Enthusiasm for science and technology, and faith in their ability to solve human problems were high. Darwin's evolutionary theory had captured the imagination of both social and natural scientists and, in the form of "social Darwinism," was being applied to the social system. His doctrine of "survival of the fittest" was interpreted to mean that cultures and individuals were successful (and therefore dominant) because they were best adapted, or "fittest." The poor—both cultures and individuals—were poor because they were less adapted, or less "fit." This ideology is congruent with, and served as a rationale for, a capitalist economic system. Free markets and competition were understood to fulfill a social and economic function by weeding out "less adapted" enterprises and individuals.

Social Darwinism proposed an evolutionary hierarchy on which every creature and culture could be ranked. It provided one criterion—evolutionary adaptation, which could be equally applied to everyone. Man, of course, was seen as more advanced, more evolved, than the animals. Western civilization was at the pinnacle of evolution, the most highly evolved form of cultural life. "Primitive" cultures were understood to be qualitatively different, simple, less evolved. Human beings in these cultures were also understood to be profoundly different: "savages," lacking many of the characteristics and qualities of "civilized" man. This is, of course, a powerfully ethnocentric view of human beings and culture. Our way—Western civilization—is seen as superior and more advanced and provides a standard by which to judge others. Because difference in social Darwinism was understood to derive from biological adaptation, superiority was believed to be genetic. To preserve superiority, racial purity had to be protected. Eugenics, which legitimated racism and anti-immigrant sentiment, flourished. There was a "compassionate" face to social Darwinism as well. It was the "white man's burden" to bring civilization and salvation to the inferior countries and races of the world. This missionary mandate was a convenient rationale for colonial enterprises in the early decades of the twentieth century.

This was the social, economic, and political climate within which anthropology emerged as a discipline in the United States. Anthropology provided a critique of social Darwinism's dominant social paradigm. As a counter to social Darwinism's biological determinism, anthropology proposed a cultural determinist view. In this view, difference arose not from genetic inferiority but from culture. Anthropology countered Darwinism's ethnocentrism with a relativist perspective. From this perspective, other cultures are not inferior, more primitive, or less adapted; they are simply different. Rather than devaluing "primitive" cultures, early anthropologists tended to romanticize them. They saw traditional cultures as providing a corrective for the excesses of technology and industrialization, as having something of value to teach Western culture. At the time, anthropology's relativist, cultural determinist perspective was seen as a radical stance and provided a powerful social critique. Until recently (Minow, 2000), relativism had been linked with liberalism, and respect for and tolerance of difference. Universalism, in contrast, had been linked with conservative social and political values.

Anthropology in the United States began with a strong relativist stance. Early anthropologists (Benedict, 1934, 1946; Boas, 1928; Mead, 1949) were interested in identifying intergroup differences, the ways in which members of different cultural groups varied in terms of personality, development, or "national character." Relativists searched for "single case examples" to disprove universalist claims. Malinowski (1927), for example, challenged Freud's claim that the Oedipus complex was a universal phenomenon experienced by all humans in all cultures. As a result of his ethnographic study of Trobriand Islanders, he concluded that in matrilineal societies the Oedipus complex described by Freud did not occur and was, therefore, not a cultural universal. He proposed that the form nuclear complexes took was determined by culture, and he described a matrilineal complex he discovered among the Trobriands. Margaret Mead (1949), a student of Boas, used ethnographic data from Samoa to explore the assumption that adolescence was a universal phenomenon. She found that in Samoa, where there were few restrictions on sexual expression, puberty occurred without the turbulence we associate with it in the West. Her relativist conclusion was that adolescence was culturally constructed, not a biological universal. Though her data have been challenged (Freeman, 1983), her conclusion has not.

Later, in the 1960s, 1970s, and 1980s, a strong universalist voice emerged in anthropology. French structuralists were interested in identifying universal structures underlying cultural variation. Lévi-Strauss (1987), for example, studied myths; he found that though the specific content of these cultural stories varied, their deep structure was the same across cultures. Mircea Eliade (1959, 1961) compared the world's great religions and found underlying universal principles and beliefs. In the early 1980s Melford Spiro, who had been a culture and personality anthropologist, disappointed with attempts to identify substantive intergroup differences, and struck by underlying similarities across cultures, shifted his focus (Spiro, 1999). He began to study cross-cultural universals and challenged Malinowski's early data refuting the universality of the Oedipus complex (Spiro, 1982). Based on a new reading of Malinowski's data, studies of marriage patterns in China, and ethnographic evidence from his own studies of Israeli kibbutzim, Spiro concluded that the incest taboo and the Oedipus complex as Freud described it were both cultural universals. During this period the early culture and personality school evolved into the field of psychological anthropology; this new approach included proponents of both relativist and universalist perspectives.

In the late 1970s and 1980s, Clifford Geertz (1973, 1979b) and proponents of interpretive anthropology reasserted a strong relativist position in anthropology. Geertz responded to issues raised by hermeneutics, a branch of literary theory, which posed serious challenges to claims of empiricism and objectivity in the social sciences. Hermeneutics, the art of interpretation, claimed that our individual and cultural filters make objective reporting of data impossible; that what had passed for objective ethnography—reporting of facts and data about other cultures—was simply interpretation. Rather than disputing these challenges, Geertz embraced them. Anthropology was an interpretive method. Anthropologists were not able to describe other cultures objectively; instead, they interpreted cultures as hermeneuticists interpreted texts. Good anthropological method consisted not of objective scientific reporting of data but of providing detailed accounts—"thick description"—and offering convincing interpretations of them. Geertz's methodological innovations are grounded in an acknowledgment that difference, between individuals and cultures, is not easily bridged; that our capacity to understand the other is limited, restricted by our culture-bound subjectivity.

Geertz's ethnographic studies, in Bali (1980) and Morocco (1979a), focused on difference in meaning as it was expressed in cultural practices, like the famous cockfight. But he was also interested in how different cultural meanings and practices shaped the self-experience of individuals. Though he is careful to delimit his interest in self

to the social self, his work begins to address questions about interpersonal and internal, intrapsychic difference across cultures.

In the 1990s, as postmodernism dominated academic discourse, "radical relativism" emerged in anthropology. Students of Geertz, such as Crapanzano (1980) and Rabinow (1977, 1987), challenged his model of textual interpretation. Cultures, they argued, were not static texts but changing systems. Informants could talk back, could verify or disconfirm one's hypotheses. Dialogue, rather than interpretation, was the appropriate mode of interaction. These radical relativists raised more serious challenges to ethnographic goals and methods, creating a "crisis of representation" (Marcus & Fischer, 1999) within the discipline of anthropology. Anthropology's goal had been to "take the native's point of view," to see the world as the "other" saw it. Radical relativists raised questions about whether this was possible. They claimed that our own cultural filters shape and distort what we see; that we are unable to escape from our cultural frames and see and experience differently. As a result, it is impossible to understand and represent the "other," to "take the native's point of view." We are constrained and confined by our cultural difference, unable to comprehend the other. According to this postmodern view, in the social as well as the natural sciences, the culturally constructed subjectivity of the observer intrudes on what is being observed and distorts our findings. This is a strong relativist position that makes difference almost absolute, and the search for understanding and commonality across cultures a very challenging one.

The idea that there is no objective basis from which to evaluate or judge cultures is implicit in radical relativism. Values are just one aspect of our distorting cultural frame—our limiting subjectivity. Our values are valid only within our cultural frame; they do not represent cross-cultural, universal "truth." From a radical relativist perspective, applying our values across cultures, judging others by our cultural standards, is meaningless at best and can be destructive at worst.

There are clear parallels between radical relativism in anthropology and constructivist and narrative approaches in clinical practice. Both emerged at the same time in response to similar, postmodern, challenges. Clinicians are charged with understanding clients across cultures; anthropologists' goal is to understand the perspective of the other. Recognizing the limitations in one's ability to listen and record objectively presented enormous challenges to both disciplines.

As this brief review of the history of anthropology makes clear, a conversation about universalism and relativism—similarity and difference—has been going on within anthropology for more than 80 years. In the early 1990s, when I began teaching a doctoral course on anthropology and social work, the relativist position dominated the field. I wondered at that time if we had heard the last of universalism, so firmly had it been rejected by the claims of radical relativism. There seemed no place left to stand to make universalist judgments or claims. Over the last 5 years, however, I have watched with interest as a strong resurgence of the universalist perspective has challenged the radical relativism of postmodernism. This resurgence has occurred across disciplines (Minow, 2000) and has had an impact on anthropology, as well as other social sciences. At present there is a debate between "liberal," "monoculturalist" universalists and "culture defender," "cultural pluralist" relativists (Minow, 2000; Shweder, 2000). This debate cuts across disciplines and is having an important impact on the social, economic, and political world beyond academia.

The Current Debate

Strong universalist claims are currently being made by an interdisciplinary group, including feminists in anthropology and other disciplines, economists, ecologists, and human rights activists. What unites these parties is an interest in "social development." Universalism, as a conceptual model, supports and parallels the move toward "globalization" in economic, social, and political realms. It is a useful rationale for a global approach. If all individuals and all cultures are essentially alike, the same economic, moral, social, and political principles should apply everywhere. The assumption that cultural differences are trivial compared with the shared species-wide similarities between human beings is basic to these universalist approaches.

Postmodernism has made essentialist, biological determinist arguments in support of universalism less acceptable (though some, for example, evolutionary psychologists, continue to employ biological models). Current arguments in favor of a universalist approach are being made on two grounds: the moral and the pragmatic. The moral argument is being advanced, for example, by human rights activists and feminists (Okin, 1999). They assert that certain values and principles should be universally applied to all human beings because they are "right" or morally superior. This position is grounded in the Aristotelian ideal of absolute good: the belief that there is one universal standard that applies to all. The pragmatic argument is being made by social developmentalists, economists, and political scientists. Their argument is that certain values work better and promote development and prosperity, and therefore should be universally applied. Both positions are universalist in that they posit a universal standard that applies to everyone in all cultures.

Feminist philosopher Martha Nussbaum (2000), for example, in her book *Women and Human Development*, makes a strong case for universal values based on a moral argument. She claims that there is one universal set of values, one moral good, one right way, which applies to all people in all cultures. She defines two "critical moral principles" that are universally binding. These are, first, the "principle of each person as an end." In her view the individual is primary, an end in him- or herself. Her second moral principle asserts that choice is a central good, essential to individual well-being. She refers both to specific choices—where to live, what work to do, who to marry—and also to choice about conforming to cultural roles and norm, for example, to conceptions of male and female, what it means to be a man or woman, in a particular culture. According to Nussbaum, all other values and rules of law should be based on and congruent with these two "critical moral principles."

Although there is much in Nussbaum's argument that is persuasive, her focus on similarity trivializes difference. She seems blind to the profound difference culture can make in the individual's experience of self and the world. In Nussbaum's view all humans everywhere want the same things. They seek "competence, mastery and control," "self-expression," and "freedom." She champions the "goods" of the autonomous Western individual, in contrast to those of cultures and individual selves who value the collective, prioritize the good of the family and the group over the individual, and value service and sacrifice over individual freedom, choice, and autonomy. She dismisses the possibility that there can be compelling, deeply held, and equally valid different points of view on these matters.

When there are apparent differences, when women from other cultures embrace and defend their traditional values and practices, she claims "false consciousness" (Minow, 2000; Volpp, 2001). According to Nussbaum, women endorse traditional cultural values only because they lack awareness of their real situation and of possible remedies or options; they lack choice. Their views are distorted by their traditional culture. If their consciousness were raised and they were given the options available to Western women—of education, autonomy, and independence—women everywhere would make the same, Western choices. In the end, Nussbaum is dismissive of what women themselves tell us.

In contrast to the radical relativists, universalists like Nussbaum, who provide moral justification for their arguments, often seem to be looking at the values and practices of others through the lens of their own values and culture. They assume the correctness of their own individualistic, Western views and are horrified by difference. In their arrogance, their self-righteous dogmatism, there are echoes of the (earlier) "white man's burden," missionary stance. As proponents of universal human rights, it is their responsibility to bring salvation and civilization to the "savages," to carry our superior Western models to the disadvantaged and downtrodden of other cultures. Missing from these arguments is an appreciation for the possible richness or value of difference, the idea that we may have something to learn from other cultures, which has traditionally been important in anthropology.

The pragmatic argument for universal values is laid out by Harrison and Huntington (2000) in *Culture Matters: How Values Shape Human Progress*. They assert that culture, and particularly the values inherent in culture, can support or obstruct human progress, when progress is defined as "movement toward economic development and material well-being, social economic equity, and political democracy" (p. xv). Certain values such as hard work, honesty, rationality, diligence, order, efficiency, individualistic achievement, self-expression, and social mobility are correlated with economic success and progress; they are understood to support progress. These are the secular/rational values of modernity and are distinguished from the values of

"traditional" cultures. Societies that embrace "good" secular/rational values achieve economic development, progress, and prosperity. Societies that fail to embrace these values, fail to progress. For example, traditional values, like a strong family or group orientation, are linked with nepotism and corruption, which are understood to retard progress.

If traditional cultural values obstruct development, then changing these values is essential to progress. According to these social developmentalists, modernization/secularization—Westernization—of values is necessary for economic growth. This is a universalist argument based not on morality but on utility; there is one set of values that works better and therefore should be universally adopted. If societies want to be prosperous, they must adopt these values. There are echoes here of the Darwinist "survival of the fittest" argument. Some values are more "fit" than others, have greater survival value, and therefore should be adopted.

Both moral and pragmatic universalists share a view of traditional culture and difference as basically negative forces that obstruct both the moral good—human rights, freedom, and equality, especially for women—and economic development. From the current universalist perspective, traditional culture and values are simply justifications for maintaining the status quo; they are being used in bad faith by those in power to legitimate gender inequality, hierarchy, and lack of opportunity (Lock, 1996). As advocates for universal human rights and universal values, they argue that cultural difference obstructs human progress and that cultural variability in values and meanings should be replaced by one universal standard. The implication is that progress and the "good" demand that we eliminate difference in cultural values. Because cultures are interactive and self-maintaining reflexive systems, as values change, meanings, practices, and ultimately experience must also inevitably change. This is a strong argument for cultural uniformity and against difference and variability.

In contrast, the current relativist position values difference. In anthropology, as "cultural psychology" has replaced "psychological anthropology" as an area of specialization, "cultural pluralism" has replaced the radical relativism of the late 1990s. There has been a shift away from, a recoil from, the extreme postmodern position that cultural difference is so profound that we cannot understand or make objective evaluations across cultures. In anthropology, as in other fields, this stance has proved to be unproductive. It has been replaced by cultural pluralism, which values and defends cultural difference (Minow, 2000; Shweder, 2000) but believes that there is common ground that makes different cultures and their members intelligible to one another. Cultural pluralists take a "both/and" approach to issues of universalism and relativism, similarity and difference. They acknowledge both an underlying universal substrate of human potentialities shared across cultures, the "psychic unity of mankind," and the richness and complexity of cultural variation, the multiplicity of ways this substrate can be developed and activated in any particular culture. They value this multiplicity and believe that we in the West may have something to learn from other cultures, that their alternate models may serve as an enrichment or corrective for our own limited cultural view (Shweder, 1991, 1998). Though cultural pluralists acknowledge the existence of "psychological uniformities" across cultures (Shweder, 1997), their ethnographic focus is on providing detailed descriptions of difference, the different ways of life, practices, meanings, and ways of being in the world, which cultures elaborate from this common substrate.

Cultural variation in values has been of particular interest to cultural pluralists. Richard Shweder (2000), a self-described cultural pluralist, wrote a chapter in the book *Culture Matters*, critiquing its universalist, cultural developmentalist position on cultural values. Though Shweder acknowledges that there are "universally binding values," he maintains that rather than one universal right way, there are a multiplicity of goods, many potential ways to lead a rich, satisfying, fully human life. These multiple goods are "diverse, heterogeneous," and "inherently in conflict with one another." He lists "justice, beneficence, autonomy, sacrifice, liberty, loyalty, sanctity and duty" as universal goods. In his view cultures select from these "goods," and "no one cultural tradition has ever been able to honor everything that is good." In this view, progress and prosperity, the good life, may be defined in multiple ways, not just in terms of Western individualism and consumer culture. Each culture provides a unique blueprint, a different model with its own legitimacy; they cannot be rank ordered or hierarchized.

Variation in emotions across cultures has also been the topic of much ethnographic study. Though early relativists focused on incommensurability in emotions across cultures (Lutz, 1988), cultural pluralists have, again, adopted a "both/and" stance. They recognize both the "strong commonalities" in emotions across cultures, based on a shared, species-wide biological substrate, and "powerful differences" (Shweder, 2000) in the ways cultures elaborate this common human inheritance. All humans are understood to be born with the same biological capacity for affect; variations are mediated by culture (and shaped, as well, by individual temperament). Cultures can elaborate and expand certain emotional potentialities or minimize and contract them. The presence or absence of language to describe affective states both reflects and constructs difference in emotions across cultures.

Cross-cultural research on families of emotions and the words to describe them (Fischer, Wang, Kennedy, & Cheng, 1998) indicates that the "social emotions," like love, shame, and respect, are most susceptible to cultural shaping and variation. Shame, for example, is present in all cultures, but in some, such as the United States, it is minimized, relegated to a small subcategory under sadness. In China, in contrast, shame is a highly elaborated emotional state. While Americans attempt to protect and minimize their children's experience of shame, in China the culture constructs frequent shame experiences as a major organizer of child development. Romantic love, in contrast, is highly elaborated and positively valued in the United States and minimized in China, where it is minimally represented in language and negatively valued. In a culture where arranged marriage and the stability of the family are highly valued, romantic love is perceived as a disruptive emotion leading to potential conflict. According to cultural pluralists, cultures may either "suppress" or "promote" specific emotional experiences; as a result, "in different societies people have distinctive emotional characteristics and simultaneously share many species-specific commonalities in their emotions" (p. 31).

Cultural pluralists, unlike radical relativists, believe that cross-cultural understanding is possible. Human beings share a common psychic substrate; cultures select from this substrate and activate different emotional and cognitive structures. Those structures that are not activated in a particular culture remain "peripheralized" (Shweder, 2000); they are not developed, they lie "dormant and un-known" (Shweder, 1997), but they remain as po-tentials within each individual. In this view, each of us retains the capacity to feel, think, and expe-rience "like" the cultural "other."

Richard Shweder (1997) provides a description of the way his field experience in Orissa, India, ac-tivated a psychic structure peripheralized in West-ern culture and previously unfamiliar to him:

> After working closely with three informants of very different backgrounds in Orissa, I decided to have a seminar in my home with the three. Food would need to be served, and as they had various and different food restrictions the only solution was to serve "prasad' " from the local temple. Prasad is the food offered to the deity who resides in the temple, and who is thought to absorb the essence of the food. Anyone, re-gardless of background can eat the god's left-overs. . . .
>
> After the seminar, there was a lot of leftover prasad. One of the informants overheard (my wife's) comment that she thought she might take what was still left and mix it with some chicken that she planned to cook for dinner. Upon hearing this, he cautioned me, saying that the rice and vegetables were prasad, not just leftover food. Since Lingaraj, the god, was vegetarian, he would be very upset. "Do not do this," he warned.
>
> Later, . . . my wife cooked the chicken, mixed it with prasad, and there it was for din-ner. I looked at it and said, "I can't eat this, Lingaraj will be very upset." Not only that, but I experienced a sense of dread. At that point, I had activated an emotional cognitive scheme that my informants had talked about. It was there in me, waiting to manifest itself once I had the proper set of concepts and experiences from long-term field work in this community.

Shweder concludes:

> It seems to me that this is one of the outcomes of participant observation. People have within themselves an enormous complexity of cogni-tive and emotional structures. Understanding others is a process by which you will find some-thing within yourself that will be the bridge to understanding difference. It seems to me that

without fieldwork it is impossible to reach that depth. (p. 162)

According to Shweder, it is possible to under-stand and feel like/with cultural others, based on unactivated but potential cognitive and emotional structures that we, all humans in all cultures, pos-sess. Activating those potential structures requires immersion in, and sustained contact with, cultural difference, the kind of immersion that occurs in the participant observation of the fieldwork process.

Implications for Clinical Practice

For clinical practitioners, questions about the pos-sibility of understanding the cultural "other" raised by relativist anthropologists are crucial. According to self psychologist Heinz Kohut (1984), empathy, which combines understanding and explaining, or interpretation, is an essential clinical skill. In cross-cultural practice empathic understanding must be cultural, as well as individual and idiosyncratic, be-cause what we seek to understand—the cognitive, affective, and experiential world of the individual client—is shaped by and varies with culture. Ques-tions about the universality of values, models, and methods, addressed by anthropologists, are also central to cross-cultural clinical practice. Clearly, the ongoing conversation or debate between rela-tivists and universalists within the discipline of an-thropology has relevance to clinical practice. Un-derstanding the strengths and weaknesses of these contrasting positions can strengthen our practice models and skills and help us avoid clinical pitfalls.

The universalist sees the other as "like me," or the same. This focus on similarity can lead to a distortion and denial of difference. For clinicians the potential danger of a universalist stance is that models and methods of practice will be misapplied across cultures. For example, as a graduate student I participated in a seminar in which the instructor, an expert in cognitive therapy, presented his treat-ment of a Mexican American woman. Applying Western values of separation and autonomy, he de-fined her cultural beliefs about her connection to and responsibility for her widowed mother as "ir-rational thoughts." His treatment goal was to elim-inate these thoughts and free the client for a more independent and "mature" adaptation. This clini-cian's failure to recognize cultural difference led him to confuse cultural values with developmental failure and individual psychopathology. His failure of empathy, his cultural misunderstanding, constituted a distorting misapplication of treatment models across cultures.

The relativist, in contrast, focuses on difference, on the ways culture shapes subjectivity. This focus on difference leads radical relativists in anthropology to question the possibility of cross-cultural communication and understanding. If the experience of the other is incommensurable, it may also be incomprehensible, impossible for us to grasp. For clinical practitioners, the relativist perspective raises doubts about our capacity to bridge the cultural gap between self and "other," worker and client, and empathically grasp the subjectivity of our culturally different clients. It can lead clinicians to fundamental questions about the efficacy of cross-cultural treatment. For example, in Santa Clara County, California, in the early 1990s, a group of social workers from the county department of social services demanded that clients be seen only by workers who shared the same cultural background and identity. In their view, successful treatment could occur only when worker and client were culturally alike. Their demand was grounded in the belief that cultural differences were so profound that they could not be bridged by clinical practice skills or treatment methods.

Clinical practitioners are challenged to find a way to heed the warnings and avoid the pitfalls of these contrasting approaches; to find a balance, an integration, or resolution of tensions between universalist and relativist perspectives. The current cultural pluralist position in anthropology suggests a possible resolution. Its both/and stance acknowledges both similarity and difference. Cultural pluralists honor the shared human potential of all members of the species Homo sapiens and recognize the diversity of subjectivity and experience selected from that potential and constructed by culture. Though radical relativists in anthropology, and postmodernists in other disciplines, raise questions about the possibility of true cross-cultural understanding, currently cultural pluralists assure us that cross-cultural understanding is possible. Because of our shared, underlying universal, species-wide potential, we retain the capacity to understand the "other" despite culturally constructed variations.

Though cultural pluralism recognizes under-

lying commonalities, its emphasis is on difference, the culturally variable ways human potentials are expressed in the different "ways of life" of different cultures (Shweder, 2000). Cultural pluralism celebrates diversity and reminds us that, as clinicians, we cannot assume that our intuitions and affective responses are congruent with or universally relevant to those of our clients. This is familiar territory for clinicians; "don't assume" has traditionally been a clinical practice dictum. Rather than assuming that our experiences are alike, we must be open to discovering the different experience of the other and to developing (new) parallel potentials within our selves. While we seek commonalities, we must recognize and respect difference, rather than denying, pathologizing, or mistaking it for "false consciousness."

An understanding of cultural difference and similarity must underlie our clinical decisions about the cross-cultural relevance and utility of theories, models, and methods of practice. We cannot assume, for example, that individual-, family-, and/or community-based models of practice will be relevant for all. Instead, we must explore cultural meanings, values, and practices and select treatment models that are congruent. The application of our individualized Western treatment models, which focus on "separation-individuation" and the "empowerment" of the autonomous individual, may be inappropriate for work with clients from cultures with collectivist values, institutions, and cultural practices. In such cultures, community-based models of practice may be more culturally congruent. But cultural difference in the meaning and enactment of "community" must also be acknowledged and accommodated. Cultural pluralism suggests that, though there may be shared underlying principles and processes of care, there are no "one-size-fits-all" models or methods of treatment.

Anthropologists' experience suggests that cultural immersion, including language learning, like that experienced in anthropological fieldwork, is one route to discovering the experience of the other in oneself. As clinicians we need to take advantage of such opportunities to deepen our cultural awareness and discover other such routes, more accessible to us in our professional lives. Perhaps the intimate contacts inherent in developing treatment relationships with multiple clients from another culture may produce similar results. As clinical practice educators we need to provide students with opportunities for cross-cultural experience. Clinical training emphasizes the importance of field-based experiential learning. Though academic learning can be an important source of insight into cultural difference, it cannot replace experiential learning about or knowledge of other cultures. If we are to prepare students to be competent cross-cultural practitioners, training must provide opportunities for cross-cultural experience for those students who enter training without them.

According to cultural pluralist anthropology, true cross-cultural understanding and the internal self-discovery it requires will be transformative for us as clinicians. As we remain open to and reverberate with the experience of the "other," we have an opportunity to "fill in the blanks," to develop the culturally unrealized potential in ourselves, to be enriched and expanded. Cross-cultural practice offers us opportunities for personal, as well as professional, growth and development. Perhaps this potential for the expansion of self (Roland, 1988, 1996) is, in part, what fuels our interest in cross-cultural dialogue and experience, and strengthens our commitment to cross-cultural practice.

References

Benedict, R. (1934). *Patterns of culture*. Boston: Houghton Mifflin.

Benedict, R. (1946). *The chrysanthemum and the sword: Patterns of Japanese culture*. Boston: Houghton Mifflin.

Boas, F. (1928). *Anthropology and modern life*. New York: Norton.

Crapanzano, V. (1980). *Tuhami, portrait of a Moroccan*. Chicago: University of Chicago Press.

Eliade, M. (1959). *Cosmos and history: The myth of the eternal return* (W. R. Trask, Trans.). New York: Harper and Row.

Eliade, M. (1961). *Images and symbols: Studies in religious symbolism* (P. Mairet, Trans.). Kansas City, MO: Sheed Andrews and McMeel.

Fischer, K., Wang, L., Kennedy, B., & Cheng, C. L. (1998). Culture and biology in emotional development. In D. Sharma & K. Fischer (Eds.), *Socioemotional development across cultures* (pp. 21–43). San Francisco: Jossey-Bass.

Freeman, D. (1983). *Margaret Mead and Samoa: The making and unmaking of an anthropological myth*. Cambridge, MA: Harvard University Press.

Geertz, C. (1973). *The interpretation of cultures: Selected essays*. New York: Basic Books.

Geertz, C. (1979a). From the native's point of view: On the nature of anthropological understanding. In P. Rabinow & W. Sullivan (Eds.), *Interpretive social sciences: A reader* (pp. 225–241). Berkeley: University of California Press.

Geertz, C. (1979b). *Meaning and order in Moroccan society: Three essays in cultural analysis*. Cambridge: Cambridge University Press.

Geertz, C. (1980). *Negara: The theatre state in nineteenth-century Bali*. Princeton, NJ: Princeton University Press.

Harrison, L., & Huntington, S. (Eds.). (2000). *Culture matters: How values shape human progress*. New York: Basic Books.

Kohut, H. (1984). *How does analysis cure?* Chicago: University of Chicago Press.

Lévi-Strauss, C. (1987). *Anthropology and myth: Lectures, 1951–1982* (R. Willis, Trans.). Oxford: Blackwell.

Lock, M. (1996). Ideology and subjectivity: Midlife and menopause in Japan and North America. In R. Jessor, A. Colby, & R. Shweder (Eds.). *Ethnography and human development: Context and meaning in social inquiry* (pp. 339–369). Chicago: University of Chicago Press.

Lutz, C. (1988). *Unnatural emotions: Everyday sentiments on a Micronesian atoll and their challenge to western theory*. Chicago: University of Chicago Press.

Malinowski, B. (1927). *Sex and repression in savage society*. New York: Harcourt, Brace.

Marcus, G., & Fischer, M. (1999). *Anthropology as cultural critique: An experimental moment in the human sciences*. Chicago: University of Chicago Press.

Mead, M. (1949). Coming of age in Samoa: A psychological study of primitive youth for Western civilization. New York: New American Library.

Minow, M. (2000). About women, about culture: About them, about us. *Daedalus*, Fall, 125–147.

Nussbaum, M. (2000). *Women and human development: The capabilities approach*. Cambridge: Cambridge University Press.

Okin, S. (1999). Is multiculturalism bad for women? In J. Cohen, M. Howard, & M. Nussbaum (Eds.), *Is multiculturalism bad for women?* (pp. 7–26). Princeton, NJ: Princeton University Press.

Rabinow, P. (1977). *Reflections on fieldwork in Morocco*. Berkeley: University of California Press.

Rabinow, P. (Ed.). (1987). *Interpretive social science: A second look*. Berkeley: University of California Press.

Roland, A. (1988). *In search of self in India and Japan: Toward a cross-cultural psychology*. Princeton, NJ: Princeton University Press.

Roland, A. (1996). *Cultural pluralism and psychoanalysis:*

The Asian and North American experience. New York: Routledge.

Shweder, R. (1991). *Thinking through cultures: Expeditions in cultural psychology*. Cambridge, MA: Harvard University Press.

Shweder, R. (1997). The surprise of ethnography. *Ethos, 25*, 152–163.

Shweder, R. (1998). Why cultural psychology? *Ethos, 27*, 4–6.

Shweder, R. (2000). Moral maps, "first world" con-ceits, and the new evangelists. In L. Harrison & S. P. Huntington (Eds.), *Culture matters: How values shape human progress* (pp. 158–177). New York: Basic Books.

Spiro, M. (1982). *Oedipus in the Trobriands*. Chicago: University of Chicago Press.

Spiro, M. (1999). Anthropology and human nature. *Ethos, 27*, 4–6.

Volpp, L. (2001). Feminism versus multiculturalism. *Columbia Law Review, 101*, 1181–1218.

10

Susan E. Donner and Joshua Miller

The Road to Becoming an Antiracism Organization

Community-based practice means, in a variety of ways, "meeting the client where s/he is." The client could be oneself, an individual, family, or organization, or a community collective coming together to address a particular issue. Because of the long and powerful history of racism as a phenomenon of American life (Frederickson, 2002), this chapter assumes that engaging issues of racism, whatever the context, will likely be a part of "meeting the client where s/he is." Social justice, equality of relationship, and the search for some sense of well-being for ourselves and others are at the heart of what we, as social workers, value. Racism, in our experience and in the experience of those with whom we work, presents a mighty barrier to those values and goals. In this chapter, we offer for consideration a broadly sketched road for human service agencies, which also assume that mitigating the impact of racism may go some distance in helping them achieve whatever their central goals are. This chapter suggests a framework for becoming an antiracism organization. We draw from the literature about institutional stages of antiracism development, offer a description of antiracism change activities for practitioners, and suggest change processes that social service agencies can pursue. Included is an organizational audit to assist in this

process. Barriers and roadblocks and ideas about responding are considered. Our ideas are also informed by work we have done as trainers or consultants to a variety of organizations.

Some of our assumptions are best put on the table, and as we do so, we invite the reader to explore her or his own. They are as follows: racism affects us all, but the impact on people of color and people who are white is very different, and because racism tends to be perceived differently, discussions about racism may be differentially useful, depending on one's racial identity (Miller & Donner, 2000). Different readings and interpretations occur with many aspects of antiracism work. One size never fits all. In a society permeated with racism, all citizens almost inescapably become racialized beings, ourselves included. Thus we believe it is important to state that both authors are white; we are embedded in the very problems we are trying to address. Reflecting on how we are situated is part of our antiracism work, as is inviting others to do the same. As we believe is the case across the spectrum of American society, individuals within an organization are likely to have very different levels of awareness about race and racism. They are likely to have differing needs in going through the process of organizational change.

A commitment to becoming an antiracism organization in a community context will likely change aspects of everything service providers do and have an impact on every person in the organization. It will also call increasing attention to the inextricably tied relationship between an organization and the community, or communities, within which it is located. Whatever changes are initially envisioned will, in all probability, take on unforeseen shapes and sizes. This is not well-charted territory. A commitment to antiracism work raises expectations that may not be realized for a long time to come. Organizations that make the commitment become accountable for actions that challenge racism. At various points along the way, the discrepancy between hopes and reality may produce disappointment and anger. And yet this important work is essential and can be transformative.

Motivations for Becoming an Antiracism Organization

Becoming an antiracism organization is apt to be neither an easy and short nor a clearly defined process. Why undertake a commitment to becoming an antiracism organization when it is such a potentially fraught project? Put simply, as Cornel West (1993) states, "race matters." Many white people, professionals, and organizations operate under an illusion without knowing how it matters, and how goals are distorted and compromised by the often insidious work of racism. A second reason is the social work profession's commitment to social justice (Swenson, 1998). A third reason is that becoming an antiracism organization is of benefit to everyone—social workers, social work students, faculty, the profession, and, most important, clients, whatever one's racial background. Michael Barak (2000), in an inclusion/exclusion model of organizational development aimed at incorporating diversity, stresses that meaningfully engaging diversity is likely to increase employee job satisfaction, commitment, and effectiveness. Though his model embraces more than antiracism efforts in organizations, it also includes them. Changing demographics is a fourth reason to become an antiracism organization. Former president Bill Clinton, in his initiative on race, stated that in 50 years, "there may be no majority race in our nation"

(Council of Economic Advisors, p. iii). Consequently, to commit to becoming an antiracism organization is to commit to a future diverse society.

Whatever the specific mission of a particular social service organization, in general it exists to improve the quality of life. As Ferguson (1996) points out, social service organizations have frequently made common cause with issues of anti-discrimination, as have many institutions of higher learning. However, through their policies and practices, they have often contributed to institutional racism. A commitment to becoming an antiracism organization is a step toward resolving this contradiction.

Perhaps the most powerful motivator is the insight that good work and racism do not mix. We will give examples later on in this chapter.

Organizations can also take an antiracism stance based on their own self-interests. Tensions in the surrounding community may negatively impact an organization's functioning. Significant unemployment rates in some urban areas for males of color (Wilson, 1996), or racism in the criminal justice system, which incarcerates disproportionately males of color, can have a devastating impact on families, individuals, and resources in the community in which an organization is based. Without addressing racism, the services an organization offers may have limited success. Antiracism work that positively affects the community may be fundamental to achieving other stated goals. If, for example, an agency addresses mental health issues and recognizes the relationship between racism and mental health, then issues of racism will become part of its agenda. It may start with its own organizational work but inexorably will be moved to work collaboratively with school systems, churches, and political bodies that influence quality of life in the community.

In a research project investigating rationales, processes, and outcomes of diversity efforts in human service organizations, Hyde (1998) emphasized two broad motivational sources for such undertakings. The first is a mainstream organizational developmental thrust focused on issues of effectiveness. The second is fueled by social justice concerns. Both are important.

Human service organizations also employ a significant part of the workforce in the United States. Focusing antiracism efforts within agencies or higher education is also congruent with the observation by the president of the National Urban League that the workplace is a prime location for potential racial healing (Price, 1999). Relative to neighborhoods, public schools, and religious institutions, the workplace is fairly diverse and more integrated than other aspects of American life and thus offers more opportunity for antiracism activities. Taking on racism within institutions, one institution at a time, can eventually contribute to a social movement to eliminate racism in American society.

What has motivated us, the authors, to do this work? We believe that in a society permeated with racism, all citizens become racialized beings. For us, being white has compromised our growth, disconnected us from parts of who we are, strained valuable relationships, increased fear, limited our access to different ways of being in the world, and constrained professional values. A part of our sense of self was founded on illusions of race neutrality and fairness. However, we have been fortunate to be part of a multicultural team of faculty in a school of social work committed to antiracism. As our own awareness and work have developed, we have come to see more clearly what we have lost by having unexamined white privilege. Simultaneously, we have recognized how vital it is for us as white people to join with people of color to actively confront racism to benefit us all. Working to dismantle that system of privilege is an essential step for all social workers. A first step may be to work within one's own institutional setting as part of the journey of taking on broader societal issues of racism. Most social workers are apt to have some limitations in their views of how racism operates. White social workers are particularly likely to have blind spots when it comes to institutional racism (Roberts & Smith, 2002; Van Soest, Garcia, & Graff, 2001). Consequently, all social workers benefit from working on issues of racism within their own organization because it leads to a much more complex perspective on how racism influences the lives of colleagues, clients, and themselves. Working within a multiracial/multicultural coalition enormously expands the multiple perspectives that are needed to inform the work and can transform it into a collaborative and collective learning process. An organization can become more unified in its purpose. Unity is likely to come only after very hard work and with the recognition that what people who are white are likely to need to learn and do

will be quite different from what people of color want to learn and do.

Nevertheless, everyone involved in antiracism organizational work might wisely anticipate that the process is likely to engender strong feelings at different points in the process. There is great potential for feeling perplexed, angry, defensive, sick of the process, lost, and wanting to maintain worldviews that orient who we are. For white people, several areas are often problematic: sorting out blind spots from genuine disagreements; distinguishing legitimate interest from unearned privilege; being able to hear that "getting it" is limited by one's own social and racial positions; hearing that friends and colleagues do not always see reality in the same way; tolerating the pain of recognizing all are implicated by racism. For people of color, there can be the frustration of seeing racism over and over and knowing their white colleagues do not always see it, repeatedly being asked to be the experts on race, feeling their perspectives are marginalized, being expected to be composed when angry, constantly encountering how little white colleagues may actually know about racism in the United States, and just living with the unfairness of it all. The temptation to flee from these issues is great. Yet when mutual understanding is achieved, and when positive action springs from that understanding, the satisfaction goes deep. Collective learning and collaborative action become possible. Conversations deepen, connections are strengthened, and organizational movement can occur. It can be as exhilarating as it is frustrating. For practitioners, to witness a better convergence between client need and services delivered becomes a powerful and reinforcing motivator.

Antiracism Organization and Racism Defined

An antiracism organization is one that assumes racism, particularly in mainstream/Eurocentric organizations, is presently inevitable and will manifest itself in a variety of ways: culturally, programmatically, personally, structurally, and functionally. Based on this assumption, an antiracism organization strives to become aware of the ways racism is sustained, and it institutes a variety of approaches to lessen and mitigate racism's impact. This is a long-term commitment, a journey often without crystal-clear maps, multiarmed, multipronged, and in this society, toward destinations heretofore unseen. Exactly what an organization that had truly and totally achieved an antiracism stance would look like can probably only be imagined in the future. In the authors' institution, which committed to becoming an antiracism institution, there is still no consensus on exactly what the institution should look like, or how it would even know if it had arrived at a final destination.

One of the foundational assumptions in the establishment of American law and in the nation's early political and civil life was an assumption "manifested [in] passionate beliefs that America was by rights a white nation, a Protestant nation, a nation in which true Americans were native-born men with Anglo-Saxon ancestors" (Smith, 1997, p. 3). Antiracism work proceeds from the acknowledgment that although the influence of this foundational assumption has definitely lessened, it has not been replaced with a multicultural, multiracial model or agenda.

When defining racism, the following areas may be considered: cultural practices and beliefs, individual attitudes, institutional and organizational structures and policies, interpersonal dynamics, group conflict, unequal power, political and economic arrangements, and white privilege. Racism is multifaceted and pervasive and has been a varying but ongoing characteristic of American society since its inception. Ayvazian and Tatum (1998) have likened it to a form of air pollution, which everyone breathes in regardless of intent. Though everyone breathes it, not everyone is aware of what is taken in. Racism is often particularly difficult to discern for those who benefit most from it. This becomes one of the tensions in antiracism work, especially in the early stages of antiracism efforts. Furthermore, the meanings of racism change with historical and sociocultural contexts. Both the forms and the manifestations of racism, as well as the goals of antiracism efforts, shift with the times (Winant, 1998). For example, today virtually no mainstream/Eurocentric social service agency would actively discriminate in its hiring practices by openly refusing to hire people of color. Yet, as is often the case, hiring practices may not include outreach into community institutions where many qualified people of color may be found, or job descriptions and qualifications may be so narrowly focused that otherwise qualified candidates of color

are excluded from consideration. These examples may not constitute active racism of the sort so easily recognized in the past, but may constitute passive racism insofar as they reinforce the status quo, which almost invariably privileges people with white skin. One of the authors, in consulting with a public school system, has been struck with how painful the stories of adolescents in the school system are. Sometimes the pain comes from blatant racism, but more often than not it comes from the persistent daily micro-aggressions enacted by white teachers and students against students of color, such as ignoring the salience of race, asking students to represent their racial group, and sharing stereotypes about a student's racial and ethnic group.

It follows, therefore, that effective efforts to become an antiracism organization require an understanding of current contexts in which issues of race and racism become meaningful. It calls for an understanding of how socially structured relations of power and privilege are constructed in both micro and macro interactions, and a critical reflexivity in coming to know one's own position in the mix (Kondrat, 1999, p. 453).

In light of these conclusions, the following definitions offer ways to recognize racism and point to directions for becoming an antiracism organization. Racism can be viewed as a system of privilege based on race, operating to the advantage of whites (Tatum, 1997). This system is predicated on contested, historically determined, and socially constructed concepts of race that are continually shifting and evolving (Omi & Winant, 1994). A consequence of racism is systematic subordination of members of targeted racial groups who have less political, social, and economic power in the United States (African Americans, Latinos/as, Native Americans, and Asian Americans) by members of a privileged racial group (whites/Caucasians/European descended) who have relatively more social power. This subordination is supported by actions of individuals, cultural norms, values, and institutional structures and practices of society (Wijeyesinghe, Griffin, & Love, 1997). Racism is manifested in organizations by staffing patterns, beliefs, policies, projects, or programs that adopt white and Eurocentric worldviews as a central norm and that marginalize those who do not accept this norm.

Though in the United States racism and skin color are intimately associated, George Frederickson, in *Racism: A Short History* (2002), both narrows and expands the content and definition of racism in the following set of ideas:

> My theory of or conception of racism therefore, has two components: difference and power. It originates from a mindset that regards "them" as different from "us" in ways that are *permanent and unbridgeable*. . . . The possible consequences . . . range from unofficial but pervasive social discrimination at one end of the spectrum to genocide at the other. . . . In all manifestations of racism from the mildest to the most severe, what is being denied is the possibility that the racializers and the racialized can coexist in the same society except perhaps on the basis of domination and subordination. Also rejected is any notion that individuals can obliterate ethnoracial differences by changing their identities. (p. 9, italics added)

Frederickson's (2002) definition, which recognizes that a belief in unchangeable racial essentialism is at the heart of racism, uses the Nazis' attempt to exterminate the Jews and America's institutionalized obsession with skin color as two prime examples in the twentieth century. His idea of essentialism as a fundamental factor highlights both the deep-seated belief systems operating in racism and the powerful political and institutional arrangements that emanate from them and reinforce them. The relationship between beliefs and structures is recursive and reminiscent of the chicken-and-egg dilemma. Frederickson also adds, "What makes Western racism so autonomous and conspicuous in world history has been that it developed in a context that presumed human equality of some kind" (p. 11). In a similar vein, Mills (1997) has observed that underlying the explicit social contract that valued equality, liberty, and justice was a racial contract that legitimized slavery, genocide, and subjugation. Individuals, organizations, and communities usually view themselves as not only valuing equality but also embodying it. As will be discussed further, one of the major obstacles to becoming an antiracism organization is the prevailing view of so many people who are white that racism does not exist, or that if it does exist, it is only in someone else. Part of this denial may be motivated by the privileges that come with being white, but part of it is embedded in the paradoxes of a society that sees itself founded on beliefs of equality. Consequently, when taking on institutional racism, addressing attitudes and beliefs is an important part of the effort, especially when the dominant group is white.

The notion of *institutional* racism has been used to mean many things: power relationships, ideologies, overt practices of discrimination, covert institutional arrangements, power inequities, political hegemony, cultural stereotypes, and more. Williams (1985) argues that it can be difficult to understand institutional racism because it is conceptually muddled. She makes a useful distinction between the creation of inequality and that which seeks to normalize and legitimize its existence. The former is expressed structurally, politically, and culturally, while the latter is an ideology and discourse. These areas of racism and inequality can be direct or indirect, intentional or nonintentional, hidden or acknowledged, yet they manifest themselves concretely in the lives of oppressed groups, such as the high rates of major disease, illness, and death among African Americans, Native Americans, and Hispanic Americans when compared to whites (Keppel, Pearcy, & Wagner, 2002). The production of inequality, often handed from generation to generation, means limited or differential access to money, employment, education, health care, longevity, power, and influential voice. The legitimatization process facilitates structural inequality through racial, class, cultural, political, and organizational ideologies. This allows those in power to assume they are participating in a natural order, and that their perspectives and practices represent the way things should be. In organizations, policies and theoretical models that guide practice can legitimize social oppression and de facto discrimination. For example, the view that the autonomous individual dependent on only him- or herself represents mental health and a preferred way of functioning can be dismissive toward cultural practices that emphasize family and collectivity. A recent article on the experiences of African American faculty in schools of social work provides a pointed example. Roberts and Smith (2002) argue that the ethic and imperative of supporting each other within the academic setting often clashes with a common goal in white-dominated institutions in which individually pushing ahead toward promotion and tenure is what is expected and rewarded. In agencies or community organizations, people of color may also attend more to the survival and well-being of other people of color than white colleagues are apt to do for each other.

Whites, much more than people of color, often think equal opportunity is not seriously encumbered by racial considerations (Akamatsu, 1998; Blauner, 1994; Bostis, 1997). Structural and racial impediments are no longer considered. These views are contrary to empirical evidence that consistently demonstrates white privilege economically, educationally, residentially, socially, and politically, forming a web of institutional racism. Despite substantial material progress by many Americans, both whites and people of color, and a narrowing of the gap in some economic areas between groups, there are still disturbing areas where "race and ethnicity continue to be salient predictors of well-being in American society" (Council of Economic Advisors, 1998, p. 2). On average, according to the Council of Economic Advisors, non-Hispanic whites (and some Asian Americans) experience advantages in health, education, and economic status relative to African Americans, Hispanics, Native Americans, and some Asian Americans. Becoming informed, particularly on the part of white workers, is thus essential to becoming an antiracist organization. Information can lead to a wish for transformation and serve as a powerful motivation to act.

People of color and whites often speak a different language when it comes to racism; whites tend to have a much narrower perspective that revolves around prejudice and egregious acts of racism, whereas people of color usually define racism in its broader institutional, social, and cultural context (Blauner, 1994). This increases the likelihood of people of color recognizing more readily than whites those policies, practices, and beliefs in an organization or community that contribute to racist outcomes. Tensions arise in the context of different assumptions. For example, white staff more typically explain underutilized services offered by an agency in communities of color either as evidence of lack of interest and motivation or by some inexplicable factor that is out of institutional control. Employees of color are apt to see more quickly the institutional barriers that inhibit access such as staffing patterns, lack of outreach, inadequate service models or educational approaches, cultural blind spots, or problematic institutional image. White staff may further resent the view of staff of color, respond defensively, and, if they have the power to do so, create a myriad of ways to minimize voices

expressing an unwelcome or threatening point of view. In the training and consultations carried out by the authors, white participants frequently get stuck early on in discussions when we, or people of color, bring up examples in which institutional racism has worked against people of color. Phenomena as well documented and common as racial profiling can quickly move whites to anger, with aggressive attempts to silence those who raise such examples, or denial that racism is a contributing factor. Many whites, particularly in the beginning stages of antiracism work, are poorly informed about the realities of racism and experience an analysis of institutional or personal racism at work as a misunderstanding of who they are or of their good intent. Stories about racism by clients may be considered exaggerations by white workers. Problems in the school system, transportation patterns, prices of goods in neighborhoods of color, town or city services in communities of color, lending practices, being watched in stores, "driving while black," and numerous other examples of ways in which people of color are discriminated against can be viewed as exaggerations or even paranoia by white listeners. For people of color, entrenched defensiveness or a sustained inability on the part of whites to recognize the impact of racial factors may produce frustration, anger, a sense of helplessness, and a reluctance to remain interested in change (Miller & Donner, 2000). Yet the numerous examples of discrimination that characterize aspects of the lives of people of color can instead provide opportunities for collaboration between people of color and those who are white.

Developmental Models for Becoming an Antiracism Organization

Antiracism work evolves from changes both in the people who are in an organization and in the organization itself, requiring what Stephan and Stephan (2001) refer to as "managing diversity." We have found it helpful to refer to theories about individual racial identity development and those that chart the stages of organizational development toward becoming an antiracism organization. Though neither provide perfect maps, both can help in orienting where one might be on an otherwise very confusing journey. During the past decade, a number of theoretical models have been posited to describe individual trajectories in establishing racial identity (Cross, 1991; Hardiman, 1994; Helms, 1990; Smith, 1991). The models assume that this is an inevitable developmental process for individuals living in a racially conscious society such as the United States, although with varying outcomes. Given the differential effects of racism, where people can either be targeted or privileged due to their skin color, this process varies for people of color and whites. Most, if not all, the models describe a process that begins with a state of naïveté about racism and one's place in a racist society, followed by a progression through increasing levels of awareness and accompanying affect, identification or underidentification with racial groups, and ultimately pride in one's racial identity and respect for other racial and ethnic groups. The models assume that because of the pernicious aspect of racism, many people will not progress to the higher stages of tolerance, inclusion, and appreciation for all racial and ethnic groups. Organizational antiracism work, however, is not likely to be achieved without addressing and facilitating the progression of individuals toward higher levels of racial identity development.

Similarly, when considering institutional racism, models have been proposed to describe organizational pathways leading to becoming multicultural, diverse, or antiracism institutions (Golembiewski, 1995; Jackson & Hardiman, 1994; Minors, 1996; Sue et al., 1998; Valverde, 1998). Despite the models having different emphases and somewhat different trajectories, all of them are developmental in approach and all stress common end goals. Although some of the models come out of higher education, the stage definitions are equally relevant for agency and community-based practices.

Valverde (1998) has focused on the culture of higher education, describing a model that leads from being a monocultural organization to one that becomes more "accommodating," and eventually to an organization that is "transformed" and truly multicultural in its people, policies, and the contents of its curriculum. Golembiewski (1995) describes an organizational developmental process culminating in an organization proactively welcoming, seeking, and incorporating diversity.

Sue et al. (1998) have compared multicultural organizational development models and have extracted common elements that can be grouped into three meta-stages. In the first stage, either overtly (through outright hostility) or covertly (through ignorance), diversity is challenged or ignored and organizations are "monocultural." The second stage involves a commitment to diversity, but there are still white (Eurocentric), male biases and assumptions. The third level is one where organizations truly embrace and value diversity.

Minors's (1996) model, like Valverde's, focuses on higher education, but with a different emphasis: rather than moving from a monocultural organization to a multicultural one, the organization moves from being discriminatory to nondiscriminatory, and eventually to an antidiscriminatory organization. His model, like Sue's, assumes that without some recognition of where an organization is, it will be hampered in its movement forward and will not have useful guides in formulating stage appropriate activities.

Both Minors's and Sue's models imply particular attitudes, uses of power, organizational practices and policies, and ideas about who should occupy the center of organizational gravity, which characterize organizations at differing stages of antiracism or multicultural work. Each also offers a very broad framework that can provide some parameters around next steps in moving toward a deeper and more advanced stage. Together they provide categories that we will use in an antiracism organizational audit. We believe that an integration of Minors's antiracism organizational change with Sue's multicultural organizational development enriches antiracism efforts. Our model operationalized in the organizational audit equates monocultural with discriminatory, Eurocentric with nondiscriminatory, and multicultural with antiracism.

As Chesler (1994) has noted, some of the models focus primarily on cultural diversity and difference, whereas others stress the importance of achieving social justice and equity. True diversity and difference do not occur in an organization without also confronting the institutional structures and power differentials that stifle diversity, as well as the values, theories, and ideologies that support institutional structures. Therefore, as will be discussed later, some conflict is inevitable as groups with less power resist their position, while those who have benefited from power resist challenges to their power. For example, a southern evangelical church was committed to changing from an extensively white congregation to one that included a significant number of African Americans (Sack, 2000). Though change has occurred, sharing power by white parishioners with African American parishioners has been, and continues to be, a stormy process. Many whites have been willing to give up power but are desperately struggling to remain in a position where it is theirs to give or keep. Welcoming people of color has been one thing, but not being able to veto a black Nativity scene has been quite another. As this example demonstrates, battles over power are inevitable in antiracism work in historically Eurocentric organizations. The struggles may revolve around whose ideas, or what services or curriculum, should prevail, over who controls the budget, or over who is chair of the board, dean, director, president, CEO, pastor, or a member of the school committee. Whatever the contested content, power struggles do occur and should be anticipated.

In our experience, both in our own institution's struggles to become an antiracism institution and in consulting with other organizations, the power struggles have taken many forms. In agencies in beginning stages (i.e. monocultural, discriminatory, or fairly uninformed about issues of diversity), power struggles often begin with contested views of reality. Many whites assert their view that discrimination and racism are simply in the eye of the beholder. For many people who are white, being able to see issues through the different experiences of people of color may be a long and frequently reworked process, one that may produce frustration and anger in people of color who have paid and will continue to pay the price for the denial of whites. If issues are more closely examined, and the influence of racism is considered, power struggles may intensify because seeing racism means doing some things differently. Initially, loss is involved for those who are white, particularly when potential gains may seem less clear. In many agencies, this may mean altering practice approaches and modes of service delivery about which staff of the dominant culture (as well as others) have strong convictions, but which may not optimally serve the best interests of the client base. As institutions evolve deeper into antiracism work and become more aware of its multifaceted nature, it will become clearer how much time and resources such work is likely to consume. Power struggles over priorities will surface inevitably because most organizations

already have a full plate, and competition for resources may already be high. Yet antiracism work clarifies the meaning of priorities to everyone in the system. This, too, often opens up space for change.

Unlike racial identity theory, models of organizational development do not specify whether the organization is predominantly a mainstream/Eurocentric organization or one that is institutionally organized by people of color. This is a significant omission. For example, the Martin Luther King Jr. Community Center in Springfield, Massachusetts, is a social service agency that was established by a predominantly black church; its mission is to serve families in its area, who are mostly African American and Hispanic. The board and staff are more than 95% people of color, and the mission statement and agency objectives articulate an overtly African American philosophy. The developmental challenges for such an organization are very different from those for a child guidance clinic, a community mental health center, or a college counseling service historically run and staffed by predominantly white boards and workers, utilizing theories of social or clinical services developed by whites. The traditional models of organizational change appear to assume the latter type of organization and are written primarily for Eurocentric systems, which are indeed the majority of social service agencies and institutions of higher education in this country.

These models can provide useful metaphors to chart an agency's progress, and we are proposing a developmental process in becoming an antiracism organization. Therefore, the developmental categories that we suggest are rough approximations and should be used as flexible concepts and tools.

The Process of Becoming an Antiracism Organization

The first step in becoming an antiracism organization or agency is engaging in open, direct, and inclusive consideration about why such a step ought to be taken. Because such a commitment has implications for all members of an organization, as well as for all its policies and activities, having broad support and agreement about purpose is very important. Such a review can address many ideas: what constitutes racism, its consequences for society as a whole, its relevance for the mission and goals of an organization, what it means in the lives of those who work in a particular agency, and the agency's clientele. Committed leadership is crucial as well (Lawson, Koman, & Rose, 1998).

For organizations that make a commitment to become antiracist, a broad-based group, endorsed and supported by organizational resources, should take on the task of concretely spelling out what this means. Comprehensively identifying the dimensions for change is an essential goal. Developing strategies for change and an action plan for implementing changes is the next stage. An assessment of which changes are possible in an organization at any point in time is important, as well as an understanding of what actions will best facilitate future steps. A grounding in general principles of organizational change is helpful in all these steps. Third, an organization must create some mechanism for monitoring and measuring change and must provide an impetus to keep the process going. As previously mentioned, becoming an antiracism organization is a long-term commitment and is not likely to progress in a straight line. As real change begins to occur, some reactivity should be expected, explored, and hopefully overcome. As has occurred in our institution, accusations that race has taken up more than its fair share of space are frequently voiced. Such assertions cannot, and should not, be silenced because if they are, resistance will go underground. They need to be explored, doubts need to surface, and the reasons for the commitment reengaged. The tensions that inevitably arise may lead to a deeper understanding and intensified movement forward, though sometimes there may be steps back before there are more steps ahead.

Bailey (1995), in a synthesis of models proposed for managing diversity in the workplace, views leadership as a salient factor in the process of organizations moving toward greater utilization of diversity. This includes striving aggressively toward pluralism in the organization by using all human potential available, valuing one's own culture and that of others, and changing the organizational culture to incorporate differences in worldviews, values, and practices.

Because issues of racism tend to flow freely between an organization and the community surrounding it, making common cause with leadership within the community is often essential. For example, an educational institution located in our community became concerned about the name of a new housing development. The name, prominently displayed on a large sign visible on a major road, is one painfully associated with slavery. The name has different meaning to different parts of the community, but its powerful association with slavery has alarmed many. A flurry of letters for and against appeared in the local newspaper, culminating in a letter by the editor requesting the developers to change the name. Charges of "political correctness" were the result. In alliance with a local religious organization, the educational institution invited prominent realtors and developers willing to discuss the issue to a meeting. All came to an agreement that the community would be better served if the development had another name. A two-pronged strategy was formulated. The first was that a very successful realtor within a community leadership role would approach the developer in a nonthreatening, nonjudgmental one-on-one conversation. The second was that the groups who had come together would offer to help with any legal, financial, or construction issues that a name change might involve. Though the issue remains unresolved, by reaching out to the broader community, and the leadership within it, the educational institution has increased the likelihood of advancing its own antiracism goals.

An antiracism audit can also serve as an important instrument for delineating the work that needs to be done in becoming an antiracism organization. The audit may also serve as a way of keeping track of where one is in the process.

An Antiracism Organizational Audit

Antiracism work and becoming an antiracism organization are inextricably linked with how one understands what constitutes racism. Appreciating that racism includes, but goes significantly beyond, issues of individual prejudice, or bias, implies that antiracism activities involve more than increasing individual or collective awareness and sensitivity, although these are valuable endeavors. Therefore, an essential component of becoming an antiracism organization is the necessity for a systematic racism "audit" of all aspects of the organization, covering all the areas identified in table 10-1 (Basham, Donner, Killough, & Werkmeister-Rozas, 1997). Another tool for agencies to consider, which takes a broad view of cultural competence similar to a comprehensive view of antiracism work, is the Cultural Competence Self Assessment Instrument of the Child Welfare League (1993). This serves as a baseline, a beginning point from where the organization hopes to move, as well as ensuring that systematic attention is paid to the organization's progress. Few organizations are starting from

scratch, and this process helps to identify areas of strength and accomplishment, as well as areas of weakness. The audit should be mapped out by all stakeholders, and it is helpful to have a representative committee established to monitor progress. As discussed previously, easy agreement is unlikely and not desirable if it is motivated by a wish for superficial harmony.

Antiracism activities in an agency may include any of the areas identified in table 10-1 (Basham

Table 10-1. Levels of Anti-Racism Organizational Development

A-Monocultural/Discriminatory   B-Eurocentric/Non-Discriminatory   C-Multicultural/Anti-Racism

Examples of activities that an organization can take towards becoming an anti-racism organization. Following each statement, indicate the level of activity for your organization as:
(A) Accomplished   (IP) In Process   (U) Unaddressed

Stage	Kinds of Activities	Progress
A	Raising awareness about the barriers to communication about race	
A	Exploring world views, biases, assumptions of staff	
B	Writing a mission statement that includes anti-racism goals	
B	Making a commitment to become an anti-racism organization in almost all organizational literature	
B	Reviewing curricula and policy relevant to anti-racism practices and diversity content	
B	Engaging in public dialogues on race and racism open to all organizational constituencies, including volunteers, boards, and trustees	
B	Examining cultural assumptions of service delivery programs	
C	Increasing financial resources allocated toward anti-racism initiatives	
C	Redistributing decision-making power to reflect the organizational diversity of people, communities, ideas, and interests	
C	Designing an appropriate and voluntary mentoring system to assist recent hires to learn the ropes	
C	Making links and alliances in the community around anti-racism efforts	
C	Establishing lines of accountability within the community about the organization's anti-racism efforts	
ABC	Hiring more faculty and/or staff of color	
ABC	Holding ongoing discussions on racism and race for staff	
ABC	Increasing training for staff on culturally informed service delivery	
ABC	Sponsoring regular seminars for faculty or staff about racism and diversity	
ABC	Providing space and appropriate context for the expression of fears, hopes, anxieties, understandings and misunderstandings that people experience in the process of anti-racism work	
BC	Giving continued attention to outreach recruitment efforts	
BC	Creating and facilitating alliances between individuals, groups, organizations to challenge policies and practices that perpetuate systemic discrimination, prejudice, and ill-treatment of people of color	
BC	Supporting practice, policies, and attitudes needed to create an inclusive environment and culture	
BC	Attending to interpersonal and inter-group relations	
BC	Creating opportunities and structures for addressing and resolving inequitable or discriminatory behavior, policies, or practices related to race	
BC	Including models of practice or service delivery that address the needs of diverse clients, students, or consumers	
BC	Supporting caucus groups or identity groups as they grapple with issues unique to them in their organization	

et al., 1997; Lawson et al., 1998). Keeping track of what an organization may have already achieved and maintaining an awareness of what is yet to be done are both important. A suggested way to monitor both is also included. As the chart indicates, some activities are more typical of particular stages of antiracism work. The three stages we have designated combine Minors's and Sue's models. The first broad stage (A) is monocultural/discriminatory, the second (B) is Eurocentric/nondiscriminatory, and the third (C) is multicultural/antiracism. The impetus for change, sometimes external pressure, sometimes an internal commitment, and often a combination of both, will influence which activities come first. For example, if an organization is monocultural/discriminatory, it may be facing legal challenges, and its hiring practice in all likelihood will be the first area of change. However, as table 10-1 indicates, the same activity may characterize all three stages. A multicultural/antiracism organization may also engage in renewed hiring efforts not out of pressure but out of an appreciation that multiple perspectives are crucial to the success of the organization.

In the training and consultative experiences of the authors, it has become clear that organizations with sincerely expressed desires to "deal with diversity" or "to become an antiracism agency" are at very different levels, grappling with very different developmental issues. Examples follow.

A large mental health organization serving a fairly diverse client base and with a relatively diverse mix of staff was just in the process of initiating diversity training. The commitment for change was coming primarily, though not exclusively, from the leadership. Having a more diverse staff was not the issue. The staff was diverse, and yet the organization was, at least in part, still monocultural. The norms of the organization and the worldviews that dictated service delivery were white mainstream/Eurocentric. The leadership, diverse itself, wanted the norms to shift and was looking for ways to engage the staff, many of whom did not see the necessity for change. For this group, simply identifying themselves as ethnic/racial individuals, particularly for those who were white, was the task at hand. For staff and leadership to begin to embrace the same goals, they needed to talk to each other about identity and issues of privilege and oppression, and what differentially that means for people. The initial conversations were risky, diffi-

cult, and heated, focusing on such basic issues as whether driving while black is or is not a real phenomenon. This is a staff that wants to do well by clients but has more talking to do before it sees the links between issues of race and mental health work. Once the connections are more firmly established, the organization is likely to have more buy-in and creative thinking from those who directly deliver the services about structural, policy, and service delivery changes.

The staff members of another organization, whose national parent group has long been working on becoming multicultural and antiracism oriented, were relatively inexperienced in talking to each other. They had not, however, regularly scheduled conversations to talk about this work, which we believe to be a necessary component of ongoing progress. In this group, issues of social identity, privilege, and oppression probably were already accepted as a part of reality relevant to the group members and their work. As mentioned previously in this chapter, for them the pressing issue was the racial, ethnic, and social matching of adult mentors with children. This task brought them squarely into the arena of the larger community from which the mostly white mentors are recruited. Though training for the mentors, who were often unaware of their judgmental attitudes toward the children of color with whom they were matched, was necessary, stronger links with salient community groups from communities in which children and mentors live were also necessary.

Conclusion

Taking the step of making a commitment to becoming an antiracism agency thrusts an organization into a momentum for change that is not entirely predictable. Though there will be moments of accomplishment, there may also be times of confusion, or a sense of not knowing where one is in the process. Expectations will rise, as they should. An organization will be held increasingly accountable for the gap between aspiration and what is at any given moment. Conflict may be more open, and disappointment more apparent. How to respond institutionally and individually is not always clear. Because whites and people of color have experienced such different realities when it comes to racism, there may be disagreements about meaningful progress or the lack thereof, as well as about the significance and meaning of differently perceived events.

Successful transformation often requires deep, ongoing alterations and a willingness to participate in affectively charged controversy, which may challenge one's sense of reality, particularly for people who are white. An antiracism commitment may also push an organization's boundaries and challenge its most fundamental practices. For example, a mental health agency might find itself immersed in issues of housing, public school, policy, or police-community relations. This requires time, expertise, commitment, and resources. It also requires that accountability for institutional change extend into the community, which is situated as a vital source of feedback and as a powerful reality check on change.

Issues around race and diversity have been, and will continue to be, increasingly complex, calling for more sophisticated and intricate approaches. Sussman (1999) characterizes the context in which the workplace takes on diversity and racism as follows:

> We have moved into a new more volatile phase of dealing with diversity. Racial, national, ethnic, sexual, religious categories are not fixed, not permanent, not stable—Just as age changes so do the other descriptions of a person's life. Labels can't keep up with the reality of people's lives. Neither can programs based on labels. (p. 5)

Two major phenomena will and must occur if an agency seriously embarks on an antiracism course (Chesler, 1994). First, whites will have to share power, formal and informal, in a real way. Second, the process will likely generate open conflict. The conflict more often than not may be a sign of progress as long as the conflicts are addressed. For staff, these inevitable occurrences may be difficult points where commitment is tested. Knowing at the start that they are inevitable, keeping in focus the pernicious nature of racism, and maintaining a guiding vision of the work can stabilize the commitment to antiracism. Racism has a very long history; surely antiracism work must have a long view. Even though the work is never over, the benefits of engaging in it are enormous. Looking back and seeing concrete change, engaging in honest, informa-

tive, and respectful conversations about race with colleagues, experiencing more attuned work with clients, and being part of work that transforms us, our agencies, and our community is deeply rewarding.

References

Akamatsu, N. N. (1998). The talking oppression blues: Including the experience of power/powerlessness in the teaching of cultural sensitivity. In M. McGoldrick (Ed.), *Revisioning family therapy: Race, culture, and gender in clinical practice* (pp. 129–143). New York: Guilford.

Ayvazian, A., & Tatum, B. (1998, August). *Racial understanding/misunderstanding: Living and learning together.* Facilitators for public dialogue on race. Smith College School for Social Work, Northampton, MA.

Bailey, D. (1995). Management: Diverse workplaces. *Encyclopedia of Social Work* (10th ed., pp. 1659–1663). Washington, DC: NASW Press.

Barak, M. (2000). Beyond affirmative action: Toward a model of diversity and organizational inclusion. *Administration in Social Work, 23*(3/4), 47–68.

Basham, K., Donner, S., Killough, R., & Werkmeister-Rozas, L. (1997). Becoming an anti-racist institution. *Smith College Studies in Social Work, 67,* 564–585.

Blauner, B. (1994). Talking past each other: Black and white languages of race. In F. L. Pincus & J. H. Ehrlich (Eds.), *Race and ethnic conflict: Contending views on prejudice, discrimination, and ethnoviolence* (pp. 18–28). Boulder, CO: Westview.

Bostis, D. A. (1997). *Joint Center for Political and Economic Studies 1997 National Opinion Poll—Race Relations.* Washington, DC: Joint Center for Political and Economic Studies.

Chesler, M. A. (1994). Organizational development is not the same as multicultural organizational development. In E. Y. Cross, J. H. Katz, F. A. Miller, & E. W. Seashore (Eds.), *The promise of diversity* (pp. 240–251). Burr Ridge, IL: Irwin.

Child Welfare League of America. (1993). Cultural competence self assessment instrument. Washington, DC: Author.

Council of Economic Advisors. (1998). *Changing America: Indicators of social and economic well-being by race and Hispanic origin.* Washington, DC: Author.

Cross, W. E. (1991). *Shades of black: Diversity in African-American identity.* Philadelphia: Temple University Press.

Ferguson, A. S. (1996). Toward an anti-racist social

service organization. *Journal of Multicultural Social Work, 4*, 35–48.

Frederickson, G. M. (2002). *Racism: A short history*. Princeton, NJ: Princeton University Press.

Golembiewski, R. T. (1995). *Managing diversity in organizations*. Tuscaloosa: University of Alabama Press.

Hardiman, R. (1994). White racial identity development. In E. P. Salett & D. R. Kaslow (Eds.), *Race, ethnicity and self: Identity in multicultural perspective* (pp. 117–140). Washington, DC: National Multicultural Institute.

Helms, J. E. (Ed.). (1990). *Black and white racial identity: Theory, research and practice*. New York: Greenwood.

Hyde, C. (1998). A model for diversity in human service agencies. *Administration in Social Work, 22*(4), 19–33.

Jackson, B., & Hardiman, R. (1994). Multicultural organizational development. In E. Y. Cross, J. H. Katz, F. A. Miller, & E. W. Seashore (Eds.), *The promise of diversity* (pp. 231–239). Burr Ridge, IL: Irwin.

Keppel, K., Pearcy, M., & Wagner, S. (2002). *Trends in racial and ethnic specific rates for the health status indicators: United States 1990-9*. Hyattsville, MD: National Center for Health Statistics.

Kondrat, M. E. (1999). Who is the "self" in self aware? Professional self awareness from a critical theory perspective. *Social Service Review, 73*, 451–475.

Lawson, K., Koman, B., & Rose, A. (1998). *Building one nation*. Washington, DC: Leadership Conference Education Fund.

Miller, J., & Donner, S. (2000). More than just talk: The use of racial dialogue to combat racism. *Social Work With Groups, 23*, 31–53.

Mills, C. W. (1997). *The racial contract*. Ithaca, NY: Cornell University Press.

Minors, A. (1996). From university to poly-versity: Organizations in transition to anti-racism. In C. E. James (Ed.), *Perspectives on racism and the human service sector: A case for change* (pp. 196–208). Toronto: Toronto University Press.

NASW Delegate Assembly. (1996). Code of ethics. Washington, DC: NASW Press.

Omi, M., & Winant, H. (1994). *Racial formation in the United States: From the 1960's to the 1990's* (3rd ed.). New York: Routledge.

Price, H. (1999, December 18). Speech to the National Urban League [on-line]. ftp://ftp.nul.org/pub/bigotry.txt.

Roberts, T., & Smith, L. (2002). The illusion of inclusion: An analysis of approaches to diversity within predominantly white schools of social work. *Journal of Teaching in Social Work, 22*, 189–211.

Sack, K. (2000, June 4). *Shared prayers, mixed blessings: How race is lived in America. New York Times* [online] http://www.nytimes.com/library/national/race/060400sack-church.html.

Smith, E. J. (1991). Ethnic identity development: Toward the development of a theory within the context of majority/minority status. *Journal of Counseling and Development, 70*, 181–188.

Smith, R. (1997). *Civic ideals: Conflicting visions of citizenship in U.S. history*. New Haven, CT: Yale University Press.

Stephan, W., & Stephan, C. (2001). *Improving intergroup relations*. Thousand Oaks, CA: Sage.

Sue, D. W., Carter, R. T., Casas, J. M., Fouad, N. A., Ivey, A. E., Jensen, M., LaFromboise, T., Manese, J. E., Ponterotto, J. G., & Vazquez-Nutall, E. (1998). *Multicultural counseling competencies: Individual and organizational development*. Thousand Oaks, CA: Sage.

Sussman, H. (1999, November). Diversity questions and answers. *Managing Diversity, 5*–6.

Swenson, C. (1998). Clinical social work's contribution to a social justice perspective. *Social Work, 43*, 527–537.

Tatum, B. (1997). *"Why are all the black kids sitting together in the cafeteria?" and other conversations about race*. New York: Basic Books.

Valverde, L. A. (1998). Future strategies and actions: Creating multicultural higher education campuses. In L. A. Valverde & L. A. Castenell Jr. (Eds.), *The multicultural campus* (pp. 19–29). Walnut Creek, CA: Altamira Press.

Van Soest, D., Garcia, B., & Graff, D. (2001). Sensitivity to racism and social work professors' responsiveness to critical classroom events. *Journal of Teaching in Social Work, 21*(1/2), 39–58.

West, C. (1993). *Race matters*. New York: Vintage.

Wijeyesinghe, C., Griffin, P., & Love, B. (1997). Racism curriculum design. In M. Adams, L. A. Bell, & P. Griffin (Eds.), *Teaching for diversity and social justice* (pp. 110–140). New York: Routledge.

Williams, J. (1985). Redefining institutional racism. *Ethnic and Racial Studies, 8*, 323–348.

Wilson, W. J. (1996). *When work disappears: The world of the new urban poor*. New York: Vintage.

Winant, H. (1998). Racism today: Continuity and change in the post–civil rights era. *Ethnic and Racial Studies, 21*, 755–766.

11

Mary E. Olson

Family and Network Therapy Training for a System of Care
"A Pedagogy of Hope"

There is a growing consensus that American graduate and professional schools have failed to keep pace with the changes in community mental health. For more than a decade, there has been a national reform of public services based on the concept of a system of care. Yet, according to a research study by Meyers, Kaufman, and Goldman (1999), new graduates of professional schools are entering the workforce without the knowledge, skills, and attitudes that reflect the values and principles of the reform. These researchers say there is an absence of knowledge among educators about the community care movement and an adherence to traditional office models. This situation also reflects the fact that the system-of-care proponents have just begun to suggest the linkages between their philosophy and clinical models. Postmodern, dialogic, and narrative approaches from the family therapy tradition represent parallel and congruent clinical advances. These therapeutic models are inspired by the same values and principles as the system-of-care framework.

This chapter will present a training curriculum that I developed. It has been taught as an advanced master's-level course at a graduate school of social work (Smith College School for Social Work). Parts of this curriculum have been the basis of presentations to community agencies and hospitals, and of postgraduate workshops and courses. Some of the material was developed originally in collaboration with Carlos Sluzki, MD, and other senior faculty at the Family Center of the Berkshires, during the years 1990–1995 when I directed the Clinical Externship in Systemic Family Therapy. This curriculum has been used successfully in a variety of settings and with trainees from a variety of clinical disciplines, including social work, psychology, psychiatry, nursing, and family medicine.

The collaborative frameworks for family therapy prepare future mental health clinicians for network-oriented therapy, also called "communal practice," a term coined by Ken Gergan, applied clinically by Tom Andersen, and mentioned by Hoffman (2000). The relevance of this training for working in a system of care has been reinforced by recent research suggesting that community practitioners are beginning to use postmodern ideas eclectically in therapy and case management (Collaborative for Community and Family-Based Practice, 2001). This way of working is consistent with the four areas of competence that Meyers et al. (1999) specify for therapists operating in a system of care: systems thinking (a postmodern conception of a system is a dialogic one, as will be explained further), family-professional relationships, cultural competence, and interprofessional education and training.

A System of Care

In the United States, the concept of a "system of care" has gained strong credibility among researchers at the Center for Mental Health Services, proponents of the Child and Adolescent Service System Program (CASSP), public health policymakers, and many clinical administrators. It is a response to the widespread and alarming absence of effective mental health services for severely disturbed children and teenagers and their families (Coffey, Olson, & Sessions, 2001; Stroul & Friedman, 1986). A recent study of nine new community-based programs in Massachusetts examines the paradigmatic initiatives that are occurring throughout the United States (Lightburn, Olson, Sessions, & Coffey, 2002).

A system of care is a service delivery system that seeks to provide a broad, comprehensive, and integrated continuum of care, in contrast to the traditional spectrum of clinic-based child and family therapy, medication, and, if these fail, hospitalization or other out-of-home placements. Ideally, the new system will help troubled children stay with their families and recover in their communities, where they will continue to live and grow. A system of care ideally comprises an integrated array of services in the areas of mental health, education, medical care, child protection, substance abuse treatment, juvenile justice, vocational training, recreational activities, and case management. It goes beyond traditional therapy by expanding the definition of mental health care and including a range of supports to the family in a variety of life domains.

Further, there are strong emphases on coordinating the responses and resources of the various helpers and giving the family a voice in the treatment process. Therefore, the network of providers meets with the family regularly to develop the care plan and discuss progress toward common goals. This approach adapts the services to fit the child and family, rather than inserting people into a preexisting menu of services (Burchard, Bruns, & Burchard, 2002). Within the system of care, the term "wraparound" is used to describe this process of tailoring the services to the particular "needs, strengths, and culture" of a family.

The system of care is not just a network of services; it is a philosophy (Stroul, 2002). The values and principles that guide this reform are known as CASSP principles. They include (1) a nonpathologizing, or "strength-based," orientation; (2) partnership with families; (3) interagency collaboration and coordination with the family; (4) the inclusion of social networks; (5) cultural competence; and (6) individualized plans with flexibility to change as families change. This philosophy is the scaffolding of the system. While it is easy to see that there are therapeutic implications of this philosophy, its developers propose a definite distinction between service delivery and treatment. Seen this way, a system of care is a proposed framework for delivering treatment; it does not constitute treatment itself.

In light of recent, renewed calls for reform of youth services (U.S. Public Health Service, 2000), Beth Stroul (2002), who originally formulated the system-of-care concept, has reexamined the philosophy. She makes the point that there are confusing myths that have grown up around systems of care, namely, that clinical interventions are not a primary focus and that nonprofessional service providers have greater value than professional clinicians. Stroul challenges these misconceptions and states that mental health treatment is still the primary service provided by the system of care. In this way, there is a clear mandate for community-based therapists to be able to operate effectively within this framework and to do treatment that draws on the naturally occurring resources of the family and social network. Traditional, expert, deficit-oriented, individual, or family models are in deep tension with this reform. The following curriculum not only provides training in clinical models that share the premises of a system of care but also introduces language practices that potentially can generate therapeutic dialogue in any part of the treatment system (Seikkula & Olson, 2003; White & Epston, 1990).

The Case for Postmodern Therapy

In the past decade, the field of family therapy has witnessed the emergence of a new template for practice based on reflection and narrative instead of strategy and intervention. There also are broader social and cultural frameworks, especially regarding gender and issues of social justice. The style of practice has evolved from a hierarchical one to therapeutic conversation based on collaboration. The intellectual movements of postmodernism and feminism challenged traditional cybernetic and systems models and provided the seeds for new forms of therapy. This evolving tradition as a whole can be traced back to the communication research of Gregory Bateson and his colleagues in Palo Alto.

One of the distinguishing features of postmodern therapy is the stance of treating the patient and family as members of a partnership within a network that includes the professionals and anyone else connected to the situation (Seikkula et al., 1995). This approach thus enacts the collaborative stance advocated by the system-of-care philosophy. From the postmodern perspective, the family is understood as a group of people who all have been through similar, difficult experiences and share the need for reconstruing these experiences in language. This kind of therapy highlights processes of communication and strives to create a language in which everyone has a voice.

The postmodern philosophical framework says language and communication are primarily constitutive of human realities (Gergen, 1999). In this way, the therapeutic conversation can be a loom on which to weave or reweave the language for a problem or symptom. This process can either dissolve the situation or reduce its larger negative effects on a person's identity and future and those of the caregivers. Creating language that gives voice and agency in relation to difficult experiences has been shown based on case studies to ameliorate many kinds of human problems and symptoms. Included are eating disorders, psychosis, depression, nonorganic somatic symptoms, chronic illness, and the effects of abuse, violence, and trauma (Anderson & Goolishian, 1986, 1991; Goldner, Penn, Sheinberg, & Walker, 1990; Griffith & Griffith, 1994; Herman, 1992; Olson, 1995a, 1995b, 2000b; Penn, 2001; Seikkula, 2002a, 2002b; Seikkula et al., 1995; Seikkula & Olson, 2003; Sheinberg & Fraenkel, 2001; White, 1995; White & Epston, 1990).

Four basic clinical applications of postmodernism are covered by the curriculum under discussion. Other material included in the course is beyond the scope of this chapter, and there is a burgeoning literature on postmodern approaches

to which students are referred (Anderson, 1997; Hoffman, 2002; Olson, 2000a). The essentials of this training are the reflecting process of Tom Andersen of Norway (Andersen, 1987, 1991, 1995); the Open Dialogue approach developed by the Finnish team of Jaakko Seikkula, Birgitta Alakare, and Jukka Aaltonen (Seikkula et al., 1995; Seikkula & Olson, 2003); the narrative therapy of Michael White (1995; White & Epston, 1990); and the linguistic turn in feminist, multicultural, and social justice models (McGoldrick, 1998). While there are important differences among these approaches, all strive to transform social worlds by fostering new language and meanings. For discussion of the differences, see Hoffman (2002), Smith (1997), and White (1995).

Recent research on caregivers' accounts of psychiatric illness in their families underscores the need for this kind of work (Stern, Doolan, Staples, Szmukler, & Eisler, 1999). According to this study, two types of caregivers' narratives tend to emerge in response to a severe psychiatric crisis: stories of "restitution or reparation" and "chaotic and frozen" narratives. The former makes meaning out of the experience, whereas the latter tends to see the episode as a series of random events, suggesting a "narrative wreckage" or "narrative chaos." Stories that bring some narrative coherence enlarge people's coping strategies, ability to find solutions, and sense of the future. As Stern et al. (1999) write,

> Befriending the incomprehensible in the psychotic experience was seen to be an important aspect of coping in restitutive accounts, placing the bizarre within a continuum of understandable human responses. Seeing the illness as an opportunity to give and receive was another significant element in these stories. (p. 366)

Both the patient and the caregivers need to participate in a therapeutic dialogue that creates positive meaning and, thus, hope. Michael White's recent work (2003) shows that this can be achieved even with young children in foster care and adoptive families who have come from situations of extreme abuse and neglect.

Alternatively, it is difficult to reconcile traditional approaches that tend to view the caregivers principally as the locus of pathology with the aim of community care, which is to support parents in learning how to become competent partners in the recovery process of their child (Seikkula & Olson, 2003). There are, of course, obvious limits to this approach when parents commit crimes of assault or incest against their children. A pathologizing discourse may weaken or disrupt the family's ability to respond to the situation. Lukens and McFarlane (2002) suggest this point when they describe how the concept of the "schizophrenogenic mother" was popular among professionals at a time when the movement toward deinstitutionalization was emptying state psychiatric hospitals of chronic patients. Many of these patients received little or no further treatment and were forced to return to their families for care. The families suffered under the conflicting injunctions that required them to take responsibility for the care of their ill member and to accept the stigmatizing blame that they were also the cause of the person's condition. The newer postmodern therapies strive to reduce blame and guilt and increase the sense of agency, thus paradoxically maximizing the resources and "response-ability" of the patient, family, and helping network.

In this way, postmodern therapy has clear differences from the earlier family therapy models that consumer advocacy groups have widely distrusted because of the seeming implicit and automatic blame assigned to the family for its situation. Indeed, it is true that two of the older, classic models—the structural approach of Salvador Minuchin (1974) and his colleagues and the systemic approach of the Milan Associates (Selvini-Palazzoli, Boscolo, Cecchin, & Prata, 1978)—propose that the problem or symptom is a product of the family system or the family-professional suprasystem. These models reconfigure the process of therapy as a deliberate intervention into the underlying organization or logic, respectively, of the network of relations. Yet this move to the social ecology has been critical to understanding people in contexts rather than as "containers" of pathology.

In fairness, there are points of congruence between structural and systemic ideas and the system-of-care philosophy. Structural therapists were the first to bring in cultural awareness and a concern for marginalized groups. Many ideas from structural therapy have been included in multisystemic therapy that fit the system-of-care concept and have been quite successful in treating juvenile offenders with an emerging evidence base for other populations (Henggeler, Schoenwald, Borduin, Rowland,

& Cunningham, 1998). Moreover, the Milan group's idea of logical connotation is integral to postmodern approaches and congruent with a "strength-based" orientation. Logical connotation describes how a problematic behavior or symptom makes sense in a particular context of action and meaning (Boscolo, Cecchin, Hoffman, & Penn, 1987). Nonlinear, contextual thinking tends to be affirming rather than pathologizing and, thus, consistent with the values of community care.

While these older approaches have contributed enduring, brilliant ideas to the field, the influence of the actual treatment models has diminished for the same reason that these models tend to be incompatible with CASSP principles. The idea of an "out-there" system that can be changed by an expert makes the family the object of therapeutic action rather than a partner in the therapeutic process (Seikkula & Olson, 2003). As Hoffman (2000) writes:

> At first, mothers were to blame. Then therapists zeroed in on parents, who were seen as triangling the child into their own conflicts. The collateral kin group was next focused on, then the other helpers who might be entangled in a case. As time went by, the lens steadily widened, but the blame remained. (p. 7)

In their original forms, it is the highly expert and authoritative nature of these earlier models and their view of the family as the source of pathology that make them dissonant with a stance of giving voice and agency and at odds with the new thinking in community practice.

Teaching Methods for Postmodern Therapy

Education and training have distinct meanings within the clinical fields (Meyers et al., 1999; Reich, 1998). Education refers to learning broader theoretical frameworks for practice and reflecting on values and principles. Although related, training tends to emphasize the development of specific skills within a particular model and developing the capacity for knowledge in action (Pakman, 1999). Because the various frameworks are often new to students, these must be taught along with forms of practice. In this curriculum, there is a combination of lecture material (education) and an interactive exercise (training), with each aspect recursively reinforcing the other. This way of structuring training is widely used in the family field.

For instance, an opening ritual accompanies the first lecture and communicates the value placed on the experiential and interactive. I typically ask participants to share a metaphor or image of transformation in the first class. This process generates symbolic language and fosters personal connections that contribute to the overall emotional atmosphere, while directing attention to a consideration of what creates positive change. In the following description of the various frameworks of the course, the first part of each section is a distillation of a lecture, and the second part describes teaching methods, other than lecture, that use film clips, role plays, cases, and experiential exercises. Thus, students can see the complex and abstract theories brought down to earth and applied to actual examples.

The optimal length of this training in terms of producing a genuine shift in perspective and transferable skills is an intensive course or externship with a minimum of 40 hours of seminar or classroom time. In an agency-based externship, the teaching seminar can be enhanced by a clinical practicum where trainees see actual families. At the same time, I have distilled these principles into 2-hour consultations resulting in an effective shift in a case. Without a much more in-depth experience of this curriculum, however, it is unlikely that trainees will be able to sustain these ideas from relatively brief workshops. In the longer curriculum, each model identifies and develops particular clinical skills. The work of Andersen is an excursion into the principles of conducting a therapeutic conversation and how to use these language and communication practices to generate new possibilities within the family and network. Open Dialogue shows how this way of working can be adapted to acute psychiatric care, when supported by fundamental changes in the organization of the treatment system. Narrative therapy is a perspective and set of skills useful for stuck, chronic, "problem-saturated" situations. The social justice therapies are crucial in applying these same clinical methods to doing therapy in a multicultural and rapidly changing society.

Bateson's Ecology of Mind

The starting point of this curriculum is the work of the anthropologist and biologist Gregory Bateson (1972, 1979), who produced the communication perspective that became the foundation for the field. The thinking of Bateson, arguably an early postmodernist, prefigured many contemporary trends and directly influenced many of the people who went on to embrace postmodern approaches to therapy (Hoffman, 2002). Even though Bateson draws on traditional systems thinking, his work anticipated the shift from the notion of an objective system to a dialogic system made and remade by words and stories.

Bateson argued that events in living systems require a different model from the scientific paradigm of linear and mechanistic causality that is appropriate for explaining the inanimate, physical world. He proposed instead to think of the living world as "mind," that is, as communicational processes constituted in the integrated network of the individual plus environment. For Bateson, this concept of mind as a communicational system is evident in all aspects of the organic universe: DNA is an informational script; the brain and nervous system operate on signals; and social processes are governed by patterns of language and communication. Bateson's analyses of social life hinge on the concept of an evolutionary ecology of communicative and recursive relationships. Communication and interaction are crucial because it is the history of joint action of organisms and environments over time that creates natural and human worlds.

Bateson's thinking addresses both structure and communication, but the early family therapists interpreted the features of a system as an objective entity—a triangle or game—that can be changed from outside (Watzlawick, Weakland, & Fisch, 1974). This form of interventionism repelled Bateson and led to a split with his early followers (Bateson, Weakland, & Haley, 1976). The publication of Bateson's articles in an anthology, *Steps to an Ecology of Mind* (1972), and of his final book, *Mind and Nature* (1979), made his ideas much more available to a broader audience who received them differently than had the early pioneers (Olson, 1984). The new generation of family therapists responded to Bateson's notion of "an ecology of mind" and his profound distrust of an instrumental epistemology based on power and control (Hoffman, 1986).

Bateson (1979) says that human beings think in terms of "stories" or "little knots of relevance" (p. 13) that shape behavior (stories projected into action). In the tradition of George Herbert Mead, he anticipated postmodern social construction theory by maintaining that the mind is social and, therefore, the way we communicate with each other becomes an essential feature of the way we think. In this way, Bateson's theory of the double bind came from a theoretical attempt to imagine the kind of interpersonal and communicational context in which psychotic ideas and symptoms would seem adaptive (Bateson, Jackson, Haley, & Weakland, 1956). It originally referred to a repeated pattern of communication within a life-important relationship where there were two different and mutually disqualifying levels of meaning about which one was forbidden to comment. (Nor could one leave the field without risking punishment.)

Subsequent writings by Bateson and his colleagues (Bateson, Weakland, & Haley, 1976) revised the original dyadic formulation of the theory. This later version is one of the central organizing ideas of this curriculum: "The most useful way to phrase double bind description is not in terms of binder and a victim but in terms of people caught up in an ongoing system which produces conflicting definitions of the relationship and consequent subjective distress" (p. 42). While looking initially at patterns of message exchange, Bateson's followers like the Milan group (Selvini-Palazzoli et al., 1978) shifted to emphasizing the larger system of relations and conflicting patterns of meaning within a social group as a whole that generate these paradoxes. To some extent, everyone in a system may be affected, although the consequences are experienced most visibly and acutely by the person(s) who develop symptom(s). From a postmodern perspective, the double-bind situation constitutes the kind of context that silences and disempowers people, resulting in loss of voice and onset of symptoms.

Film clips from the movie *Shine* (Scott & Hicks, 1996) have been used effectively to illustrate the double-bind theory. *Shine* is the story of David Helfgott, a gifted pianist who had a psychotic break in late adolescence. The scenes of David's childhood and adolescence portray the intense and conflicting injunctions tied to gaining outside recog-

nition and leaving home in a Jewish family with parents who view the outside world as dangerous, having lost close family members in the Holocaust. Sketching this legacy of trauma and loss humanizes the parents by placing their behavior in context, while showing the dilemmas emanating from their tragic experiences. Analyzing this film teaches implicitly the principle of logical connotation: the story of David renders his experience meaningful and supports the significance of narrative in making sense of his deterioration. Appreciating the entire context, including the cultural position of the parents, can foster an understanding of everyone involved and reduces the blame assigned to David or his family. Finally, David's recovery, although idealized in the film, shows how he builds an adult life despite its painful opening chapters, thus conveying a sense of personal agency in the face of enormous difficulty.

Another useful classroom exercise is reading transcript interviews as scripts. Excerpts from the clinical work of James Griffith and Melissa Elliott (Griffith & Griffith, 1994) form a useful bridge between Bateson's double-bind theory and postmodern therapy. Participants play the different parts and can learn how an experienced therapist conducts a therapeutic conversation. Griffith and Elliott draw on a variety of important formats and ideas: the reflecting team, collaboration, a network orientation, techniques from narrative therapy, and an awareness of how culture, gender, race, and ethnicity can influence the problems people bring to therapy. Their emphasis is on life stories rather than diagnostic categories or pathogenic systems, with special attention to double-bind communication, or what they call "unspeakable dilemmas." A gender premise, a family myth, or a religious system can produce an unspeakable dilemma, while silencing the kind of conversation needed to resolve it. The heart of this therapy is the telling of a person's story and giving expression to what was felt to be unspeakable in the presence of others.

Published interviews of this work read in class have included "When Patients Somatize and Clinicians Stigmatize: Opening Dialogue Between Clinicians and the Medically Marginalized" (Griffith & Griffith, 1995). This example focuses on an isolated, homebound 12-year-old girl and her depressed, divorced mother, who participated in a joint meeting conducted by Griffith, Eliott, and other medical colleagues. The girl had been evaluated for a sleep disorder, rheumatoid arthritis, and a variety of other health problems that the mother kept bringing to doctors but were not found to be present. This sensitive interview, however, opened up a conversation about the daughter's unvoiced feelings of emotional paralysis. After listening to a reflecting team, both mother and daughter were able to see their situation differently, dissolve the medical focus, and express their concern for each other in a new and more constructive way that supported the daughter's desire for more independence.

It is important to teach the ideas and their applications, while simultaneously encouraging trainees to develop their own perspectives and creativity. In an academic setting, one way of doing this is to ask students to keep journals on the readings and classes. Students are encouraged to write about how they would apply the ideas to cases from their field placements. I also invite students to imagine applications outside the therapy office, for example, in schools or a case management situation. Critiques of the ideas are also encouraged. The journals can serve as a set of written assignments for the course that helps students find their voices. Freire's (1971) concept of the midwife-teacher is one who engages the potential, creativity, and imagination of students. I strive to incorporate this model both in the journal assignments and by encouraging collaborative dialogue in the classroom.

The Reflecting Process

The work of the Griffiths introduces the reflecting process of Tom Andersen (Andersen, 1987, 1991, 1995). Originally using a format inspired by Bateson's ideas and advanced by the Milan Associates (Boscolo et al., 1987), Andersen moved from a hierarchical structure to a more horizontal one. The reflecting team is a simple and extremely important idea in the contemporary family field and has been adapted, in creative ways, to work with children and adolescents (Friedman, 1993). In its original formulation, a three-person reflecting team made up of professionals, sitting with the family or behind a one-way screen, listens to the conversation between the therapist and the family. The therapist then asks the family if they are interested in hearing from the team. If so, the team members reflect on what they have heard and have this conversation in the presence of the family. After the reflections, the interviewer asks the family to comment on what the team has said. The family respond to the ideas that fit and thus gain a voice in their own evolution. The reflections of the team are speculative and non-pejorative and tend to be comments that address, for instance, the family's dilemmas, emotional atmosphere, or future possibilities.

The reflecting team also draws on the contribution of the late psychologist Harry Goolishian, who, with Harlene Anderson, argued that, above all, human systems are language based, created in and through dialogue (Anderson & Goolishian, 1988). Thus, therapy is a conversation, where new stories arise from the exchange. Alternating conversations foster "depth perception," an atmosphere of learning that allows the family to consider other perspectives. The reflecting process provides a format where the family can stand outside its situation and listen to different ideas about it. A new picture can develop with a new sense of alternatives (Andersen, 1987). Videos illustrating Andersen's approach include *Dialogue and Dialogue About Dialogue* (Andrew & Clark Explorations/Masterwork, 1992), *Reflecting Elder Stories* (Andrew & Clark Explorations/Masterwork, 1998b), and *Dialogues and Postmodern Connections: 3 Part Series*, with Harlene Anderson (Andrew & Clark Explorations/Masterwork, 1998a). The reflecting process is an important feature of both the Open Dialogue approach and narrative therapy, thus becoming a thread throughout the curriculum (Seikkula et al., 1995; Seikkula & Olson, 2003; White, 1995).

One way to teach the basic mechanics of a reflecting team is to do a role play based on a family invented by the participants. One group plays the family, and another group forms a reflecting team. The remaining students listen "as-if" they are family members who provide comments at the end (Andersen, 1997). It can be useful for the instructor to be the therapist in the first interview, so students can learn from an experienced person. An alternative is to have a trainee rotate through the position of therapist with the instructor, it is hoped, as "an angel on their shoulder." That is, the "therapist" can stop the interview at any time and consult with the instructor about what to say next.

In his recent work, Andersen (this volume) has come to emphasize "open reflecting talks" in a variety of contexts, while also sketching the evolution of the "northern network" and the principles of the training program in the European Nordic North.

This kind of open-ended and participatory dialogue can be adapted easily to a classroom, workshop, research evaluation (Andersen, 1997), or other settings relevant to community care. Throughout this curriculum, we use the reflecting process with case presentations and the cultural genogram described later in this chapter. The most effective experiences with the reflecting process seem to be when a trainee presents an actual clinical dilemma and other members of the class or workshop reflect on this real situation. An example of this kind of reflecting consultation is provided at the end of this chapter. What has been impressive about this process is the way it changes the nature of our conversations about families. The collaborative format seems to energize participants and to make then conscious of the effects of their language, respectful of families and of each other, and capable of hearing and sustaining multiple perspectives, thus inhabiting what Gregory Bateson (1972) called an expanded "ecology of ideas."

Open Dialogue

Drawing further on Bateson's legacy and, in particular, Andersen's idea of reflecting process, Open Dialogue is a network-based language approach for severe, acute psychiatric crises. Pioneered in Finland, it is close to the idea of wraparound used in the United States (Seikkula et al., 1995; Seikkula, Alakare, & Aaltonen, 2001a, 2001b). Although VanDenBerg (VanDenBerg & Grealish, 1996), the originator of the wraparound, does not define his process as therapy, therapeutic ideas, such as "reframing" and "the strengths assessment," are incorporated in its design. Open Dialogue explicitly merges the distinction between planning and therapy and makes the "treatment meeting" the main therapeutic forum. There is a blending of dialogue and disposition in acute care. The implications of this model for a system of care are wide-ranging. Open Dialogue shows that "transformative dialogue" may be possible in various kinds of settings not traditionally defined as hosting clinical interventions (Gergen & MacNamee, 2000). In the United States, there is growing interest in Open Dialogue as the equivalent of a "wraparound" crisis intervention model within a system of care.

Open Dialogue was developed at Keropudas Hospital, a traditional, combined psychiatric inpatient and outpatient setting in western Lapland.

Following Alanen (1997), the Keropudas group began to have a treatment meeting in advance of any kind of therapy when earlier attempts to do family therapy failed in the hospital system. Its basic format is to bring together the person in acute distress with the team and all other important relations—relatives, friends, and other professionals—connected to the crisis. Dedicated to giving immediate help, the meeting occurs within 24 hours of the initial contact. It is organized by a mobile crisis team composed of outpatient and inpatient staff and takes place, if possible, at home.

The treatment meeting was conceptualized initially by the Keropudas group as a way to minimize the occurrence of double-binding transactions in acute settings (Seikkula & Sutela, 1990.) A brief excursion into a separate, ethnographic study of the experience of patients with head injuries (Krefting, 1990) will make this point clearer. Krefting's research illuminates the kind of communication difficulties that the Finnish team independently noticed occur in the treatment system of youths with psychiatric problems. There tend to be repeated patterns of conflicting messages from different sources: the family, the social network, the professional health care system, and the vocational rehabilitation system. There also tend to be pervasive social directives for independence and the contradictory messages of dependence. In what we can see as an analogue to psychiatric care, Krefting writes: "[Many] of the double binds experienced by the head injured are created by pressures from community norms and expectations, rather than specific people" (p. 864). Even so, professionals can be powerful generators of conflicting meanings. With the organic impairment of the head injured, they often have little chance of accommodating, cognitively, their complex set of contexts. As a result, "common behavioral problems noted . . . include concrete thinking, angry outbursts, paranoia, and loss of trust of caregivers" (p. 861). The double-binding transactions appear to exacerbate emotional difficulties and preclude the occurrence of more positive alternatives. In contrast, the team operating in Open Dialogue coordinates and integrates the participating systems formed by a severe psychiatric crisis. It serves to maintain psychological continuity (e.g., a coherent and consistent treatment team and plan) until there is a resolution of symptoms, thus reducing the iatrogenic effects of the patient's involvement with multiple systems.

As the work of the Finnish team has evolved, the idea of "dialogism" by Bakhtin (1984) became central. The aim of the treatment meeting explicitly became defined as that of dialogue, in which the patient can find voice, thus reducing the person's sense of isolation. This approach emphasizes the process of finding language for psychotic experience that previously was inexpressible and creating a shared understanding of the crisis within a network. The use of ordinary words and creation of joint meanings tends to generate a collaborative set of relationships and to open up an avenue to people's own knowledge, skills, and capabilities.

The two other key principles tied to dialogism are "tolerance of uncertainty" and "polyphony" (Seikkula & Olson, 2003). Tolerating uncertainty means establishing a climate of safety and intense support, with daily meetings, if needed, so that the solutions can emerge from the dialogue itself rather than be imposed prematurely by experts. Polyphony, an interplay of multiple voices, allows for the process of exchange by which new words and new stories enter the common discourse and give voice to the previously incomprehensible suffering of the patient. The reflecting process among the helpers is a crucial part of this polyphonic conversation.

One of the effects of these language practices in the treatment meeting is to create a transparency in psychiatric care—indeed, the "openness" of Open Dialogue. The deleterious effects of contradictory injunctions originating from different contexts can be countered by making the confusing messages open for discussion during the meeting. There are no separate staff meetings to talk about the "case," so all "case management" issues, including medication, hospitalization, and psychotherapeutic options, must be addressed in the meeting with everyone in the network present.

In teaching Open Dialogue, there is a combination of lectures describing the principles, the impressive outcome research (Seikkula et al., 2003), and reading (Seikkula & Olson, 2003). The author describes her own experience doing an ethnographic study of Keropudas Hospital and the acute team in Tromsoe, Norway, where, under the guidance of Tom Andersen and Magnus Hald, this way of working has become well established, with some slight differences from the Finnish approach. Students practice learning to conduct "a dialogical dialogue" in small groups by discussing an ordinary problem that they feel comfortable disclosing (Seikkula, personal communication). Observers within the groups are invited to give reflections on the dialogue. Role plays of severe psychiatric crises are not performed. Alternately, transcripts of published sessions can be read aloud. The story of Pekka and Maja, an interview conducted by the Finnish team at Keropudas Hospital (Seikkula & Olson, 2003), shows the resolution of a psychosis in Open Dialogue. This transcript has been read and analyzed in class discussion.

Externalizing Conversation

While the Open Dialogue approach was developed in the context of acute care, the narrative therapy of Michael White and David Epston (1990; White, 1995) was invented for "problem-saturated" situations with difficulties of longer duration and chronicity, in which people have experienced more "identity damage" as a consequence. Drawing on Bateson and poststructuralist Michel Foucault, Michael White shows how to "reauthor" the problem-saturated stories that clinicians often encounter in public agencies and outpatient community-based settings. In contrast to Open Dialogue, narrative therapy is not designed for the acute crisis phase of severe psychiatric problems.

White argues that one of the most oppressive effects of the dominant mental health discourse is the identification of the person with the problem, rather than identifying the social contexts and discursive practices in which problems are embedded. The technique White invented, called "externalizing," creates a linguistic separation of the problem from the person. Externalizing the problem helps locate "unique outcomes," or exceptions to the problem. Those experiences that fall outside a dominant, negative script provide the stuff for creating alternative, more hopeful stories. The idea is to find and develop a new story based on unique outcomes that have not been given significance because they do not fit in with the person's self-narrative of inadequacy or failure that has become the "receiving context." A self-critical narrative often has roots in the larger, oppressive normalizing "truths," or socially constructed cultural narratives about personhood, sexual orientation, class, gender, or racial identity. Narrative therapy attempts to counteract the effects of these demoralizing "truths" in people's lives.

White and Epston have created a rich and imaginative repertoire of questions, rituals, letters, archives, and other written documents, and much of this work has been developed for children and adolescents. These techniques and skills make visible the effects of problems and bring forward the skills, knowledge, and agency of the person in counteracting them. Narrative therapy represents one of the most compassionate therapies for chronic, long-term problems. The early critics of narrative therapy raised concerns that the therapists do not listen enough to people's suffering or respond to their desire to find meaning in it. In the last decade, by incorporating the influence of the reflecting process, narrative therapy has become more collaborative, participatory, and flexible. Videos for teaching narrative therapy include *Escape From Bickering* (American Association for Marriage and Family Therapy, 1989), *Re-authoring a Life in the Face of Lost Dreams* (Andrew & Clark Explorations/Masterwork, 1994b), *The Best of Friends* (Andrew & Clark Explorations/Masterwork, 1994a), and *Interview With Harassment* (Educational Media Centre, 1999).

In teaching narrative therapy in an academic setting, one option for the final assignment is to ask advanced students to construct a narrative of professional development based on "sparkling facts" (White, 1989/90). "Sparkling facts" are the unique outcomes, or successful learning experiences and effective negotiations of difficulties within their professional education. The students first do this exercise in small groups of four to five people consisting of the interviewer, the interviewee, and the other students, who reflect on the person's experience as "outsider witnesses." An outsider witness is a person whose words can enrich the preferred story and help give it weight. Not all students will be able to be interviewed in class, so they are encouraged to form pairs and meet outside of class to have the same dialogue.

A successful example of this learning exercise comes from Samantha Smith (2003), a graduate student in social work, who discussed in class and then wrote about doing therapy with Javier, an 8-year-old Puerto Rican boy, whom she saw in an urban school-based mental health program called Partners for Success. The boy was referred for significant obesity, depression, poor social skills, academic struggles, absenteeism, and concerns over

his history of broken bones. He had had several prior therapists and was on his way to becoming a chronic case. Samantha, who was already familiar with narrative therapy from this field placement, creatively wove the idea of "unique outcomes" together with other ideas and techniques from different approaches.

While it is beyond the scope of this chapter to describe all that went into this therapy, one ingenious idea was that Samantha facilitated a noncompetitive basketball team that provided Javier with his first tangible experience of being an athlete. When Javier first met Samantha, he expressed a strong interest in basketball and told her about the 75 trophies he had already won for outstanding competitive play. Samantha did not challenge this make-believe but was inspired to give him an experience of actual basketball, thinking it might help this boy initiate a new narrative about his identity. This activity was combined with play therapy in which the therapist created a sensitive connection that allowed Javier to give expression to the many painful things in his life. Soon this boy began to change and started to laugh and smile on a regular basis. Teachers saw dramatic improvement in his schoolwork and attendance. Javier also began making friends and losing weight. Samantha worked actively with his mother and teachers to reinforce this new identity as the "real Javier," who previously had been eclipsed by his problems.

Finally, another student, Lynne Anderson, who interviewed Samantha in class during the small-group exercise, suggested the parallel process between Javier and Samantha where both emerged feeling like "the real thing." Samantha wrote:

> We both entered the therapy feeling somewhat like "frauds": he having to lie about his relationships and athletic abilities and me identifying as a completely inexperienced therapist who was not likely to make a difference in this kid's life. [By the end], Javier now had genuine friendships and basketball skills and I now had some pride in my work and could feel justified in being paid for such services in the future!

Samantha's account of this "sparkling fact" in her professional development helped to solidify a confident identity as a child therapist and gave her a direct experience of a narrative technique that increased her understanding of its therapeutic effect.

Unspeakable Dilemmas of Social Identity

Narrative therapy is among various distinct strands of family therapy that have attempted to address the political and social contexts of people's lives. From the outset of the curriculum, there is an emphasis on these contexts not only as they shape human life but also in terms of the social and political ingredients of theory building itself. Starting in the mid-1980s, the impact of the feminist critique altered American family therapy by showing that there were gender biases built into the traditional models that privilege autonomy and power. Once the objectivity and neutrality of the dominant theories were thus challenged, the use of a postmodern, collaborative stance assumed a compelling logic. That is, basing therapy on a collaborative process of inquiry, rather than a theory of structural reality, makes sense in a rapidly changing world where, as Judith Stacey (1996) states, "contemporary Western family arrangements are diverse, fluid, and unresolved" (p. 7). The convergence and tension between postmodernism and the critical implications of feminism and other social justice movements—or two kinds of thought, deconstructive and political—is an important subdimension of the course.

The clinical work of the Gender and Violence Project at Ackerman shows the relevance of a language-based approach to gender dilemmas of various kinds, including violence and abuse (Goldner et al., 1990). Unlike prior family models, this group includes the moral and ethical considerations about safety and responsibility of the persons caught up in these situations. Gender prescriptions are addressed in clinical practice through the use of specific techniques like "deconstructing violence," developed for work with couples where the man wants to stop being violent. Deconstructing violence is a slow-motion analysis of a violent episode that takes place between the therapist and the male partner. It surfaces the gender premises, feelings, memories, and images that converged in the violence, thus finding words and making a narrative for the person's otherwise fragmented experience. These clinical discussions can be supplemented with Sut Jhally's educational video, *Tough Guise* (1999), examining the rise of hypermasculinity in America and its effects on different racial groups. Jhally's work deciphers the stories told by the larger culture about masculinity as evident in the media and media imagery.

I use my clinical work and research on anorexia to explore the idea of gender-linked unspeakable dilemmas and how these are built into the social experience of girls growing up in our culture. Introducing Grimms' fairy tales (Hunt & Stern, 1944/1972) is useful in looking at a traditional Western gender discourse. Students read aloud "The Beam" and "The Shepherd Boy" and contrast the representations of female and male knowledge. There is a convergence among this gender discourse, the double-bind theory, and Gilligan's "relational paradox," where young adolescent girls learn to silence voice and body to gain acceptance and protect relationships (Brown & Gilligan, 1992; Olson, 2000b). The story of a young woman with bulimia shows how collaborative formats of therapeutic conversation and writing can give voice to, and thus address, the unspeakable dilemmas tied to gender prescriptions (Olson, 1995a). These ideas converge with Mahmoud's (1998) excellent article on the double binds of racism. It becomes clear that the double-bind situation goes beyond the family and can be an artifact of cultural narratives about social identity. In tandem, the film *The Joy Luck Club* (Stone & Wang, 1993) shows the intergenerational transmission of double-binding premises rooted in culture, gender, and race as refracted through mother and daughters confronting the tragic circumstances and legacies of immigration (Tan, 1989).

As Charles Waldegrave (1998) observes, the influence of postmodernism opened space for and legitimated other diverse voices. In the 1990s, more presentations at conferences and more articles began to appear from wider social and cultural perspectives. The multicultural movement became the recognition of difference and how differences are socially constructed and politically inflected. Even the term "multicultural" became critiqued for obscuring the link in the United States between "different" and "less" (Akamatsu, 1998). A cultural thread had developed in the 1960s in family therapy, but these earlier models lacked the explicit political analysis of difference that emerged in the late 1990s. By now, class, culture, gender, race, and sexual orientation can define all families not just marginalized ones.

As the gender critique challenged theories of

therapy as biased, a cultural perspective has shown that these same theories are culture bound. According to the anthropologist Clifford Geertz (1983), the concept of a separate, autonomous self is a rather peculiar notion in most parts of the world where self is conceived as embedded in relationship and community. Conceptions of emotion, identity, communication, and cognition are all shaped by culture. The concept of family itself is culturally determined. Cross-cultural comparisons of legal marriage afforded to gay and lesbian couples and access to reproductive options and adoption illustrate this point. This awareness is imperative for American therapists operating in a diverse, multicultural society.

The cultural genogram developed by Ken Hardy and Tracy Laszloffy (1995) is one way of learning how to enter a therapeutic conversation about difference. Trainees are invited to do a cultural genogram, following Hardy and Laszloffy's guidelines of identifying the "organizing principles" and "pride/shame issues" of the family's particular cultural group. The group is asked to join in by reflecting on the cultural question about the family posed by the trainee presenting the genogram. Here the emphasis is on both multicultural knowledge and the ability to conduct an inquiry that does not impose stereotypes. The aim is to facilitate a context for self-definition and agency.

Voice and authorship are political shifts that emerge from methods of collaboration. The curriculum examines many examples of giving voice, with special attention given to social justice therapy, a model in which families participate in the organization of the treatment context itself (Waldegrave, 1990). The same principle is upheld by the system-of-care framework, namely, that to create a socially just framework, there must be a commitment to partnership with families in the building of services.

An Example of a Postmodern Education in Action

The following account, which provides an example of a consultation using dialogic, reflecting, and narrative ideas in a mental health agency that serves a poor community on the outskirts of Boston, illustrates how postmodern clinical practices can be hand in glove with the system-of-care philosophy.

Although this consultation occurred in a mental health agency, the exact same format can be used in classroom settings and postgraduate workshops to teach community-based mental health practice.

Chris O'Rourke, MSW. who had been trained in this curriculum and worked at this agency, asked me to provide training to the staff. I organized the consultation around an actual case where the clinicians were feeling stuck. The consultation began with a 30-minute introduction sketching the idea of dialogue, the format of the reflecting process, and the narrative technique of finding exceptions, or unique outcomes, to shift away from problem-saturated stories. These therapeutic principles produced both a process and an outcome compatible with the system-of-care movement. Specifically, this clinical consultation promoted a nonpathologizing framework, a partnership with the family, interdisciplinary collaboration, cultural awareness, and the inclusion of natural supports from the person's own relatives to stabilize the crisis rather than turning to an institution.

Rose, the person at the center of concern, and her family did not attend the consultation, even though she and her children were invited to participate. The reason for this may have been that this way of working was new and unfamiliar, both to the professionals and to the client. While this mother reportedly benefited significantly from this consultation, her presence in the actual conversation would have been highly valued. At the same time, this example shows that working even with part of the therapeutic network can produce a significant shift that helps people who are unable to attend. Obviously, in an academic setting, it would be highly unusual for families to attend, and as in this situation, the primary contact with the network would be the treating therapist.

The consultation took 2 hours. Chris presented, with insight and compassion, the case of a 32-year-old African American woman who was the mother of four children, ages 7 to 11. Rose originally came to the clinic after the death of her beloved grandmother and in the aftermath of her boyfriend's infidelity with a neighbor. She was depressed, poor, and unemployed, and was living in dangerous public housing. Rose also had a complicated history of childhood sexual abuse by an adult outside the family. Her marriage had been violent, and she left the children's father because he beat her. This mother also had a history of alcoholism but stopped drinking because, she reckoned, "I can either be an alcoholic or a mother." It was evident that she loved her children and that these relationships had a positive, stabilizing effect on her life. Her children had an array of difficulties for which Rose sought help at the clinic, including a concern for her eldest son, who had once been suicidal.

Chris had been seeing Rose individually for more than a year, and another therapist, Helen, had been working with Rose and her children. Both therapists were present at this meeting and described excellent work assisting Rose in handling repeated crises in her life. Their primary concern about Rose was a continued weight loss during the past year. Rose, who was 5 feet, 3 inches tall, was not eating much, and her weight had fallen to about 85 pounds. To help Rose eat, Chris had arranged for her to attend a psychiatric day treatment program that she had attended sporadically the previous summer. Rose also took medication, with mixed results. For the therapist, the question looming over the consultation was whether Rose had to be hospitalized on an inpatient unit, thus jeopardizing her ability to take care of her children. The hope of the consultation was to generate new possibilities for Rose to stay in the community. This proposal also protected her children, since they would not have to be separated from their mother.

The consultant started by thinking how we might together create a safety net around Rose and counteract the larger shared sense of being overwhelmed by her problems. Without minimizing or downplaying her difficulties and symptoms, the consultant's goal was to find alternate perspectives and possibilities that might help everyone feel safer and more hopeful. The consultant organized the staff into three groups. The first group included Chris, Helen, the family therapist, and the consultant. The second group was the reflecting team, which included the members of the staff who were the child and family specialists. The third group was the larger group of other staff members, many of whom volunteered to listen "as if" they were family members. The same structure can also be created in a classroom.

The consultant continued by listening to the first group and drawing a genogram that included a question that brought forward exceptions to the story of Rose not eating. This part of the consultation began with the two questions posed to Chris, as the person requesting the consultation, and were

first proposed by Andersen (1995): "What is the history of the idea to have the meeting?" and "What would be a good outcome for the meeting?" The consultant based her subsequent response on the answers provided to these questions,; thus, the meeting became an evolving dialogue. Being respectful to all participants by acknowledging their responses was key.

The themes of this initial conversation emerged as concerns about Rose's safety and her prior experiences of abuse and danger. The first thing the consultant did was to create a protective protocol around the weight loss. Chris agreed to ask the primary care physician to define the weight Rose needed to maintain to be medically safe. Should Rose decide to go below this weight, then a hospitalization would be pursued. This clarity brought a sense of safety and relief to everyone.

After Chris and the other therapists presented the case, the reflecting team commented. The team honored Rose's suffering and also highlighted aspects of her story that held new possibilities. After listening to the team, Chris said that he was filled with emotion because it was the first time that he did not feel alone with this frightening case. Helen, the family therapist, also felt the team's support and compassion.

After the initial set of reflections, we continued the conversation and developed the idea of building a network of care around Rose and her children that included not only the professionals but also Rose's mother, her sister, and the other women in her life. From the genogram, we had learned that there were strong women in Rose's family who had been the only people capable of getting Rose to eat. In the past year, she had become separated from these family members when she had to move to a different neighborhood because of a change in her housing subsidy.

Following the consultation, Chris shared two ideas with Rose that seemed to help her to change. The first was to comment on her competence as a mother, the love she had for her children, and how much she wanted to keep them safe. The second was to share our appreciation for Rose's connection to the women in her family and to tell her how important these relationships were. Chris asked her how she could continue to draw on these relationships to help her manage. Who else could she identify as support? The main clinical outcome of the consultation was to create a network around Rose by calling attention to the women in her family as life-important sources of nurturance and care. In this way, the staff found a natural way to help Rose diffuse the crisis.

As a postscript, Chris added that over the next months, Rose developed a stronger sense of personal agency and purpose and was taking care of herself and eating more adequately. Rose responded deeply to the acknowledgment of her abilities as a mother. She was empowered by this recognition and in the months ahead began looking for a new place to live. Chris was impressed by Rose's determination to move herself and her children from where they had been living and into a safer apartment closer to her own family. Although he left the agency during Rose's search for housing, he felt strongly that he saw a different person emerging—a person capable of taking the action she needed to get to a better place.

In a brief period this consultation accomplished several things on multiple levels. First, by sharing ideas, the team created a much richer description of this woman's life that led to new possibilities and ultimately kept Rose in the community, out of a hospital, and out of a possible inpatient career. Second, the consultation built support and safety around the therapists, who had felt isolated and alone. Third, the consultant provided training for the staff and facilitated teamwork, rapport, and supportive interactions among them. In this way, the reflecting process helped the staff to work together effectively in a crisis. The dialogic and narrative practices that come out of the family therapy tradition offer formats that can serve to generate creativity and connection. As this example shows, by introducing opportunities for inquiry and reflection, this capable staff came up with a solution without recourse to more costly measures.

Basic Guidelines for Doing Clinical Consultation in Community Care

The following is a summary of guidelines for doing clinical consultation with a community-based orientation that reinforces the principles of the system-of-care philosophy:

1. Present clear, brief guidelines for the reflecting process. The interested practitioner

should consult this literature for a more extensive description: Andersen, 1991, 1995, and Griffith & Griffith, 1994, pp. 160–162, for their succinct distillation of Andersen's principles of the reflective position.

2. Focus on an actual clinical situation. In a world of limited time and resources, this will be experienced as real help.

3. Present two or three clinical ideas and keep this part relatively brief (20 to 30 minutes in a 2-hour consultation). If this consultation is part of a longer course, it is still important to review for students the ideas in use.

4. Describe why these particular ideas are useful in this particular situation. For instance, in community agencies, reflecting conversation can help build clinical teams in which people can share ideas and find solutions, in contrast to the isolation and fragmentation professionals often experience. Finding exceptions in problem-saturated stories can create an effective difference when this is extremely hard to do.

5. Begin with the following two questions: "What is the history of the idea to have the meeting?" and "How would you like to use this meeting?" The first question addresses the immediate context and the ideas people are bringing to it. The second question constructs agency and launches people in the direction of their hopes and best intentions. Refer to Andersen's (1995) own in-depth discussion of these questions as starting points.

6. In most agency contexts, professionals are not used to having clients present for staff training, so it is unlikely that they will have enough trust, at first, to bring them. It is possible to constitute the missing voices in the network and gain a more fully polyphonic conversation by doing a genogram and asking reflexive questions (Seikkula, personal communication). For instance, "If Rose were here, what would she say has been helpful to her?" "If Rose's sisters and mother were here, what would they say about her not eating?"

7. Hypothetical, future-oriented, or externalizing questions engage the imagination and introduce reflexivity, or the capacity to stand outside the situation and view it from a different experience, for example, "What does Rose's ability to leave an abusive marriage and stop

drinking tell us about the person she is becoming?"

8. Do not outlaw other points of view. Embrace differences. All ideas can be in the service of dialogue and reflection.
9. Listen for the emergence of a new sense of possibilities, exceptions, meanings, and naturally occurring resources. Let the solutions come from the dialogue itself.
10. Conduct the consultation with a spirit of improvisation, compassion, and hope.

Conclusion

The postmodern curriculum trains clinicians to do therapy in a way that integrates the values and principles of a system-of-care approach. The new clinical practices in the service of the community movement look for ways to reduce suffering and foster recovery by drawing on the possibilities within the existing professional and social networks. In this endeavor, the use of language and the establishment of dialogue are living elements that can be garnered in helping to reconstruct the terms on which the people live their lives. A genuine dialogue can create a different future by generating new meanings and new, more helpful relationships within a social network. Such practices lend themselves to being more culturally, racially, and gender sensitive because they steer clear of objectifying the other and attempt to provide the tools for claiming a sense of control over one's destiny.

In his book *Pedagogy of Hope,* Freire (2002) makes the point that "teaching is not a simple transmission" (p. 80). Echoing Bateson, he goes on to say that "teaching someone to learn is only valid . . . when educands *learn to learn*" (p. 81). One of the mandates of his pedagogy is to learn to learn how to have "critical hope" rather than a naive hopefulness (p. 8). In training clinicians in community-based practice, critical hope lies in teaching them how to embrace suffering without creating pathology; to listen and generate dialogue in the face of the incomprehensible; to ask questions that surface people's ideas, skills, capabilities, and prospects; and to understand the power of language as a world-making, identity-making activity. It is always difficult to say exactly what a particular consultant did to shift a desperate situation: there is no single intervention, but a collaborative process

that happens between people—shaped by reflection, dialogue, and certain kinds of questions—that creates a context where the new can emerge. It is in the magic of human interchange that we find freedom where we were stuck, that we are joined with others in shared responsibility, and that instead of the weight of pathology, we are lightened by solutions that make care a new experience of hope.

References

Akamatsu, N. N. (1998). The talking oppression blues: Including the experience of power/powerlessness in the teaching of "cultural sensitivity." In M. McGoldrick (Ed.), *Re-visioning family therapy: Race, culture, and gender in clinical practice* (pp. 129–144). New York: Guilford.

Alanen, Y. (1997). *Schizophrenia: Its origins and need-adapted treatment.* London: Karnac Books.

American Association for Marriage and Family Therapy (Producer). (1989). *Escape from bickering* [Videorecording]. (Available from American Association for Marriage and Family Therapy, www.aamft.org)

Andersen, T. (1987). The reflecting team: Dialogue and meta-dialogue in clinical work. *Family Process, 26,* 415–428.

Andersen, T. (1991). *The reflecting team: Dialogues and dialogues about dialogues.* New York: Norton.

Andersen, T. (1995). Reflecting processes: Acts of informing and forming: You can borrow my eyes, but you must not take them away from me! In S. Friedman (Ed.), *The reflecting team in action: Collaborative practice in family therapy* (pp. 11–37). New York: Guilford.

Andersen, T. (1997). Researching client-therapist relationships: A collaborative study for informing therapy. *Journal of Systemic Therapies, 16,* 125–133.

Anderson, H. (1997). *Conversation, language, and possibilities: A postmodern approach to therapy.* New York: Basic Books.

Anderson, H., & Goolishian, H. (1986). Systems consultation to agencies dealing with domestic violence. In L. Wynne, S. McDaniel, & T. Weber (Eds.), *The family therapist as systems consultant* (pp. 284–299). New York: Guilford.

Anderson, H., & Goolishian, H. (1988). Human systems as linguistic systems: Preliminary and evolving ideas about the implications for clinical theory. *Family Process, 27,* 371–393.

Anderson, H., & Goolishian, H. (1991). Thinking about multi-agency work with substance abusers and their families. *Journal of Strategic and Systemic Therapies, 10,* 20–35.

Andrew & Clark Explorations/Masterwork (Producer). (1992). *Dialogue and dialogue about dialogue.* (Available from the Andrew & Clark Explorations/Masterwork Web site, http://www.masterswork.com)

Andrew & Clark Explorations/Masterwork (Producer). (1994a). *The best of friends.* (Available from the Andrew & Clark Explorations/Masterwork Web site, http://www.masterswork.com)

Andrew & Clark Explorations/Masterwork (Producer). (1994b). *Re-authoring a life in the face of lost dreams.* (Available from the Andrew & Clark Explorations/Masterwork Web site, http://www.masterswork.com)

Andrew & Clark Explorations/Masterwork (Producer). (1999a). Dialogues and postmodern connections: 3 part series (Available from the Andrew & Clark Explorations/Masterwork Web site, http://www.masterswork.com)

Andrew & Clark Explorations/Masterwork (Producer). (1999b). *Reflecting elder stories.* (Available from the Andrew & Clark Explorations/Masterwork Web site, http://www.masterswork.com)

Bakhtin, M. (1984). *Problems of Dostoevsky's poetics: Theory and history of literature* (Vol. 8). Manchester, UK: Manchester University Press.

Bateson, G. (1972). *Steps to an ecology of mind.* New York: Ballantine.

Bateson, G. (1976). A note on the double bind: 1962. In C. Sluzki & D. Ransom (Eds.), *Double bind: The foundation of the communicational approach to the family* (pp. 39–42). New York: Grune and Stratton.

Bateson, G. (1979). *Mind and nature.* New York: Dutton.

Bateson, G., Jackson, D., Haley, J., & Weakland, J. (1956). Toward a theory of schizophrenia. *Behavioral Science, 1,* 251–254.

Bateson, G., Weakland, J., & Haley, J. (1976). Comments on Haley's "History." In C. Sluzki & D. Ransom (Eds.), *Double bind: The foundation of the communicational approach to the family* (pp. 39–42). New York: Grune and Stratton.

Boscolo, L, Cecchin, G., Hoffman, L., & Penn, P. (1987). *Milan systemic family therapy: Conversations in theory and practice.* New York: Basic Books.

Brown, L., & Gilligan, C. (1992). *Meeting at the crossroads: Women's psychology and girls' development.* Cambridge, MA: Harvard University Press.

Burchard, J. D, Bruns, E. J., & Burchard, S. N. (2002). The wraparound approach. In B. J. Burns & K. Hoagwood (Eds.), *Community treatment for youth: Evidence-based interventions for severe emotional and behavioral disorders* (pp. 69–90). New York: Oxford University Press.

Coffey, E. P., Olson, M. E., & Sessions, P. (2001). The heart of the matter: An essay about the effects of managed care on family therapy with children. *Family Process, 40,* 385–399.

Collaborative for Community and Family-Based Practice. (2001). *Innovations/dilemmas/reflections/recommendations.* Unpublished manuscript.

Educational Media Centre. (Producer). (1999). *An interview with harassment* [Motion picture]. (Available from Educational Media Centre, University of Auckland. Private Bag 92019, 23 Symond St., Auckland, New Zealand)

Freire, P. (1971). *Pedagogy of the oppressed.* New York: Seaview.

Freire, P. (2002). *Pedagogy of hope: Reliving pedagogy of the oppressed.* New York: Continuum.

Friedman, S. (1993). *The new language of change: Constructive collaboration in psychotherapy.* New York: Guilford.

Geertz, C. (1983). *Local knowledge: Further essays in interpretive anthropology.* New York: Basic Books.

Gergen, K. (1999). *An invitation of social construction.* London: Sage.

Gergen, K., & MacNamee, S. (2000). From disordering discourse to transformative dialogue. In R. Neimeyer & J. Raskin (Eds.), *Constructions of disorders* (pp. 333–349). Washington, DC: American Psychological Association.

Goldner, V., Penn, P., Sheinberg, M., & Walker, G. (1990). Love and violence: Gender paradoxes in volatile attachments. *Family Process, 29(40),* 343–364.

Griffith, J. L., & Griffith, M. E. (1994). *The body speaks: Therapeutic dialogues for mind-body Problems.* New York: Basic Books.

Griffith, J. L., & Griffith, M. E. (1995). When patients somatize and clinicians stigmatize: Opening dialogue between clinicians and the medically marginalized. In S. Friedman (Ed.), *The reflecting team in action: Collaborative practice in family therapy* (pp. 81–99). New York: Guilford.

Hardy, K. V., & Laszloffy, T. A. (1995). The cultural genogram: Key to training culturally competent family therapists. *Journal of Marital and Family Therapy, 21,* 227–237.

Henggeler, S. W., Schoenwald, S. K., Borduin, C. M., Rowland, M. D., & Cunningham, P. B. (1998). *Multisystemic treatment of antisocial behavior in children and adolescents.* New York: Guilford.

Herman, J. (1992). *Trauma and recover: The aftermath of violence—from domestic abuse to political terror.* New York: Basic Books.

Hoffman, L. (1986). Beyond power and control: Toward a "second-order" family systems therapy. *Family Systems Medicine, 4,* 381–396.

Hoffman, L. (2000). A communal perspective for relational therapies. *Journal of Feminist Family Therapy, 11*(4), 5–17.

Hoffman, L. (2002). *Family therapy: An intimate history*. New York: Norton.

Hunt, M., & Stern, J. (Trans.). (1944/1972). *The complete Grimm's fairy tales*. New York: Pantheon.

Jhally, Sut (Director). (1999). *Tough guise: Violence, media, and the crisis in masculinity* [Motion picture]. (Available from the Media Education Foundation, 26 Center Street, Northampton, MA 01060)

Krefting, L. (1990). Double bind and disability: The case of traumatic head injury. *Social Science and Medicine, 30*, 859–865.

Lightburn, A., Olson, M., Sessions, P., & Coffey, E. (2002). Practice innovations in mental health services to children and families: New directions for Massachusetts. *Smith Studies in Social Work, 72*, 279–301.

Lukens, E. P., & McFarlane, W. (2002). Families, social networks, and schizophrenia. In W. McFarlane (Ed.), *Multifamily groups in the treatment of severe psychiatric disorders* (pp. 18–35). New York: Guilford.

Mahmoud, V. M. (1998). The double binds of racism. In M. McGoldrick (Ed.), *Re-visioning family therapy: Race, culture, and gender in clinical practice* (pp. 255–267). New York: Guilford.

McGoldrick, M. (Ed.). (1998). *Re-visioning family therapy: Race, culture, and gender in clinical practice*. New York: Guilford.

Meyers, J., Kaufman, M., & Goldman, S. (1999). Promising practices: Training strategies for serving children with serious emotional disturbance and their families in a system of care. In SAMHSA (Eds.), *Systems of care: Promising practices in children's mental health, 1998 Series* (Vol. 5). Washington, DC: Center for Effective Collaboration and Practice, American Institutes for Research.

Minuchin, S. (1974). *Families and family therapy*. Cambridge, MA: Harvard University Press.

Olson, M. E. (1984). *Form, difference, and change: A study of Bateson, the Milan Associates, and second-generation family theory*. Unpublished master's thesis. Smith College School for Social Work. Northampton, MA.

Olson, M. E. (1995a). Conversation and writing: A collaborative approach to bulimia. *Journal of Feminist Family Therapy, 6*(4), 21–45.

Olson, M. E. (1995b). The family-therapy perspective. In S. Donner and P. Sessions (Eds.), *Garrett's interviewing: Its principles and methods* (4th ed., pp. 113–119). Milwaukee, WI: Families International.

Olson, M. E. (Ed.). (2000a). *Feminism, community, and communication*. Binghamton, NY: Haworth.

Olson M. E. (2000b). Listening to the voices of anorexia: The researcher as an "outsider-witness." *Journal of Feminist Family Therapy, 11*(4), 25–46.

Pakman, M. (1999). Designing constructive therapies in community mental health: Poetics and micropolitics in and beyond the consulting room. *Journal of Marital and Family Therapy, 25*, 83–98.

Penn, P. (2001). Chronic illness: Trauma, language, and writing: Breaking the silence. *Family Process, 40*, 33–52.

Reich, J. (1998, June). Do we know what students are getting from their education? *American Psychological Association Monitor*, 41.

Scott, J. (Producer), & Hicks, S. (Director). (1996). *Shine* [Motion picture]. Australia: South Australian Film and Film Victoria.

Seikkula, J. (2002a). Monologue is the crisis—dialogue becomes the aim of therapy. *Journal of Marital and Family Therapy, 28*, 275–277.

Seikkula, J. (2002b). Open dialogues with good and poor outcomes for psychotic crisis. Examples from families with violence. *Journal of Marital and Family Therapy, 28*, 263–274.

Seikkula, J., Aaltonen, J., Alakare, B., Haarakangas, K., Keränen, J., & Sutela, M. (1995). Treating psychosis by means of open dialogue. In S. Friedman (Ed.), *The reflective team in action* (pp. 62–80). New York: Guilford.

Seikkula, J., Alakare, B., & Aaltonen, J. (2001a). Open dialogue in psychosis I: An introduction and case illustration. *Journal of Constructivist Psychology, 14*, 247–266.

Seikkula, J., Alakare, B., & Aaltonen, J. (2001b). Open dialogue in first-episode psychosis II: A comparison of good and poor outcome cases. *Journal of Constructivist Psychology, 14*, 267–284.

Seikkula J., Alakare, B., Aaltonen, J., Holma, J., Rasinkangas, A., & Lehtinen, V. (2003) Open dialogue approach: Treatment principles and preliminary results of a two-year follow-up on first episode schizophrenia. *Ethical Human Sciences and Services, 5*, 1–20.

Seikkula, J., & Olson, M. (2003). The open dialogue approach to acute psychosis: Its poetics and micropolitics. *Family Process, 42*, 403–418.

Seikkula, J., & Sutela, M. (1990). Co-evolution of the family and the hospital: The system of boundary. *Journal of Strategic and Systemic Therapies, 9*, 32–42.

Selvini-Palazzoli, M., Boscolo, L., Cecchin, G., & Prata, G. (1978). *Paradox and counterparadox*. New York: Jason Aronson.

Sheinberg, M., & Fraenkel, P. (2001). *The relational trauma of incest: A family-based approach to treatment*. New York: Guilford.

Smith, C. (1997). Introduction: Comparing traditional

therapies with narrative approaches. In C. Smith & D. Nylund (Eds.), *Narrative therapies with children and adolescents* (pp. 1–52). New York: Guilford.

Smith, S. (2003). *Sparkling facts in the case of Javier.* Unpublished manuscript.

Stacey, J. (1996). *In the name of the family: Rethinking family values in the postmodern age.* Boston: Beacon.

Stern, S., Doolan, M., Staples, E., Szmukler, G., & Eisler, I. (1999). Disruption and reconstruction: Narrative insights into the experience of family members caring for a relative diagnosed with serious mental illness. *Family Process, 38,* 353–369.

Stone, O. (Producer), & Wang, W. (Director). (1993). *The joy luck club* [Motion picture]. United States: Hollywood Pictures.

Stroul, B. A. (2002). *A framework for system reform in children's mental health.* Washington, DC: Georgetown University Child Development Center, National Technical Assistance Center for Children's Mental Health, Child Development Center.

Stroul, B. A., & Friedman, R. M. (1986) *A system of care for severely emotionally disturbed children and youth.* Washington, DC: Georgetown University Development Center.

Tan, A. (1989). *The joy luck club.* New York: Putman.

U.S. Public Health Service. (2000). *Report of the Surgeon General's conference on children's mental health: Developing a national action agenda.* Washington, DC: Author.

VanDenBerg, J. E., & Grealish, E. M. (1996). Individualized services and supports through the wraparound process: Philosophy and procedures. *Journal of Child and Family Studies, 5,* 7–21.

Waldegrave, C. (1990). Social justice and family therapy: A discussion of the work of the family centre. *Dulwich Centre Newsletter,* no. 1, 1–47.

Waldegrave, C. (1998). The challenges of culture to psychology and postmodern thinking. In M. McGoldrick (Ed.), *Re-visioning family therapy: Race, culture, and gender in clinical practice* (pp. 404–413). New York: Guilford.

Watzlawick, P., Weakland, J., & Fisch, R. (1974). *Change: Principles of problem formation and problem resolution.* New York: Norton.

White, M. (1989/90). Family therapy training and supervision in a world of experience and narrative. *Dulwich Centre Newsletter,* Summer, 27–38.

White, M. (1995). *Reauthoring lives: Interviews and essays.* Adelaide: Dulwich Centre Publications.

White, M. (2003, August). *Constructing stories of empowerment.* Paper presented at Smith College School for Social Work. Northampton, MA.

White, M., & Epston, D. (1990). *Narrative means to therapeutic ends.* New York: Norton.

12

Martha Morrison Dore and Anita Lightburn

Evaluating Community-Based Clinical Practice

Program evaluation as a distinct field of professional practice was born of two lessons. . . . First, the realization that there is not enough money to do all the things that need doing; and second, even if there were enough money, it takes more than money to solve complex human and social problems. *As not everything can be done, there must be a basis for deciding which things are worth doing.* Enter evaluation.

(Michael Quinn Patton, 1997a, p. 11)

As this passage from Michael Quinn Patton indicates, evaluation of social programs and clinical practice has become an essential component of our collective efforts to solve, ameliorate, or prevent the problems and difficulties that negatively impact our communities and erode the lives of the people living in them. Beginning in the Great Society years of the 1960s, when evaluators sought to convince legislators and the general public that federally sponsored social programs were an effective approach to dealing with the problems of the poor and disenfranchised, evaluation has increasingly played a critical role in program development, as well as in assessing program outcomes (Cronbach, 1980). Indeed, the evaluation enterprise now wears multiple hats: (1) as facilitator in the development and implementation of new programs and services; (2) as a key source of understanding and direction in the revision of established programs; and (3) as the identifier, interpreter, and disseminator of program results. Contemporary evaluation is not only about accountability but also about knowledge building and program management. It is not an event that occurs at the end of the trail of program design and implementation but an ongoing process that starts with engaging practitioners and participants in identifying community needs and potential

means of addressing those needs. The life of an evaluation is the life of a program, existing simultaneously and bound inextricably in a dance of learning and change toward achieving a well-defined end: affecting systems change.

In this chapter, we will present a constructivist approach to evaluation that we believe honors the principles of community-based clinical practice. This approach is context for the three broadly defined roles of evaluation just described. It is our purpose to present a model of evaluation that is synchronous with these principles. We hope to enable those involved in implementing community-based clinical practice models to view evaluation as an essential tool in building their programs and practice.

Interestingly, over the past two decades, as the conceptualization of evaluation has evolved from focusing solely on demonstrating program effectiveness, the discourse has paralleled the emerging notion of community-based clinical practice. This is not to suggest that the evaluation field has abandoned its emphasis on accountability. Indeed, the discussion in this field reflects the divisions in epistemology in general between those who wholly embrace the positivist hypothetico-deductive approach to knowledge development, or, in this case,

153

to demonstrating the impact of a social initiative (see Boruch, 1994, for further discussion of this paradigm in program evaluation) and those who ascribe to a more constructivist approach to understanding program, process, and impact (Reichardt & Rallis, 1994). Those in the positivist group are inclined to focus on demonstrating program effectiveness by statistically testing a hypothesized causal relationship between program outcomes and the program elements aimed at achieving these outcomes. Those in the second, or constructivist, group believe that such an approach is too limiting, that the criteria for implementing a cause-effect approach to program evaluation are too restrictive and do not reflect the realities of community-based clinical practice. They see social programs as continually evolving entities that require an approach to evaluation that recognizes and captures this developmental process (Connell, Kubisch, Schorr, & Weiss, 1995; Schorr & Kubisch, 1995). Instead of focusing on explaining cause and effect, constructivist evaluators focus on understanding the process of program development and implementation as viewed by those intimately involved in that process. This understanding occurs through ongoing and in-depth contact and relationships with those involved, as opposed to the distanced objectivism of the positivist perspective.

Constructivist Evaluation Synchronous With Community-Based Clinical Practice

It seems clear to us that the constructivist perspective is closer to the principles of community-based clinical practice, even though there is room for both perspectives in evaluating these programs (Datta, 1997; Greene & Caracelli, 1997). Like this approach's emphasis on culturally responsive services, the constructivist perspective on evaluation calls for intimate knowledge of the characteristics of the systems in which a program is located in order to better shape the evaluation and interpret its implementation and outcomes. Community-based clinical practice reflects conceptualization and actualization of the concept of "self-in-community," which recognizes how the individual is shaped by community-level factors such as power relations, privilege, exclusionary criteria and

beliefs, racism, and other forms of oppression. Similarly, constructivist evaluation approaches attend to the impact of context on program design and implementation, as well as on program evolution and outcomes. In Dore's chapter in this volume, for example, she interprets the impact of the Family of Friends program, aimed at creating supportive communities for families in three day care centers, within the context of the history and administration of each center and within the context of the larger sociodemographic community surrounding the center, thereby increasing understanding of the barriers encountered in implementing the program model, as well as its outcomes. A positivist evaluation that looked simply at whether the intervention resulted in the intended outcomes would fail to capture the role of context in shaping how the intervention was actually implemented (differently in each center, as it turned out), as well as how context affected the program's effectiveness in achieving its proximal goals of increasing parent involvement, knowledge of child development, and use of age-appropriate methods of child discipline.

Constructivist approaches to program evaluation have given rise to particular evaluation models that also reflect principles of community-based clinical practice. These include participatory evaluation (Ayers, 1987; Whyte, 1991), stakeholder-based evaluation (Bryk, 1983; Greene, 1988), utilization-focused evaluation (Patton, 1997b; Patton, 2001), and empowerment evaluation (Fetterman, 1996; Fetterman, Kaftarian, & Wandersman, 1996; Schroes, Murphy-Berman, & Chambers, 2000; Scriven, 1997). As their titles convey, each of these models calls for inclusion of program participants (clients, clinicians, administrators, funders, community resources, etc.) in the development and implementation of program evaluation, albeit to varying degrees. The key issue is the role of the "expert" evaluator in the evaluation process, similar to the debate over the authority of the "expert" clinician in the processes of community-based clinical practice models (Stufflebeam, 2001). In the empowerment evaluation model, for example, Fetterman (1996) characterizes the relationship between evaluator and program participants as a collaborative partnership in which the participants, not the evaluator, control the evaluation process, formulating the evaluation questions, selecting the data collection instruments, designing and implementing the data collection process, and interpreting and disseminating the results. The evaluator may act as midwife, collaborator, mentor, or consultant, depending on the circumstances, but the evaluation is essentially an internally driven one controlled by program participants themselves.

We agree with Stufflebeam (2001) that constructivist evaluation models have a number of advantages. Implementation of each constructivist model is highly dependent on open communication among all parties to the intervention. Thus, they are all based on the ethical foundation of full disclosure, of both the evaluation process and its findings. Gone are mystical data collection processes imposed on participants, findings that present an abstraction of numbers gleaned through unintelligible statistical procedures, and final reports that serve only as collectors of dust on shelves, far out of reach of those for whom they are intended. Constructivist evaluation is based on the well-established clinical principle that individuals are more likely to engage in a process of change when they understand the process and feel included in its development. This principle is reflected in community-based clinical practice in its emphasis on strategies to involve both the service-providing community and individuals and families in the community in a collaborative process to build their collective capacity to promote the social and emotional well-being of all its members.

Constructivist approaches to evaluation focus on eliciting a variety of ideas and opinions from participants as precursor to reaching consensus regarding the questions to be answered through the evaluation. In this way, constructivist evaluation, like community-based clinical practice, acknowledges divergent perspectives and points of view, some of which may be culturally determined and others of which may be influenced by the location of the participant in the community's power structure, or by aspects of privilege conferred by the larger social context based on race, gender, or ability.

Involving Multiple Voices

The notion of the role of multiple voices in evaluation was introduced to the broader evaluation world by Robert Stake in the 1970s (Stake, 1983)

and has since been developed and refined by others in the field (see particularly Greene & Abma, 2001, for a compendium of papers on responsive evaluation, the term given to the evaluation process that deliberately seeks inclusion of multiple, often-silenced voices). Stake's notion of responsive evaluation is that it is informed by varying perspectives with differing values and expectations, such that the evaluator's initial conceptualization of the evaluation task is challenged and changed in response. Although Stake does not advocate actively including program participants in the evaluation process, he was among the first to recognize the differing perspectives that can inform (and inhibit) that process (Abma & Stake, 2001). Responsive evaluation is a flexible, dynamic process that embraces the inclusion of diverse perspectives. In addition to informing the evaluation, the responsive approach also interprets the evaluation findings according to the diverse perspectives and values of the participants. This not only recognizes the variety of participants' values in interpreting evaluation findings but also acknowledges the potentially diverse perspectives of the various audiences for evaluation results.

It is widely accepted that knowledge is situational, bound by context. To truly understand a program or social intervention, the evaluator must understand the beliefs and experiences of all involved and must honor and represent these in reporting evaluation results. Those who are invested in the outcomes of community-based clinical practice include not only program participants but also a wide variety of professional contributors who make up a multidisciplinary team: teachers and principals, physicians and nurses, social workers, psychologists, and guidance counselors. While these professional contributors may collaborate together in community programs, their professional training may be from different traditions, beliefs, and frames of reference such that priorities and practice agendas collide or compete. For example, many professionals focus on individual change rather than system change through work with transactions between individuals and their community. Understanding such differing professional perspectives is an important step in defining factors that may influence outcome. For example, a child mental health program that seeks to be family-centered may have very different outcomes if it employs clinicians trained in individual child therapy.

Responsive Evaluation Methods Honor Culture

Like community-based clinical practice, the responsive approach to evaluation recognizes and honors culture as an essential factor in shaping participants' responses and determining their value stances vis-à-vis a particular intervention and its evaluation (Madison, 1992). According to Hood (2001), it was not until Stake's groundbreaking explication of responsive evaluation, which recognized the value of qualitative methods for gathering data such as interviews, observations, and document reviews in the evaluation process, that mechanisms were present for capturing the cultural context of social interventions and for interpreting outcomes in that context. The priority of responsive evaluation is to provide the audience for its findings with a "vicarious experience" so that it can understand the "essence" of the program in all its dimensions, including that of culture (Hood, 2001, p. 37). For example, the description in this volume of the South Bronx programs provided by Levine and Eismann, and by Coffey and her colleagues of their work in Kosova, develops context as the central factor that shaped these interventions, responding to place, language, and tradition and beliefs.

In the evaluation process, concern about the role of culture in designing, conducting, and presenting the evaluation should be center stage for the research advisory committee and the evaluator. Culture should be acknowledged and responded to in determining what questions are asked, how outcomes are identified, what outcome measures are used, and how data are collected and interpreted. As Hoagwood and her colleagues (1996) point out from cross-cultural studies, "Culture constitutes more than a source of variation, it determines the conditions . . . of studying mental health" (p. 1057). The research advisory committee should be responsible for reviewing and evaluating the cultural accuracy and responsiveness of the evaluation design, implementation, and interpretation of findings. It should be clear to all consumers of the evaluation that culture has been a major informant of all aspects of the study.

The lived experience of the evaluator is also not separate from interpretation of program processes and evaluation findings. According to the constructivist perspective, it is central to that interpretation. As in community-based clinical practice, it is essential that evaluators, like clinicians, are aware of their own lived experiences, including culture, which colors understanding and interpretation of program events and evaluation findings. Exploration of the evaluator's cultural perspective through constant comparison with the values and understandings of a wide variety of program participants gleaned through in-depth interviews and observations allows the evaluator to gain new insight into how her own perspective enters into and colors her work.

The Challenges of Participant Involvement

The constructivist evaluator's belief in the importance of participant involvement in the evaluation process or, at the very least, in accurately representing participants' experiences in the social intervention under study, has challenged the field of evaluation practice to find ways of collaborating with those who were formerly objects of study. This is similar to the community-based clinical practice principle of engaging community members in identifying service needs, as well as ways to meet those needs that are syntonic with accepted and acceptable ways of communicating, relating, and helping within the context of community norms and values. Engagement of participants in both endeavors has meant relinquishing the "expert" position, with its accompanying privilege and power. A true collaboration between evaluator and participants as called for in most constructivist evaluation models suggests that both have critical expertise to bring to the endeavor and that one is not more valued than the other. While the evaluator may possess special training in the principles and techniques of evaluation, without the contextual and experiential knowledge of participants, the evaluator's tools are without essential materials with which to craft an appropriate evaluation design.

This process of mutual collaboration is not without its challenges, however. It is often a lengthy and demanding process to solicit multiple perspectives and to integrate competing personal and political interests into a rational model for evaluating a particular program or intervention. Warren-Adamson (2002) describes extensive negotiation with six UK family resource centers to implement a parenting scale, where administrators were concerned that they demonstrate positive outcomes, since services were in danger of being cut. The evaluation findings raised more questions than were answered, partly because the family center participants had not been involved in evaluation planning and because the parenting scale was externally imposed. Subsequently, the evaluator and stakeholders reexamined how the selected outcome measures had been negotiated with attention to the power politics within the centers themselves. The complexity of that negotiation process became apparent to all, and reexamination of that process provided the impetus to bring all family service center stakeholders (including parents) together to determine what influenced outcomes in this complex ecosystem, what services mattered most to parents, and what measures would be sensitive enough to capture important outcomes within a relatively short time period. Parents clearly voiced the difference the program had made in their lives, despite the lack of strong positive results from the outcome measure that had been used. Fortunately, political leaders listened, and the programs were not defunded.

Bringing participants such as agency administrators, supervisors, clinicians, clients, agency board members, and agency outsiders such as community collaborators to the table to forge agreement on program goals, desired service outcomes, and the essential questions to be answered in the evaluation regarding program design and implementation, as well as benefits to clients, is a daunting task indeed. Meezan and McBeath (2004) recently completed a study of capitated child welfare services in Wayne County, Michigan, in which they gathered together personnel from nine private, not-for-profit child welfare agencies that contracted with the county to provide services to children and their families entering the child welfare system. According to Meezan, the team at the table often numbered 30 to 40 people from the nine agencies. The agency roles of working group members ranged from administrator to frontline staff. The initial purpose of this group was to design an evaluation of the impact of capitation on service delivery. Meezan and McBeath believed that, unless the participants in the study were also responsible for the de-

sign and collection of data, any adverse findings would be rejected by the participating agencies as an artifact of the evaluation design. When it was found that capitation resulted in severely truncated service delivery to children and their families when compared with agencies providing noncapitated services, the agencies embraced the study's findings and used them to explore reasons for this effect, rather than fighting the findings themselves. Meezan admits, however, that gathering representatives from nine agencies with very different histories, funding sources, and treatment philosophies, and creating a collaborative working group was a long and sometimes arduous process—and this group did not include agency clients or outside collaborators.

Research Advisory Committees to Guide Evaluation

One mechanism that we have used to good effect in past evaluations is to create a Research Advisory Committee for each project. This mechanism was first suggested by Peter Pecora, research director at Casey Family Programs, where it has worked well in that multisite, multistate agency's extensive research and evaluation endeavors. The research advisory committee is composed of the evaluation team, agency personnel, including administrators, supervisors, and line staff, agency clients, and representatives of community groups with whom the agency closely collaborates. Members of the research advisory committee are usually program specific, that is, they are closely involved or will be involved in the program for which the evaluation design is being created. Again, the initial steps in creating a truly collaborative working group are to elicit the multiple perspectives of group members concerning the purpose and goals of the program or intervention to be studied. We have found that the time invested in the discussion of program goals and the mechanisms designed to reach those goals is valuable in establishing both the tenor of the collaboration and the conceptual model of the program's theory of change. Too often in social programs, the theory underlying the relationship between a program's intended users, the activities intended to bring about change, and the program's proximal and distal goals is unarticulated. Spending time exploring why it is that the particular activities or interventions offered by a program are believed to be efficacious in addressing a problem or condition presented by the targeted client group is critical to designing an evaluation plan that will truly capture the program's intent.

Theory-Driven Evaluations and Reconciling Different Theories of Change

Along these lines, theory-driven evaluation has come to the fore as an approach to evaluation that responds to the lack of well-articulated relationships between program activities and outcomes so often seen in social programs (Bickman, 1987; Chen, 1990; Connell et al., 1995; Weiss, 1995, 1998). The usefulness of a theory of change in community-based clinical practice programs has been summed up by Chaskin (2002) as a means to "tame the initiative's complexity, reduce its uncertainty and harness its evolutionary nature in order to make it more evaluable" (p. 32). The challenge in these programs is that often multiple perspectives and different theories of change must be reconciled. An exploration of the basis for different perspectives is an important dialogue that evaluators can facilitate. Research may be required to support different perspectives through reviewing the available evidence.

A case in point concerns evaluations of integrated family support programs that provide a positive alternative to current child welfare practice in the United States and United Kingdom that often separates children and parents. However, randomized and experimental studies of family support programs have shown mixed results because of oversimplification of the program model, failure to adequately describe or measure the treatment provided, and the "paucity of good measures to assess the effect of these programs on parents, families and communities" (Weiss & Greene, 1992, p. 137). Evaluators have also expressed concern about the limited attention given in these evaluations to how context mediates program outcomes (Bond & Halpern, 1988; Lightburn, 2002; Weiss & Halpern, 1990; Weiss & Jacobs, 1988). These early efforts to evaluate family support programs taught researchers in community-based programs to appreciate program complexity and the role of context in shaping evaluation implementation and out-

comes. They recognized that a sound theoretical framework is required to do justice to the potential of a community-based program, like family support centers, as a robust alternative for families and children who are at risk for poor long-term outcomes.

Warren-Adamson and Lightburn (this volume) have worked toward building a theory of change grounded in case examples drawn from evaluations of integrated family support programs over the past two decades. These authors appreciate the evolutionary nature of family support programs (Lightburn, 2002; Warren-Adamson, 2002) and the challenge of developing program evaluations that capture the positive outcomes that staff and participants report in their narratives of individual and program success. This experience highlights the urgent need for sensitive quantitative outcome measures (Warren-Adamson, 2002; Wigfall & Moss, 2001).

Developing Theories of Change That Involve Community

Program staff can benefit from evaluators' assistance in identifying theories that support interventions in community settings and that dynamically use community in the therapeutic process. In our experience, when staff members are asked to elaborate on their reasons for choosing a program design or a particular method of helping, they quickly become engaged in thinking carefully and often creatively about the fit between client need and capacity and the realities of community-based clinical practice. Staff involvement in identifying a theory of change is particularly important in the development of community-based practice, as clinicians frequently have not considered the various meanings of community that are important to their own work and their clients' well-being (see Swenson, this volume; Saleebey, this volume). The complex realities of community must be represented in the processes of practice, as well as its outcomes. It is helpful to map how various definitions of community may influence change for the purpose of understanding need, as well as capacity and assets, so that the ways in which context mediates outcome can be fully considered. In this respect we value Chaskin's (2002) perspective that:

> it is important to consider the "community's social fabric" as both an outcome goal and as a

mediating variable that influences how—and to what extent—community change can occur. These community-based interventions thus seek both to work through the infrastructure of communities in order to achieve particular outcome objectives (e.g., reductions in child abuse, improvement in school achievement, . . .) and to strengthen the social infrastructure itself; they seek to "build community" by strengthening community resources, enhancing social interaction among members and promoting "social capital" as a collective good available to community members. (p. 28)

The evaluator can ask key questions that enable staff members to consider more fully the realities and impact of community, thereby stretching their notion of the boundaries of practice and opening up new possibilities that should be considered for more effective community-based practice. If this review is done at the outset of the evaluation, at the very least there is opportunity to focus and refine the program design, and at best it helps staff rethink priorities and gives new direction to their work.

We agree with Stufflebeam (2001) that the evaluator should not usurp the responsibility of staff to define theory, avoiding the potentially awkward position of evaluating a theory of his or her own creation. However, we join with others in suggesting that identifying the theoretical models of change that underlie community initiatives is an essential first step in developing appropriate evaluations and in understanding and interpreting evaluation outcomes (Connell et al., 1995). We have observed in collaborating with staff that the theoretical framework of a program or social initiative is often an unspoken assumption, lying just below the surface of program staffs' consciousness and simply awaiting the probing of the evaluator to bring it to life. In general, staff members can be readily engaged in exploring questions about why certain activities or interventions were selected for the program over others to effect the desired changes and achieve the outcomes sought. The evaluator's expertise facilitates staff in bringing to the surface latent assumptions about change in the program's focal problems or issues.

The work of Argyris and Schön (1974) on the use of theory in practice, as well as current research on the unconscious use of Baysian logic by athletes to anticipate future outcomes and shape their responses accordingly (Wolpert & Körding, 2004), assures us that a logic model always underlies the choices made in designing social programs or initiatives. Evaluators do not carry responsibility for inventing a program theory but, rather, should engage program staff and others in recognizing and articulating this framework.

Logic Models and a Learning Organization Approach to Theory Development

The use of logic models offers another means of assisting staff in discovering their theory of change, as it relates to activities and outcome. Wright and Paget (2002) report from their experience as evaluators helping agencies work on systems change that a learning organization approach using logic models engages staff in making connections between goals and objectives and the process of change. Such an approach can be integral to the development of effective community-based clinical practice models, as clinicians are challenged to examine underlying assumptions that may lead to shifts in their thinking about how they practice.

Evaluations over the last two decades of the system of care approach to meeting the needs of children and adolescents with severe emotional and behavior problems illustrate the difficulty of assessing a model whose theory of change is not shared by policymakers and clinical staff (Lightburn, 2002; Stroul, 2002). Clinicians working in programs that are part of the child mental health system of care model are often unaware of the theory of change that supports their work. A tenet of the system of care model is the centrality of family in the life of the child and the need to work holistically with the child in the family context to effect change in the child's psychosocial functioning. In contrast, clinicians frequently focus treatment on the child alone, without attention to the importance of the family in the therapeutic process (Green, Johnson, & Rodgers, 1998). A more beneficial approach to meeting the needs of children and adolescents with severe emotional and behavioral disorders would engage clinicians and administrators together in developing a logic model for their particular program context. Clinicians may be unaware of the theory of change that supports how they work within the system of care to achieve positive outcomes. For example, the system of care philosophy emphasizes family involvement at the clinical, program, and policy levels, which means that families are seen as collaborators and partners in working on solutions to their children's problems (Stroul, 1996). This laudable principle is not often implemented in practice. Instead, a traditional emphasis on child-centered individual change is used, a treatment approach that minimally engages the family and that certainly does not view families as partners (Green et al., 1998; Lightburn, 2002).

A beneficial approach to this disconnect between policy and practice involves working with clinicians to review their logic models to identify the theory of change that informs their practice with children with severe emotional disturbance. This necessarily includes reviewing current research that supports the centrality of working with families who are the enduring caretakers of their children. As collaborators in the evaluation process, clinicians can review their practice theories and explore and negotiate divergent theoretical understandings with the goal of coming to agreement in order to work in concert with system of care policies (Lightburn, 2002; Schön, 1983; Stroul, 1996, 2002).

A Grounded Theory Approach to Identifying a Theory of Change

In their work on grounded theory, Glaser and Strauss (1967) suggest another approach to identifying the theoretical base for a program. Unlike the dialogue we advocate with program participants, their approach is based on a systematic process of observing program activities, interviewing participants, and reviewing program documentation, leading to an inductive understanding of theorized relationships between client, intervention, and outcomes. The process described by Glaser and Strauss for developing a grounded theoretical understanding of a program model is very like the methods used in a formative or process evaluation, which we will describe later in this chapter. Combining these two approaches and using the formative evaluation process to confirm or revise a program's logic model as developed through discussion with program participants would help ensure that interpretation of findings regarding pro-

gram outcomes is solidly grounded in a well-defined theory base.

Integrating Constructivist Approaches With the Essential Program Evaluation Functions

In the beginning of this chapter, we identified three essential functions of program evaluation. These, in brief, were to (1) facilitate the development and implementation of new programs and strategies for addressing social and community problems; (2) support the ongoing review and revision of existing programs to meet changing participant and community needs; and (3) assess a program's ability to achieve its intended outcomes. These three functions are reflected in formative, process, and outcome evaluations. In the next section of this chapter we will examine these three types of evaluation, discuss their implementation in community-based clinical practice programs, and provide some examples of their utility in achieving their desired ends.

Formative Evaluation

As the name suggests, formative evaluation is focused on the development of new programs or strategies for addressing social problems. For this type of evaluation to occur, the evaluator must be engaged from the beginning in the design and development of the intended initiative. A formative evaluation includes two key elements: the needs assessment and the pilot study. The concept of needs assessment is well known to community-based practitioners, who are likely to conduct a such an assessment with individual clients or client groups as part of the treatment planning process. The needs assessment in formative evaluation is broader in scope but serves a similar purpose of identifying the extent and characteristics of a problem, issue, or concern, factors contributing to the problem, and resources currently available to ameliorate it, and the impact or potential impact of the problem on those who are likely to participate in the program or intervention designed to address the problem. In an evaluation approach designed to involve participants from the beginning, the needs assessment would be carried out by potential program participants in collaboration with agency staff.

One example of such a collaboration was a needs assessment carried out at the Lowell, Massachusetts, division of Casey Family Services, a multistate agency that addresses the needs of families who are at risk of problems in parenting and poor developmental outcomes for their children. The agency sought to develop a family support center in a public housing project in downtown Lowell serving a predominantly immigrant population of Cambodians and Latinos, primarily Puerto Ricans. Agency staff members engaged with residents in the housing project who spoke English to design a brief interview questionnaire that could easily be translated into other languages and would elicit residents' ideas regarding community problems, needs, and possible solutions. They used this questionnaire as a guide to interview as many residents of the housing project as possible. The residents who were interviewed proved to be most concerned about their children. These concerns included the failure of the local school to provide English as a second language (ESL) services to children and their parents or to address immigrant children's special learning needs, the parents' inability to help their children with homework, and fears about how their children were spending their free time, especially in light of the rampant drug dealing in the streets just outside the project. Parents universally wanted their children to succeed in their adopted country but did not understand enough of the language or culture to be of help to them in that process. With the results of this community needs assessment in mind, the Casey staff and community residents designed a family support center that would offer an after-school homework club and Saturday and holiday activities for children, youth, and families, as well as employ native-speaking staff to help non-English-speaking parents advocate for their children's needs at the local school. Once community residents saw that the family support center staff was responsive to their concerns about their children, more families became involved in the center's activities, suggesting additional programs and services such as ESL and computer classes for adults, which were added in response.

This example not only documents the importance of the needs assessment as a first step in the formative evaluation but also illustrates the iterative process of program development, which must be taken into consideration when designing any type of evaluation. Most social interventions are fluid, shaping services in response to the changing needs of participants. This is especially true in community-based clinical practice, where part of what sets these programs and services apart is their responsiveness to community concerns and their commitment to community development. Communities, no matter how these are defined, are constantly changing and in flux as changes occur in the larger political, economic, and social systems that affect them. The Ayers and Lyman chapter in this volume aptly describes the evolution of one agency's program in response to changing community needs over time. Trying to capture an evolving program with only standardized outcome measures is a little like trying to hit a moving target; no matter at what point the outcome data are gathered, by the time they are analyzed and the final report is produced, the program itself is often no longer what it was at the time it was measured. A community needs assessment as part of program planning, and as part of a periodic program review, can begin to help identify changing community conditions and priorities and inform services in a preventive rather than reactive way.

Pilot Testing a Program's Design

A pilot test of a program model can also be part of the formative evaluator's tool kit. Those designing and implementing new programs and services can plan to collect data for a specific period: long enough so that a program will have had time to provide a full complement of services to participants, but not so long as to become institutionalized in a particular way of doing things. This makes it possible to revamp and revise as understanding grows of how the program is unfolding. A pilot period in rolling out a new program or initiative can also provide the evaluator an opportunity to test out methods for collecting process and outcome data on the program. This can help avoid the costly discovery later that a carefully chosen instrument does not adequately capture the changes the program is intended to bring about, or that participants' progress in the program is different than initially believed so that the designated data collection points are inadequate or irrelevant in relation to the process of change.

In one family reunification program with which

we are familiar, the initial evaluation design, based on the program model, called for collecting data on the return of children in foster care to their biological families at 6 months after entering care. It quickly became clear in the program's pilot period that, for most families, 6 months was too early for reunification to take place, so that measuring this event at that time point made the program appear to be failing its participants. However, measuring family reunification 12 months after foster care entry demonstrated that most families in the program were able to adequately address the problems and conditions that had contributed to child placement by that time. Those families who were unable to respond to the opportunities offered by the family reunification program by 12 months after placement were observed to be unlikely to do so no matter how much time elapsed. Revision of the evaluation design on the basis of the pilot study allowed for a more responsive and reflective data collection schedule and thereby ensured more accurate assessment of the program's effects.

Revising a program design or its approach to service delivery as the result of a formative evaluation pilot study is not cheating; it is good business. In fact, one model of evaluation, known as developmental evaluation, emerged from the management consulting and organization development literature (Patton, 1994). In this model, according to Patton (1997a), "the evaluator becomes part of the [program] design team helping to shape what's happening, both processes and outcomes, in an evolving, rapidly changing environment of constant interaction, feedback, and change" (p. 106). Patton contrasts developmental evaluation with what he calls more traditional models of evaluation that are based on theories of change, incorporate well-specified treatment approaches, and establish clear outcome goals. We would disagree that these two approaches to evaluation are different or mutually exclusive, but we suggest that there is always a developmental aspect to any evaluation. Like the stages of therapeutic intervention, which require different techniques, the formative and process stages of program development require different approaches to evaluation: more developmental in the early stages and more traditionally outcome oriented in later stages. Although, as noted earlier, social programs and initiatives are always in some state of flux, the literature on organizational development suggests that all systems, whether they are

organizations or programs within organizations, seek some level of stasis over time and are most open to influence and change in the early stages of their development (Kanter, Stein, & Jick, 1992).

Process Evaluation

Although some experts on evaluation use the terms "formative evaluation" and "process evaluation" interchangeably, we separate them here to emphasize their different roles and functions in the evaluation process. The formative evaluation, occurring as it does at the very beginning of the program development process, focuses on generating information to aid in program design and implementation planning; process evaluation helps program participants understand the actual operations of the program once it is up and running. The overarching question for the process evaluator is, Is this social program or initiative being implemented as designed? If not, What are the contextual and systemic forces that are reshaping the program over time? In other words, simply put, What is happening and why? For, unless we understand what happens to our program models on the ground, so to speak, our understanding of their impact and outcomes is greatly limited.

This is the primary difference between intervention research, which takes place in tightly controlled settings where the context has little impact on the implementation of the intervention, and program evaluation, which occurs in real-world settings where anything goes, and even the most well-thought-out, well-designed program is constantly shaped and buffeted by forces that cannot be controlled. Stories in the evaluation literature are legion about well-funded demonstrations of program effectiveness, designed to adhere to all the tenets of scientific rigor, that were sabotaged in one way or another by some unforeseen force in the environment. Often this has to do with failure of the treatment to be implemented as designed because of lack of training of clinicians in the model. Treatment manuals are now de rigueur for any implementation of a particular intervention model, though it is unclear if reading a manual is sufficient to ensure adherence to a particular treatment approach without ongoing training and supervision of clinicians. There is also concern that manualized treatments are too narrowly focused and do not allow for the intuition and creativity that are part of the armamentarium of any good clinician. One response to concerns over fidelity in program implementation is the process evaluation, which uses a variety of strategies and techniques to answer the question, What's happening and why?

Process evaluation employs a variety of data collection strategies and techniques to capture the program implementation process, often including qualitative methods such as observation, interviewing, and analyzing written documents. Observation of meetings of program staff, clinical case conferences, meetings with community partners, and even individual and group treatment sessions may be carried out to help create a picture of how the program or initiative is actually functioning. One strategy that has been effectively used in a process evaluation carried out by Everett, Homstead, and Drisko (2004) is to employ diarists, or individuals who are familiar with the community but are not a part of the program or its sponsoring agency, to act as local observers at all program-related program related activities and events. These diarists are trained in advance to look for particular elements in the program's implementation that are identified in advance by the participants and are reflective of the program's purpose and goals. Examples of such program elements would be the level of client input into ongoing program planning, or the degree to which program staff recognize and respond to community residents' culturally determined beliefs about seeking help and communicating personal problems. Diarists could capture the number of times clients serving on the program's planning committee offered specific suggestions regarding program enhancements or changes or, in the latter case, how often program staff mention cultural beliefs or concerns in program planning meetings or in individual case conferences. If a program is designed as a collaboration among participant groups, including clients, clinicians, supervisors, administrators, and community partners, observing who attends planning meetings and whose voices are heard and ideas attended to would be an essential aspect of a process evaluation.

Effective process evaluations depend on the knowledge and skills of the evaluation staff. It is difficult for evaluators unfamiliar with frontline practice to provide the rich observations that capture the essence of clinical interventions. Clinicians trained as participant observers increase the likelihood that critical information will not be overlooked. The practice experience of clinician/observers provides an invaluable point of reference for exploring details of their experiences with the program under study with other clinicians and clients, as well as administrators. There is the potential for a more nuanced understanding when clinician/observers evaluate programs similar to those in which they have worked. Observer training, validity checks, triangulation of data, and member checking all help to ensure the reliability of observational data gathered by clinician/observers.

Informed Consent: An Ethical Concern in Evaluation

A word of caution: ethical considerations regarding the use of human subjects are of utmost importance in implementing any kind of program evaluation that gathers data on living individuals, no matter whether it is via observation, interviewing, or reviewing (nonpublic) case records. The individuals who are being interviewed or observed or read about must know that this is taking place and why, and have the option of refusing to participate in the evaluation. Written consent must be obtained from all evaluation participants. The federal government has issued very specific guidelines for consent forms, which must describe (1) the purpose of the program and of the evaluation; (2) how the evaluation is to be carried out; (3) what will be expected of the participant in the evaluation; (4) any potential ill effects that the participant may suffer from participating in the evaluation; (5) the benefits to the participant from participating in the evaluation; (6) the participant's right to refuse to participate and how to express that right. Participants who are receiving services from a program or intervention must understand that their services will not be affected in any way if they choose not to participate in the evaluation process. A paragraph at the end of the consent form must indicate that the individual signing the form has read it and has had the opportunity to ask questions about any part of it that he or she does not understand. This paragraph also gives the name and contact information (usually a telephone number) of the person carrying out the evaluation in case the participant has further questions about the evaluation or later wishes to withdraw consent. The consent form is signed by both the participant and a witness, usually whoever is explaining the evaluation process to the participant. Often this is a clinician or other staff member in the program. The original copy of the signed consent form is kept in the agency's records, and a photocopy is given to the participant. The consent form should be consistent with principles of community-based clinical practice in reflecting the language, reading level, and forms of expression of program participants. A well-constructed and sensitively presented consent form expresses respect for the privacy concerns, as well as the altruistic impulses of participants.

If the program being evaluated is part of, or is funded by, a larger agency or organization, that entity may have, as part of its organizational structure, an institutional review board (IRB). This is a group of people well versed in research ethics who review all proposals for research and evaluation to be carried out under that particular organization's auspices. The purpose of this review is to ensure that all necessary efforts have been made to protect research participants from any harm. If the program is being evaluated by an outside evaluator, that individual may have access to an IRB review through a university or other affiliation. Though not required by law unless the agency undertaking the evaluation receives government funding for research, an IRB review helps to authenticate the ethical legitimacy of the endeavor.

Developing Qualitative Data

Interviewing the multiple layers of participants in a program or social initiative is a common way to inform a process evaluation. It is important to elicit a variety of perspectives from those inside and outside the program because each category of participant—client, clinician, supervisor, administrator, board member, community collaborator—will have a different perspective on the program and a different point of view regarding its implementation. In our experience, those most removed from the actual day-to-day work of the program are likely to describe a more conceptual understanding of its implementation, whereas those such as clients and clinicians who are closest to daily practice tend to report on elements of the program as it is operating on the ground. Administrators focus on evidence of actualization of the program's overall phi-

losophy, whereas clinicians cite practical concerns such as timely response to referrals or difficulties in involving external collaborators in case conferences. Integrating these perspectives to develop a complete understanding of the program as implemented requires matching them against the program model as originally conceptualized to locate similarities and differences. This underscores the importance of spending time up front developing a complete program description to provide criteria for the process evaluation.

Another technique frequently used in process evaluations is extracting data on program implementation from written records, including meeting minutes, client case records, agency management information system (MIS) printouts, billing records, and other program-level documentation. Agency MIS data often capture client demographics, referral information, treatment planning, including treatment goals and actions to be taken to attain those goals, community collaborations, case activity, and length of treatment. These data are essential to understanding whether the program is actually serving the client population it was intended to serve; who the sources of referral are and whether additional cultivation of referral sources needs to be done; whether treatment planning is occurring as described in the original program description (i.e., goals are clearly specified, time limited, and achievable; actions to achieve those goals are consistent with the program's theory of change); whether community resources are actively sought and collaborations with external providers developed; what the level of case activity is and where these activities are taking place (in the agency, in the community, in the client's home); and how long clients are participating in the program. Process data are essential to guide program administration and staff in refining program components. They are also critical in explaining outcomes that can have far-reaching implications for policy and practice decisions. In the first instance, an example drawn from the second author's work with a comprehensive early childhood program—the use of management logs at chosen representative intervals—helped staff understand how they used their time, described what services were provided, and identified barriers to service provision. Staff members were excellent consultants on developing categories that had meaning to them, based on their experience and expectations of what was involved in fulfilling the program's mission. This type of process information enabled staff and administration to gain a perspective on what it took to do their work, what tasks they were actually able to do, the realities of time invested in travel and networking, and how to predict future workload. This information was also used to rethink the focus of the program based on initial goals.

Process evaluation data are equally invaluable in interpreting final evaluation outcomes. An example of an outcome evaluation that poses serious concern for policymakers, practitioners, and evaluators alike can be seen in the findings of the Fort Bragg systems of care study that compared strategies for improving outcomes for children and adolescents with serious emotional problems. Wide discussion and debate have been given to the evaluator's conclusion that the considerable investment in providing community-based services with a system of care approach did not merit that investment when compared with other systems that were not as costly and that produced similar outcomes (Bickman et al., 1995). Hoagwood's (1997) rigorous review of the Fort Bragg study findings shows how process variables were key to understanding outcomes. She challenges the conclusion drawn by Bickman and colleagues that a system of care approach does not improve clinical outcomes based on her observation that process variables were neither sufficiently developed in the research design nor adequately addressed in the analysis. This critical omission should be heeded by all who are involved in community-based evaluation studies.

Community-based clinical services that work across multiple service systems require complex networks to support clinical goals in new ways. An example would be wraparound services for seriously emotionally disturbed youth that often require collaboration and sharing of resources across various domains such as education, mental health, child welfare, social services, and physical health care. It is therefore essential that evaluators and program administrators invest time in defining terms that describe accurately the service network, relationships between providers, and service linkages. Development of a network of services in community-based programs is an ongoing activity that should be tracked over time, with special attention to quality of service provision. These are important data in the interpretation of distal outcomes such as reduction in psychiatric hospitalization or placement in foster care.

Refining and Ensuring Quality Interventions

In our experience, a process evaluation can be instrumental in identifying additional staff training needs. In one early childhood intervention program evaluated by the first author (Dore), the process evaluation quickly identified gaps in clinicians' knowledge of how to set clear, achievable, incremental goals with clients as a mechanism for helping participants advance their parenting skills. In another program, this one a family-based intervention with children with serious emotional disturbances and their families, it became clear that clinicians required ongoing training and case consultation in the ecosystemic/structural approach to family treatment that provided the program's theory of change. Without continued support and supervision, clinicians often reverted to the psychodynamic therapies in which they had been trained, focusing on the treatment needs of the child rather than taking a holistic view of the family system as articulated in the program model. Treatment "drift" is, in fact, one of the greatest threats to implementing community-based clinical practice models. As Ayers and Lyman describe so well in their chapter in this book, helping clinicians embrace and implement a new approach to treatment, particularly one that challenges their previous training and practice and requires new behaviors on the clinicians' part, is a significant challenge in developing community-based programs.

The goal of the process evaluation, then, is to understand and document the day-to-day reality of the program or initiative under study. It uses information gleaned from personal observation, participant interviews, and documentation of program-related events to develop a picture of how the program as designed is working in reality. It recognizes that community-based programs are open to influences from various elements in the social, political, and economic environment and are shaped by the skills and deficits of their various participants. Although a detailed description of a program model in all its various dimensions can aid in ensuring its implementation as originally conceived, there is no program or initiative that is implemented exactly as initially intended. Indeed, part of what makes a program community based is its flexibility in responding to changing community and participant needs. The results of a process evaluation must be considered to be a snapshot at a point in time, designed to inform participants of how the program looks at that moment, not how it will look at some time in the future. With this in mind, it is important to engage in periodic process evaluations, or "checkups," of programs that are in existence over a long period to ensure that they are continuing to respond to community need and are reflective of the various dimensions, including population characteristics, of the communities in which they are located. Communities change over time, and one role of process evaluation is to enable programs to respond to that change in an informed way. Good process evaluations are also substantive resources for strategic planning. It is in the ways we have outlined above that evaluation fulfills the second function noted in the opening paragraph of this chapter: as a key source of understanding and direction in revising established programs. We now turn to the third function of program evaluation: the identifier, interpreter, and disseminator of program results.

Outcome Evaluation

When many people think of a formal program evaluation, the first word that comes to mind is "judgment." The popular conception of an evaluation is about judging the worthiness of a particular program or social intervention in relation to its effectiveness in addressing some social problem or issue. Although as we hope we have demonstrated here, there is much more to evaluating a program than simply judging its worthiness, there is no question that a summative or outcome evaluation allows for judgments to be made regarding the program's effectiveness in achieving its goals and making the changes it intended to make in whatever problem, issue, or concern it was designed to address. As the quotation from Patton at the beginning of this chapter indicates, when there are limited resources and many community needs, it is absolutely incumbent on agencies and organizations to identify the

most effective and efficient ways of meeting those needs. As we know, demonstrating program effectiveness is often a complicated endeavor, one that siphons precious resources away from providing direct services to clients to spending them on proving that programs actually do what they claim. This can be particularly difficult when the evidence that is demanded is costly to gather and provide, or when the demands for rigor in collecting this evidence are dysynchronous with the values and beliefs of the service providers. An example of the latter is the expectation that the only truly valid and reliable method for evaluating program outcomes is the gold standard of research design, the randomized experimental study.

During the 1960s and 1970s, as a result of the work of Campbell and Stanley (1963), Cronbach (1980), and others, the true experimental design in which program applicants were randomly assigned to treatment and no-treatment groups was held out as the only way to evaluate social programs (Stufflebeam, 2001). The difficulties in conducting true randomized outcome evaluations became quickly apparent as they require not only substantial funding but also widespread agreement among program participants to be implemented effectively. Participants, including clinicians and clients, have often objected on ethical grounds to assigning persons with particular problems or needs to a no-treatment control group. Believers in the power of experimental design to demonstrate causal relationships between program activities and treatment outcomes respond that assigning clients to receive an unproved treatment may not be any better than assignment to a no-treatment group. Such a perspective does not reassure those who believe that a treatment program is effective based on their own clinical intuition and experience, mechanisms that are increasingly recognized as playing important roles in building knowledge for practice (Schön, 1983).

It is incumbent on those invested in demonstrating the effectiveness of community-based clinical practice to join with evaluators, consultants, and research scholars to develop better strategies for capturing the complexity of these interventions (including mediating factors), as well as more sensitive measures of proximal outcomes that can identify progress toward the distal outcomes sought by the program. Using current methods, only about one third of rigorous randomized studies of community-based programs show positive outcomes, whereas studies done in controlled research settings support significant beneficial effects for the same interventions (Hoagwood, 1997). Each new evaluation of community-based clinical programs provides an opportunity to advance the quality of evaluation design, to improve program development and implementation, and ultimately to increase knowledge about what works with whom and why. As we work to develop more effective ways of evaluating community-based clinical practice, substantial guidance can be gleaned from the national evaluations of family service centers reviewed by the second author (Lightburn, 2002) and the recent system of care evaluations of the Comprehensive Community Mental Health Services Program (Friesen & Winters, 2003; Holden et al., 2003).

Quasi-experimental Outcome Evaluations

As a result of the difficulties in implementing randomized experimental designs in outcome studies, alternative methods, including quasi-experimental designs, are commonly used to test program effectiveness. The question to be answered is, What are the results of this program or intervention for those who are expected to benefit in some way? Quasi-experimental designs, though not as powerful as the randomized experimental design in controlling for threats to the validity and reliability of findings, are somewhat easier to implement and less objectionable in ethical terms for many program participants. One form of quasi-experimental design that is frequently used in outcome evaluations is randomly assigning participants to one of two different programs so that every participant receives some form of treatment. Often one of the treatments represents the customary treatment for a particular problem or issue, and the other treatment represents an alternative to, change in, or enhancement of the customary treatment.

An example of this type of quasi-experimental outcome evaluation is the first author's study that tested the effectiveness of adding a mental health component to an early home visiting program. The original program was designed to address the need for parenting information and instruction on the developmental needs of infants by first-time ado-

lescent parents. The intervention consisted of periodic home visits by a paraprofessional who was trained to observe parent-infant interaction and give advice to new parents on infant stimulation activities. After this program had been up and running for a while, the home visitors began to convey to their supervisors concerns about certain clients who seemed listless and unable to respond to their infant's behavioral cues, even with support and instruction. After a needs assessment, which included a standardized depression scale for the mothers, showed that a substantial portion of the very young mothers in the program had elevated depression levels, program staff decided to add a mental health component to the program in the form of a trained clinician who would carry those cases in which the mother was determined on the basis of the depression assessment to be at high risk of mental health problems and insecure infant attachment. The mental health clinician would do the parenting education and infant development instruction that were customarily done by paraprofessionals but would address the emotional needs of the mothers through counseling as well. Unfortunately, there were many more first-time young mothers with elevated depression levels than could be handled by the mental health clinician; therefore, some continued to be seen by the paraprofessional staff, providing opportunity for a naturally occurring quasi-experimental outcome evaluation. There were three groups in the evaluation: (1) nondepressed adolescent mothers receiving home visitation by paraprofessionals; (2) depressed adolescent mothers receiving home visits by this same group; and (3) depressed adolescent mothers receiving home visits by a trained mental health clinician. Results of the outcome evaluation, which looked at indicators of mother-infant attachment and infant social and physical development, indicated that outcomes for the group treated by the trained clinician far exceeded outcomes for both of the other groups, even for those in which the mothers were not depressed according to the screening instrument. Since this study was done, other such studies have found that outcomes in early intervention programs are better across the board when the home visiting is done by a professional such as a social worker or nurse as opposed to paraprofessional staff. (Olds et al., 1997).

Many types of community-based clinical programs and interventions lend themselves well to quasi-experimental evaluations. Another example from the first author's experience is the study of a school-based group intervention directed at latency-aged children from drug- and alcohol-involved families living in high-risk neighborhoods in Philadelphia (Dore, Kauffman, & Nelson-Zlupko, 1999). In this study, because many children were identified by school personnel and self-identified as eligible for the group-based intervention, which could accommodate only 10 to 12 children at a time, the groups were implemented sequentially across the school year; thus, children who were eligible but on the waiting list for a group served as the naturally occurring control group for those receiving the experimental treatment. Four groups were run simultaneously in two public elementary schools over a 2-year period, resulting in slightly more than 100 children in each of the control and experimental conditions over that time, a sufficient number with which to make statistical comparisons on the selected outcome variables. This form of quasi-experimental design, sometimes known as a wait-list control group design, assumes that those who are on a waiting list for services share similar characteristics with those who are actually participating in a program or receiving services. This was probably true in the Philadelphia study, since children who participated in the first series of groups during the fall semester were selected at random from the entire list of eligible children. It is important in using this design to ensure that those selected for treatment from the wait list do not have some particular characteristic, such as a certain kind of presenting problem or more emergent treatment needs according to the referral source, that would automatically set them apart from the total pool of eligible participants. The idea in using an experimental or quasi-experimental design for evaluating outcomes is to be able to demonstrate that the differences between the treated and untreated group were caused by the treatment and not something else. Selecting those clients with a particular problem or urgent need automatically makes the treatment group different from the wait-list control group, and that difference can account for differences in outcomes as well.

Other types of quasi-experimental designs, such as the time-series design, are also frequently used in evaluating program outcomes. This approach involves measuring the same group of participants on the same criteria over time before, during, and after program participation. For example, Dore used a time-series quasi-experimental design in a study of family-based mental health programs for children (Lindblad-Goldberg, Dore, & Stern, 1998). When families with seriously emotionally disturbed children entered this program, clinicians obtained extensive histories of the prior mental health treatment both of the child and of others in the family. This history included inpatient and outpatient services in the mental health system, as well as services and placements in other child-serving systems such as child welfare, juvenile justice, and substance abuse. A primary outcome goal of this program was to prevent crisis-driven psychiatric hospitalizations of the child, as well as to build supports and services for families in the community and thereby prevent long-term child placements in residential care. Families were followed for 12 months after completing the program, and data were gathered on service system involvement and out-of-home placement at treatment completion and at three points after treatment. By comparing the seriously emotionally disturbed child's service history 1 year prior to, during, and 1 year after family-based treatment ended, we were able to show that the number of psychiatric placements decreased dramatically. Those that did occur were planned rather than crisis-driven, were often for medication adjustment or further psychiatric assessment, and were of significantly shorter duration.

The time-series design, while useful, particularly if pretreatment data are readily available, are not as robust as other quasi-experimental designs because they are vulnerable to external events. For example, if changes in funding for psychiatric care of Medicaid-eligible children had occurred at some point during this study, making hospitalization of children for psychiatric reasons more difficult, this might account for the lower rates of hospitalization after family-based treatment, rather than the treatment itself. Adding a control or comparison group of children with similar diagnoses and treatment histories who did not receive family-based treatment, and comparing the placement histories of the two groups over a 12-month period that coincided with the posttreatment 12 months of the treated group would have added significantly to claims that the family-based treatment was the factor responsible for lower hospitalization rates in the treated group.

The seeming difficulty and expense of employing experimental and even quasi-experimental methods to evaluate community-based clinical programs can present a daunting obstacle when resources are few and time and skills for data collection even more limited. Increasingly, however, as Ayers and Lyman, and Meyers point out in this volume, federal, state, and local funders of community-based programs require empirical evidence of their effectiveness in meeting program goals and in addressing the problems, issues, or concerns intended. This is why, as indicated earlier, building in both time and resources from the beginning to conduct a responsible program evaluation is key. This is money well spent in the long run if the outcome evaluation is positive and can be used to support requests for additional funding for the program. As Ayers and Lyman suggest, it can also demonstrate to funding sources that this is a responsible agency that is committed to developing and mounting effective programs. If instead the outcome evaluation demonstrates unequivocally that the program is not meeting its identified goals or helping participants make the intended changes, then agency administrators and others have an ethical responsibility to seek other ways to ameliorate the problems, issues, or concerns the program was intended to address. However, if the evaluation has also included formative and process components, there have been prior opportunities to identify and address deficits in the program model before these are revealed by the outcome evaluation.

Goal-Driven Evaluations

Goal-driven evaluations take one of two forms, one based on program goals, and the other on the goals of individual participants. Program goals are, of course, what the program is aiming to achieve for all clients: stabilize persons with severe and persistent mental illness in the community; prevent the out-of-home placement of children with severe emotional and behavior problems; increase the parenting skills of first-time adolescent parents; decrease the social isolation of children from substance-abusing families; increase the capacity of parents of children in a preschool day care program to create a nurturing and supportive community for families. The potential goals of community-based

clinical programs are endless. The point here is that they must be clearly stated and universally agreed to by all program participants in order to provide an overarching framework for both program implementation and evaluation. The first author (Dore) once had the experience of trying to work with the staff of a program aimed at preventing something—no one was quite sure of what—for families and children in the community. Some thought the goal of the program was to prevent child abuse and neglect; others thought it was to prevent family breakdown and out-of-home placement of children; still others believed it was to enhance the skills of family members to live together; and still others thought the goal was to meet the needs of families in distress, however the families defined them. With such different ideas about the goal of the program, gaining consensus on intervention methods and staff training needs was nearly impossible. Each staff member functioned according to his or her own therapeutic orientation and training. Some did individual psychotherapy with family members, others drew on various family therapy models and techniques, and still others used a more systemic approach, bringing together various community collaborators to create a network of supports for each family on their caseloads. Treatment lengths varied enormously, but most cases were never closed because, without well-defined program goals, there was always another problem or issue in the family to be addressed, another crisis to attend to.

When the funding source for this program began to demand accountability, the first author (Dore) was brought in to help staff members evaluate the program's outcomes. After two days of listening to the program staff—administrators, supervisors, and clinicians—debate the goals of the program with no observable movement toward consensus, I employed a strategy to good effect to bring participants to consensus on program goals. At the beginning of the third and final day, all those present were asked to write down on a piece of paper in 20 words or less what he or she envisioned the goal of the program to be. Forcing this very verbal group of skilled debaters to limit their goal statements to 20 words focused and clarified their thinking. When their statements were shared, there was more unanimity than had been previously apparent. We were then able fairly quickly to come up with a single goal statement to which all were willing to agree. There is something about forcing participants to put their thoughts in writing that changes the dynamics of the process. Once we had determined the program's distal goal, designing an appropriate intervention model and determining staff training and implementation needs was fairly straightforward.

Evaluability Assessment

Having clear, measurable program goals is such an essential part of the evaluation that a name has even been given to the process of determining whether these exist or can be clarified: *evaluability assessment* (Monette, Sullivan, & DeJong, 2002; Patton, 1997b). Dore's experience with the program described earlier in this chapter is not unusual. According to Weiss (1972), who has written extensively on the evaluation process, evaluators often encounter what she calls "fuzzy" program goals, which she suggests may result from clinicians' intuitive, rather than analytic, approach to program development. Patton (1997b) argues that this fuzziness may be an unspoken attempt to avoid conflict among program participants if there are competing or conflicting perceptions or interests; however, he ultimately believes that fuzzy goals are most often a function of conceptual difficulties in developing the program framework rather than a deliberate effort to avoid confronting differences. One example of a fuzzy program goal given by Patton (1997b) is as follows: "Clients will receive services which they value as appropriate to their needs and helpful in remediating their concerns" (p. 155). This goal statement would drive a stake through the heart of any evaluator. It says nothing about what the program is trying to achieve except for satisfied clients, which, though a noble aim, is not generally sufficient to satisfy funders who seek concrete results for their dollars. Another example of a program goal quoted by Patton (1997b) could have been taken directly from a brochure describing the program Dore discusses earlier: "Develop a supportive, family-centered, empowering, capacity-building intervention system for families and children" (p. 155). Goal statements like this one that are filled with jargon and describe a process (develop an intervention system) rather than the intended outcomes for program participants (in this case families and children) are all too common. An evaluator would ask, "What is the 'supportive, family-centered, empowering, capacity-building intervention system' intended to do?" "What kinds of changes will participating in such an 'intervention system' bring about in families and children?" Clarifying the conceptual thinking, including the theory of change, that lies behind fuzzy goal statements like these is the first task of the evaluator in conducting an evaluability assessment.

Conclusion

If, after reading this chapter, you have concluded that evaluating community-based clinical practice, while not for the faint of heart, is absolutely essential to the advancement of this treatment approach, we have done our job well. We also hope that we have conveyed the essence of a constructivist approach to evaluation that sees programs and services that address problems in living as developmental in nature, constantly evolving in response to community and participant needs, as well as social change. It is the mandate of program evaluators to capture this process at the point in time the program is implemented through a process evaluation. This process evaluation then informs the findings of the outcome evaluation with regard to achievement of program goals.

It is also our intention that the reader of this chapter recognize the importance of having a well-defined and clearly articulated theory of change, informed by current research on human behavior and treatment effectiveness, that, in turn, informs the program design. This theory, as we have discussed, forms the basis for the program's logic model, which describes the problem or issue the program is designed to address, the characteristics of those whom the program is intended to serve, the services they will receive and the characteristics of those providing these services, and, finally, the outcomes that the program is intended to achieve. Program goals are both proximal (sometimes called program objectives), representing immediate program effects such as a change in a particular behavior (e.g., increased mother-infant interaction), and distal or sought-after outcomes (e.g., secure attachment). A program's logic model provides a visual road map for the implementation activities required to get the program up and running as designed. It also provides the evaluator with information to guide observation of the implementation process and allow for more nuanced understanding of the program's functioning at a particular point in time. The logic model and its underlying theory of change also guide the evaluation of program outcomes and the selection of outcome measures that will capture the program's intended effects.

If we have focused more heavily in this chapter on the process of evaluating a program's implementation rather than its outcomes, it is because we strongly believe that (1) this is an often overlooked, but critically necessary component of adequately capturing the effects of community-based clinical programs; (2) without understanding what a program *is*, any attempt to understand what it *does* is meaningless. If a program does not achieve its intended outcomes, is it because the model itself was inadequate, or because the model was not implemented as intended? Did the program actually service the participants for whom it was originally designed? Were the intended services delivered in the manner in which they were intended, or did drift occur in which the method of service delivery changed in some significant way during the implementation process? These are the questions the process evaluation is intended to address and whose answers allow us to better interpret program outcomes.

This is not to say that identifying appropriate, measurable outcomes is not critically important to establishing the effectiveness of community-based clinical services as well. We hope that we have stressed the importance of selecting program goals that are consistent with the program's theory of change and are readily captured in the program's logic model. The measurement of outcomes should reflect community expectations of how the changes sought through the program would be manifested in the participants served. An essential element in community-based clinical practice is cultural awareness and competence in service delivery. Likewise, evaluation of specific outcomes should reflect this same attention to culture in the methods and strategies selected for measuring change, and in interpreting program effects.

Our advocacy of including representatives of all participant groups—clients, clinicians, administrators, and community partners—on a research advisory committee to ensure that a variety of perspectives is represented is one way to address the evaluator's possible limitations regarding cultural

competence. Dore's recent experiences in helping to develop an evaluation plan for a Baltimore family resource center, which included the insights and input from a wide variety of program participants, staff members, and community volunteers, confirmed this belief in the richness of multiple voices in designing and implementing program evaluations. These participants, whose cultural experiences were very different from those of the evaluator, pointed the evaluator to aspects of the program that would have remained unrecognized but which, according to participants, were crucial to their engagement in the programs of the center and their attainment of personal developmental (proximal) goals—eventually leading to achievement of the program's distal goals of family economic self-sufficiency, child safety and permanence, and family well-being.

Community-based clinical practice, integral to an increasing number of innovative approaches to helping, will benefit from thoughtful evaluative methods that describe how practice is developed and implemented and how outcomes are mediated by community. We have described evaluation as a dance of learning for all involved, leading to a complex understanding of the change process and accountability for clinical work made possible through attentive formative and process evaluations. Clinical practice that is situated in the community and that involves the community as essential in therapy and recovery will benefit from clinicians' and consumers' collaboration in evaluation to increase effective practices within a system of care. To this end, we advocate for a constructivist approach to evaluation, so that multiple perspectives will enable us to understand the complexities of systems change, the desired outcomes, and the most useful ways of measuring these outcomes. As we understand the generative force in our communities, fundamental in supporting change and our culture of care, we will be clearer on what is possible for us to achieve together.

References

Abma, T. A., & Stake, R. E. (2001). Stake's responsive evaluation: Core ideas and evolution. In J. C. Greene & T. A. Abma (Eds.), *Responsive evaluation*. New Directions for Evaluation, 92 (pp. 7–22). San Francisco: Jossey-Bass.

Argyris, C., & Schön, D. A. (1974). *Theory in practice*. San Francisco: Jossey-Bass.

Ayers, T. (1987). Stakeholders as partners in evaluation: A stakeholder collaborative approach. *Evaluation and Program Planning, 10*, 263–271.

Bickman, L. (Ed.). (1987). *Using program theory in evaluation*. San Francisco: Jossey-Bass.

Bickman, L., Guthrie, P., Foster, E. M., Lambert. E. W., Summerfelt, W. T., Breda, C., & Heflinger, C. A. (1995). *Managed care in mental health: The Fort Bragg experiment*. New York: Plenum.

Bond, J. T., & Halpern, R. (1988). The cross-project evaluation of the Child Survival/Fair Start Initiative: A case study of action research. In H. Weiss & F. Jacobs (Eds.), *Evaluating family programs* (pp. 347–370). Hawthorne, NY: Aldine de Gruyter.

Boruch, R. F. (1994). The future of controlled randomized experiments: A briefing. *Evaluation Practice, 15*, 265–274.

Bryk, A. S. (Ed.). (1983). *Stakeholder-based evaluation*. San Francisco: Jossey-Bass.

Campbell, D. T., & Stanley, J. C. (1963). *Experimental and quasi-experimental designs for research*. Chicago: Rand McNally.

Chaskin, R. J. (2002). The evaluation of "community building": Measuring the social effects of community-based practice. In A. N. Maluccio, C. Canali, & T. Vecchiato (Eds.), *Assessing outcomes in child and family services: Comparative design and policy issues* (pp. 28–47). Hawthorne, NY: Aldine de Gruyter.

Chen, H. (1990). *Theory-driven evaluation: A comprehensive perspective*. Newbury Park, CA: Sage.

Connell, P. J., Kubisch, A. C., Schorr, L. B., & Weiss, C. H.(1995). *New approaches to evaluating community initiatives: Concepts, methods, and contexts*. Washington, DC: Aspen Institute.

Cronbach, L. J. (1980). *Toward reform of program evaluation*. San Francisco: Jossey-Bass.

Datta, L. (1997). A pragmatic basis for mixed-method designs. In J. Greene & V. Caracelli (Eds.), *Advances in mixed-method evaluation: The challenges and benefits of integrating diverse paradigms* (pp. 33–46). San Francisco: Jossey-Bass.

Dore, M. M., Kauffman, E., & Nelson-Zlupko, L. (1999). "Friends in need": Designing and implementing a psychoeducational group for school children from drug-involved families. *Social Work, 44*, 179–190.

Everett, J., Homstead, K., & Drisko, J. (2004, January). *Local observers: An innovative method of data collection for community-based research*. Paper presented at the Society for Social Work Research annual conference, New Orleans, LA.

Fetterman, D. M. (1996). Empowerment evaluation: An introduction to theory and practice. In D. M.

Fetterman, S. Kaftarian, & A. Wandersman (Eds.), *Empowerment evaluation: Knowledge and tools for self-assessment & accountability* (pp. 3–48). Thousand Oaks, CA: Sage.

Fetterman, D. M., Kaftarian, S., & Wandersman, A. (Eds.). (1996). *Empowerment evaluation: Knowledge and tools for self-assessment and accountability*. Thousand Oaks, CA: Sage.

Friesen, B., & Winters, N. (2003). The role of outcomes in systems of care. In A. Pumariega & N. Winters (Eds.), *The handbook of child and adolescent systems of care* (pp. 459–486). San Francisco: Wiley.

Glaser, B. G., & Strauss, A. L. (1967). *The discovery of grounded theory: Strategies for qualitative research*. Chicago: Aldine.

Green, B., Johnson, S., & Rodgers, A. (1998). Understanding patterns of service delivery and participation in community-based family support programs. *Children's Services: Social Policy, Research and Practice, 2*, 1–22.

Greene, J. C. (1988). Stakeholder participation and utilization in program evaluation. *Evaluation Review, 11*, 341–351.

Greene, J. C., & Abma, T. A. (2001). *Responsive evaluation*. San Francisco: Jossey-Bass.

Greene, J., & Caracelli, V. (1997). Defining and describing the paradigm issue in mixed-method evaluation. In J. Greene & V. Caracelli (Eds.), *Advances in mixed-method evaluation: The challenges and benefits of integrating diverse paradigms* (pp. 5–18). San Francisco: Jossey-Bass.

Hoagwood, K. (1997). Interpreting nullity: The Fort Bragg experiment—A comparative success or failure. *American Psychologist, 52*, 546–550.

Hoagwood, K., Jensen, P., Petti, T., & Buena, B. (1996). A comprehensive conceptual model. (Outcomes of mental health care for children and adolescents, part 1). *Journal of the American Academy of Child and Adolescent Psychiatry, 35*(8), 1055–1063.

Holden, E., Santiago, R., Manteuffel, B., Stephens, R., Brannan, A., Soler, R., Liao, Q., Brashears, F., & Zaro, S. (2003). System of care demonstration projects. In A. Pumariega & N. Winters (Eds.), *The handbook of child and adolescent systems of care* (pp. 432–458). San Francisco: Wiley.

Hood, S. (2001). Nobody knows my name: In praise of African American evaluators who were responsive. In J. C. Greene & T. A. Abma (Eds.), *Responsive evaluation* (pp. 31–44). San Francisco: Jossey-Bass.

Kanter, R. M., Stein, B. A., & Jick, J. D. (1992). *The challenge of organizational change*. New York: Free Press.

Lightburn, A. (2002). Family service centers: Lessons

from national and local evaluations. In A. Maluccio, C. Canali, & T. Vecchiato (Eds.), *Assessing outcomes in child and family services: Comparative designs and policy issues* (pp. 153–174). New York: Aldine de Gruyter.

Lindblad-Goldberg, M., Dore, M. M., & Stern, L. (1998). *Creating competence from chaos: A comprehensive guide to home based services for children with serious emotional disturbances and their families.* New York: Norton.

Madison, A. M. (Ed.). (1992). *Minority issues in evaluation.* San Francisco: Jossey-Bass.

Meezan, W., & McBeath, B. (2004, January). *Managed care in child welfare: An overview, process and outcome study of an incentive based contracting model in Wayne County, Michigan.* Symposia presented at the Society for Social Work Research conference, New Orleans, LA.

Monette, D. R., Sullivan, T. J., & DeJong, C. R. (2002). *Applied Social Research* (5th ed.). Fort Worth, TX: Wadsworth.

Olds, D., Eckenrode, J., Henderson, C. R., Kitzman, H., Powers, J., Cole, R., Sidora, K., Morris, P., Pettitt, L. M., & Luckey, D. (1997). Long-term effects of home visitation on maternal life course and child abuse and neglect: Fifteen year follow-up of a randomized trial. *Journal of the American Medical Association, 278,* 637–643.

Patton, M. Q. (1994). Developmental evaluation. *Evaluation Practice, 15,* 311–320.

Patton, M. Q. (1997a). *Practical program evaluation.* Newbury Park, CA: Sage.

Patton, M. Q. (1997b). *Utilization focused evaluation: The new century text* (3rd ed.). Thousand Oaks, CA: Sage.

Patton, M. Q. (2001), Evaluation, knowledge management, best practices, and high quality lessons learned. *American Journal of Evaluation, 22,* 329–336.

Reichardt, C. S., & Rallis, S. F. (1994). The relationship between the qualitative and quantitative research traditions. In C. S. Reichardt & S. F. Rallis (Eds.), *The quantitative-qualitative debate: New perspectives* (pp. 5–12). San Francisco: Jossey-Bass.

Schön, D. A. (1983). *The reflective practitioner: How professionals think in action.* New York: Basic Books.

Schorr, L. B., & Kubisch, A. C. (1995, September). *New approaches to evaluation: Helping Sister Mary Paul, Geoff Canada, and Otis Johnson, while convincing Pat Moynihan, Newt Gingrich, and the American public.* Presentation at the Annie E. Casey Foundation Annual Research/Evaluation Conference. Baltimore, MD.

Schroes, C. J., Murphy-Berman, V., & Chambers, J. M. (2000). Empowerment evaluation applied: Experiences, analysis, and recommendations from a case study. *American Journal of Evaluation, 21,* 53–64.

Scriven, M. S. (1997). Empowerment evaluation examined. *Evaluation Practice, 18,* 165–175.

Stake, R. E. (1983). Program evaluation, particularly responsive evaluation. In G. F. Madaus, M. S. Scriven, & D. L. Stufflebeam (Eds.), *Evaluation models: viewpoints on educational and human services evaluation* (pp. 312–335). Boston: Kluwer-Nijhoff.

Stroul, B. (1996). (Ed.). *Children's mental health.* Baltimore: Brookes.

Stroul, B. (2002). Systems of care: A framework for system reform in children's mental health. Washington, DC: Georgetown University Child Development Center, National Technical Assistance Center for Children's Mental Health.

Stufflebeam, D. L. (2001). *Evaluation models.* San Francisco: Jossey-Bass.

Warren-Adamson, C. (2002). Applying a parenting scale in family resource centers: Challenges and lessons. In T. Vecchiato, A. Maluccio, & C. Canali (Eds.), *Evaluation in child and family services: Comparative client and program perspectives* (pp. 120–134). New York: Aldine de Gruyter.

Weiss, C. (1972). *Evaluation research: Methods of assessing program effectiveness.* Englewood Cliffs, NJ: Prentice-Hall.

Weiss, C. H. (1995). Nothing as practical as a good theory: Exploring theory-based evaluation for comprehensive community initiatives for children and families. In J. Connell, P. J. Kubisch, A. C., Schorr, L. B., & Weiss, C. H. (Eds.), *New approaches to evaluating community initiatives: Concepts, methods, and contexts* (pp. 65–92).Washington, DC: Aspen Institute.

Weiss, C. H. (1998). *Evaluation: Methods for studying programs and policies* (2nd ed.). Upper Saddle River, NJ: Prentice Hall.

Weiss, H., & Halpern, R. (1990). *Community-based family support and education programs: Something old or something new.* New York: National Center for Children in Poverty.

Weiss, H., & Jacobs, F. (Eds.). (1988). *Evaluating family programs.* Hawthorne, NY: Aldine de Gruyter.

Weiss, H. B., & Green, J. C. (1992). An empowerment partnership for family support and education programs and evaluations. *Family Service Review, 5,* 131–148.

Weiss, H. B., & Halpern, R. (1989). *The challenges of evaluating state family support and education initiatives: An evaluation framework.* Cambridge, MA: Harvard Family Research Project.

Whyte, W. F. (Ed.). (1991). *Participatory action research.* Newbury Park, CA: Sage.

Wigfall, V., & Moss, P. (2001). More than the sum of

its parts? The story of a multi-agency child care network. London: National Children's Bureau Enterprises.

Wolpert, D. M., & Körding, K. P. (2004). Bayesian integration in sensorimotor learning. *Nature, 427*(6971), 244–247.

Wright, L. & Paget, K. (2002). A learning-organization approach to evaluation. In A. Maluccio, C. Canali, & T. Vecchiato (Eds.), *Assessing outcomes in child and family services: Comparative design and policy issues* (pp. 127–140). Hawthorne, NY: Aldine de Gruyter.

Yin, R. K. (1989). *Case study research: Design and methods* (Rev. ed.). Newbury Park, CA: Sage.

The Leadership Journey in Community-Based Clinical Practice: Practice, Theory, and Policy

13

Tom Andersen

The Network Context
of Network Therapy

A Story From the European Nordic North

A network of mental health teams providing alternative, community-based psychotherapeutic interventions was first started in the north of Norway in the late 1960s and blended in 1988 with a similar network in the north of Finland that had started in the very early 1980s. Therapists from northern Sweden joined the northern Norwegians in 1988 and became part of their training program. The network, then consisting of Finns, Swedes, and Norwegians, invited the northwest Russians to join in 1994; later these four nationalities collaborated on a training program in Arkhangelsk, in northwest Russia. Because these countries have at least three very different linguistic traditions, English is the shared language for the network. From this northern Nordic network a larger network has emerged, including groups from eight countries: Denmark, Estonia, Finland, Latvia, Lithuania, Norway, Russia, and Sweden. All want to develop alternative psychotherapeutic practices when psychotic crises occur and share an interest in the principles of "open talks" and "network therapy."

In this chapter, the history of the Nordic northern network will be outlined. Basic principles for the practice of Open Talks, in the network, particularly those that integrate reflecting team practices, the organization of such practices, and the corre-

sponding philosophies are described. A training program for northern Sweden and northern Norway that corresponds to these practices and philosophy is also discussed.

Now

The networks are rather extensive at the moment, and many teams participate in them and keep them alive and flowing. It has not always been so. Often something starts with only a few persons, or even only one, and then it takes off. However, although only one voice, my own, was heard at first, that voice did not come from nowhere. My voice was generated from many voices that had not been heard or had not yet spoken. Those voices belong to the patients and their relatives, and to the assistants who work at the bottom of the treatment systems, those who spend the most time with patients. Their position at the bottom of the hierarchy makes their voices easily become muted. My formal position, high up in society, came to me as a gift. While I certainly had done something to achieve it, it was mostly given as a gift. Being in such a powerful position, I had to accept the responsibilities and obligations that accompany it, namely, to speak the voices that have not yet been heard and the voices that have not yet spoken. Sometimes voices are not spoken because the words have not yet been found, or a person feels too fearful to speak the words.

Before

I used to be a general medical practioner in remote places in north Norway in the early 1960s. That experience gave me the understanding that diseases and their cures generated networks of interested people who wanted to help out. I felt the presence and the need for such networks in my body. When, in the mid-1960s, I turned from medical practice to psychiatry, I noticed that when a troubled person was taken out of his community and admitted to the mental hospital in Tromsø (English spelling is Tromsoe), it was often very difficult for that person to reconnect with the community, including family, work, and neighborhood. The psychiatric care at that time was centered in the hospital in Tromsoe that served the two northernmost counties, Troms and Finnmark, with 200,000 inhabitants. This area consists of rough coastlines, rough mountains, and often rough weather, and is quite large: 600 by 100 miles. The roughness is balanced by the beauty of nature and the special changes in light and colors, with two summer months that have sun all day and night, and two winter months without any sun.

I was stimulated by an interest to reach out to do something "out there," in the community. I approached Lester Libo, a professor in psychology from New Mexico, who came to Tromsoe in 1969 and told us how he and his colleagues had set up services in their communities. One hundred fifty professionals from Troms and Finnmark attended this event and were enchanted. Shortly after, we, hospital-based professionals, started the first small attempts to go out and collaborate with the local providers. To our surprise, we often could prevent admissions to the mental hospital without too much effort, and it seemed that changing the perspective from central to local was what created the effect.

After affiliating with the newly established University of Tromsoe, I then went to New Mexico to stay for a year to pursue the question of the necessity of mental hospitals. When I came home and

hoped to reconnect and work with friends and colleagues at the mental hospital, the door was closed. Perhaps they felt that I had betrayed them by leaving them and going to the university, a baby cuckoo flying from the nest.

However, the ideas of family therapy that had reached the north of Norway in the early 1970s made us ready to work in and with the context and to let time be our working friend. We set up training programs, very homemade and blended people from the cities with people from the communities in our groups. Some of our meetings were in the city "in here"; some in the community "out there."

In 1976, I was offered a professorship in social psychiatry at the University of Tromsoe, and we launched a 3-year project from 1978 to 1981. The aim was to decrease the admissons to the mental hospital. Seven mental health professionals, including three psychiatric nurses, one psychologist, and three psychiatrists, met the patients, together with providers working in the "first line" of Tromsoe's social and medical services. The seven mental health professionals had no treatment facilities of their own. If a governmental agency in Oslo, the capital of Norway, had not supported the project, it would never have happened. The psychiatrists at the mental hospital, themselves working in the "second line" (psychiatric outpatient services) and "third line" (services inside the hospital) did not favor it. The project was successful in at least four senses: (1) the first line liked the availability of the mental health group and the opportunity to learn from them; (2) their confidence was increased by being able to contribute much themselves; (3) they learned what psychiatry can and cannot do; and (4) the admissions to the hospital went down. When the group offered to continue after 1981, the county authorities asked the psychiatrists at the mental hospital for their opinion. Not surprisingly, they advised that the group be disbanded, which is what happened. I learned that a system cannot be changed from outside; it can only be changed from inside by itself.

Before it split, the group of seven had been part of a 2-year systemic oriented family therapy training program led by Philippe Caillè from Oslo. Through that program we met Lynn Hoffman from New York and Luigi Boscolo and Gianfranco Cecchin from Milan. We even visited northern Italy in 1982 to learn more of the Milan approach that was so much "in the winds" at that time. In Italy we met Peggy Penn, and these new connections strengthened our bonds to the network of ideas that were evolving.

Leave the Mainstream and Go to the Margins

I have always based my life on the idea that if change does not happen one way, there must be another way. Since the established psychiatrists preferred to close the doors on systemic thinking and practices, I organized 3-day meetings in June every year, way out in the communities. They were so far out and so basic that the only people who came were those who were genuinely interested. The first conference in 1983 was in a small fishing village, Gryllefjord, on the Arctic Ocean. Lynn Hoffman and Peggy Penn came and enchanted the participants. The next year, in June, Luigi Boscolo and Gianfranco Cecchin came to another remote village. We have subsequently met every year in June, at a new place each year. Many have been invited: interesting people from the "big world." Two of them were Harry Goolishian and Harlene Anderson, who then returned many times, just as many of us traveled to visit them in Galveston and Houston, Texas. It was important to invite international speakers and to bypass academics in Oslo. Academics in the capital have traditionally thought of themselves as "first-class," while thinking of people from the North as "second- or third-class." Some of us got tired of that definition of ourselves and went our own way.

These events attracted many people and became important meeting places. Some people have come every year, some now and then, some only once. Those who came and continue to come understand that they can choose either to participate in the seminar discussions in the daytime or converse during the sunny nights. That has been an important first principle for all invited participants. The second principle has been to bring in good speakers. The third has been to locate the seminars in the margins, outside of traditional cultural centers. People from all disciplines and all agencies have come and constituted a complex society with different wishes, meanings, and beliefs.

Since these June seminars were so well attended, we started a January seminar in Tromsoe in 1988. Symbolically, we met in the center of the networks in the middle of the dark time. These conferences followed the same two main principles: including everybody and inviting good speakers. They also gave us a chance to launch an annual meeting at which we could discuss how this growing network was to go on. No votes by participants have ever been necessary. We talk until we agree. If we cannot reach consensus, we continue the discussion the following year.

March 1985

In the middle of all this growing activity and turmoil of different kinds, one of the teams in Tromsoe that until the fall of 1984 had tried to work in the Milan systemic way started to comment differently on the families' situations. From saying to families, "This is how you shall see the situation" and "This is what you shall do," they now said, "In addition to what you see, we see this" and "In addition to what you have tried to do, can you consider doing this?" The team had moved from an either-or position to a both-and position, which was a big leap, practically, rationally, philosophically and ethically. This helped to prepare for the next leap, namely, to let the team members speak among themselves with the families listening to the teams talk. We called it "reflecting team" at that time, as we now call it "reflecting process(es)." The principles are simple: when the listening team receives the story that the family wants them to hear, the team members usually become moved by the story. What happens to them when they become moved, such as having an idea or a question or an emotion, is then given back to the family. The story has touched the listener, and the listener returns what happened to her or to him. This simple method quickly spread in northern Norway and is now also practiced in many countries. Its simplicity makes it applicable to many professional areas and in many kinds of problematic situations.

The simplicity of our approach is that the therapist concentrates on receiving what the other wants her to receive. The therapist then returns to the other what happens with her when she receives it. What she might receive and respond to include all the other's expressions, such as words, smiles, looks, handshakes, emotions, and so on. This simple therapeutic model leaves out all kinds of instructive activities that are common in other therapeutic models.

Our philosophy is that we, as human beings, first of all live as participants in relationship with others. What we do as participants, such as talking, not only connects us with others but also creates meaning, and it informs us and others. Most of all, what we express forms our lives and our understanding. This philosophy is rather different from the traditional assumption that what a person says and does comes from inside the person, from an "inner core," and that language passively transfers thoughts from one person to another.

Because both this mode of working and its philosophy have been applicable in so many different circumstances, I now prefer to call it "open reflecting processes." At first I was surprised that countries that had been under oppressive regimes were so attracted to open reflecting talks. Now I understand that these open talks comprise not only openness but also equality and solidarity, which have political elements. In contrast, many other therapies comprise control and power, which are quite different political elements.

The therapists who engage in open reflecting talks are first of all encouraged to develop abilities to feel relationships in their bodies. Abilities to understand and explain rationally are also necessary, but they come second and third. To learn to feel in the body, I have emphasized cultivating awareness of the body while in dialogue. Reading and doing research are also important but are of secondary importance.

Training: Shall We or Shall We Not?

Many individuals from the North took family training in programs in the South, in Italy. However, travel and fees were so high that only a few people from each agency could be given this opportunity. In the early 1980s came the idea of a training program. The network included two groups: those who needed the credential of such education and those who worried that a formalized program would constrain our freedom. It took us 3 years to determine to go for it. The training program started January 1, 1987, and we created two possible tracks: to go through it and reach a "diploma," or

to go through it without reaching a "diploma." The program consisted of five parts: (1) The participants applied as a group. They constituted a local group first, and the various groups could be composed of people from different agencies and different educational backgrounds. They met a half day every week to work together and were supposed to bring in their ongoing daily work, for instance, to meet a family of one of them together with the group. This required that the groups have permission from the chiefs of the agencies to do this. (2) The groups selected their supervisor from a list of available supervisors. That supervisor came to the group once a month. The group did *not* go to the supervisor. (3) The participants were expected to read six books written in Nordic languages. (4) The participants were expected to participate in four larger gatherings: the June and January seminars, or other similar and approved seminars. (5) The groups were expected to produce and present a written text (paper) or spoken text (videotaped discussion). Those who went through all five parts received the "diploma." Those who preferred only the first two parts did not. Therefore, the groups could be composed of both "diplomates" and "nondiplomates."

Organizing Principles

The network had, until 1987, been very loosely conducted. One secretary at the university and I managed everything. But with the training program, we had to establish an "approving body" to review applications from groups, choose supervisors, and organize and approve the big gatherings besides the January and June seminars. At first, a group of four was established as the leading group. Each of the three northernmost Norwegian counties had one representative, and the fourth came from the University of Tromsoe. When the Swedes joined in 1988, one representative from the northernmost county in Sweden joined as the fifth. The leading group has had telephone meetings once a month over all these years. Minutes from these meetings are distributed to all groups and supervisors.

The annual meeting in January in Tromsoe has functioned as a general assembly. All who are or have been students or supervisors can take part and speak. If there were to be a vote, every one of them would have one vote. Voting has not yet occurred.

We have talked until we have agreed. The network has had no memberships, fees, presidents, goals, bylaws, or budget. Every seminar has its own budget. Such elements have not been necessary for us, and we have seen that the introduction of them elsewhere easily creates divisive opinions and distancing tensions. It was therefore safest to keep them out.

Two Significant June Seminars

One June seminar was held in Sulitjelma in 1988, and the other in Svolvaer in 1993. The first belonged to the ideas of constructivism, the second to social constructionism. Six epistemologists and three clinical groups were invited to the seminar in Sulitjelma, called "A Greek Kitchen in the Arctic." The epistemologists were Lynn Hoffman, Heinz von Foester, Ernst von Glasersfeld, Fredrick Steier (all of the United States), Humberto Maturana (Chile), and Stein Braaten (Norway). Three groups presented four videotaped sessions: (1) Harlene Anderson and Harry Goolishian, Galveston Institute, Houston; (2) Luigi Boscolo, Milan; (3) Gianfranco Cecchin, Milan; and (4) Anna Margrete Flåm and Tom Andersen, Tromsoe. All videos were fully transcribed and distributed to participants and invited speakers beforehand.

The six epistemologists were asked to point out where and how constructivist ideas appeared in the films. That did not happen; instead, the six became clinical "semisupervisors," sometimes with strong opinions based on feelings. That we did not come close to what we hoped for did not matter. The seminar, which has become a marker in the field of family therapy, both within and beyond northern Europe, opened up for discussion and debate the value of the language of cybernetics versus the language of daily social togetherness. Harry Goolishian later stated that his mind had been working day and night for 3 months after that meeting. He subsequently abandoned the language of cybernetics that had so strongly prevailed in the field of family therapy through the 1980s. His and Harlene's breakthrough article appeared in *Family Process* 6 months later (Anderson & Goolishian, 1988). The name of the seminar was my idea. I had visited a Greek island in the mid-1960s with my family and friends, and the local citizens would greet us by serving dinner in a big kitchen. As guests, we were

seated around a big round table, and two women cooked on an open fire in a corner, and they sang and danced. As we ate, townspeople came in and sat along the walls to watch our happiness around the table. After a while they left, and new people entered, and still later new ones entered. Those moments were so incredibly thrilling that I thought, "I must make a Greek kitchen in the arctic one day." It happened to a considerable extent when we moved the six epistemiologists and the six clinicians toward the center of the room, where they were surrounded by the participants sitting in big circles.

In 1993, the seminar "Constructed Realities: Therapy, Theory and Research" in Svolvaer, a fishing village in Lofoten, attracted 350 people. It was the the biggest venture ever in the village and the biggest June seminar so far. It was meant to be big, with many participants and with many big names as speakers. Many academicians who had recently received positions at the tiny University of Tromsoe attended. Many from the academy came up from Oslo as well. The academicians tended to have more traditional views of knowledge and research. Many of them challenged our work and thinking, saying, "This is rather speculative! You have to prove its use! You have to document! Let us see the results! When you have done double-blind experiments we can start to listen to you!"

These strong voices, which seemed, in Wittgenstein's words, to be bewitched by the dominant language in academia, were both challenging and frightening. And they were right. We could not "prove" it. Good experiences from practical work had encouraged us to go on. However, experiences and stories were not good enough in the early 1990s. At that time, I felt, and have continued to feel, that this seminar was done in part for our survival. Harry Goolishian, my close collaborator in preparing it, and I started it in May 1991. A great disaster struck us when Harry died on November 10, 1991. His death was disastrous in many senses: he still had so much to do and to formulate, and he was so meaningful for many individuals. Uneasily, I went to Kenneth Gergen, who generously stepped in immediately. We planned the seminar overnight.

The well-known invitees were Harlene Anderson, Brent Atkinson, Ron Chenail, Tom Conran, Kenneth Gergen, Mary Gergen, John Lannaman, Sheila McNamee, John Shotter, Peggy Penn, and Donald Polkinghorne (all United States); Margareth

Wetherell and Johnathan Potter (both United Kingdom); Steinar Kvale (Denmark) and Hanne Haavind, Magnus Hald, Anders Lindseth, and Sissel Reichelt, Åge Wifstad (all Norway). The eight issues to guide presentations were: Knowledge, One or Many?; Multiple Realities and Therapeutic Process; Human Understanding; Language and Construction of the Self; Research Alternatives; Qualitative Research in Clinical Work; Feminist Issues in Theory and Research; and Power, Ethics, and Practice. Each well-known presenter had written one article for this conference, and all participants received them beforehand. In the conference, four to five of the important presenters spoke on the eight issues, and two selected "voices of the people" discussed responses with the presenters. Occasionally some voices of the people said, "I understood nothing!" Thereafter the audience was included in the discussion.

The June seminar turned out to be the demonstration I had hoped for. We showed that these ideas are well formulated and well-founded philosophically, that practices that correspond to these philosophies have been developed, and that social constructionsim is a strong and new ideology of our time that challenges traditional ideologies and clinical practices.

A Growing and Merging Network

In the middle of all these gatherings, much happened in daily life. In 1988 some Swedes from Gaellivare came to the January seminar. They wanted to join the training program as the first from outside Norway, and they were certainly welcomed. Many other Swedish groups have followed. In March 1988, five Finns came. Jaakko Seikkula and colleagues started out in the very early morning from Tornio, in north Finland, drove 8 hours by car through the winter storms and arrived at noon in Tromsoe. They had heard that something called a "reflecting team" had happened in northern Norway, and they wanted to know more. They themselves had, to our great interest, much to tell. They spoke softly and modestly about "meetings on the borders." We quickly understood that major developments had occurred in their work with psychotic crises. We felt immediately connected and have been since. They left in the afternoon to drive 8 hours back.

Actually we have gotten used to traveling, and many of our hours are spent this way. Tornio-Tromsoe is 8 hours by car, and Gaellivare-Tromsoe is 6 hours. However, on such long trips we can let our eyes rest on the beautiful landscape and let our minds go; much good thinking is done under such circumstances. North Finland has long, sloping hills with many rivers and lakes and quiet birch and pine woods; north Sweden is more hilly, with big pine and spruce woods and many reindeer along the roads; north Norway is filled with high mountains divided by many fjords and has only small birch trees.

Four Northern Areas

Even though much is similar in thinking and practice in the four northern countries, there definitely are differences, shaped by geographic, political, and economic distinctions. The following section presents a closer look at one agency in each of the four areas.

Keropudas Hospital (in Finnish: Keraputaan Sairaala)

This is the name of the mental hospital in Tornio, western Lapland, north Finland. Jaakko Seikkula has written extensively about the work in this area, as have his colleagues Jyirki Keraenen, Kauko Haarakangas, and Birgitta Alakare (Seikkula et al. 1995). The hospital used to be a boarding home for 300 "burned-out" psychiatric patients whose treatment had been terminated in the big mental hospital in Rovaniemi far away. There were academically educated people on the staff, and the area had no therapeutic tradition or ideology from before. The doctor in chief, Jyrki Keränen, was a friend of Jukka Altonen, who is a professor in family therapy at the University of Jyväskylä. Jukka, who used to be a student of the well-known Yrjö Alanen, professor in psychiatry at the University in Turku, was willing to visit on a regular basis. In the very early 1980s, they approached the six municipalities they served to ask if some of these elderly patients could return to their home communities. Many patients went home, and the free space inside the hospital created the possibility of receiving the acute cases, not sending them to Rovaniemi. Shortly thereafter, they took care of all psychiatric cases in the area of six municipalities, with 72,000 inhabitants.

Between 1981 and 1984, the Finnish team tried to engage the families when somebody was to be admitted, but few families were willing to come. When they stopped planning the family meeting beforehand and met the families more informally, the families came. When they reviewed the work in 1988, they saw that 50% of patients with first-episode psychoses could return home. That encouraged them to make a big change. Instead of starting the crisis work at the hospital, they did it in the patients' homes. They established five crisis teams out in the communities that were available 24 hours every day of the year. Anyone—the patients, relatives, neighbors, or the authorities—can call and ask for assistance. A meeting is then arranged within 24 hours in the home of the patient with the network that had been created by the crisis. These meetings, which often are very emotional, concentrate on the question, What shall be the next step? They also try, with communal effort, to find meaning in what seems meaningless, such as psychotic expressions. Even though the meetings are filled with uncertainty and fear, the professionals avoid making conclusions or summaries too soon.

A central principle of the work is to have tolerance for uncertainty. Everybody who wants to speak can speak, and everyone who wants to be heard is heard. These meetings are repeated the next day and the day after that, and may go on for 10 to 15 days. If the patients are uneasy or agitated or cannot sleep, they are given mild tranquilizers but not neuroleptics. Two or three providers constitute a team that follow the case as long as needed, and if the patient is admitted to the hospital, which seldom occurs, the team continues their work inside the hospital. Continuity is another central principle. To be able to do this work, many professionals must be available. Therefore, all the 90 employees, mostly nurses and nurses' aides, have gone through a 3-year family therapy training program and are licensed psychotherapists in Finland. Keropudas Sairaala has developed its own training program with basically its own psychologists and psychiatrist as teachers. Three of these, Jaakko Seikkula, Jyrki Keränen, and Kauko Harankangas, have been granted PhDs at the University of Jyväskylä.

The Finnish team have done a 2-year and a 5-year follow up of 86 new first-episode psychotic crises between April 1, 1992, and April 1, 1997. They met with 80 families after 2 years and 73 families after 5 years. The results were stunning: 85% of the patients were without symptoms, 85% were working or studying, and 77% did not use any neuroleptics. The number of days in hospital was very minimal compared with what happens elsewhere in the world.

Gaellivare Outpatient Clinic for Children and Youth

Gaellivare is a small settlement in the northernmost part of Sweden. This public outpatient clinic for children and youth serves four municipalities with 60,000 inhabitants. The area is scarcely populated and makes up one eighth of all Sweden. The huge mining activities of the last hundred years are now in decline. Compared with the rest of Sweden, the unemployment rate is now high, as are the crime rate, alcohol use, and suicide.

The clinic, until 15 years ago, worked from an individual perspective, but after joining the northern Nordic network, it has changed to a communal network perspective. The Gaellivare clinic, which has had no competing ideology in its area, has until now had seven employees, all females: three social workers, three psychologists, and the chief, a child psychiatrist. Recently one male psychologist has been added to the staff. The clinic has to receive all kinds of cases because it is the only service in the area. It has never had a waiting list. There are no inpatient services for children and youth in the area, and they are not needed; everything is done on an outpatient basis. Anyone, such as a mother, a teacher, an anynomous neighbor, police, and so forth, can call. The secretary forwards the telephone call to one of the staff immediately.

That first phone conversation, which usually constitutes a situation of crisis, can last 1 or 2 hours, and the staff member often ends the talk by saying, "Do you want to continue the talk tomorrow? We can come to you." The clinic has approximately 200 new registered cases each year and approximately 100 such "telephone cases." Interestingly enough, when they go out to the network and talk about the critical situation, the problem often dissolves before a child is defined as a patient. One could say it is network therapy without a patient. The goal is to avoid referring cases out, which means that when somebody brings a case, two of the staff go together to where the problem has appeared and work there. Meetings may take place at a school, kindergarten, social welfare office, or medical hospital. They always work in pairs: one talks with those who are engaged in the crisis, and the other listens. After a while the two have a reflecting talk between themselves with those in crisis listening to that talk.

The Gaellivare clinic has also developed open reflecting talks in cases when the families are mandated by the authorities to be investigated, such as when somebody suspects neglect or abuse of the children. The social worker at the children's protective services is asked to bring the parent at once. When the family comes, the accusations are shared openly, and all, including the parents, are invited to find what will be the best for the children. When the authorities expect a certain investigation, the parents are invited to be part of the planning of that investigation. The law in Sweden says that the report shall be finalized within 4 months. Here it takes longer, since the families, during the period of investigation, change for the better so that the authorities often withdraw their concern. Ten years ago the Gaellivare clinic was engaged in approximately 20 such cases each year; the number now is much lower than that. This decline is most probably a consequence of the open collaboration with the social worker from the protective services. The social workers now intervene in families earlier, before everyone has gone into "the trenches," and they can do the work now on their own.

The work with 174 families during 1 year was evaluated. Teams met with 58% of them one to four times, 22% five to eight times, and 20% nine times and more. Six months to 1 year after therapy ended, more than 80% of the families reported that the situation was better or much better compared with what it was at the start, 10% said it was the same, 3% said it was worse, and no one said much worse. Only one child was admitted to the psychiatric ward. Talking with the families from 6 months to 1 year after therapy ended indicates that the children are well. The problems may still be there, but the parents know to handle them. The parents say that it goes well because, they, the parents, "fixed" the situation. The families are particularly thankful that the staff members were willing to talk about what the families wanted to talk about, and nothing more. This is possible because staff members avoid

any diagnostic procedures. Such procedures so easily define the problems in professional terms, not in the families' terms. Diagnostic terms, which may be alien to the families, often produce distance between the families and the professionals.

Staff at the agencies that the Gaellivare clinic collaborates with have been through the training program that is common to north Sweden and north Norway. That has most probably contributed to the high level of collaboration between the different agencies. Actually, this clinic has been noticed by the central authorities in Sweden, who want to apply these modes of collaboration in other parts of Sweden as well.

A particular part of the Gaellivare clinic's work must be mentioned. The leader and child psychiatrist Eva Kjellberg, trained by the Swedish art therapist Janet Swensson, has asked the families to paint when they cannot talk (Kjellberg, Edwardsson, Niemelä, & Öberg, 1995). That happens when fighting and no listening occurs, when words became dangerous, or when words just disappear. The members of the families are in the same room and do their individual painting as they are standing. They themselves determine the size of the paper and where to place it on the wall, and they select the colors for painting freely. They are not instructed what to paint or how. They are only encouraged to start with a nice color and enjoy themselves. All families have appreciated this proposal, and they quickly become engaged in deep concentration. Once in a while they walk over to one another in the family and speak in a connected, friendly manner.

When they finish the painting Eva says, "You own your painting, and you can determine what to do with it. However, we might all of us look at one painting at a time, and tell what happens with us when we see it." Most amazing changes occur: tensions disappear, and the words come slowly back. The expression through painting is very personal, but at the same time it is protected. Nobody beside the painter him- or herself understands the emotional content of the painting. But to share it with others and witness their responses has a strong positive connecting power. The problems that disconnected people vanish. Eva proposes that all human beings carry unfinished pictures, and when they are given to the paper, and seen and received by others, they are completed. A new picture emerges, which can be painted and conceptualized. The mystery of this healing process is far from understood. However, even if it is not understood, it can be used to help the families.

Psychiatric Center for Tromsoe and Karlsoy: Psychiatric Services for Adults

Magnus Hald, the psychiatrist in chief for this center, and his colleagues have over the last 10 years worked on converting the hospital-based and specialist-oriented services from individual treatment based on pathology perspectives toward community-based services based on relational and networks perspectives. They are in the middle of this process, which can be compared to making an ocean wave move the opposite way. Because this conversion is far from finished, it will be mentioned only briefly here.

At first these services were provided in an integrated outpatient clinic of the larger mental hospital in Tromsoe. Being part of this big organization constrained every attempt to make changes, since changes had to be approved from above. The hospital has been not only a traditional psychiatric hospital but also very conservative. When the mental hospital was integrated as a part of the university hospital of north Norway in Tromsoe, an organizational change linked the outpatient clinic directly to the director of the university hospital. This separation from the rest of the psychiatric hospital allowed the freedom to make changes.

One important step was to establish an acute team to take care of all crises. That team has been willing to immediately assist the general practitioners, public health services, and social services in the two municipalities it serves. Professionals in the community services participate with the team members and the patients' networks in crisis work. This move has been highly appreciated by the community services. Earlier, when hospitalizations were needed, the acute team had to admit its patients to the wards in the mental hospital. The acute team, which is network oriented, and these wards, which as indicated earlier worked from individual-, pathology-, and control-oriented perspectives, did not always find it easy to collaborate. When the outpatient clinic was designated by the hospital to become the crisis center's own ward, new possibilites arose. Now the whole center can coordinate what happens in the whole network, and in a smoother way develop continuity for the patients between their stay in the hosptal and the treatment in the community. While in the middle of this new big step, Jaakko Seikkula comes regularly to work with them and uses his experiences in western Lapland in north Finland to assist them.

Archangelsk: Experiences in Connecting With Northwest Russia

Shortly after Russia opened to the West after the fall of Communism, we invited two Russian guests to our annual seminar in June 1994. The meeting was of such value for them and for us that they came back to the next year's June seminar. From then on, we felt connected with the Russians, and six of us went to Archangelsk in September 1995. Since then, we have visited frequently. When the Russians wanted us to implement a 2-year training program, seven of us traveled to Archangelsk twice a year: one Finn, three Swedes, and three Norwegians. The program provided practical training in language- and network-oriented psychotherapeutic talks; we often call them "open reflecting dialogues." After that program ended in 2001, four of us continued to come—one Finn, two Swedes, and one Norwegian—to help the Russians develop their own training program.

It was important for us that the Russians defined what kind of assistance they wanted and how we should give it. That means that we, beforehand, had no ideas of what and how our collaboration should be. That had to be determined by a discussion between the Russians and us. The Russians wanted to work clinically with us on their ongoing daily work challenges. We therefore visited four locations: hospital I for adult patients and the children's department; the outpatient clinic in Archangelsk; and hospital II for adult patients.

We always met and worked with patients. Most often we, the visitors, talked with a patient and sometimes his or her family, and the young Russian psychiatrists listened to that talk. Then the Russian psychiatrists talked among themselves about what was invoked in them as they listened. While that happened, the patient and family listened. At the end the patient and family gave their responses. What I have appreciated the most during these visits have been the psychotherapeutic interviews that included the young Russian psychiatrists. The meetings have always been very emotional. What else could one expect in Fyodor Dostoyevsky's country? We, as well as the patients at the hospital, were filled with shifting emotions.

The work with painting, described earlier in this chapter, was implemented in the psychiatric department for children (Kjellberg et al., 1995). The "family" the children painted with were the other children on the ward. That work created a very special new community where fights and competition between the children decreased drastically. When they once tried to show us a videotape from a painting session, the video screen they had did not work. Therefore we had to move to another ward with older children. When the young persons on this ward saw the film, they got very quiet. We asked them what their thoughts were. One said quietly, "I thought of my whole life!"

Though some of the patients we met with were quiet, all were emotionally engaged, such as an old man, Vladimir, who had stayed at the hospital for years and did not talk anymore. When the focus in the conversation turned to a statement in his records about his previous interests in mathematical formulas, he started talking. His excitement then made it impossible for him to stop. Other patients were passionate and intense and could make us feel we were engaged in a talk with Fjodor Karamasov. A young man, Ivan, who had committed crimes, was willing to talk only if he could bring his priest, an Orthodox father, with him. In the presence of the father, he excused himself for being a man who acted as soon as a thought came to his mind. We discussed for a while if there was any possibilty to put in some time between the thought's arrival in his mind and his actions. The priest, in sincere emotional engagement, gave his opinion of such a possibility from a biblical perspective, and the man was willing to accept and continue his religious thoughts. All of us in the room were in some kind of trance as the discussion unfolded.

Some patients were fearful of words and could not speak. As a young girl, Irina had been raped. In an attempt to assist the girl to find words and thereby find a meaningful way to continue her life, the young psychiatrists were willing to share with her their own experiences of being unjustly oppressed. It was of particular help for the young girl to hear how they had overcome both shame and hatred, so that they could proceed in life without acting on their first thoughts of revenge. Other patients were artistic and eloquent. A young man, Pavel, on the closed ward, had listened to radio and

thereby learned to speak English fluently. He volunteered as translator in a consultation, and it was hard to know who was most filled with joy, he for delivering his very useful skills or us for being guided by such a talented man. Yes, all the psychotherapeutic talks were always filled with emotions.

There have also been difficulties. The open and democratic modes of network therapy have often clashed with the traditions that still prevail in Russia, namely, static hierarchical structures (information shall flow from down, up, and instructions shall come from the top, down) and fragmentation (a person does a small bit of the whole process and nothing more). As Russia needs time to restore its economy, it also needs time to find ways for people to live together differently. During this waiting time, we have made a northern collegium of eight persons, with two from each of the four countries where we have training programs. When the Russians need help in their own training program, they can call on assistance from the other six; either someone will come to them, or they can travel to one of the other three countries. That way, they can regulate the connection with the other three countries without being subjected to colonialism. Most probably there will be a day when we travel to them and learn. This connection has actually produced a book: *Open Talks Between East and West.* Some of the chapters are written by Russians, the others by a Swede, a Finn, and a Norwegian. The book is printed in Russian on the left page and in English on the right page.

An International Network on the Work With Psychotic Crises

Since 1996, groups from eight countries, Sweden, Finland, Estonia, Lithuania, Latvia, Denmark, Russia, and Norway, have come together once a year to share experiences with psychotherapeutic work with psychotic crises. This meeting, which moves from country to country from year to year, comprised 17 groups at first; now there are 30. All attendees are groups that belong to the public services within geographically defined areas. The groups come from very different cultural, geographic, and economic contexts. These meetings can therefore only consist of the sharing of experiences, not instructing each other. Somebody might have an interesting situation to mention; others might want to discuss organizational, clinical, philosophical, or ethical dilemmas. Other issues include sharing of how training programs are set up in the various contexts, and discussions of successful or failed cases.

A common design to investigate clinical outcome has been developed and recently implemented. Because the 30 groups altogether serve a population of more than 3 million people, such studies might yield very interesting findings if we can continue to find the support to operationalize them.

An Educational Program for North Sweden and North Norway

Now we have a 2-year training program in relational and network therapy for north Sweden and north Norway. North Finland has its own program, as mentioned previously. Our present training program is administered by the University of Luleaa in north Sweden and the University College of Tromsoe and the University of Tromsoe, north Norway. It gives credentials in the college and university system. The college and university accepted all the principles from the previous training program, namely, that the students are assigned to groups that meet and work practically together once a week, and meet with their supervisor once a month. In addition, the reading list is much extended; students meet in six 1-week gatherings during the 2 years, and they produce a written group report and pass an examination. Other features of the educational program include the following:

1. Admissions requirements: Most of the students have formal educational competence, but some enter the program based on real-life competence. Even if students do not have the normally requested education, they are accepted if they have had 5 years of practical work and are over 25 years of age.
2. Group composition: The groups can be composed differently. The members might come from the same agency, or more commonly from different agencies.Usually the members have very different backgrounds. No one from the police force has yet been a student, but we hope they soon will come. This mixture in

the groups is in itself a way to let people learn what other agencies do, how they think, and what society expects of them. Being acquainted this way makes it easier to collaborate later in the same community. In their practical work with families, group members will encounter the work from different perspectives. They will feel in their bodies the reality that different descriptions coming from different perspectives are not only normal but very useful. They will therefore not only increase their tolerance for differences but also appreciate them. Much original, local work has been developed by the local groups.

3. Supervision: The supervisors try to follow the flow of the groups and avoid instructions. The supervisors are assistants, and the students know very well if they need assistance, and eventually what kind at which time.
4. Readings: The current reading list includes greater attention to networks and the philosophies of collaboration. We certainly have a special part on the history we have in common with the other countries along the same latitude of the North.
5. Teaching methods: In the six 1-week gatherings we try to make the students' own practical experiences and thinking the basis for the "teaching." I put this word in quotation marks because our "teaching" tries to avoid instructive tendencies. In these weeks, we let live supervision of a group's practical work at home be a prominent part, the group's report on its own training process is discussed, and each group presents a dilemma or critical situation it has confronted. This dilemma is the basis for clarifying philosophical points of view, utilizing, for instance, the ideas of Wittgenstein or Levinas.
6. Content: Many of the issues addressed are practical, including various forms of reflecting processes, kinds of questions, ways to collaborate with families, and applications to different kinds of presenting problems, such as psychotic crisis or domestic violence. There are theoretical discussions on various kinds of knowledge, and we include consideration of various texts: the spoken, the written, and the filmed. We discuss the philosophy of the notion that "we first have to talk with those with whom we meet about how we shall collabo-

rate before we start collaborating." The various practices of language and the corresponding philosphies are central. We try to elucidate these questions through the help of certain philosphers such as Aristotle, Kant, Wittgenstein, Levinas, Loegstrup, Bakhtin, and Vygotsky. This is done with the help of our local philosophers. We explore the contributions of constructivists like Bateson and Maturana, as well as social constructionists like Gergen and Shotter.

7. Student responsibilities: We emphasize the need for students to be a part of the planning of the six 1-week gatherings. A new class of students arrives in September. They are together in a 1-week gathering with the students who started a year earlier. The written group report is intended to let the students investigate their own development and eventual change during the training program. There is a home examination, in which the student explores and discusses the particularities of a situation or a program or therapeutic process or an ethical dilemma. We do not want students to repeat what they have heard or read, but to think, investigate, and formulate their own opinions or questions.

Conclusion

I have tried to write this chapter on behalf of all who belong to the networks that are mentioned. Here I take the privilege to write for myself and to say a few words about meetings and the body's participating in meetings. John Shotter (2003), who has visited us frequently, writes about a person's "spontaneous expressive activities" and says that they are central in life (in my words they *are* the activities of life), that they are bodily, and they are responses to the spontaneous expressive activities of others with whom we meet. Talking is a very powerful expression. Shotter agrees with Voloshinov (1986), who says, "It is not experience that organizes expression, but the other way around— *expression organizes experience*. Expression is what first gives experience its form and specificity of direction. . . . *The organizing center of any utterances, of any experience, is . . . in the social milieu surrounding the individual being*" (pp. 85, 93). Shotter is also excited by the word "chiasmic," meaning activities

of intertwined and reversible nature. With a smile, he says that he does not fully understand the word, but he likes it. Those words have made me think of meetings of "chiasmic" nature, as one shifts from one's own perspective to another's, and then back to one's own. We see both with our own eyes and with others' eyes. It has been important in the meetings that have been mentioned in this chapter that we have strongly held on to the principle that nobody needs to fear that their eye or perspective will be stolen or lost. These will always remain with the individual person as long as the person wants to hold on to them.

I feel that I have been very bold to end with such "big words." Please forgive me. The meetings I have spoken of have been organized around the following issue: How can we be helpful *with* others in ways that protect their identity and their feeling of being valuable? The experiences that have come out of all these meetings, which we hopefully have been able to express to ourselves and others, have been that we must protect solidarity, the cornerstone of democracy. The networks and meetings that have been mentioned here are some (small) contributions to that endeavor. We live in a time in which solidarity and democracy are threatened by anarchy, and the anarchy we can see in our world today is paradoxically based on two opposing but still mutually dependent pillars; militant fundamentalism and market fundamentalism (Barber, 2001). We will keep our meetings going, our small contribution to solidarity.

Acknowledgments

Gunn Eva Andersen and Gerd Furumo, secretaries at the Institute of Community Medicine, University of Tromsoe, have, by their skillful contributions, made it possible for these networks to survive. We owe them many thanks for that. The Swedish Eastern European Committee has financed the Russians' participation in meetings in our countries and our participation in the training programs in Arkhangelsk. We are also very thankful for that.

References

Anderson, H., & Goolishian, H. (1988). Human systems as linguistic systems. *Family Process, 27*, 371–394.

Barber, B. (2001). *Jihad vs Mcworld*. New York: Ballantine.

Kjellberg, E., Edwardsson, M., Niemelä, J., & Öberg, T. (1995). Using reflecting processes with families stuck in violence and child abuse. In S. Friedman (Ed), *The reflecting team in action: Collaborative practice in family therapy* (pp. 38–61). New York: Guilford.

Seikkula, J. Aaltonen, J., Alakare, B., Harankangas, K., Keränen, J., & Sutela, M (1995). Treating psychosis by means of open dialogue. In S. Friedman (Ed.), *The reflecting team in action: Collaborative practice in family therapy* (pp. 62–80). New York: Guilford.

Shotter, J. (2003). Being "moved" by the embodied, responsive-expressive "voice" of an "other." http://pubpages.unh.edu/~jds/

Voloshinov, V. N. (1986). *Marxism and the philosophy of language* (L. Matejka & I. R. Titinik, Trans.). Cambridge, MA: Harvard University Press.

14

Edward P. Eismann

Unitas: Therapy for Youth
in a Street Society

In the midst of the street was the tree of life. . . . And the leaves of the tree were for the healing
of the nations.

Apocalypse 22:2

This is Hunts Point, South Bronx, New York City. It is a vibrant, bustling community in metamorphosis. For decades now it has been a high-risk, multiproblem environment where crime, unemployment, broken homes, rampant drug dealing, failing schools, neighborhood deterioration, smog, pollution, and the chronic high-decibel noise of traffic and aircraft have impacted peoples' lives in alarmingly stressful ways. It is also a community where cultural ties and loyalties, deep religious sentiment, hope for a better future, and neighborly kinship abound. It was into this context that Unitas, a community mental health organization addressing the needs of hard-to-reach youth, was born and has continued to flourish over 35 years. Originally a part of a larger organization, the Lincoln Community Mental Health Center, Unitas first tried to provide a traditional, office-based array of clinical services of an individual, group, and family nature to an unserved, neglected population of severely at-risk youth. The response to this traditional service was disastrous. A statistical analysis of the time indicated that among four clinicians, 1.8 children were being seen per month through intake. Born of such frustration, Unitas took clinical thinking and practice from the office setting and applied it to the open setting of community life, developing

therapeutic linkages between older and younger neighborhood youth in a network of social support. It did this through developing, maintaining, and supervising a large cadre of older youth who bought the idea that they could serve as special friends or parent figures to troubled neighborhood children in a new kind of family focused on mutual helpfulness. Using the language of "symbolic kin" and "symbolic families," an alternative system of mental health care was born, one where youth became engaged in learning to have a collective pro-social influence on each other and the younger children as they might experience in real functional family life where life was not chaotic. In addition to the personal relationships formed in these local "symbolic kin" dyadic and family groupings, a "symbolic extended family" community session was created, composed of some 100 to 150 "symbolic families" meeting daily or weekly in street or school settings to discuss and resolve interpersonal tensions and problems related to life, street, and family. The therapeutic model is a radical departure from traditionally conceived office-based mental health services, but one that offers therapy in the clients' own life space and in the company of their own influential network. Unitas aims to teach its youth to find positive affirmation, supportive resources, and mastery of the tasks of living not from the individual therapies of formal mental health systems but through the influence of the already naturally existing network of family, friends, and each other and, in this neighborhood system, through the persuasion of teenage role models who live with them right here—the caretakers found so conveniently in their own backyard.

This chapter describes community mental health theory as the clinical rationale underpinning the creation of this neighborhood caretaker system, then demonstrates how such theoretical concepts were applied in practice to a local neighborhood, and finally concludes with a reflective analysis of my own transformative journey in creating this therapeutic street society. Who I have become in this process is no more than the person I am by nature and nurture in unity with the environmental wisdom that has formed me.

Community Mental Health: The New Paradigm

It is 1967, a time of tremendous national social unrest and exciting potential for change on social, political, racial, and economic levels. It is the Great Society of Lyndon Johnson, the War on Poverty, model cities, civil rights, and the recent assassination of a president. It is the time of militant groups such as the Black Panthers and Young Lords and their attempts to establish equitable treatment and social justice for the poor by either peaceful collaboration with white power structures or separatism. It is the time of the burgeoning of the community mental health movement, whose ideology, in synchrony with the social, economic, and political thrust of the times, emphasized the impact of systemic forces, in addition to the biological and psychological, as causative in mental illness.

Community mental health as a theoretical construct evolved from a one-dimensional medical model of the nineteenth and early twentieth centuries into a systemic model based at least equally in the social sciences. This evolution, which was a radical departure from the exclusive one-to-one psychoanalytic and biological model of its remote and recent past, represented a new ideology in clinical perspective. The shift in perspective away from the exclusivity of biological and psychodynamic reductionism to explain mental illness to systems

thinking was considered psychiatry's "third revolution" (Whittington, 1965) and was the theoretical underpinning of the new paradigm called community mental health. It particularly had its roots in Lewin's (1948, 1976) field theory, which emphasized that people operate in a social field that to a significant degree determines behavior and that human behavior cannot be understood apart from ongoing interpersonal relations.

Social Work as Community Mental Health in Practice

This concept of behavior being systemic or multi-determined and emphasizing the reciprocal interchanges between the individual and the environment in which he or she is embedded is the most fundamental postulate of social work theory and practice. The community mental health movement, without intending it, actually brought social work thinking back to center base from its decades-long preoccupation with the primacy of intrapsychic determinants of behavior. But it was actually short-lived, and some critics have alleged that community mental health support of the innovation of outreach into communities became a "new and more efficient superstructure for the distribution of the same old services" (Shatan, 1969, p. 318). Ralph Nader, evaluating the community mental health movement in 1974, reported that community mental health centers had done most poorly in the development of a concern for a total population, the development of preventive services, and the enhancement of community strength, and that these centers had done best in those endeavors most similar to traditional clinical service activities (Bloom, 1977). As the community mental health movement within a decade or two of its inception lost its own identity and reverted to functioning once more in a traditional clinic mode largely under the auspices of Medicaid, the social work profession was pulled back once more to the medical model, with its emphasis on biological and individual explanations for disordered behavior. Social work students and practitioners now thought and spoke of themselves as "therapists" and of fieldwork as "internship." Managed care within medical contexts and the emphasis on symptoms being the result of "an imbalance in brain chemistry," requiring an infusion of brand medications to change chemical imbalances, further distracted from the social work wisdom of seeing the client as a unity of person within context. A solid wave of systemic thinking and practice, however, continued undaunted to permeate the field of practice, with mounting empirical evidence accumulating that supported the basic Lewinian postulate that human behavior is significantly determined by the characteristics of one's social field, and that profound changes can be effected in behavioral functioning by influencing the environmental field one is embedded in.

Social Work as Social Psychiatry in Practice

Of particular note in operationalizing systems thinking in the original community mental health paradigm, as well as in its subsequent applications, was the seminal work of Caplan in America and of Jones in England (Caplan, 1964, 1974; Jones, 1973, 1976). Caplan wrote extensively on the contribution made by ordinary citizens as effective treatment agents to their neighbors, emphasizing the informal affective and instrumental support function they serve, or potentially can develop through encouragement and consultation. But, he asserted, it was in the quality of support from one's social network that people's mental health was impacted in substantive ways. Destructive behavior was seen as a breakdown in attachment to significant others in one's natural network, or at least a deficiency in one's primary group ties. The solution for Caplan was to rebuild or reinforce those positive ties that did exist or to create new ones to replace the influence of negative network responses. In this sense, social support was considered a primary goal in community mental health practice, enabling people to have an experience of connectedness and belonging to offset the social disintegration resulting from alienation.

Jones's impressive work in the 1940s under the discipline of social psychiatry grew out of his work with combat victims from the war who had to be returned promptly to the battlefield after "treatment." His observations of their interactions with, and mutual aid to, each other in the hospital setting led him to develop his principles of a therapeutic community, an organizational structure that allowed him to take advantage of the natural healing that combatants were already offering to each

other. Systematizing such natural phenomena, Jones developed the concept of therapeutic community, which he described as synonymous with social psychiatry, where the goal was "to utilize natural social relationships in the social organization of the program as the primary source of therapeutic change" (in Filstead & Rossi, 1973, p. 11). Jones's (1973) systemic thinking in England dovetailed with the developing paradigm of community mental health in the United States and led him to comment: "The ideas originally developed in a hospital setting have equal applicability to any social system, whether it be in institutions such as prisons, subcultures such as religion or the school system, or political system on a local or national scale" (p. 336).

In sum, community mental health, as the new paradigm, stressed the influence that social forces in which people were embedded had on their individual behavior and aimed to alter peoples' lives through influencing the dynamics contained in these forces.

Focusing on the influence of context in the treatment and prevention of dysfunctional behavior, Langston (1970) reviewed relevant literature of the time and described five directives essential to implementing the practice of community mental health. There would be:

1. A need to focus on all members of a designated community, functional as well as dysfunctional;
2. A need to address primary prevention through interventions aimed at intercepting potential disturbance in the normally well;
3. A need to establish social treatment goals aimed at promoting social adjustment in ordinary life rather than reconstruction of personality;
4. The need to provide continuity of care through seeing that people in one's care are integrated in a comprehensive network of care; and
5. A need to use oneself together with other community caretakers to extend one's effectiveness by working through and with other people.

The Application of the New Paradigm to a Street Society

Unitas operationalized this new paradigm as a preventive and alternative system of mental health care for a high-risk population of inner-city youth. It was initiated in those early years of the community mental health movement's growth and sustained without interruption over three decades and into a new century. In keeping with its systemic paradigm, and consonant with Langston's (1970) review, Unitas focused on a designated community of functional and dysfunctional youth. It initially developed the therapeutic potential of its own community caretakers of youth, its own "citizens" (Caplan, 1974), by engaging and then coaching them to wield influence on each other and the neighborhood children by creating a supportive social structure to promote social adjustment in one small influential context of all their lives, namely, the open system of the street. It was the street where one found the most alienated, hard-to-reach youth, the most needy, and eventually the most responsive to attachment. It was on the street where one found the street heroes and heroines who responded to the call to service. Together they needed each other. It was on the street where power and influence could be informally leveled and negotiated. The program eventually moved into schools and settlement house systems as well, coaching teachers and recreation workers to develop their personal capacities to serve as therapeutic change agents to youths in their own systems. That aspect of Unitas is the story of its interventions as applied to formal organizations and is not reported here.

Entry Into Street Culture

Armed with these notions of community mental health theory emphasizing systemic interventions and community caretaking, I decided to get as close as possible to the lives of the children of the South Bronx and their potential caretakers by immersing myself in their street culture (Eismann, 1996). However, the decision to become enmeshed in this culture, first as participant observer and then as active practitioner, was not just the result of my theoretical persuasion. It was born of my terrible frustration sitting as an office-based clinician at the local Lincoln Community Mental Health Center, whose services few youth were responding to. Driven by such frustration, as well as by intense curiosity regarding this clinical conundrum, I walked the streets for months, sitting in school yards, on tenement stoops, curbs, and car fenders, and "hanging out" in alleyways, bodegas, and social clubs. I made connections and "friendships," as did the friendly visitor of the bygone settlement house days. People wanted to know who I was. I explained that I was Dr. E. from Lincoln Health Center and that my (self-defined) job was to hang out and talk to youngsters who had problems or worries. The floodgates opened. Children poured out their hearts about family, bullies, violence, and drugs; teens accepted my mediation in street conflicts. I talked the language of therapy, but now in their systems and networks. There was no dearth of customers; in fact, it was difficult to hold back the tide. From this experience, I saw that this population of youngsters not only was not resistant to mental health interventions in their lives but sought me out with undaunted motivation as long as two elements were present in this engagement: *my immersion in their social setting* and *in the company of their social network*. That was the design that made the difference. So I began to dream about developing an intervention that would serve as an alternative form of mental health care whereby the influence of the naturally existing network in one's social setting would be recognized, organized, and then cultivated for healing purposes. Noting that children often hung around groups of teenagers, their natural role models in this street system, I slowly engaged these streetwise teenagers as my "consultees" in this networking venture. Clueing into the emphasis on family relationships prevalent among the heavily Hispanic and African American population, and over time setting myself in the symbolic role of "grandpa," the court of last appeal, enlisted these neighborhood young men and women to serve as caretakers, co-padres, co-parents, symbolic "mothers and fathers," to the children of their own street. I began meeting with these teens to provide structure and training to them in their child-caring work while also giving them direct help with their own concerns. I arranged for these young caretakers to meet with children in schools, libraries, recreation centers, and church settings. This brought me into contact with the larger network of agencies serving youth so that my ability to open doors for children and the teen caretakers themselves was effected with minimal bureaucratic constraints. And everywhere I went, I was met with openness and support. But all this is another story. For expansion of the detailed steps in this initial journey, only summarized here, I refer the reader to other sources (Eismann, 1996; Farber & Rogler, 1981; Procidano & Glenwick, 1985).

Street Society as Tribal Council

It is 1:30 of a hot summer afternoon as I pull into Fox Street in the South Bronx, gutted buildings and trash-strewn streets announcing the neighborhood's stature as the worst of New York City's slums. I am surrounded by kids chattering in English and Spanish, all wanting something from the beat-up van that serves as the play closet of my "traveling clinic": bats, balls, paper, crafts, ropes, games. Play: the natural language of childhood, the link, the bait, to communication and relationship in a child's world. More on this later.

It is now 2:30 P.M. Continuing a daily ritual, I take my place cross-legged on the asphalt, in the gutter, the first point of a circle that falls into place without any further announcement. We are to begin the "tribal council," the "family circle," the therapeutic community session that kicks off each day. Within a few minutes, some 75 to 100 children and teenagers have followed suit, arranging themselves in their own little family groupings in a circular format around me, radiating up to 30 feet in diameter. They know the rules: we begin when all are quiet. And so around the group can be heard, "sh-sh-sh" as the children shush each other, anxious to get on with the meeting and the play to come.

And so I begin. "Hello, my friends. As you know, this is Unitas, and Unitas is a wonderful community of boys and girls, young men and young women, and some older men and women who meet like this each day to play together and talk together about better ways of getting along and settling problems peacefully. If you have anything you would like to say today, just raise your hands as I come around so I can see how many have something to bring to the family today." I make eye contact, at least momentarily, with each child as I go around the circle. A number of hands dance up and down in the air in response to my question. Group interaction follows around the concerns aired. Mundane or trite, one might say, but reflective of the worries of childhood: "He broke my toy," a ball that was "roofed," "she took my quarter," "he hurt my brother," "why can't we play ball, too?" and so on. All concerns are golden nuggets inviting the thinking of the group with follow-up support and

rational collective decision making. Affirmation of each response and much "reframing" create a net of safety for all. That is the hope, the intent. Success in achieving this is modified by humble failures as well.

From the corner of my eye I detect a conflict emerging between caretaker Felix and two of his oppositional "sons," Antonio and Adam. Felix has been trying to control their disruptive behavior in the group, and they in turn have been increasingly defying his power over them. Taking authority into his own hands, he starts to physically remove them from the group. It threatens to develop into a real fracas. I quickly intervene: "What is happening over there?" "These stupids are not listening to me," Felix responds, "so I'm kicking them out." Felix has overstepped a community rule, which is that whenever a caretaker cannot handle a problem alone, he or she is to ask the community for help. I say: "You need some help. Thank you for making that known." I rise from my community space and enter the circle's psychodramatic space and say to Antonio and Adam, "I don't want you to leave. Would the two of you be willing to come to the middle of the circle and tell us what went on that you were asked to leave, so you have a chance to speak your heart? And you, Felix, would you come over here to speak your heart to your sons so they know what it is clearly that you expect of them as their caretaker? Have a seat here and you over there. Is there anyone else who has some thoughts on this matter?" Diana raises her hand and is invited to join the inner circle of protagonists and antagonists. I turn around and say to all: "Listen up, all of you, there was this problem between Antonio and Adam and their caretaker, Felix. Also, Diana, who is a caretaker in a nearby family, has something to say, too. Felix was telling these two brothers to be quiet, but they were not listening to him. That was the problem. So, let's find out more about this. Felix, what happened, and what did you actually say to them?" Felix recounts his words: "I said 'please shut your mouth,' but they did not listen, so I said it again, 'shut your mouth.' They still paid me no mind, so I finally shouted 'shut up' to them." "You finally became forceful after nothing else seemed to work, and then when I questioned what was happening, it was then you asked for help by stating the problem. That is where the rest of us come in, is that it?" "Yeah, that's it," he says. "Thank you."

Turning to Adam, I invite him to tell us what happened from his point of view. Adam says he remembers being yelled at to "shut up . . . shut up." I comment that he seems to say this with a lot of anger; what actually was he feeling at the time? He shrugs. "Who thinks they know how Adam might have felt?" A child raises his hand and is invited to come into the psychodramatic enactment as well. "Sit next to Adam," I tell him, "and make out you are Adam himself, although I will call you Adam II." Adam II comments strongly that he would have felt very mad to be talked to that way. Adam I agrees with bobbing head. "Antonio, how about you, why didn't you quiet down when asked? What is your story?" Antonio states that it is the same, and that he didn't think it was right to be cursed at that way. I summarize: "Do you all see now what went on? The caretaker of the family was responsibly doing his job in making sure his sons around him were paying attention in the circle. He exercised his rightful authority in his own way of speaking. The sons here are saying we hear him, but we don't like being told to 'shut up, shut your mouth.' How many of you here like it when people say 'shut up' to you?" The group is awake. The question has landed on empathic ground. "So you know how the brothers felt?" I have neglected Diana. She has been bursting at the seams to speak as I have tediously labored to bring focus to this confrontation in the middle of the street. Containing herself no longer, she says with passion: "It is not just how they felt; they were talking constantly. I saw them and even motioned to them to quiet down, but they sneered at me, and (looking directly at them) I don't like that kind of disrespect." I comment, "So this was your observation from sitting nearby, and you were feeling as frustrated and annoyed as Felix; you know through your own anger how the caretaker might also have felt." In defending Felix, Diana has loyally implemented another community rule, namely, that caretakers should support and back each other up as an "executive system." I turn to the community and say, "This is getting more and more interesting. There seem to be two sides to this story, as in all stories. Let's see how the story will unfold." I look firmly but in an engaging manner at Antonio and Adam and say: "You have heard what Felix said, backed up by Diana. I am going to push you a little bit to continue this wonderful cooperation you are showing by asking you if you

could, and I hope you would, talk to Felix in such a way as to win his attention to what you have to tell him, but in a respectful manner. Tell him that you don't mind being told what to do but the kind of words he uses makes a big difference. Talk to him now about this." Both boys respond to the direction, and Adam, taking the lead, says squarely to Felix, "We don't like it when you curse at us to make us do something. That's not right." I say, "Good words, nice way of directly talking to someone you have a gripe with . . . very manly." Felix says back, "You don't want me to say 'shut up,' right? Well, then, when I tell you to be quiet, I expect you to do that . . . ok? I don't want to keep telling you to always do that. Be quiet when I tell you. I did ask you nice but then you gave me no choice." I comment, "You want them to respect you as much as they want you to respect them with the words you use." Diana, undaunted in her support of Felix, adds: "You know he's right, and so do I, so remember what he is saying to you." Adam and Antonio each say, "Sorry for talking." "Thanks for apologizing," Felix says. "Next time I won't curse at you, but you have to listen to me the first time." I look with admiration at Felix and say, "Listen, these brothers had a lot of courage to get up here and voice their problem, and Felix, you did too, together with Diana's backing. Great . . . wonderful work, all of you." As all return to their place in the outer circle, a round of applause gives recognition to their courage. "Thanks all of you," I say. "This is not easy; it is our work together." It is almost time to close the meeting, so I conclude: "Listen up, all of you, especially you caretakers. Next time take care of things the way we did here, speak up sooner and respectfully to each other whether on a trip or right here in this circle. I want you to remember that problems are opportunities to learn from, not excuses to slug things out. If you don't act on this thinking, how will your children ever learn to get along with others?" Having rationalized my advice giving as a psychoeducational intervention, I conclude the session: "As we finish up, what do you think of the courage shown here today by Ada and Chico and then Elena and Maria, a while back, and then Felix, Diana, Adam, and Antonio? They were the ones here who had the courage to speak up and help this group." A chorus of yeas and a hearty round of applause resound around the circle, clear as the grin on my face, as the heroes and heroines in today's minidrama of life enacted in this thera-peutic theater beam and bask in their deserved rec-ognition.

A Dynamic Perspective on Therapeutic Community and Developmental Need

An afternoon of play follows. Play! The work and language of childhood. In simple moment-to-moment interactions of play, children's perceptions of and engagements with the world are expressed for communication, reinforcement, and benign cor-rection. And so Unitas enlists the influence of com-munication from this already existing network and uses the peer voices to bring about behavioral change in each other's lives. So when Bobby, a hy-peractive, attention-getting, disorganized child, breaks impulsively into a line, demanding, "I want the ball," I turn to Renee, a waiting child, and say, "Renee, will you talk to Bobby about his behavior?" She responds quickly and says: "You know, Bobby, you have to wait your turn. This is like going to lunch in school. You'll get your lunch, but you have to wait your turn." Without a word, Bobby takes his place and waits. Because the power came from a peer, Bobby took the comment, and because Renee is a normal child with no defensive axes to grind, she knew just what to say in a child's idiom. All I have to do is to be a sensitive navi-gator. The troops do the work as long as I believe in them.

This theme of the troops doing the work is the core idea in the support community. I carry it into every area of Unitas, relying mainly on these care-takers, the teenagers, as its healthy, giving com-ponents. It is the teenagers who, with my guidance, deal almost solely with even the most disturbed of the Unitas children, taking them for extra one-to-one sessions during the day, talking with their par-ents, even feeding them at times to give the angriest youngsters an opportunity to recapture some of the early nurture they have missed. This was just the case with Ernesto and eight other oppositionally defiant children whose presence reminded me daily of war on a battlefield, each child strategically plan-ning what was necessary in the service of survival, and questioning always on which side the victory would eventually fall. It was always the ancient story: good guys versus bad guys. Of course, I was the good guy.

The battlefield being a given, one strategy I pro-posed was to be psychodynamic in specificity, aimed at the need to address early deprivation by providing "symbolic realization" (Secheheye, 1951) and a "corrective emotional experience" (Alexan-der, 1948; Bowlby, 1966). And so, armed with these theories and with metaphoric imagery, I linked these youngsters with selected caretakers who would provide them with milk in the quietness of the fire escape in the back of the church lot car-ingly in a one-to-one relationship. Equipped with part of a crate of milk saved from the city lunch program for each day, at a prescribed time in the afternoon consistent with regularity and predicta-bility to inculcate security and expectation, I insti-tuted the "nursery of the street." This attempted treatment intervention aimed at providing devel-opmental stimulation by a "relationship through feeding" experience that was dyadic, instinctively pleasurable, relational, kinesthetic, and predictable in the interest of behavioral change. Though ini-tially supported by classical drive theory, subse-quent developments in object relations, self psy-chology, and social systems theories have placed an emphasis on the primacy of significant others in affectional bondedness and continuity of rela-tionship. It is how I explain things now. This ex-pansion of psychodynamic theory and the integra-tion of social systems thinking does appear to be a richer way of explaining why "these boys do seem better."

Street Society Caretakers Speak for Themselves

As I make my way to the noise and activity of the street itself, I scan all the caretakers with their sym-bolic sons and daughters and I think, "Why is ab-senteeism so rare among these caretakers, these symbolic 'mothers and fathers' and their symbolic children?" I conclude that for the caretakers partic-ularly, it must be a hunger for the purpose it gives them in terms of inclusion, belonging, nourish-ment, affirmation, and last but not least, a hunger for connection with a nurturing, symbolic parent of their own, expressed in their relationship with me. Through transferential dynamics, that relation-ship provides them with a corrective experience to help heal the abuse and neglect so many of them suffered in their real lives. And while this reflection applies to all, children and caretakers alike, it seems that the caretaking teens are among the biggest gainers in this picture. For Miguel, who by his own admission "made a habit of not talking" (an elective mutism) until 3 years before when he became part of Unitas, the desire to be a symbolic father became the wedge to opening communication with the world. For Juan, a teen lost in the middle of a large multiproblem family, it was the personal attention that alleviated his loneliness and engaged his constant presence. As he said, "It was the way I was treated here that made me want to treat someone like that, too. I experienced a lot here and to one who never got that, you are a brother to him" (Eismann, 1996). For Luis, who came to Unitas as a withdrawn child of 12, only to grow into the open, outgoing leader he has become, "Unitas is kind of a perfect place. I was the quietest one when I first came, I didn't want to do anything, just sit and watch TV. But now," grins the lanky teenager, rakish with an orange comb jammed in his short Afro, "I'm the busiest, noisiest one of the lot." Jorge, an overanxious and overachieving caretaker, speaking of Mark, who was his symbolic father, says, "If it weren't for Mark in my life . . . I was full of anger and wanted to hurt people because I was hurting and did not feel right for anyone else to be happy. I hated everyone and Mark took that hate away from me" (Shapiro, 1988). And Mark, sullen and uncommunicative, a boy who eventually grew into the model caretaker, touching the lives of innumerable youth, reminisces:

> I will never forget the experience of not having a father. I would never want anyone else to have that experience. It is like my quest in life is to be available to anyone who missed a mother or father in their life. I was lucky, though, because I had a special experience with Doc, Miguel, and the other brothers who nurtured each other, and that is what made me strong and able to go on.

As I reflect on my decades of listening to the needs, hopes, and dreams of thousands of youth in school, church, settlement house, and street settings, the message is the same: the cry for inclusion, personal empathic attention, and relationship with an accepting father (I specify father rather than parent in general because of a repetitious theme in the verbal dialogues of both boys and girls related to the longing for and anger at the absent father; being male, I am more directly the object of positive or negative transference) who provides reason and

constancy in their chaotic lives. When offered these three experiences, not so far removed from the essential taste of treatment itself, it appears they internalize these dispositions for their own maturation. Doing so enables them to provide the same experience, in turn, to their symbolic children, who again, in turn, become caretakers to the next generation of symbolic children. The call to youth, in 1968, to serve as community caretakers remains unbroken into 2004. What remains equally unbroken is the realization of one of the dreams of the community mental health movement, namely, that prevention on primary, secondary, and perhaps even tertiary levels can be actualized when mental health professionals, believing in this vision, use themselves to organize any social setting to enlist, support, and develop the potential influence of the already existing social network to bring about changes among its members and to modify the environment itself.

Reflections of a Community Clinician: The Person, Not the Technique, as Essential Variable

Every enterprise begins with a person with an idea. The person applies this idea to practice and then develops a method for transmitting that idea and its practice to others; selection is made of those most capable and responsive to the idea and its application, and who are helped to internalize it. Finally, a method is developed to ensure a way of transmitting the idea and its practice to subsequent descendants. Maintaining an idea in a sustained way and institutionalizing a methodology for passing the idea on is extremely difficult. The original mission of an enterprise and its expression as taught and practiced by a founder are always subject to evolutionary developments, manipulative opportunism by those in power, constructivist viewpoints that reframe and even subvert the original idea, and the victory of mediocrity and bureaucratization over a founder's innermost passionate vision. These are compelling topics too vast to consider in this chapter. What I can consider here is a reflection on the variable of myself as person, the dynamics of my own life, and the thinking of other minds that profoundly influenced me, all of which made possible the creation and sustenance of the work of Unitas. I hope that such reflection may be useful to others, particularly clinicians, inclined to create or found new services. I share reflections of my own journey in this quest to make some difference in this faltering but glorious world.

Much of the literature on healing emphasizes that rather than any technique or mere adherence to a particular school of psychological thought, it is the strength of a therapist's belief in a specific worldview, his or her specific perception of reality, the philosophical conviction underpinning the very meaning he or she makes of the purpose of life that, when conveyed to others in the therapeutic relationship, brings about change. And so, here I am on Fox Street in the South Bronx, a clinical social worker by professional definition in this context. But who I am will make the difference, not what I am or how I define my credentialed identity. I come with an ideology already formed about life, a worldview, a weltanschauung that I had developed from the influence of my own family and cultural experiences in response to the needs and struggles of my own life. Clinical formation had to find a way of being in sync with who I was. This mind-set, this worldview that I brought to practice was reflected in three beliefs: first was the belief in the innate desire and capacity of all people to be helpers, healers to each other, and not restricted to a healing caste, either priestly or clinical; second was the belief that empathic communication breaks the barriers of alienation, enabling personal development to emerge, as well as community to be built and their interpersonal effects transmitted to others; third was the passion of a belief I had in envisioning and creating a more loving place in some small part of the world. These beliefs encompassed the "who I am" that I brought with the "what I am."

The Person

The personality and way of thinking of any leader, political, therapeutic or religious, is vital to the achievement of any venture. I am a friendly, outgoing, gentle person. I am empathic, hurt easily, and am basically shy. I take things to heart, too seriously. In this seriousness I become easily discouraged and thereby prone to depression. Time, dogs, good friends, and the grace of God pull me over to the side of sanity again. A creative bent, egged on by my childhood shyness, took my early social cravings and sublimated them into deeply felt artistic expressions in music, art, and drama and

then organized to entertain and serve others. I transformed the basement and yard of my house into a puppet theater, a hospital for stray dogs and cats, an amusement park complete with rides, a restaurant, a school. I had a passion for music and immersed myself in adolescence in musical groups wherever they were, in school, in church, in volunteer organizations. These activities brought me into a world of friendship that satisfied the passion I felt for music, as well as my cravings for social connections. In the context of this passion, my overarching goal was to become a concert pianist, but I gave up this quest during my late teens and early manhood to pursue the priesthood in the Roman Catholic Church. This latter quest was consistent with my cumulative seriousness of purpose, for in my adolescent years I made a decision to find a meaning to life and to live for a purpose beyond myself. It was born of the deaths of two people: an uncle and a grandfather. When I gazed in grief at them in their coffins, I asked the age-old questions: "Why did you have to die?" "Is this all life is about?" "What is life, anyway?" "Does God exist?" "What is my relationship with other human beings supposed to be?" Thus began my quest for meaning, the search for an "ideological identity" (Coles, 2000). To me, the priesthood offered the epitome of meaning, namely, not only to be of service to others in the needs of this life, but to be for others an instrument of grace into the next. The experience of the 9 years in this monastic formation was a profound one, deepening and solidifying the social and philosophical questions I was struggling to answer. The eventual answer was found neither in priesthood nor even in social work but in the person of myself, which these noble vocations helped develop and enrich through their teachings and influence and which eventually found their ultimate expression in Unitas.

Philosophical introspection and sublimated social hunger were always, and continue to be, my most deeply felt inner experiences. The valuation of ideology to satisfy my introspective questions, and deep friendships and creativity to satisfy my social hunger were the chief expressions of this inner experience. These expressions of ideology, creativity, and friendship eventually found their culmination in the creation of Unitas, rooted as it is in a clearly defined spiritual ideology, in the creative use of psychological theory, and in a celebration of the love of friendship, the friendship of agape, as well as the friendship of mutual need or, as it is formulated now, the friendship of "instrumental and affective support." Such concepts as the love of friendship and its variations find their expression in psychodynamic theory, with its own esoteric language, but have their underpinnings in the philosophical writings following the thinking of Plato, Aristotle, Cicero, and Thomas Aquinas. Philosophy establishes the wisdom of loving; psychodynamic practice teaches how to develop our loving selves, and using such love, develop this love in others.

The effectiveness of Unitas cannot be divorced from these philosophical and social beliefs that I, as originator, deeply held and through which I attempted to influence the minds, hearts, and behaviors of the original core group of teens, who through the years passed on these beliefs to subsequent numbers of children who grew up in Unitas and became its cadre of leaders in due time. (I have no objective knowledge of myself that could specifically pinpoint those qualities, those variables that were outgrowths of my personal beliefs, which touched a neighborhood of teens enabling them to respond to my "call" to them.) My ability to reach out to neighborhood teens, even from another cultural world, to form a working alliance with them, and as such create a core group, came from the deep caring they personally felt from me as a result of my beliefs in their goodness, power, and basic altruism, which flowed from my own perception of life and human nature. As Miguel, now age 45, but only age 10 when Unitas began, said, "The only thing not evaluated is you, Doc. But for something like this to work, the person has to be right, and the chemistry, and the situation. The basic thing was you, Doc, that made the difference and then the other things you did." Miguel distinguishes between me as a person and what I did. But what I did to form alliances with these young people at the very beginning contained the expression of me to them as a person at the same time as I "did things." This "person variable" that Miguel speaks of is difficult to measure but essentially transcends all theories and techniques underlying practice. You really cannot measure this "person variable" accurately but can only describe it anecdotally. The very person of the therapist is at the core here. Interventions and techniques from clinical practice must be in sync with this personality core and must flow with it naturally. There are pianists who play the notes and fill the air with sound, and there are pianists who play the same notes and fill the air with music. By just listening, you know the one from the other. You know the firefly from all other beetles by its glow. You discover in life where your spark is, your Midas touch, and by using it, the world around you changes. It is the essential you, born of genetics merged with cultural influences. And that still does not capture the essential you but may come closer. You must know your spark, and then others around you who are touched by your influence validate it. Some are not touched by your influence. That is the client-person variable, a variable equally complex to isolate for analysis and beyond theoretical musings in this chapter. I speak here only of the therapist-person variable, a subject in itself of essential understanding that transcends the study of all other variables undertaken in the research of psychotherapy.

> Strip away a therapist's orientation, the journals he reads, the books on his shelves, the meetings he attends—the cognitive framework his rational mind demands—and what is left to define the psychotherapy he conducts? Himself. The person of the therapist is the converting catalyst, not his order or credo, not his spatial location in the room, not his exquisitely chosen words or denominational silences. . . . The dispensable trappings of dogma may determine what a therapist thinks he is doing, what he talks about when he talks about therapy, but the agent of change is who he is. (Lewis, Amini, & Lanuan, 2000, pp. 186–187)

My reflections here speak in depth of four ideological dispositions that have infused and underpinned my clinical practice and constitute my very personhood: faith, hope, love, and purpose.

Faith and Hope

It was Jerome Frank (1973) who, reviewing much of the literature on healing, concluded that regardless of any specific theory, the essential curative elements in healing resided in faith and hope, and explained that it was the belief or hope that a person had in a power that could heal, human or spiritual, that set healing energies in motion. For purposes of healing, Frank said, the matter of objective reality is insignificant; it is a specific belief in a certain way that influences us. So, as one person can inspire another to perceive reality differently, reality changes for that person whether or not it actually is that way. In fact, psychotherapy appears to do just that: to help a person break through crippling perceptions of reality or distortions and view the same reality through a different frame. However, the ability of a therapist to influence such a change of perception would depend, according to Frank, both on the strength of a therapist's own belief in the perspective of reality he/she offers and on the confidence that he/she is able to inspire in a patient to see reality similarly. These abilities of the therapist in turn evoke faith and hope in the patient. The stronger the therapist believes in and persuasively conveys his ideological understanding of the problem to the patient, the stronger the healing forces of faith and hope are stirred up in that patient. The expectation of cure, fostered by such faith and hope, is itself curative. Thus, strengthening a belief in an ideology, an alternate perception, and conveying this to the other persons with the confident expectation that they too will believe in it are the basic common elements in all psychotherapies, according to Frank.

These thoughts from Frank had a profound meaning for me because they so accurately described a perception and conviction I had, an ideology derived from my religious beliefs and introspective reflections, namely, that people were meant to live in loving cooperation and mutual helpfulness with each other and in partnership with a higher power. In fact, this perception provided the very substratum on which my practice was built and around which my therapeutic interventions and techniques were organized. The power of this belief enabled and impassioned me to have the zeal and courage to set out confidently to organize and mold a neighborhood of children and adolescents into a therapeutic community, a symbolic family through which troubled psyches could be influenced. The strength of this belief and its transmission remains for me the very foundation of Unitas, the reason for its accomplishments, as well as, in its absence, its dips into mediocrity. Such assumed achievements or failures are essentially related to the personhood and impassioned belief system of the organization's personnel at any time, and the motivation this inspires to serve others.

Love

I was also aware that my belief that this loving community could be created out of the naturally existing relationships in that community needed to be communicated to the children and teens with a conviction that was contagious, for through the confidence that I could inspire in my young friends, their faith and hope in me, and the "reality" I was proposing to them, would be awakened. The communication of my belief and the invitation to partake of it with me were to be done through empathic love. From the writings of Carl Rogers (1951, 1964, 1968; Rogers & Wood, 1974) and his followers who deepened and expanded his thinking, I came to understand how to communicate love in a disciplined way so that the building of this "reality" I was proposing to my community of youth would evoke their belief in the desirability of building this same reality and the confidence that they had the powers to accomplish this. The Rogerians spoke of loving relationships as containing three essential ingredients: accurate empathy, respect, and authenticity, which when communicated from one person to another, would have a profound effect on that person in terms of healing for the troubled and reaffirmation for all. Such empathic love, for Rogers, was the heart of psychotherapy. And so, when I took to the streets to invite the first teens to work with me in starting to build the Unitas community, and when I first met with a stoop-side group who traipsed in from other streets to meet with me daily to satisfy their social hunger, it was the empathic understanding, respect, and genuineness I communicated to them that enabled their faith and hope in themselves to be awakened. The belief that they could build a caring community among themselves and their little street brothers and sisters followed upon that awakening.

What particularly impressed me about the Rogerian philosophy and method of healing that I used to "operationalize" empathic love was its universality. Rogers was speaking of a loving disposition that all people needed to receive in order to achieve harmonious relationships. This thinking has had far-reaching effects not only in psychological treatment but also in humanistic education and a diversity of human relationship training programs throughout the world. The universality of Rogers's approach to people in general, including those in therapy, had particular appeal to me, since I was building a community of healing in its own right, composed of both normal and maladjusted youth, not just a therapeutic model for referral of those diagnosed in need. Here was a man who spoke of the curative element of love to heal the broken and strengthen the unbroken, and implicitly asking for a belief in the power of love to do this for all. Extending this thinking into a community context was a natural and theoretically valid extension of Rogers's ideas.

Purpose

The question has been asked of me repeatedly: "Why have you stayed for 35 years in a poverty-stricken community in the South Bronx whose social-psychological characteristics are so staggeringly notorious that they rate among the most problematic in New York City?" The question is no different than that asked of many people: Why do they stay faithful in a relationship, or loyal to their country, or work in underdeveloped countries, or raise a severely handicapped child? The answer usually has to do not only with faith, hope, and love, as reflected on earlier in this chapter, but equally with purpose, all of which qualities are found in people all around us.

My own answer is that working in an abandoned section of the city with people who could be numbered among the most neglected fills for me a deep need to be wanted, useful, and significant and satisfies for me a sense of ethical rightness. In this, I was touched and affirmed by the "social feeling" concept of Alfred Adler (Ansbacher & Ansbacher, 1967), who said, "Every human being strives for significance, but people make mistakes if they do not see that their whole significance must consist in their contribution to the lives of others" (p. 156). The extent to which purpose energized my belief in my vision with such fire as to stick with the growth of Unitas through all the setbacks was all-pervasive. It meant living for a purpose beyond myself. Victor Frankl (1973, 1975, 1992) taught me how to transcend my immediate frustrations through defining a purposeful goal to aim at, to envision a dream. Frankl learned how to survive the atrocities of Auschwitz and help his fellow sufferers to do so, too, by keeping alive in himself and

others the meaning of their lives to the people outside who loved them and awaited their return or envisioning a passionate mission they needed to accomplish by staying alive, which only they could do. As Frankl (1992) said, "He who has a 'why' to live for, can bear almost any 'how' " (p. 30).

When Bruno Bettelheim (1974) studied the socialization processes in an Israeli kibbutz, he was impressed with the cohesiveness of the collectivity in carrying out its work and child-rearing tasks, and he concluded that it was purpose that gave these people the psychic energy to maintain their way of life against great odds: "I am convinced that communal life can flourish only if it exists for an aim outside itself. Community is viable if it is the outgrowth of a deep involvement in a purpose, which is other than, or above, that of being a community" (p. 307). I did not conceive of Unitas as a community of children and youth who would just be friends with each other as in a community center, but as a community of youth who would be bonded with each other in relationships of deeply felt friendship and mutual helpfulness, a modern-day version of being their "brothers' keepers." Their willingness to do this, as well as their belief in their own power to do so, would be transmitted to them through my belief in the vision and in their capacity to achieve it. Although they would meet with frustrations and setbacks with the children and each other, they would need to remember and believe in the purpose of this community: to bring mutual aid and a sense of agape to troubled children and each other. Remembering that they were recipients of the communities' bounty as well as givers was essential in maintaining their membership. This therapeutic community was understood as a community of reciprocal exchange and could be most accurately described by Cobb (1976) in his classical definition of social support: "Social support is information leading the subject to know he is cared for and loved, esteemed and valued, and that he belongs to a network of communication and mutual obligation" (p. 300).

For me, creating and maintaining a loving community of children and teens who cared for each other in this "network of communication and mutual obligation" had a deep natural and spiritual meaning. I found natural meaning in the sense of being able to create a more loving world. But above all else, I found spiritual meaning in the sense I had of finding God, however to be conceived, in this community of love, for I remembered the hymn I sang as a child: "Ubi Caritas est. . . . Where Love is, there is God. . . ." And so, an ideology rooted in faith, hope, love, and purpose that I had developed in response to the needs of my own life became the basis for the creation of Unitas. My faith and hope in the inherent capacity and desire of people to be healers, helpers to each other; the love of agape that I believed could be, and would be, transmitted to others as sparks that kindle other sparks; and the spiritual vision of creating a more loving place in some small part of the world formed the unshakable foundation of Unitas, without which underpinning this vision never would have soared with a life of its own and been sustained over the decades into a new millennium. The question of Unitas's future existence is contained in the impassioned belief system of its contemporary organization at any point of its present life.

It was 1967. It is now 2004. I was a younger, energetic man 37 years ago. I am now a septuagenarian. The belief in the vision and in the capacities of youth to find their significance in contributing to the lives of others is as strong in me as ever it was. My mind is still sharp and I still sit in tribal council, but my energy level makes me move more slowly now. Unitas has been my life's work together with raising a family and taking care of elderly parents. People say to me that Unitas was possible in its own day, but life and the changing circumstances of our times, including violence, rampant drug dealing, child abuse, homelessness, racism, managed care, funding restrictions, and a host of such variables, make an outreach approach into neighborhoods and schools to build connections between people informally, as reflected in the story of Unitas, a naive, unrealistic, and even dangerous paradigm to follow in our present world. I could not disagree more with these defensive critiques. The "dangerous" circumstances and social ills were as much a part of the reality then as they are now. If I were to be again a young clinician with a dream, I would take exactly the same journey whatever the context: whether Fox Street in the South Bronx or an analogous Fox Street in any other social environment. The spiritual vision and the scientific wisdom from psychological and sociological thought that informs my practice are the guiding lights unaltered by the alleged changing circumstances of our times. We stay the same as human

beings, with our needs for attachment, connectedness, and belonging. To organize any social setting in such a way as to evoke the faith, hopes, love, and purpose of that setting's people to make a better world among themselves is a therapeutic objective as viable today as ever it was. It is the noble practice of our social work profession. It is ultimately a spiritual vision of the dream of a more loving world.

References

Alexander, F. (1948). *Fundamentals of psychoanalysis*. New York: Norton.

Ansbacher, H., & Ansbacher, R. (Eds.). (1967). *The individual psychology of Alfred Adler*. New York: Harper and Row.

Bettelheim, B. (1974). *A home for the heart*. New York: Knopf.

Bloom, G. (1977). *Community mental health: An introduction*. Monterey, CA: Brooks/Cole.

Bowlby, J. (1966). *Maternal deprivation and the growth of love*. Baltimore: Penguin.

Caplan, G. (1964). *Principles of preventive psychiatry*. New York: Basic Books.

Caplan, G. (1974). *Support systems and community mental health*. New York: Basic Books.

Cobb, S. (1976). Social support as a moderator of life stress. *Psychosomatic Medicine, 38,* 300.

Coles, R. (2000). *The Erik Erikson reader*. New York: Norton.

Eismann, E. (1996). *Unitas: Building healing communities for children*. New York: Fordham University Press.

Farber, A., & Rogler, L. (1981). *Unitas: Hispanic and black children in a healing community*. New York: Fordham University Press.

Filstead, W., & Rossi, J. (1973). Therapeutic milieu, therapeutic community and milieu treatment. In W. Filstead & J. Rossi (Eds.) *The therapeutic community* (pp. 3–13). New York: Behavioral Publications.

Frank, J. (1973). *Persuasion and healing*. Baltimore: John Hopkins University Press.

Frankl, V. (1973). *The doctor and the soul*. New York: Vintage.

Frankl, V. (1975). *The unconscious God*. New York: Simon and Schuster.

Frankl, V. (1992). *Man's search for meaning*. New York: Simon and Schuster.

Jones, M. (1973). Therapeutic community concepts and the future. In W. Filstead & J. Rossi (Eds.), *The therapeutic community* (pp. 325–336). New York: Behavioral Publications.

Jones, M. (1976). *Maturation of the therapeutic community*. New York. Human Sciences Press.

Langston, R. (1970). Community mental health centers and community mental health ideology. *Community Mental Health Journal, 6,* 387–392.

Lewin, K. (1948). *Resolving social conflict*. New York: Harper and Row.

Lewin, K. (1976). *Field theory in social science: Selected papers* (Dorwin Cartwright, Ed.). Chicago: University of Chicago Press.

Lewis, T., Amini, F., & Lanuan, R. (2000). *A general theory of love*. New York: Random House.

Procidano, M., & Glenwick, D. (1985). *Unitas: Evaluating a preventive program for Hispanic and black youth*. New York: Fordham University Press.

Rogers, C. (1951). *Client centered treatment*. Boston: Houghton Mifflin.

Rogers, C. (1964). *Psychotherapy and personality change*. Chicago: University of Chicago Press.

Rogers, C. (1968). *Man and the science of man*. Columbus, OH: Charles Merril.

Rogers, C., & Wood, J. (1974). Client centered theory. In Arthur Burton (Ed.), *Operational theories of personality* (pp. 211–258). New York: Brunner/Mazel.

Secheheye, M. (1951). *Symbolic realization*. New York: International Universities Press.

Shapiro, S. (1988). *Unitas: Ties that bind* (video documentary). New York: Channel L Working Group and Unitas Therapeutic Community.

Shatan, C. (1969) Community psychiatry: Stretcher bearer of the social order? *International Journal of Psychiatry, 7,* 312–321.

Whittington, H. G. (1965). The third psychiatric revolution—really? *Community Mental Health Journal, 1,* 73–77.

15

Judith C. Meyers

Pathways to Reforming Children's Mental Health Service Systems
Public and Personal

This chapter weaves together reflections on two journeys, one quite public and the other more private. The public journey is the evolution of services for children with serious mental health problems in America over the past century and how the experience of one state—Connecticut—provides a more in-depth look at what has and has not occurred. The private journey is the evolution of my own thinking about children's mental health service systems, informed by my education as a clinical and community psychologist, my training in the world of public policy, my experience working in leadership positions in federal, state, and local settings over the past 20 years, and my most recent work in Connecticut. I will explore how these journeys have intertwined and what might be learned from each.

In 1983 the United States Congress appropriated $1.5 million to the National Institute of Mental Health to create the Child and Adolescent Service System Program (CASSP) to address the needs of children and adolescents with serious emotional disturbances. These needs had been recognized from the earliest years of the twentieth century. Despite a series of efforts, most of which ended in failure, they had been inadequately met. With the creation of CASSP, the concept of a "system of care"

became part of the lexicon, and the tide turned (Stroul & Friedman, 1994). Over the past 20 years there has been tremendous growth in systems of care, with expanding resources, research, and services to respond to children whose emotional, behavioral, and cognitive disorders make it difficult for them to succeed in their own homes, schools, and communities.

In an article about the creation of CASSP, as part of a history of the federal government's efforts to improve services for children and adolescents with mental health problems, the authors noted that the CASSP appropriation was but a short phrase attached to the legislation for the continuation of the then 6-year-old Community Support Program for adults with chronic mental illness. The phrase was "placed by an aide in the congressional report that described Congress' intent that $1.5 million be expended on a similar program for children and adolescents with serious emotional disturbances" (Lourie, Katz-Leavy, DeCarolis, & Quinlan, 1996, p. 104). I happened to be that unnamed aide. At the time I was a Congressional Science Fellow in the House of Representatives working in the office of David Obey (D-WI), who served on the Appropriations Subcommittee responsible for funding for the Department of Health and Human Services, and who was an avid supporter of the Community Support Program.

Sixteen years later, having worked in several policy and academic settings related to children's services, I moved to Connecticut to direct the Child Health and Development Institute of Connecticut, a new not-for-profit organization created to promote long-term systems change to improve the health of children throughout the state. One of the first projects I was asked to undertake was a review of the publicly sponsored children's behavioral health services in Connecticut. What I found out was that 16 years after the advent of CASSP, Connecticut was still struggling with many of the same issues that the program was intended to remedy.

Connecticut's Journey

When I arrived in Connecticut in 1999, there was an increasing concern among state policymakers, practitioners, and parents about children with serious behavioral and emotional problems. This, however, was by no means the first time that policymakers in that state had recognized the need to attend to the difficulties in meeting the needs of children with emotional disorders. In fact, three decades of reports about children's behavioral health reveal striking consistency in articulated goals and in the descriptions of the difficulties attaining them (Geballe, 2002). In 1975 Connecticut established a consolidated state children's agency (Department of Children and Families [DCF], including child protection, children's mental health, and juvenile services), which had as one of its goals a well-functioning children's mental health system that connected all Connecticut children and youth who have mental health problems to appropriate care in a timely manner (Geballe, 2002). Connecticut had even gone so far as to frame a systems of care orientation in legislation passed in 1997 that articulated the principles and mandated a systems of care approach (Public Act 97-272), and as many as 18 communities had developed local systems of care collaboratives by 1999.

Despite these significant milestones, little had been done to reorient a system based in institutional and residential treatment and traditional modes of practice to put the principles of a system of care into practice. Unlike many other states, Connecticut had neither a history of investing in building community-based services to meet the needs of children nor a strong family advocacy and support system—two key ingredients for building and sustaining a community-based, family-centered approach to serving children and their families. By 1999 the state was investing more than $200 million in mental health services for children, but five separate state and local child-serving systems administered these services, including child welfare, mental health, mental retardation, education, and Medicaid. The resulting system, such as it existed, was complex, fragmented, and difficult for families to access and maneuver. The situation had reached the point where large amounts of state funds were being used to maintain children in psychiatric hospitals far beyond the time necessitated by their clinical conditions. This budget drain captured the attention of the highest officials, who were facing a severe budget shortfall as an economic downturn was beginning to result in declining revenues.

Shortly after I arrived, the Child Health and Development Institute of Connecticut (CHDI) was asked to conduct a study for the Department of Social Services (DSS) in fulfillment of a legislative mandate (Section 36 of Public Act 99-279). The study resulted in the report *Delivering and Financing Children's Behavioral Health Services in Connecticut* (2000), which included a review of the service utilization and expenditures for behavioral health services by the state Departments of Social Services, Children and Families, Mental Health and Addiction Services, Mental Retardation, and Education and a set of recommendations to improve the quality and integration of children's behavioral health services.

CHDI is a nonprofit organization created in 1998 by the board of the Children's Fund of Connecticut, a public charitable foundation focused on community-based primary and preventive health care initiatives. The board created the institute to serve as a mechanism for promoting long-term change in the systems that have the greatest impact on children's health in Connecticut. Connecticut's two leading medical universities—Yale and the University of Connecticut—play a leadership role in CHDI's development and work, contributing their resources to bring the best information from research and best practice experiences throughout the country to help inform, train, and support policymakers and practitioners.

CHDI was likely perceived by state leaders to be a good fit for carrying out the study for several reasons: it was perceived as neutral and objective (not affiliated with one branch of government, one particular state agency, or a particular political point of view); it was affiliated with both of the state's two major universities, and thus there was no need to pick one over the other; it was a new organization with no history or baggage, which can accumulate very quickly in a small state like Connecticut; and its new director, namely, me, had expertise in program, policy, and financing with regard to children's mental health systems. The study was conducted in partnership with DSS and the DCF (Child Health and Development Institute of Connecticut, Inc., 2000). I hired Carl Valentine, a national consultant with expertise in financing children's systems, to assist with collecting and analyzing the state data. We developed a state implementation team with representatives from DSS and DCF to assist with the study and created a Children's Behavioral Health Task Force as an advisory committee with representation from other state agencies, family advocates, and providers, to review and discuss the findings along the way.

The study's findings were derived based on the following: financial and service utilization data provided by state agencies; a review of the literature on the organization and financing of children's behavioral health services; review of case studies; deliberations of the Children's Behavioral Health Task Force; interviews with service providers, consumer families, and advocacy groups; and extensive discussions with staff of state agencies.

Delivering and Financing Children's Behavioral Health Services

Key findings of the study included the following:

- Of the 184,000 children enrolled in Connecticut's Medicaid managed care program (HUSKY A), approximately 12% used one or more behavioral health services during the 12-month period studied (April 1998–March 1999).
- The state spent approximately $207 million from five different child-serving systems (Medicaid, child welfare, education, mental health, and mental retardation) for behavioral health services during this time (the juvenile justice system, which spends additional dollars for mental health services for court-involved children, was not included in this study).
- Twenty percent of the dollars ($41.1 million) was spent on acute psychiatric hospitalizations for 1,067 children (5% of the population receiving services).
- Fifty percent of the dollars ($104.2 million) was spent for residential treatment serving another 13% of the children.
- The remaining 30% was available for home and community-based services serving the largest proportion of children.
- Bottlenecks in the system were keeping children in psychiatric hospitals and residential treatment settings long beyond the time they needed to be there. More than half of the children in the state's custody who were in private psychiatric hospitals were ready for discharge to a less intensive and less expensive setting but in many cases were hospitalized for more than 3 months because of inadequate community-based services.
- Seventy-two percent of the funds expended were state dollars, 20% were federal dollars, and 8% were local funds through the school systems.
- Children in custody of the state's child protection system through DCF accounted for a large share of the expenditures. Although only 5% of children enrolled in HUSKY A were in the custody of DCF during the reporting year, they accounted for 60% of all behavioral health expenditures on behalf of HUSKY children.

With regard to service delivery, the study reinforced what was already known by many: that the high number of children who remained in psychiatric hospitals and residential treatment settings for increasingly long periods of time when such care was no longer considered appropriate was a direct result of the combined lack of care coordination and lack of alternatives in the community. Children remained in these settings because of a lack of "step-down" and other appropriate transitional services that could provide less intensive care when a child's family, the school, or the community was unable to provide adequate support and services. This lack of available step-down services not only kept children in these out-of-home settings for longer periods than was necessary and at high cost but also prevented other children from quickly accessing these services when needed, leaving children backed up in emergency rooms and in the community awaiting care.

For services to be more responsive, appropriate, and effective, supporting the best possible developmental outcomes for children with behavioral health disorders, reform in the children's behavioral health system was needed, including significant restructuring in the way that services were organized, financed, and delivered for children with serious and complex behavioral health problems. The solutions rested on capacity building at the community level, using community-based, family-centered, culturally competent, systemic approaches to treatment rather than a "bricks and mortar" approach through building more institutional settings or adding beds.

The study recommended the following actions:

- Expand and enhance local systems of care as the mechanism for coordinating and delivering behavioral health services for children with severe emotional disturbances and their families;
- Build a richer array of community-based services;
- Develop a statewide family support network;
- Develop and implement a blended funding approach to support the comprehensive integrated community-based systems;
- Develop measurable outcomes to assess the effectiveness of services;
- Conduct training to support the implementation of the system of care;
- Improve information systems;
- Conduct a thorough evaluation.

The timing of the study was critical, resulting in the state's readiness to adopt the recommendations rather than have them shelved. The status quo was becoming increasingly unacceptable. There were the mounting costs to the state of children remaining in hospitals as the result of a reinsurance agreement whereby the state picked up a larger portion of the costs after a child had been hospitalized for more than 15 days. There was pressure from the hospitals, whose emergency rooms were overflowing with children with mental health problems for whom there were no open beds. There

were predictions that it was only a matter of time before a child died unnecessarily as a result. Connecticut Community KidCare was the outcome of this planning process.

The commissioner of DCF, Kristine Ragaglia, became a strong proponent of the reform agenda. In her first several years as commissioner she had been an advocate for increasing the number of residential beds, but soon she came to recognize this was an expensive and not particularly effective way to fix the problems in the system. Her counterpart at the DSS, Patricia Wilson-Coker, had a background in child welfare and law and was also supportive from the start.

The study produced by CHDI lent credence to a direction that key state agency staff and advocates were already supporting by documenting objectively and irrefutably the problems in the system and the need for change. The proposed reforms were further supported by the General Assembly, which, in June 2000, charged the commissioners of DCF and DSS to develop the elements of a plan to reform the current system, and by a July 2000 report issued by the Governor's Blue Ribbon Commission on Mental Health.

Connecticut Community KidCare was designed over the next 8-months to a year by an implementation team of state agency staff working in concert with the Behavioral Health Advisory Group. CHDI continued to provide technical assistance and facilitation to the process but moved to a behind-the-scenes role as the state agencies took increasing ownership of the process.

The details of the plan were presented in January 2001 in a report to the General Assembly (Connecticut Department of Children and Families and Department of Social Services, 2001). The plan at that point represented a far-reaching vision, incorporating all the elements of the systems of care values and principles. As written in the first paragraph of the implementation plan submitted to the legislature in January 2001:

> The Department of Children and Families and Department of Social Services are preparing to embark on a sweeping reform of the public child behavioral health service system. The new Connecticut Community KidCare initiative is designed to eliminate the major system gaps and barriers that have plagued child behavioral health in recent years. The proposed initiative

will allow children with behavioral health problems to grow and develop within nurturing family environments, increasing their ability to succeed in their homes, schools and communities. The new system will be family driven and family focused, giving families choice and helping families to care for children who have behavioral health challenges. The new system will emphasize the strengths of individual families and children and be culturally responsive. (p. vii)

The state agencies recognized that their vision was a tall order, but they firmly believed that it could be realized. As the report further states:

Building this new system is an evolutionary process that will require time for planning, training and capacity building, and a gradual phase-in of fully working systems. It will also require changes in structure, organization, management, financing, practice, and philosophy, affecting those involved at every level, from families to providers to State agencies. (p. vii)

The key elements of the Community KidCare plan at that point included the following:

- A full carve-out from managed care of children's behavioral health services for all children enrolled in HUSKY;
- A comprehensive benefit package, including outpatient, day program, home-based, care coordination, nonmedical support services such as respite care and therapeutic recreation, as well as out-of-home services, including residential, therapeutic foster care, and hospitalization;
- Integrated funding streams, including Medicaid, S-CHIP, Title IV-E, and state general funds;
- Support for family involvement through funding for a family support organization, and involvement of families at all levels of policy and planning;
- A new administrative structure to include an administrative service organization (ASO), regionally based lead service agencies, and community collaboratives (formerly known as local systems of care);
- Training and staff development;
- A comprehensive evaluation of the reform.

Phase-in of KidCare was scheduled to begin in July 2002 with the selection of an ASO to administer a full carve-out followed by the selection of two lead service agencies with access to the enhanced benefit package. The intent was for KidCare to be operational statewide within 1 to 2 years after that.

In spite of a few setbacks that slowed down the rate of progress, the implementation of KidCare continued on track over the next 18 months. More than $23 million in new funding was committed to community services, including emergency mobile services, care coordination, day treatment, intensive home-based treatment services, and respite services. Twenty-seven local collaboratives were engaged in developing individual treatment teams, with the support of more care coordinators and more services from which to draw. Family organizations had been invigorated through state and foundation support with a thriving network of parent support groups, including several focused on the needs of Afro-Caribbean and Hispanic families. More than 2,000 people in state and provider agencies and family members came together in 4-day workshops to learn about how to work in a community-based, family-centered, strengths-based approach through the KidCare Institutes. There was an increasing effort to support evidence-based interventions such as multiple systemic therapy and functional family therapy.

The values and principles of a system of care approach had been deeply embedded in legislation, policy standards, and guidelines in Connecticut, as indicated by the following statement included in DCF's 2002 System of Care Status Report to the legislature:

The federally defined System of Care Model underlies the paradigm shift in financing and service delivery in which KidCare is founded. Like the System of Care model, KidCare is based upon a philosophy in which service planning is driven by the needs and preferences of the child and family. Both KidCare and the systems of care model provided through the Community Collaboratives seek to prevent children's problems from escalating by offering an array of flexible, individualized services that will maintain children in their homes and community. KidCare and Connecticut's Community Collaboratives espouse quality, comprehensive, community-based service provision through partnerships, interagency agreements, and key-stakeholder associations. While KidCare is the materialization of systemic service restructuring, the system of care approach has been the solid foundation created a decade ago in which to frame the core tenets of Connecticut's reform initiative. (Connecticut Department of Children and Families, Division of Mental Health, 2002).

As a participant, witness, advocate, and possibly even one of the catalysts to the beginnings of a major transformation in Connecticut's mental health system for children, I found this a thrilling time. There was a readiness for change that had been building for years. I was one force among many that converged at that time, and I felt tremendously lucky to have been in the right place at the right time to be able to make a difference. I also had had enough experience to understand that such transformative change in public systems is not linear and never easy. As the first 6 months of this fiscal year (January–June 2003) unfolded, that reality came home to roost. Connecticut's journey in the past 3 years mirrors the nation's journey of the past 20 years.

The Nation's Journey

Building Systems of Care in Connecticut

Connecticut was not alone in its history of having years of concern for children with serious mental health problems—recognizing the need for action yet experiencing the slow pace of reform. Nationally there has been a consensus on the nature of the problem that has not changed much for decades. The awareness of a need for comprehensive coordinated services for children with emotional disturbances was articulated as far back as the 1909 White House Conference on Children, which recommended new programs to care for "mentally disturbed children," and again in 1930 when another White House Conference echoed these recommendations. It was not until 35 years later that attention was again focused on the need for improved mental health services for children. The Joint Commission on the Mental Health of Children was convened and delivered its report to Congress in 1969, stating that large numbers of emotionally, physically, and

socially handicapped children did not receive necessary or appropriate services and that the mental health service system for children and youth was wholly inadequate (Joint Commission on the Mental Health of Children, 1969). The report stated: "It is an undesirable fact that there is not a single community in this country which provides an acceptable standard of services for its mentally ill children, running a spectrum from early therapeutic intervention to social restoration in the home, in the school, and in the community" (pp. 6–7). The report called for complete diagnostic, treatment, and preventive services available to all children and youth and a child advocacy program at all levels of government, including an adviser in the White House. It also recommended funding to provide incentives to states and communities to establish a range of coordinated services providing interrelated, continuous care and treatment for children in need.

As Nicholas Hobbs aptly summarized in 1975:

> Countless commissions, committees, and conferences, including White House conferences, have addressed the problem of providing services for children and have been appalled by the confusion they find. Report after report stresses the absence of any overall design for the delivery of services, the dispersion of responsibility among dozens of agencies, the fragmentation of effort, and the frequency with which children in need of assistance get lost in the system. (p. 180)

With the advent of CASSP in 1983, however, there has been remarkable progress. With CASSP as an impetus, the concept of a system of care to serve children with serious emotional disturbances was defined and continues to this day. Children's mental health services received another significant boost when the Children's and Communities Mental Health Services Improvement Act of 1992 created a new federal program to support the expansion of community-based systems of care for children with serious emotional disturbances and their families. This program, the Comprehensive Community Mental Health Services for Children and Their Families Program, began in 1993 with initial funding of $5 million. From 1993 to 2002, grants to 67 communities in 43 different states to improve and expand their systems of care have been awarded, with $107 million projected to be available in fiscal year 2004. According to the national evaluation of these programs, the approach was more effective in helping children and adolescents with serious emotional disturbances (Friesen & Winters, 2003).

The troubling news is that despite the recent progress after almost a century of attention of one kind or another, we still have a long way to go. Although the values and principles that are the foundation of a systems of care approach seem widely accepted and adopted, the full translation of these principles into practice still eludes us, and the call to attend to the problems continues to be sounded at the state and national levels. In a review of reports addressing children's mental health issued by 10 states between 1997 and 2001, a strong and consistent concern about the inadequacy of efforts to address the mental health needs of children and their families was evident. In a familiar-sounding theme, these reports were consistent in favoring the values, principles, and beliefs of a system of care framework—interagency collaboration, individualized, comprehensive, and culturally competent care, and support for a strong family role. The range of recommendations also had a familiar ring: create more flexible and less categorical funding; integrate and coordinate planning and improve accountability; improve the quality of services through increased attention to the recruitment, training, and retention of staff; make greater use of evidence-based treatments; expand provider networks; establish professional standards; and reduce stigma and increase support for children's mental health through public education (Friedman, 2002).

The Surgeon General's landmark report on mental health in 1999 observed: "The system for delivering mental health services to children and their families is complex, sometimes to the point of inscrutability—a patchwork of providers, interventions, and payers. Much of the complexity stems from the multiple pathways into treatment and the multiple funding streams for services" (U.S. Department of Health and Human Services, 2000, p. 179). The report also concludes that most children in need of mental health services do not receive them.

Even more recently, President Bush established the President's New Freedom Commission on Mental Health. The commission's goal was to recommend improvements to enable adults with serious mental illness and children with severe emotional disturbance to live, work, learn, and participate fully in their communities (New Freedom Commission on Mental Health, 2003). Once again, a national report cites fragmentation and gaps in care for children with serious mental illness and calls for replacing unnecessary institutional care with efficient, effective community services and integrating programs across levels of government and among many agencies. Once again, a report calls for services and treatments that are individual, family centered, and culturally competent rather than oriented to the requirements of bureaucracies. Once again, a report calls for creating flexible financing strategies to support the use of the most effective treatments and services. Once again, a report calls for early identification, screening, and treatment.

Challenges to Change

Connecticut's journey mirrors the nation's journey in developing systems of care, and while much progress has been made, the challenges remain, leading to continued calls for transformations in how services are organized, financed, and delivered (Glied & Cuellar, 2003). There has been an expansion in federal, state, and local funding, but our public systems continue to spend most of their resources on crisis situations. When dollars are as short as the political horizons, it is hard for elected officials to invest in the long haul. In Connecticut the first part of the reform to bite the dust were the lead service agencies. As the economy turned downward in 2000–2001, a time in which Connecticut, one of the wealthiest states in America, was hit hard by the loss of revenues from declining capital gains, those who controlled budgetary decisions in the Office of Policy and Management determined that money needed to be spent on services, not infrastructure. While it is not hard to recognize the political appeal of that decision, and perhaps even the short-run humanitarian appeal, it was also clear to those of us who had helped design the reform that if the system was going to be successful, it needed to be operated and administered as close to the communities as possible, rather than centrally out of Hartford. Connecticut does not have counties that serve as governing units; it has a state government and 169 cities and towns, with nothing in between. Pulling away the lead service agency model was a major setback for building a community-based system.

The implementation of KidCare became seriously stalled 6 months ago. One major aspect of the reform, the creation of a Behavioral Health Partnership whereby funds would be pooled, and three state agencies would partner to contract with an ASO to manage a full carve-out of the system, hit a snag. The inevitable resistance resulting from major change efforts is coming, not surprisingly and perhaps understandably, from providers who are concerned about the impact on their reimbursement rates and whether enhancements to the children's system will result in diminished resources for the adult system. Ostensibly as a result of a disagreement between several key legislators and the executive branch regarding rate setting for providers and oversight of the system, the implementation came to a halt.

There has been no KidCare training for the past 6 months, the evaluation has been put on hold, and while the community-based services continue to be developed, the system as envisioned is still a long way off. In Connecticut, as is true nationally, while there is progress in developing a broader ranges of services, the majority of children with serious mental health problems are involved with multiple systems associated with poor treatment planning and outcomes. The greatest portion of public dollars for children's services continues to be spent on the fewest children—to pay for institutional and residential placements for children with the most serious problems. The least amount is spent for prevention and early intervention.

One positive development has been a burgeoning interest in and attention to the mental heath of young children that accompanies the increased focus on young children being better prepared to succeed when they enter kindergarten. As noted in the Surgeon General's report:

> The wider human services and law enforcement communities, not just the mental health community, have made prevention a priority. Policymakers and service providers in health, education, social services, and juvenile justice have become invested in intervening early in children's lives: they have come to appreciate that mental health is inexorably linked with general health, child care, and success in the classroom and inversely related to involvement in the juvenile justice system. It is also perceived that investment in prevention may be cost-effective. (U.S. Department of Health and Human Services, 1999, p. 133)

The President's New Freedom Commission also devotes one of its six goals to early detection and intervention, and includes among its recommendations that we promote the mental health of children. It remains to be seen whether there will be a shift in resources to move the rhetoric to reality.

Reflections on Why Sustainable Change Is Difficult to Achieve: My Personal Journey

No one has the definitive answer to why lasting change is difficult to achieve, but as someone whose professional journey over the past 22 years has given me the opportunity to observe and engage in the efforts to improve children's mental health systems at the federal level and in several states, including the most recent work in Connecticut, I can offer my own reflections, routed in a paradigm of systems change that stems back to my earliest days as a clinical and community psychologist.

Although I did not have a name for it when I first chose to become a clinical and community psychologist more than 30 years ago, I came to learn that the theoretical underpinnings of much of what I believe and do have been guided by general systems theory. This theoretical orientation, first articulated by biologist Ludwig Von Bertalanffy in the 1920s, is a framework that highlights the complex relationships and interconnectedness among the biological, ecological, social, psychological, and technological dimensions of our increasingly complex lives. The key characteristics of systems thinking are as follows:

- A shift in focus from the parts to the whole— a system as a whole cannot be reduced to its parts—or, as more commonly stated, the whole is greater than the mere sum of its parts;
- Thinking in terms of connectedness, context, and relationships—the properties of the parts can be understood only within the context of the larger whole;

- Objects are embedded in a world of relationships from which they cannot be separated;
- Organisms as a network of relationships exist within societal relationships within social systems and within ecosystems. Each system is nested within other larger systems (Senge, 1994).

Systems thinking clearly underlies the values and principles of a systems of care approach, which is based on the recognition that children are part of families, families are part of communities, and that to improve outcomes for individual children, one has to understand the connectedness of the child to all aspects of community life, including groups, organizations, agencies, institutions, and neighborhoods. All are separate entities but also parts of related networks, such that intervention in one part of the system has repercussions for the whole system.

I was first introduced to general systems theory while a postdoctoral fellow at the Yale Department of Psychiatry, working on a psychiatric unit of a community hospital. The director of the unit, Dr. Irwin Greenberg, was steeped in systems theory and used it to shape the clinical service and clinical teaching. Case consultations under his direction involved seeing individuals in the context of their biological, intrapsychic, familial, community, and larger world systems, as well as along the time dimensions of past, present, and future. This theory has informed my thinking and work ever since.

During that time I was working as a clinician with individuals and families and had little opportunity to focus on community-level change. In working with adults diagnosed as chronically mentally ill, I often felt frustrated and ineffective, like Sisyphus pushing the proverbial rock. Individual, group, family, and milieu therapy along with psychotropic medications may have helped relieve symptoms or helped people adjust to their conditions, but they did little to pave the way for productive participation in the economic and social aspects of their so-called community, the place where they resided and called home. One patient would leave only to be replaced by another with similar concerns. I observed that conditions such as neighborhood efforts to prevent zoning for halfway houses, rejection of applications for Social Security Disability Income, and lack of job training and supported employment were much more powerful in keeping people out of a community than any of the therapeutic approaches we were providing to keep them in the community. At best we were helping people adjust to bad situations over which they had little control.

The combination of my roots in community psychology, with its focus on primary prevention, social change, and understanding of individual, organizational, and societal behavior, experience in clinical settings, and exposure to systems thinking led me to depart from the traditional role of a psychologist to seek preparation to engage at a broader level with the issues I saw as much more determinant in affecting the lives of people with serious mental health problems. I completed a 2-year postdoctoral fellowship at Yale's Institute for Social and Policy Studies, during which time I became affiliated with the Bush Program in Child Development and Social Policy at Yale. I learned a great deal more about economics, political science, policy analysis, epidemiology, and public health than had ever been broached in my graduate training in psychology. During that time I changed my focus from adults to children, for it became apparent to me that if one was going to have an impact on reducing the consequences of mental illness in our society, it made most sense to focus on prevention and early intervention beginning in the earlier years of life. A 1-year Congressional Science Fellowship sponsored by the American Psychological Association in conjunction with the American Association for the Advancement of Science followed.

Since then I have served in various settings and locations in the arena of children's mental health and child welfare services. I have worked in university-based programs focused on linking research and policy for children at the Bush Program in Child Development and Social Policy both at the University of Michigan and at Yale; served as the administrator of Iowa's child welfare system, where I was responsible for administration of the state's services for children, including foster care, adoption, child protection, child care, home-based services, and the state's juvenile institutions; was a senior program officer overseeing the Mental Health Initiative for Urban Children at the Annie E. Casey Foundation (King & Meyers, 1996); and worked as a consultant to several states and communities largely through my affiliation with the National Technical Assistance Center for Children's Mental Health at Georgetown University. These and other experiences have given me a broad perspective on the challenges in instituting systemic reform on behalf of children with mental health problems and their families as I have grappled with how one supports, prods, catalyzes, facilitates, promotes, and advocates for change, both from within as the administrator of a state system and from without as a consultant.

I gave up my career as a clinician because I thought I could make a greater difference by working at the systems and policy level. Within a few years time, I went from an inpatient unit of a community hospital to the halls of Congress, and since then have been many places in between. I have come to appreciate that it takes many people at all levels—policy, systems, practice, families—who share a common vision and goal to push for systemic change. No one place or position has more power than any other to make it happen. The power in one position comes mostly from being in a position to stop the movement temporarily, but the movement will eventually find its way around the resistance if the cause is right.

What Will It Take to Support and Sustain Systems Reform?

The reform of children's mental health service systems as envisioned is clearly no easy task or it would have succeeded by now. In a review of the factors necessary for maintaining children's mental health systems over the long haul, Koyanagi and Feres-Merchant (2000) stated, "Adopting the systems of care approach promoted in federal law requires a sea change in policy, clinical practice and administration. States and localities are expected to reorient, re-design and re-finance child mental health services into true 'systems' of care" (p. 11). As they noted, and I have observed repeatedly, this rarely is a linear process, and it can be easily sidetracked by changes in leadership, funding commitment, and the inevitable pockets of resistance that arise when major systems changes are being undertaken.

A systems perspective teaches us that pressing for change threatens stability, increasing the power of forces resisting change and thus maintaining the status quo, preserving the integrity of the existing system. Reforms always encounter resistance. This stability is important to us as biological organisms

and as a nation that has survived as a democracy without the threat of revolution beyond the one that created us. This stability can be a detriment when it preserves a way of operating that has far surpassed its usefulness. As noted in a monograph summarizing the lessons learned from the Annie E. Casey Foundation's New Futures Initiative, as the reform agenda threatened the stability of the current system, "Vested interests in current practice, fiscal constraints, and political risks created a constant force capable of minimalizing system change" (Annie E. Casey Foundation, 1995, p. 2). Perhaps in understanding the forces of resistance to the changes inherent in moving from an institutional- and residential-based system that is focused on the individual child, excludes the family, and is not rooted in the community and schools to a systems of care approach, those who are committed to change can overcome the status quo.

In moving a children's mental health system toward a community-based, family-centered approach, pockets of resistance to change may occur in a variety of places. Providers and their agencies may see the changes as threatening their sources of funding or requiring them to change their deeply embedded theoretical orientation and methods of practice. Often these are groups that have an organized and strong presence in the legislature and executive branch. Others fear the unknown and do not want to leave the comfort of the familiar. If a practitioner is used to the comfort and safety of his or her own office as the locus of treatment, leaving that confine and venturing out into the community or homes of children and families can be daunting. Inertia is another powerful force for keeping things as they are, as exemplified by the statement "That's the way it's always been" as a common refrain to explain why things occur as they do in a bureaucracy even when they make no sense. One can usually look for which groups or individuals may lose power, influence, status, a sense of identity, or earning power to locate the strongest resistance to change, regardless of its broader benefit.

Elements of Change

My experience, both in Connecticut and nationally, further informed by the observations of others, suggests that key elements must be in place if we are to overcome resistance to change and support and sustain all the elements of a system of care. These elements include (1) leadership; (2) a broad-based commitment at all levels; (3) mechanisms to build the capacity of practitioners and support and sustain the presence of family advocates; (4) increased attention to quality improvement and accountability through solid data and evaluation; (5) adequate and sustained funding; (6) the integration of mental health principles and practices into all child-serving systems; (7) the expansion of the use of evidence-based practices that have demonstrated that clinical interventions in the right context will result in better outcomes for children and families; and (8) building public will and support. If these elements are left unattended, the next generation of policy-makers and practitioners will be repeating the same tired litany 20 if not 100 years hence. I will elaborate on each of these elements.

Leadership

For a reform of state policies and services to succeed, leadership from both within government and without is necessary. Leaders are needed who can articulate the vision, manage the complex process of change, and help keep sustained commitment through the political shoals. A commitment from the top leadership, ideally in both the executive branch and the legislature, is important. Change of this magnitude requires legislative and fiscal initiatives to sustain the reform over time. At the same time, leadership of a different sort, sometimes referred to as leadership from behind, or servant-leadership, is needed (Spears & Lawrence, 2002). Such leadership can exist in a variety of settings, but these are usually people committed to the cause who are invested in the betterment of community, working collectively for social change, often behind the scenes.

A turnover in top leadership can lead to a loss of momentum, of commitment, and of memory and understanding. The history of the children's mental health movement has taught us that a reversal in political will, especially with changes in leadership, can easily lead to the demise of a major reform effort. In Connecticut, KidCare had the support of the commissioners of the two key state agencies involved. They became public spokespersons, championing it each step of the way, sometimes in the face of less than full support from legislators, providers, and others in their own administration who were concerned about the fiscal liabilities. One of those commissioners has since left, and it falls to her successor to pick up the sword and continue the fight. Since it was not her initiative to begin with, it remains to be seen how effective and committed a voice she will be, particularly as the reform has begun to meet some of the inevitable resistances.

Broad-Based Commitment for the Reform Effort

Champions of the reform are needed not only from key legislators but also from private sector leaders, across multiple state agencies, and among staff at many levels within state agencies at the state and community level to keep an effort at systems reform moving through political and funding setbacks. As I wrote in an earlier publication about sustaining reform, "Ownership by one individual, one party, one agency, or even one branch of government cannot sustain a reform agenda over time. Broadening the base of support at the earliest possible time with deliberate inclusion strategies is important" (Meyers & Davis, 1997, p. 98).

Because of the many political and bureaucratic constraints on elected and appointed officials, and because they inevitably come and go before the work of a movement such as transforming a children's mental health system is sustained, leadership from without is needed. Organizations such as the Child Health and Development Institute, which are more independent and objective, can help serve as a catalyst to the process and maintain a consistent voice about the direction that needs to be maintained over the long haul, through efforts that vested interests can too often derail.

Leadership from among parent advocates is another important source of external pressure. In my experience the most powerful voices to sustain change are those of family advocates. Family members of children receiving services are committed to their children over the long haul. They are most invested in seeing change that will benefit the lives of their children and will be the most passionate advocates if brought into the process. When Connecticut committed to its KidCare reform, the family advocacy movement was weak to nonexistent across the state. Part of the reform has been an investment both by the state and by private foundations in building and supporting a family advocacy movement. As noted earlier, there are now several such organizations serving different populations and working collaboratively under one umbrella, called FAVOR. They represent a strong and independent voice. In recent setbacks to the reform, their calls and visits to their legislators have had the most powerful influence in sustaining the commitment to and support for KidCare. While theory, research findings, and data and evaluation help shape the minds of decision makers, the voices of families sharing the experiences of their children speak to their hearts.

Building Capacity

Moving from an institutional to a culturally competent and family-centered community-based approach is a major philosophical shift that requires new attitudes, beliefs, skills, and values. If government is to fundamentally change the way its service systems operate, workers from managers to frontline staff need to understand and act on this new approach in all aspects of their work so that the new systemic thinking permeates all they do. This requires a comprehensive approach to workforce development and training that cuts across discipline and agency boundaries at both the graduate preprofessional and in-service levels, instills a focus on the system of care concept, philosophy, and treatment approach, and trains providers to apply effective prevention and treatment services within that context (Meyers, Kaufman, & Goldman, 1999).

In Connecticut, with the assistance of Cliff Davis and Sheila Pires at the Human Service Collaborative, CHDI designed a 5-day competency-based institute to begin to address the attitudes, knowledge, and skills needed to provide strengths-based training that emphasizes individuals and families as partners in community-based planning and behavioral health care of children and families in support of the implementation of Connecticut Community KidCare. The curriculum addressed the basics of a system of care approach; the strengths and needs of children with serious mental health disorders; how to develop individualized strategies of treatment and support; how to build partnerships between providers and families; and how to collaborate with other systems and communities. Using a train-the-trainer model, more than 120 trainers were prepared to train groups of 25 that included a mix of parents, community service providers, and staff from the DCF, judicial, and education systems. More than 2,000 people were trained over a 2-year period. While that was successful, we never believed it would be sufficient to

change practice. The challenge has been in sustaining the commitment to training necessary to move beyond this initial exposure so that all those involved have the opportunity for ongoing supervision, learning, and support to translate what they have learned to a sustained change in practice. One way this has been accomplished is by incorporating the curriculum into the preservice training for all new staff hired at DCF, while we continue to work to establish a plan for ongoing workforce development training and to work with the graduate schools of social work to infuse this material into their curricula.

Attention to Quality Improvement and Accountability Through Data and Evaluation

One of the key roles that CHDI has played in the implementation of KidCare has been to advocate for and oversee an evaluation of the reform. We were successful at the start in making the case that it would be important to document how the initiative was being developed, what was working, what was not, and why. Such information was invaluable for several purposes: improving services, marshaling public support, informing management, and sustaining involvement in service systems. A multiyear evaluation would provide information to policymakers to help sustain their investment in the initiative by addressing their key concerns about cost-effectiveness of the system; it would provide important feedback to stakeholders about how the process was developing so that adaptations could be made. Also important to me, it would document how the process was unfolding so that in the event that the initiative was derailed, there would be clear information to explain what happened so that the initiative would not be held accountable if expected results were not achieved.

DCF contracted with CHDI to manage the evaluation, and we selected the Human Services Research Institute and its partners, the Technical Assistance Collaborative and the University of South Florida, to design and carry it out. The first year of this multiyear evaluation has focused on how the reform was implemented and began to establish baseline measures. It is addressing four questions:

1. Are the new services being implemented as planned?
2. Are services family and child centered?

3. Are families satisfied with the services they are receiving?
4. Are system capacity and responsiveness improving?

In subsequent years, the evaluators will analyze trends in the capacity of the system, the responsiveness of the system over time, and changes in children's outcomes. What we have learned in conducting the evaluation is that accessing quality data is very difficult. There is a lack of technology in state agencies, leading to poor-quality data and difficulty in sharing data across state agencies. The requirements of the new federal Health Insurance Portability and Accountability Act of 1996 (HIPAA), which went into effect in 2003, only add to the challenge.

The state of the art in evaluating the effectiveness of systems of care is still quite limited. Systems of care are complex and evolving processes. The Surgeon General's report on mental health (U.S. Department of Health and Human Services, 1999) summarized what we know from national evaluation studies with the following statement:

> Collectively, the results of the evaluations of systems of care suggest that they are effective in achieving important system improvements, such as reducing use of residential placements, and out-of-state placements, and in achieving improvement in functional behavior. There also are indications that parents are more satisfied in systems of care than in more traditional service delivery systems. The effect of systems of care on cost is not yet clear, however. Nor has it yet been demonstrated that services delivered within a system of care will result in better clinical outcomes than services delivered in more traditional systems. (p. 133)

My commitment to conducting a comprehensive evaluation in Connecticut is not only about supporting the work in one state but also about making sure that we use this opportunity to contribute to the national knowledge base and evolving learning about developing children's mental health systems of care. In examining the factors that helped support and sustain the Comprehensive Community Mental Health Services system sites after the termination of federal funding, those with the strongest prospect of continuing and growing following the termination of federal funds were noted to have made excellent use of data and evaluation of outcomes (Koyanagi & Feres-Merchant, 2000). I believe this is true not only at an individual site level but also for states and for the movement as a whole.

Sustained and Adequate Funding From a Variety of Sources

In my 20 years in this field, I have seen the federal commitment to building children's mental health systems grow from just over $1 million in 1984 to over $100 million expected this year. In my 5 years in Connecticut, $23 million new dollars were appropriated to build a community-based service system. Clearly, these are substantial increases, but just as clearly it is not enough.

When Connecticut Community KidCare was first designed, we knew it would take at least 5 years to build the community-based capacity sufficiently to reduce reliance on the more expensive out-of-home services, allowing for the redirection of resources. My biggest concern was and continues to be that the state would not invest sufficiently to build and sustain the changes. Change of this magnitude takes a long time and requires a long-term investment, sufficient to have it succeed.

As an example, the plan for Connecticut Community KidCare initially called for more than 400 care coordinators, enough to cover the estimated 4,000 children with serious and complex mental health disorders, with a caseload of 10 per coordinator. To date, funding has been sufficient to hire 60 care coordinators, who have served 400 children, with no current plans for expansion.

The problem, however, is not solely one of inadequate new resources to do the job but the constraints on existing resources, with Medicaid being the chief example. Many of us in Connecticut have been working to expand the use of Medicaid to support some of the essential services for children to remain in their home communities. Connecticut has not made full use of options within Medicaid that are available for this purpose. Achieving this within an environment where cutting budgets to address state deficits includes proposals to charge families at 50% of the poverty level for their use of Medicaid has been especially difficult.

When exploring alternative sources of funding, philanthropic foundations should not be overlooked. In Connecticut several foundations have contributed substantial resources to Connecticut Community KidCare, helping to fund the elements of the system seen as most important to keeping the reform moving against odds. The Connecticut Health Foundation and the Children's Fund of Connecticut have made significant investments in evaluation, training, promoting evidence-based practices, and supporting the development of the local collaboratives. Although the amounts contributed may be small relative to the public resources, they can help sustain the work through the patches when the public funding is held back or reallocated for political reasons.

Integrating Family-, Child-, and Youth-Centered Mental Health Services Into All Systems That Serve Children and Youth

The systems of care approach is based on the understanding that one cannot address the mental health of children, particularly those with more serious disorders, without attending to many other service systems that affect their daily lives. Many of these children come into contact with the child protection system and the juvenile justice system. Whether they do or not, the schools, the health system, social services (Temporary Assistance for Needy Families [TANF] and Medicaid), and the early care and education service system are important touch points for serving the needs of these children and their families.

It is clear to any of us who have worked in this field that the children's mental health agency cannot go it alone. Looking at the experience of sites that participated in the federal Comprehensive Community Mental Health Services Grants, it was clear that funding from multiple sources was necessary to sustain the programs once the grant money was no longer available. Mental health and Medicaid dollars were not sufficient. Resources were drawn from myriad federal, state, and local sources from many different systems (Koyanagi & Feres-Merchant, 2000). Our own initial study of the system in Connecticut corroborates this.

Connecticut is one of a small number of states that has an integrated children's agency that is responsible for child protection, children's mental health, and juvenile institutional services. Even with Connecticut's structural advantage, it has still been a significant challenge to integrate planning,

funding, and service delivery across systems. One of the hallmarks of progress in the development of KidCare was the establishment of a Behavioral Health Partnership Agreement whereby three state agencies (DCF, DSS, and the Department of Mental Health and Addiction Services) agreed to work together, committing both their programs and their dollars to an integrated service system, but it has taken 2 years of deliberations to reach this point, with many starts and stops. Efforts to work with the schools and the juvenile justice system are ongoing but not easy.

Expansion of Evidence-Based Practices

To achieve better clinical outcomes, we know that there is clearly a need for more attention to the effectiveness of services delivered within systems of care that includes the relationship between changes at the system level and changes at the practice level. What happens in the interaction between the therapists and the child and family is the ultimate determinant of how well the systems reforms work. We have seen marked progress in the increase in use of community-based clinical interventions that are demonstrated to be effective with specific populations of children with mental health and substance abuse problems in real-world settings. These interventions include multisystemic therapy, functional family therapy, multidimensional family therapy, and Oregon Treatment Foster Care (Ford, Gregory, McKay, & Williams, 2003).

In Connecticut we are actively seeking to expand the use of evidence-based interventions. We have developed a unique partnership to promote the use of evidence-based practices in public systems. The Connecticut Center for Effective Practice (CCEP) is a public-private partnership that includes DCF, the Court Support Services Division of the judicial branch, the Department of Psychiatry at the University of Connecticut Health Center, the Yale Child Study Center, and CHDI, which serves as its administrative home. CCEP's purpose is to enhance Connecticut's capacity to improve the appropriate diagnosis and treatment of children with serious and complex emotional and behavioral conditions by supporting the development, evaluation, training, and dissemination of effective prevention and treatment services. The initial focus of the work has been on children and youth with behavioral health needs who are in, or at risk for placement in, the juvenile justice system, and on multisystemic therapy (MST).

CCEP partners also worked together to continue the state's effort to deliver other evidence-based services, including Functional Family Therapy, Multi-dimensional Family Therapy, and Intensive In-Home Child and Adolescent Psychiatry Service (a model developed by the Yale Child Study Center and now being delivered in 16 sites throughout Connecticut under contract with DCF).

We are learning, however, that even the most well-developed models, those with defined treatment manuals and methods of quality management through training, data collection, quality monitoring, and evaluation, are difficult to replicate. As well developed as MST is, it still relies on the capabilities and commitment of provider agencies and their staffs to adhere to the model, and for the state agencies as purchasers of the service to hold firm in setting standards and requiring accountability for performance.

Our state public systems are eager to transform their systems so that their resources are used to purchase treatments that are known to be effective. This eagerness, while a tremendous opportunity, also presents a challenge in that they are moving to implement some of these practices more quickly than there is the capacity to support. A survey of providers with whom state agencies contracted to provide intensive community-based behavioral health services to children involved in the legal system in Connecticut indicated that although programs, providers, and advocates have goals that are consistent with the findings of scientific research on treating delinquency, they typically do not have access to the materials, training, or funding required to implement evidence-based practices (Ford et al., 2003).

Likening what happens when there is divergence from an evidence-based model as prescribed to what happens when physicians reduce the dosage of psychotropic medications below clinically desirable levels, Glied and Cuellar (2003) note the reduction in the efficacy of the intervention. That has been our experience to date, but we are attempting to address this challenge through the academic-public partnership, which will enhance the collection, analysis, and dissemination of evaluation and research findings and thus put us in a position to advocate for the policies and practices that support adherence to effective clinical practices.

Promote Public Awareness and Public Will

Ultimately the success of building community systems that will support the mental health of children requires ownership from the community as a whole. When it comes to mental health, we well know this is a challenge because of the stigma associated with mental illness. To build a broad understanding that a system of care approach is different and can make a difference requires helping people understand and accept new ideas. In business parlance this is known as social marketing. Among the graduates of the Comprehensive Community Mental Health Program, those sites that understood the concept of marketing were more successful in achieving sustainability. As noted by Koyanagi and Feres-Merchant (2003):

> Sites should expect to have to "sell" the system of care to staff of other agencies, to market its potential to community leaders and describe it clearly and concisely to local and state politicians. Many policymakers, and certainly many staff in other agencies, are jaded about reform in children's services. Too many attempts have been made and too many failures have occurred for them to have faith in this new approach, unless they can be shown some concrete results. (pp. 31–32)

A Journey, Not a Destination

I have spent the better years of my career devoted to a movement to build community-based, family-driven, culturally competent systems of care for children with, or at risk of having, serious mental health problems. This chapter has been an attempt to weave my own experience and perspective with what has occurred nationally over the past century and more recently in the state of Connecticut.

There are clearly lessons learned, and I have done my best to share those. In my own development I have resonated with the tenets of systems theory and servant-leadership. Both have provided conceptual frameworks that allow me to stay the course over many years while the efforts at change confront the inevitable roadblocks and challenges. As noted by Robert Friedman (2002), who along with Beth Stroul pioneered the concept of a "system of care" in children's mental health, there is an increased recognition of the complexity and difficulty of implementing the values and practices of systems of care. He states, "Given the challenge of developing and implementing systems and services for a diverse population of children and families, many with co-occurring conditions, we need to have realistic expectations to expect gradual, incremental progress, and be prepared to be in it for the long haul" (p. 47).

Systems are slow to change. That is their beauty and their curse. It takes a commitment to a vision and values, patience, and a cadre of committed people who share in the cause. While the research is not yet conclusive, an accumulating body of evidence reinforces the work. Underlying all this is the experience of children and their families, who provide the passion and the reason to continue. Occasionally someone in Connecticut will pronounce that "KidCare is dead." I look around and remind them that there has been incredible progress, even if we are not where we hoped we would be. This is true on the national scene as well. We have come a long way. We have a long way to go.

References

Annie E. Casey Foundation. (1995). *The path of most resistance: Reflections on lessons learned from new futures*. Baltimore: Author.

Child Health and Development Institute of Connecticut, Inc. (2000). *Delivering and financing children's behavioral health services in Connecticut*. Farmington, CT: Author.

Connecticut Department of Children and Families and Department of Social Services. (2001). *Connecticut community KidCare: A plan to reform the delivery and financing of children's behavioral health services*. Hartford, CT: Author.

Connecticut Department of Children and Families, Division of Mental Health. (2002). *Annual system of care status report for community collaboratives*. Hartford, CT: Author.

Ford, J., Gregory, F., McKay, K., & Williams, J. (2003). *Close to home: A report on the behavioral heath services for children in Connecticut's juvenile justice system*. Farmington, CT: Connecticut Center for Effective Practice of the Child Health and Development Institute of Connecticut.

Friedman, R. (2002). *Child and adolescent mental health: Recommendations for improvement by state mental health commissions*. Tampa: University of South Florida, Department of Child and Family Studies, Louis de la Parte Florida Mental Health Institute.

Friesen, B., & Winters, N. (2003). The role of outcomes in systems of care. In A. Pumariega & N. Winters (Eds.), *The handbook of child and adolescent systems of care* (pp. 459–486). San Francisco: Wiley.

Geballe, S. (2002). *The state of children's mental health in Connecticut: A brief overview*. Farmington, CT: Connecticut Health Foundation.

Glied, S., & Cuellar, A. (2003). Trends and issues in child and adolescent mental health. *Health Affairs, 22*(5), 39-50.

Hobbs, N. (1975). *The futures of children: Categories, labels, and their consequences*. San Francisco: Jossey-Bass.

Joint Commission on the Mental Health of Children. (1969). *Crisis in child mental health: Challenge for the 1970s*. New York: Harper and Row.

King, B., & Meyers, J. (1996). The Annie E. Casey Foundation's mental health initiative for urban children. In B. Stroul (Ed.), *Children's mental health: Creating systems of care in a changing society* (pp. 249–261). Baltimore: Brookes.

Koyanagi, C., & Feres-Merchant, D. (2000). For the long haul: Maintaining systems of care beyond the federal investment. Washington, DC: Center for Effective Collaboration and Practice, American Institutes for Research.

Lourie, I., Katz-Leavy, J., DeCarolis, G., & Quinlan, W. (1996). The role of the federal government. In B. Stroul (Ed.), *Children's mental health: Creating systems of care in a changing society* (pp. 99–114). Baltimore: Brookes.

Meyers, J., & Davis, K. (1997). State and foundation partnerships to promote mental health systems reform for children and families. In C. Nixon & D. Northrup (Eds.), *Evaluating mental health services: How do programs for children "work" in the real world?* (pp. 95–116). Thousand Oaks, CA: Sage.

Meyers, J., Kaufman, M., & Goldman, S. (1999). Promising practices: Training strategies for serving children with serious emotional disturbance and their families in systems of care. Washington, DC: Center for Effective Collaboration and Practice, American Institutes for Research.

New Freedom Commission on Mental Health. (2003). *Achieving the promise: Transforming mental health care in America*. Final Report (DHHS Publication No. SMA-03-3832). Rockville, MD: Author.

Senge, P. (1994). *The fifth discipline fieldbook: Strategies and tools for building a learning*. New York: Currency/Doubleday.

Spears, L., & Lawrence, M. (2002). *Focus on leadership: Servant leadership for the 21st century*. New York: Wiley.

Stroul, B. A., & Friedman, R. M. (1994). *A system of care for children and youth with severe emotional disturbances* (Rev. ed.). Washington, DC: Georgetown University Child Development Center, Child and Adolescent Services System Program Technical Assistance Center.

U.S. Department of Health and Human Services. (2000). *Mental health: A report of the Surgeon General*. Rockville, MD: U.S. Department of Health and Human Services, Substance Abuse and Mental Health Services Administration, Center for Mental Health Services, National Institutes of Health, National Institute of Mental Health.

Susan C. Ayers and D. Russell Lyman

The Development of a Community-Based System of Care

"Where Were You When I Was 16 and Needed You?"

Shirley, a 33-year-old African American mother of seven children, asked this compelling question in 1992 during a home visit with Peggy, her family support worker, a key member of the clinical team that had been working with the family for 4 years. Agency clinicians became involved with Shirley and her children in 1988, after all the children had been removed from her care multiple times by the state's child protective agency. Shirley, who had become a mother at 16, was about to lose them permanently. More than a decade later, in 2003, Shirley remains involved with the Guidance Center, Inc., a community agency serving the comprehensive developmental, mental health, and family support needs of children and families in Somerville and Cambridge, Massachusetts.

Today Shirley is a psychologically stronger woman who has developed more effective parenting skills. She uses weekly center-based therapy, family support, and group work with other mothers who have similar backgrounds. Two of her children have been in college, another is in high school, and the youngest is an emotionally healthy, achieving

seventh-grade student in the Cambridge public schools. Because the right kind of help was not there for Shirley when she first needed it, her three oldest children have not fared as well. Shirley has participated with us in telling her story, hoping it will help others build on their strengths so they can better walk their complicated life paths.

The Guidance Center's community-based clinical practice model evolved in response to the needs of parents like Shirley. Our model and practice were crafted through the creative mix of visionary leadership and active, experienced, flexible staff, who worked with Shirley and other courageous families and children needing mental health intervention. Our goal[1] in this chapter is to weave Shirley's story throughout the chapter to put the Guidance Center's model and the development of its integrated service continuum into a historical context and reflect upon lessons learned from those we have endeavored to treat. We will also illustrate how a combination of descriptive clinical research, knowledge of best practice, and dynamic advocacy can be used to secure resources, facilitate change, and ultimately create a comprehensive continuum of care for troubled children and families.

Roots of Our Model

The Setting

The Guidance Center serves the communities of Cambridge and Somerville, Massachusetts, contiguous cities just across the Charles River from Boston. When Shirley first came to the Guidance Center, it was the child and family outpatient mental health clinic component of the local community mental health center serving about 300 families. Today, the Guidance Center is an independent, private, nonprofit agency with a broad range of programs that begin at the earliest moments of life and include services for the most vulnerable of children and families challenged by developmental disabilities and child protection and mental health issues. Serving well over 3,000 families and children, we are able to identify needs of parents like Shirley before their first child is born and then be a partner and resource throughout the family's development.

The Guidance Center's mission is to be a leader in providing comprehensive prevention, developmental, and mental health services to Cambridge and Somerville children, including our youngest and most vulnerable infants, in respectful partnership with their families and our community colleagues. We offer families, children, and our colleagues the integrated programs, resources, and expertise they will need to meet the developmental challenges involved with raising healthy children in safe and loving families, child care settings, classrooms, or after-school programs. Our continuum of care begins before birth with pregnant mothers and includes universal home visiting for newborns; early intervention for infants and toddlers in their homes and child care settings; Cambridge Head Start; a classroom-based violence prevention program; and groups and counseling work in schools, youth centers, and other places where children spend time. Outpatient mental health and cross-cultural services are provided in a clinic setting and at home.

We are actively engaged in family outreach and support services for families coping with domestic violence, parental estrangement, and developmental disabilities. The needs of high-risk children and their parents or caretakers are met through a family-focused after-school program and intensive around-the-clock wraparound services designed to keep emotionally challenged young people at home. Infused in our work is a consistent striving toward cultural competence. The Guidance Center, with its array of services, stands in great contrast to the agency at its inception.

The Beginnings of a Continuum of Care

In 1954, the Cambridge Mental Health Association (CMHA), the Guidance Center's historical birth parent, was founded in response to a group of concerned citizens who through their research established the need for community-based mental health services. The CMHA was founded as a nonprofit organization, and its directors decided to give first priority to children's services, "because of public demand and in the belief that preventive work should start at a young age" (Glasscote, Fishman, & Sonis, 1972, p. 55). In 1955, financial support from the Division of Mental Hygiene of the Massachusetts Mental Health Act was obtained, and the association established its first program, the Cambridge Guidance Center. In 1968, an application for federal funding led to the creation of the Cambridge-Somerville Mental Health and Mental Retardation Center by establishing specialized nonprofit agencies. A comprehensive array of inpatient and outpatient services was developed for children and adults in both communities.

The director of the agency felt strongly that most children in the community, regardless of level of need, could be successfully served with their family in outpatient services rather than in institutions. While other communities were building hospital units for troubled children with the same funding stream, he oversaw the development of the components of the "Cambridge-Somerville Mental Health Center Without Walls." He ensured that programs designed to meet the broader developmental needs of children were also part of this community-based system.

Thus, the Guidance Center's services in those early years were limited to outpatient treatment for children and families and consultation to community agencies. The first consultation efforts were directed to the settlement houses and community centers. In 1962, a day program was started that served developmentally delayed preschoolers, for whom there were no related services available. It was not until the mid-1960s that the Guidance Center would become part of a larger system of care.

In 1963, President John F. Kennedy's Comprehensive Mental Health Act prioritized federal spending for community mental health. This set the stage for the 1965 Massachusetts Mental Health Act, which would bring new support for those services in the state. This was in contrast to the common practice of using government funds to build large, comprehensive community mental health centers with the expectation that consumers come to the centers, as opposed to providing services in agencies throughout their communities. The CMHA was designated to operate the Cambridge Guidance Center as the child ambulatory service for the city of Cambridge. At this time Shirley was just 12 years old and suffering severe abuse and neglect in her family's home in Boston, where such centers existed.

Early Community-Based Philosophy

An early brochure for the Cambridge Guidance Center describes the children's service as an outpatient community organization designed and staffed to help children who experience more than the usual difficulty in growing up. The Guidance Center staff held the philosophy that the center owes service to the entire community. Charles Hersch, assistant director and chief psychologist at the agency, said,

> It is incumbent upon us to extend ourselves where possible to provide service. Every child in town is to one degree or another our responsibility, for whatever kind of problem he may be experiencing. One can't always translate this concern into clinical activities, but the viewpoint is reflected in our thousands of hours of consultation to agencies in the community and the considerable investment we've made in community planning. (Glasscote et al., p. 56)

The director of the agency, Robert Reid,[2] felt strongly that most children in the community, regardless of level of need, could be successfully served with their family on an outpatient basis. He ensured that programs designed to meet the wider developmental needs of children were part of this system. As he oversaw the development of the components of the Cambridge-Somerville Mental Health Center Without Walls, the Cambridge Head Start, early intervention, and a respite program for developmentally disabled children in time became components of the continuum of the community mental health center.

The seeds for a broad, developmentally comprehensive, community-based, systemic vision were sown early and embedded in the agency mission. The system had a long way to go, however, because the components of the Center Without Walls, while bound by their association with each other, nonetheless operated as independent and sometimes competing agencies. Many of the important parts of the system were there, but they stood side by side, much like silos.

A Child Guidance Model Detour

On the practice front, the Cambridge Guidance Center got detoured from the early systemic community service by the implementation of the child guidance model. Embraced by the Boston psychoanalytic community of the 1960s and 1970s, this model consisted of center-based services, in which a psychiatrist saw the child weekly and the parents were seen by a social worker at less frequent intervals. For children seen at the center, activities with the Cambridge schools in the late 1960s and early 1970s were sporadic, limited to classroom observation and an interview with the teacher. Eventually in the 1980s some program/classroom consultation in the schools developed that was a first step back to the earlier vision of using our clinical expertise to address the social and emotional needs of the child and family in their community context.

As Shirley began to have her children in 1976, in agencies like the Guidance Center there was growing recognition that many children who needed mental health services were not getting them, and often services were not effective (Stroul, 2002). Studies by the Joint Commission on the Mental Health of Children (1969) and the President's Commission on Mental Health (1978) had concluded that in addition to problems with service access, children were in more restrictive settings than necessary. This was certainly true of Shirley's children during their periods of removal from home. Major reasons for this were that only a limited range of service options were available for seriously emotionally disturbed children and their families, and collaboration between service systems for children was poor. By this time, systems of care principles were being articulated (Stroul, 1996; Stroul & Friedman, 1986), but funding streams and service system change had not yet caught up. By 1986, Shirley had six children under the age of 10, who had been removed multiple times by child welfare but had never had comprehensive family-based treatment.

What Was Missing

Two key ingredients were missing from this early association of community-based services. First was a family-centered treatment model. Breaking away from the child guidance model, which isolated the treatment of the child from the parents, and moving toward a family-centered practice would prove to be a long and difficult process. There had been sporadic progress in this area, including providing an initial home base to emerging leaders in the family therapy movement, but the resistance to the shift to a family-centered model was intense. The progressive family therapy practitioners stayed briefly with us. They left choosing to spend their careers developing newly emerging theories and practice with like-minded clinicians. The agency had not yet fully developed the vision or resources to create and support the immense change that family-centered practice would bring to the Guidance Center.

Second, a cohesive and shared vision of a system of care for families had not yet been fully articulated. There was a lack of integrated knowledge, coordination, and collaboration between the clinical and community components to ensure that a comprehensive, family-centered plan was developed to support the needs of the identified child, parent(s), and the other children in the family. Service providers, including the many involved with Shirley's family, were not communicating adequately. Often they were unaware of who else was involved with the family, and what other community resources were available.

In 1988, when she was 28 years old, Shirley tried to take her life. Shirley's desperate act was emblematic of the growing acuity of mental health problems in the community. This acuity called for the implementation of the community-based vision set by early agency leaders. The Guidance Center was at a turning point in its development. This challenge, to create an integrated system of care that would address the developmental, social, and emotional needs of all children in families like Shirley's, was to be faced by new leadership.

Evolution of a Continuum of Care

New Leadership

In 1988, new leadership was brought to the CMHA and its sole program, the Cambridge Guidance Center, which continued to operate as the child and family outpatient component of the Cambridge-Somerville Community Mental Health Center. The new executive director[3] came with 10 years of clinical social work experience and many lessons learned from developing and directing the family program on a child inpatient unit in a local community hospital. This unit, which was quite unique in the late 1970s and 1980s, operated with the core understanding that parents' involvement in their child's diagnostic workup and treatment was critical to the positive outcome of the hospitalization and discharge. This was the single most important lesson learned. The unit developed an innovative, family-centered model, which included parent-child therapeutic activity groups targeting enhanced positive parenting and parent-child communication skills (Ayers & Colman, 1987). Many of the parents involved in the 12-week program emerged with improved limit-setting skills, a greater capacity to identify and process their own feelings and those of their children, and a stronger sense of themselves as capable and caring parents. The program served as a model for what later became the Guidance Center's family-focused therapeutic after-school program.

Another lesson was recognition of the need to support the family in telling its own "family story." As each child's clinical records were collected at the beginning of the hospitalization, it became evident that various reports and evaluations reflected differing and often isolated perspectives on the family's experience. The perspectives of the various authors, including pediatricians, therapists, child protective workers, school personnel, and psychologists who had done testing, were limited in scope and often represented differing professional or agency agendas. In all the reports, a common theme was blaming parents for their children's problems. One of the most important outcomes of each hospitalization was the ability of the family to understand and then tell their own story to the host of helping professionals involved in their lives. The hospital evaluation process deliberately brought the community players together so they could share their perspectives and begin to hear the family life story. This set the stage for the family to create a community-based team that understood their story, had a shared agenda, and supported them in their efforts.

A third lesson learned through inpatient work was that community-based practice has the opportunity to be innovative and flexible, with the capacity to make adjustments and realign resources to meet the needs of families and children. Because the unit served a wide geographic area, it offered a broad view of how the larger child-caring "systems" did (and did not) work to support the healthy social, emotional, and behavioral growth of children and their families. It became apparent that the pockets of practice and program innovation often had as much to do with community leadership and collaboration as with resource allocation. This led to a profound commitment to metasystemic thinking and a host of wide-ranging relationships with many of the community leaders who were developing new models to meet the clinical complexity found throughout our communities. The new director was known and trusted by many Cambridge and Somerville families and community leaders outside the Guidance Center. The challenge was to gain that same respect inside the Guidance Center.

Shaping Community-Based Clinical Practice, Taking on the Challenge

New leadership found some real strengths at the Guidance Center, including signs of a shift in the clinical culture to more family involvement in their child's treatment, a diverse multicultural clinical team working with Spanish-, Portuguese-, and Haitian Creole–speaking families, a strong clinic-based group program for boys and girls, and a clinically supervised therapeutic mentor program for children seen in outpatient treatment.[4] There was also a rich array of existing resources in the Cambridge community.

A step in the right direction was the Guidance Center's collaboration in the Family and Youth Assistance Program (FYAP), a 3-year demonstration grant from the U.S. Department of Health and Human Services, conceived in 1988. Key city and state funders were brought together with local child and family agencies to begin to disseminate and apply the systems of care work being done in other parts of the country to the Cambridge-Somerville area. The FYAP initiative never took full root in our community, as evidenced by the lack of any lasting coalitions or the implementation of redesigned, collaborative, and systemic models. This model had a number of bureaucratic layers involving agencies that had not spent enough time together to develop a fully articulated vision of community-based services. FYAP was top-heavy, and turf issues drained energy away from developing a unified sense of direction. The model was also designed as a 3-month intervention, whereas project clinicians struggled for permission to work with families like Shirley's for as long as 2 years.

The financial model in 1988 also presented significant challenges to implementing change. As the child and family outpatient component of the Cambridge-Somerville Community Mental Health Center, the clinic was staffed by long-term state psychiatrists, psychologists, and clinical social workers. A fundamental problem with this public-private partnership was having the locus of control and direction of the staff resting with state staff outside of the agency, meaning substantive change in the organization had to be accomplished by persuasive vision and leadership. In fact, most Guidance Center staff had been in the agency for as long as two decades. It was the responsibility of the CMHA's board of directors to hire the executive director to oversee the fiduciary and operational aspects of the CMHA and the Cambridge Guidance Center. The 17 state employees at the Guidance Center were supervised and paid by the state at a cost of $700,000, so the CMHA's actual budget was about $350,000, generated through insurance billings, a small school consultation contract, and donations. This revenue supported some administrative and clinical staff, paid the operating costs of running the clinic, and gave some room for program development.

Many children and families who were being treated at the clinic were experiencing significant psychiatric acuity, but the staff had few clinical strategies or flexible resources to enable family members to live safely together. The extensive needs of Shirley and her family challenged agency leadership to support the staff to explore new clinical models that address complex, interdependent needs. The clinicians were about to be pushed well beyond their medical model training and practice and into the exciting work that the systems of care research was beginning to articulate (Stroul, 1996). We were determined to create a vision of a new family- and community-focused practice model that the clinicians would want to embrace.

It was a delicate and slow process that required establishing trust by building on staff strengths and developing a shared concept and passion for community-based work. The process of change seemed to compel clinicians to cling tenaciously to their identities within their professional disciplines. Helping them recognize the value of teaming with community partners and new nontraditional supports vital to a family support model seemed to come only after they experienced a positive process or outcome with a child or family. Some staff members were aware of new models, but most were distinctly unenthusiastic about the prospect of actually going out into the community to find and work with such troubled families, especially without more flexible resources and support.

Shirley's Story Informs Our Model

Shirley was born in 1960 and raised in Boston's urban neighborhoods. Her parents were deeply troubled, especially her father, an alcoholic who violently abused his wife and their eight children. Shirley's post–traumatic stress disorder left her with an intractable depression and poor executive functioning, making it impossible for her to create a stable home environment for her own children. She found herself trapped in controlling, abusive relationships with the men who fathered her children. The four oldest children were severely abused by these men and were removed from Shirley's custody, some more than once. When the children were removed, she lost her public financial support, leaving her with limited options. Shirley lived in battered women's shelters, with family members, or with boyfriends prior to her 1988 suicide attempt and hospitalization. When Shirley was hospitalized, her six children, ages 2 to 12, were placed in separate foster homes, and the oldest, age 12 headed to his third residential placement. Shirley began to be seen by a therapist at the local hospital outpatient clinic. The four older children in foster placements were referred to the Guidance Center.

The development of Shirley's children was punctuated by repeated placements and hospitalizations depending on her ability to care for them. The effects of these disruptions affected the children differently depending on their age, and if or when they were able to receive effective, family-centered services that included Shirley. This history is depicted in figure 16-1 to provide a visual encapsulation of the history of disruption, displacement, and reunification that Shirley and her children experienced. It also illustrates how different the outcome was for her first three children, who did not benefit at an early age from comprehensive, community-based, family-centered services, compared with our involvement with her subsequent children, who were still very young or not yet born.

Throughout 1989, Shirley's children were seen in a sibling group at the Guidance Center, and an attempt was made to have the foster parents also seen. All efforts were directed at keeping a family connection among the children and creating some unified parenting strategies among the foster parents. As the negative behavior of Shirley's 10-year-old son continued to escalate, the executive director at the Guidance Center convened a series of key case consultation meetings. Attending the meetings were several child protective workers and their supervisor, four therapists from the Guidance Center working with the siblings and foster parents, several school personnel, and no representative for Shirley. It was readily apparent that few of the people in the room knew each other. There was little accurate information among the players, and no systemic understanding of the family. No unified strategy had been developed, nor was the anticipated outcome that the children would be in their family context. For Shirley and her children to be seen and served as a family, we needed to get all the key players, including Shirley and her therapist, into partnership with each other, on the same page and on the same team.

The Guidance Center's effort to achieve this team approach was the beginnings of what was becoming known as "wraparound." By this time, calls to action around the escalating unmet mental health needs of children and families had begun to influence social policy (Knitzer, 1982), and principles of systems of care were being articulated (Stroul & Friedman, 1986). The wraparound movement had not yet taken a firm hold at the

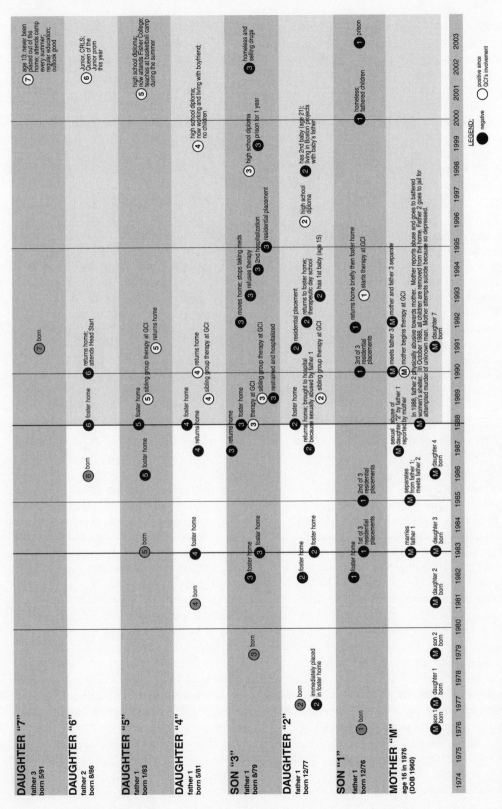

Figure 16.1. Shirley's story

227

community level. This vision of wraparound services needed a central person, agency, and team to nurture and implement the model. The model is relationship-based and must be accessible to families over time. For more than a decade, Shirley and her children had been struggling through repeated failures, traumas, and disappointments with each other and their helpers. It would take a great deal of trust building and communication to create a network of support for them. The resulting coalition of helpers came to be known at the Guidance Center as the "therapeutic network team."

Building a Therapeutic Network Team: Obstacles and Opportunities

In the late 1980s and early 1990s, building consensus among the many community agencies to create a family-centered plan with Shirley was daunting, yet essential. Indeed, there was no public policy expectation among state agencies and local schools that such a plan would even need to exist. Without it we were doomed to continue the cycles of family disruption, shame, and blame, doing greater damage to Shirley and her children with each removal to foster care. Thus the central goal of our case consultation meetings was to build consensus around a family-centered plan for Shirley and her children with the array of professionals, who had disproportionate power and multiple agendas. Crafting a unified action plan for the children, ages 13, 12, 10, 8, 6, and 3, who were desperate to be reunited with their mother, involved a delicate balancing act over time. We needed to develop true partnerships with the most central agencies, each with their respective challenges, described later, to build an effective therapeutic network team.

Each public agency involved with the family saw only a piece of the puzzle—its area of concern. It was common for the multiple players involved with the child or children in a family to have different opinions about interventions, placement, and disposition. Parents, especially isolated ones like Shirley, were rarely at the table for the discussion. For instance, the primary focus of school personnel was on the educational needs of the children, and in the most troubling family situations, if it appeared that the child needed to live outside of the home to learn, they could make that happen. Education was their primary mission, not keeping

a family intact. Indeed, if they made the judgment that a parent was not capable of executive functioning, they could take the initiative to pick up the full cost of a residential placement. When the school paid, school personnel were in charge of that decision. This meant they could avoid having discussions with the child welfare agency about the child's readiness to return home (which might not necessarily improve the child's school functioning).

Perhaps most discouraging was the profound pessimism of the local state child protective leadership, which held out little hope for Shirley's rehabilitation. Like many parents, Shirley was often blamed by child-serving professionals for shortcomings in parenting, when in fact she was suffering in a system that added to her burden by taking her children away from her rather than putting in place the community supports she needed for her family to survive. Having lost custody of her children so many times in her 28 years portended a permanent loss of custody, unless some dramatic changes could occur.

Central to the implementation of a successful, family-centered plan was having Shirley's treatment transferred to the Guidance Center from hospital-based services, so that her family could all be seen in one place. This provided us with firsthand knowledge of Shirley, both her strengths and her challenges. It also enhanced work with protective services. For example, she was having weekly supervised visits with her children at the time (1989), yet the young child protective workers doing the supervision inadvertently made the visits more difficult by reminding the children that if they did not behave, they would never return to their mother. Given the children's natural distress when they had to end their visits, this message often exacerbated their acting-out behavior. Providing some basic education to the workers so they could understand the negative impact of this message and giving them other strategies to support the children's positive behavior was another key intervention. We needed the protective workers and their leadership as allies, since they held immense decision-making power over the lives of the children. Their view also needed to become more inclusive of a family focus. We needed to work with child protection in a way that would supportively open doors to the family. One answer to this was the development of our outreach model.

Developing the Outreach Model

In 1990 we acquired the first "flexible" support component for our evolving clinical model, a family outreach worker. We knew that this was our first big break, and we took full advantage of it, based on what we knew we needed to create a wrap-around capacity. At this time (1990) wraparound models were being used experimentally in demonstration projects such as those at Fort Bragg (Bickman, 1996) and Ventura County (Hernandez & Goldman, 1996). Our state's child welfare office also was beginning to contract for short-term home-based family services. Shirley's story had already taught us that what was often missing in those early models was the "glue" to hold their services together, which began for us in the form of outreach.

The Guidance Center had been advocating with the state mental health authority to develop a therapeutic after-school program for latency-age children and their families, and to that end was given a state paraprofessional worker from the local early intervention program named Peggy.[5] Obviously we could not get an after-school program started with just one person (it took another 4 years for that program to become a reality), but we knew that Peggy could become a partner with the clinical staff to do outreach work to families whose children have been referred for treatment. Though the clinical staff questioned her credentials and at first did not know how to partner with her, it did not take long for Peggy, an experienced parent who had run her own therapeutic child care center, to engage with a handful of the more systemic-thinking staff to create our outreach model.

Gradually Peggy was accepted as a member of the clinical team and blazed the way for our distinctive model of outreach that is thoroughly integrated into the clinical work. Peggy, as a parent, made parent-to-parent mentoring possible. We came to realize that recruiting and training outreach staff from the diverse bilingual, bicultural communities we serve enables them to use their understanding to cement partnerships with parents that are inclusive of family background, beliefs, and traditions. The outreach model also provided a window into the daily life of a family, thus offering a rich perspective for the entire clinical team.

Shirley's door was the first one Peggy knocked on. Shirley's treatment had been transferred to the Guidance Center when her hospital therapist left her position, yet due to her severe isolation and depression, she had not connected with her new Guidance Center therapist and was deteriorating at home.

In developing the outreach model, Peggy and her subsequent colleagues created the strategy known as "Dunkin Donut therapy." When the licensed clinician is unable to make any headway with a parent, or the family's need far exceeds what a clinical hour can provide, an outreach worker joins the clinician, and they become a team. When the outreach staff goes on a home visit to begin the engagement with a "resistant" parent, bringing coffee and doughnuts is a surefire strategy to get in the door. Once inside, staff are able to begin to build a relationship, which over time often reveals that the "resistance" is in fact a debilitating depression, a well-earned mistrust of professionals, or even a fear of going outside the apartment, all of which were true in Shirley's case. Peggy and her colleagues offer concrete support with practical matters, making sure food is on the table, managing a household budget, or getting children to their doctors' appointments. Over time a relationship with the whole family develops that supports the more formal therapeutic work. It frees up families to invest in the therapeutic work because they have begun a partnership with a member of a clinical team that promptly addresses their daily living needs in tangible ways.

Clinicians began to understand what a handful of families knew already, that Peggy could make their lives much easier and the therapeutic work more meaningful. School personnel, child protective workers, probation officers, and of course the local Dunkin Donut franchises know our outreach staff as partners for parents and children.

In Shirley's situation, Peggy became a lifeline and the glue for the Guidance Center's evolving clinical model. Often too depressed to even open the door, Shirley found that once she let Peggy into her home, they began to build a partnership. Her spirit had been broken through years of abuse and shame, and formal learning has been difficult for her. Shirley also carried a burden of suffering created by the caregiving system, that had worked with a deficit model and lacked understanding of her situation and therefore also failed to provide critical coordination for services. Consequently, service providers fragmented her family by repeatedly taking her children away. Often, as in Shirley's case, the children were taken away as newborns, thus doing permanent damage to parent-child attachment. The friendship and mentoring of an outreach worker began to change this for Shirley. Part coach and part cheerleader, Peggy provided enough support to see Shirley through four therapists, with whom she had highly productive, healing relationships.

The Therapeutic Alliance Supported by Outreach

Shirley's reflections about the roles each therapist played in her Guidance Center experience are simple, instructive, and compelling. While we knew Peggy offered continuity, connection, and trust, Shirley also experienced Peggy as a surrogate parent for her own children. Indeed, her kids called her the "donut lady," and even though they gave Peggy a hard time, whenever they needed something, they would ask their mom to call her for help. Peggy, who always had the whole family in focus, helped Shirley begin to see what more positive parenting was all about.

In partnership with Shirley, Peggy helped her learn little things like having milk instead of soda in the bottles of her toddlers, and more significant things such as the importance of going to the school and child protection meetings. "She was the one," explains Shirley, "who held everything together over the years. Peggy introduced me to my first therapist, and said I would like her, but I didn't want to go." Peggy persisted and provided the foundation that Shirley needed to make the significant therapeutic transitions that were ahead.

Shirley began to cry as she talked about her relationship with this first therapist. She opened her door to a social work intern named Mary in 1990. "She was spunky, warm . . . like a sister and friend. She brought me my very first birthday cake. . . . I had never got nothin' for birthdays or holidays, so I never celebrated anything." That began to change as she let Mary into her life. "She focused on me and the kids. We had no furniture, so somehow she got some chairs so we could sit on them when she came to visit. She made me get out of the house and go for walks. One time when we had no food she took me shopping, and instead of buying just one of everything, she bought two. I told the kids it was Mary who put the food that I cooked on our table that night." Shirley talked about how Mary made her think about her future, her dreams. What she marveled at most was that Mary gave Shirley her home phone number in case of an emergency. "I didn't believe she really gave me her number, so I called and when she answered, I was so shocked that she was telling me the truth, and then I hung up."

By 1991, Shirley had given birth to her seventh child. Her youngest three children had been returned by the child protective agency to her care, but her oldest three children continued to cycle between foster care or residential placement with regular family contact. This same year the state began changing the way it purchased services in mental health, giving the Guidance Center its next big opportunity to make more changes that would support our vision for a more flexible, comprehensive family-centered practice, tailored for and accessible to our most challenged families.

Privatized Purchase of Neutral Services

On July 1, 1991, Massachusetts "privatized" its community-based state purchasing system. The drive behind privatization was the belief that services purchased by the state would be more efficient and of higher quality if they were put out as contracts for competitive bid by private, community-based organizations like the Guidance Center. That meant that the state employees were transferred out of the Guidance Center to work in state institutions, and the Guidance Center was given a contract to provide mental health services and community support for children and families driven by specified target outcomes. This created the opportunity for the Guidance Center to set our sights on the development of a fully articulated community model with newly hired senior leadership and staff, who shared our vision and now were fully employed and supervised by the Guidance Center management.

Together with knowledge gained in community outreach practice with families like Shirley's, the flexible dollars contracted by our state mental health authority enabled us to embed the outreach model into our core clinical system. Outreach became part of our culture and a valued component of clinical teamwork; it meant that we had a greater capacity to treat and support the diverse needs of very challenging families. State funding also enabled us to pay salaries to clinical staff (as opposed to paying them on a fee-for-service basis for only the reimbursable services they delivered) and keep the expectation for billable hours reasonable. By expecting 21 billable hours per week, we could support the expectation that clinical staff would also travel to engage and work with families and children in their homes, schools, or after-school programs, or wherever there was a need. The flexible dollars also paid for the critical collateral time that is essential for this work and allowed progressive clinicians like Mary to make strategic therapeutic use of their time in activities such as grocery shopping with a struggling parent or working with the outreach worker to find furniture for impoverished or disorganized families.

Creating a Bridge and Providing Continuing Support

Shirley's therapist Mary left the Guidance Center in 1993 after four years of committed work, which had begun to bring Shirley out of what she described as her "fog." This work laid the foundation for a new but fragile perspective of herself as a parent and woman worth caring about. "When she left, she really hurt me, and I cried and cried," said Shirley. "I knew she had to get on with her life, but it took me a really long time to get over her. She drove a red car, and every time I saw one go by, I looked to see if she was inside." Peggy remained Shirley's mainstay, continuing to oversee the family's functioning and making sure that the youngest child got enrolled in Head Start and the others had therapists and school plans as needed. She visited Shirley weekly, making sure there was food in the house and bringing her to her medication appointments so that her depression, which had deepened since Mary's leaving, would not overwhelm her.

It took Shirley at least 6 months to open the door to her next therapist, Amie, who rode her bicycle across town every week to see her. Amie would knock on the door, and Shirley would not answer. "I knew it was Amie knocking on my door, but I wouldn't let her in. But you know, she kept coming on her bicycle every week in the rain and snow, and finally when I saw her standing there in a really bad storm, I just opened the door." That was in 1994. Taking the time to travel by bicycle

for repeated nonreimbursable no-shows was of course possible only with committed staff in a flexibly funded community service delivery model, working in tandem with Peggy's outreach work, which maintained the family connection.

Shirley said of Amie, "She focused on me. She made me get out of the house every week, and we would go outside and sit or walk and talk. She would never let me stay inside. She'd say, 'This is your therapy time, and we are going to use it for you.'" Amie's notes reflect that they were able to do a tremendous amount of work together over the next 2 years. Shirley was gaining some confidence with her parenting; she rebounded from her depression and despair more rapidly; she was feeling better about herself and began to come out of her profound isolation and make some new friends. Her referral to the state to get job training finally came through, and Amie and Peggy supported her through several tries at this. They also continued the work of building Shirley's confidence to bolster her ongoing desire to get her high school equivalency, helping her with finding resources, completing applications and homework, and developing the skills to do this work on her own. Shirley reports that when Amie left for a new job in 1996, "I could let Amie go."

In 1996, Leslie was the next therapist who came into Shirley's life. Peggy introduced them. Leslie was the first African American woman Shirley had ever met with, and they worked together for the next 6 years. "Leslie would never come to my house. She would call me in the morning and say in that warm voice of hers, 'Get up, baby 'cause I am expecting you here today.' And she'd call back later just to check to see that I was up. . . . Leslie was like a mother, sister, and aunt to me. She taught me about African American history and all the great things women have done. I looked up to her. She was so smart, she came from the South and lived in the projects, and she made it! She inspired me and made me believe I could be someone, too." Shirley sought out employment and worked part-time on and off at several jobs. Leslie also helped her have expectations for her children, to do chores and schoolwork and be part of a family team. "She always wanted to know what I had cooked for them, and at the holidays she made sure I did something good for myself. She'd say, 'You deserve something too, even if it's something small.' I always have her in my head."

With Leslie's good-bye, Peggy, the anchor of the clinical team, helped Shirley through the next transition. Currently Shirley is working with a senior Guidance Center clinician on the most practical matters—tutoring so she can pass her high school equivalency exam, not taking the bait when her teenage daughter wants to draw her into an adolescent struggle, taking care of herself in her relationships. Shirley no longer remains home refusing to open her door to anyone. While remarkably improved in her ability to have relationships, work, and be a good mother, Shirley is not completely trouble free. Each developmental challenge she faces with her children is made more difficult by their shared history of fragile attachments and repairs, so Shirley continues to use targeted Guidance Center support. Now that her oldest children are having babies of their own, she is very excited about her grandmother role and is grateful for the opportunity to "give my grandchildren what I couldn't give my children."

State Changes Begin to Support Community Systems of Care

Over time, state leadership, given the flexibility of the contract structure, was able to buy innovative community-based models. Our Family After School Program (FASP), which was one of these innovative outreach models, had come to be known in the community as an effective way of holding fragile families together. This helped to convince state payers that the same principles could be applied with children and families involved in a milieu after-school service. In 1993, child welfare dollars were used to purchase slots for 6- to 13-year-olds at risk for being placed outside of their homes. Shortly thereafter, Department of Mental Health dollars were used to purchase more slots, which meant that families like Shirley's, with protective issues, mental health issues, or both, could benefit from the highly structured, skill-building activities for both children and parents in the therapeutic milieu, with built-in carryover to the home.

The FASP Model: A Milieu After-School Program

Program clinicians work with state case managers to identify those 6- to 13-year-old children and families most in need of support after school so that they can avoid hospitalization or out-of-home placement. Children's educational needs are addressed during the day in school, and after school they are able to work on improving their communications, peer relations, homework, and family relationships. Structuring the child's after-school hours also gives struggling parents like Shirley some respite and the chance to attend to some of their own life improvement needs. The program includes intensive case management and operates in close collaboration with the children's school placement (often a special needs school). Every 6 weeks all the key players meet with the family to ensure that the therapeutic network team is working toward shared goals. In FASP each family (16 in all) has a social worker who coordinates care, as well as an assigned family support/milieu worker who does home-based outreach and accompanies children home on a van service. Parents are invited to join therapeutic and skill-building groups in activities such as art therapy, social skills work, violence prevention, and computer literacy instruction. A parent support group is offered one afternoon a week, and whole families are invited to special events such as Thanksgiving dinner and holiday parties.

Wraparound Care

By 1995, wraparound continuums of care for families had taken hold in many states, some of which were pooling dollars from multiple state agencies to develop a broad range of intensive family support services for at-risk children. Wraparound models were being presented with great excitement at national conferences, and reviews of the effectiveness of systems of care were appearing in the literature (Bruns, Burchard, & Yoe, 1995). Senior staff had been attending these conferences since 1990, bringing back new knowledge and relationships with state agency colleagues, who were also looking for opportunities at their purchasing level to create local systems of care.

The Family Advocacy, Stabilization, and Support Team

For the Guidance Center, the wraparound movement brought with it the opportunity for us to develop the Family Advocacy, Stabilization, and Support Team (FASST). This is our home-based intervention and intensive care coordination model for highly challenged families. Children ages 3 through 19 with serious mental health issues (69% of those referred have been hospitalized previously, and 29% have lived in residential or foster home settings) are referred by the state's Department of Mental Health. Ancillary services are either purchased by the program from flexible funds or are supported by insurance. This program has been another catalyst for change in the agency by demonstrating to staff and the community that the whole family must have a network of community supports wrapped around them. More than 50% of these families have experienced some form of abuse or neglect, and in more than half of the families, members other than the "identified patient" suffer from serious mental illness.

Our Department of Mental Health presented the opportunity to create our wraparound program by transferring the dollars that it used to purchase residential care for 10 seriously emotionally disturbed children in our area and putting the funds out to bid in 1995 for a home-based wraparound program. Moving contract dollars in this manner was a way of funding local 24-hour-a-day, 7-day-a-week wraparound teams. Our growing understanding of wraparound systems of care and our early commitment to outcomes work were definite assets for the Guidance Center in the proposal process. We were awarded $550,000 per year in a flexibly funded cost reimbursement (as opposed to fee-for-service) model. In addition to going anywhere families needed them, the team also had flexible dollars to purchase whatever goods or services families needed, from Tae Kwon Do lessons to sexual abuse evaluation or short-term residential diagnostic assessment. Peggy now had a full-fledged wraparound mobile team behind her. Now we could intervene in time to prevent the loss of children like Shirley's to the residential system. Though the eligibility of one child as seriously emotionally disturbed was the gateway to the system, we intervened with the whole family. If siblings really needed residential care, the team could provide the support to step them back down to less intensive levels of care as each was able.

The well-researched, well-documented, and remarkable success of our FASST model[6] has kept 87% of children with their families in the community. Our success with FASST has given state leaders valuable information indicating that very troubled children can be sufficiently supported in safe families to get well in community settings, rather than being sent off to a residential placement. Our track record with FASST was a factor in the recent decision of the state child welfare agency to pilot a similar initiative with the Guidance Center. The Family Intensive Reunification and Stabilization Team (FIRST) program provides intensive levels of home- and community-based intervention and support for children returning to their families following protective custody. In this program a full-time social work clinical case coordinator and a full-time family support worker work with just four families. Had they been available when Shirley needed them, such teams could have saved Shirley and her children tremendous suffering, avoiding state expenditure of hundreds of thousands of dollars in residential and foster placements.

Children With Voices and Meeting Place

In 1999 the state child welfare agency also sought bids for domestic violence services, and the Guidance Center developed a collaborative model that could provide assessments, advocacy, and services for mothers and children witnessing and experiencing situations similar to what Shirley had been through. In Children with Voices, program staff work actively with other agencies to ensure that families receive services tailored to their needs. Shirley continues to use her "Mothers in Action" group at the Guidance Center for survivors of domestic violence as a support.

It took almost a decade of operation for our supervised visitation program, Meeting Place, to achieve state support. Meeting Place provides a safe place, with trained visit supervisors, for children from broken homes to visit with their noncustodial parent. Meeting Place which had come on board in 1991 supported only by foundation and donor dollars, achieved child welfare funding in 2001 by proving its worth in fostering healthy child development and preventing family violence. With the change in the state purchasing system, the program used hard demographic and outcomes data to convince the state that supervised visitation was a remarkably effective way to protect children from high-conflict families, 70% of whom have witnessed domestic violence and experienced emotional trauma, child abuse, and neglect.

The Needs of Early Intervention Programs (From Birth Through Early Childhood)

The tragedies Shirley and her children lived through exemplify both the crushing challenges families face and the ways that systems designed to help such families often fail them. Especially for a young mother like Shirley, family isolation, survival instincts, and a transgenerational history of destructive family patterns set up dependence on any source of income, housing, and "protection," which ends up enabling domestic abuse in the name of survival. Mothers who have survived trauma often have compromised brain functioning, and they may live in poverty, without adequate education or work skills. They are confronted with multiple problems among nuclear and extended family members, often bringing them in contact with child welfare. The stigma involved with seeking help for social and emotional problems contributes to avoidance of services, even if they are known to be available. When combined with culturally imbued perceptions of "mental health," this can add up to mistrust of authorities, including child welfare, school, and mental health providers. This is exacerbated by deficit model treatment driven by problem-focused payers seeking quick solutions. Parent blaming adds to the mistrust, and parents like Shirley often come to us with a long history of inadequate, disjointed, and disrupted clinical treatments that have come hand in hand with the repeated removal of multiple children. Essential attachments are compromised or destroyed at critical moments in a child's development, which for Shirley included the removal and placement of a newborn child because the father had abused some of the older children. In Shirley's case the child welfare personnel believed that she would never get her children back. To their credit, a senior manager about 12 years later offered, "I don't know what you all did with Shirley, but as far as we are concerned, your staff worked a miracle."

No one had taken the time to know Shirley and her children, to determine their strengths and understand their culture, both in terms of how interventions should be adjusted to be helpful and in terms of how cultural values and assets could support growth. Shirley's family was "lost" in the system because early childhood services, the schools, and mental health care systems did not talk or plan together using family-centered, strength-based models. Shirley encountered repeated rubber fences in the system, in which families either cannot gain access to services for eligibility reasons or must sacrifice critical rights to obtain desperately needed services. For example, some parents have been forced to relinquish custody of their children to obtain residential care. Above all, we failed Shirley and her first children because we were not in a position to intervene in her teen years, when she first faced the challenge of motherhood.

Early Intervention as a Core Element of the System of Care: A Definitive Organizational Decision

During the course of Shirley's time with Leslie, senior management at the Guidance Center developed a deepening conviction that being there when Shirley needed us meant being able to identify problems and intervene at the earliest moments of life. The stage is set for the development of a child's social and emotional wellness even before birth. Yet so many families, child protective workers, or teachers bring their children to our clinic long after the problems have begun, when their difficulties have become so severe that no one could ignore them. Our awareness of this led us to develop Infant-Toddler Services, a range of prevention and developmental programs for children under 3 years of age, and to manage Head Start, an early care and family program for children 3 to 5 years of age living in poverty.

When a separate corporation in the area, the Center for Mental Health and Retardation, Inc., which operated Early Intervention and Cambridge Head Start services, began looking for a home, we jumped at the chance to provide it. Though this affiliation proved to be labor-intensive and costly, it was worth the investment. Our early intervention program, which provides developmental therapies to infants and toddlers with developmental delays or risks for delay, served as a platform from which to develop other community-based early childhood programs. One of these, Healthy Families (funded locally by the Children's Trust Fund), provides home visiting for teenage mothers until their first child reaches 3 years of age. Maternal and child health nursing assessments and service linkage for at-risk mothers before birth are now available in our newest program, Early Intervention Partnerships. In addition, our FIRST Link initiative, funded largely by grants and donor dollars, enables us to provide a welcome screening and linkage visit to every consenting parent giving birth in our area.

In addition to vastly improving our clinical knowledge about how best to intervene during pregnancy and early childhood, our affiliation experience taught us two important lessons. The first is that bringing together separate corporations with programs that provide different services to distinct age-groups is a long-term process of building trust and awareness. Perhaps even more challenging than encouraging early childhood developmental specialists to attend to the mental health needs of the whole family is educating mental health clinicians to recognize and address the needs of infants and toddlers. Since the referred client of a clinician in children's services is usually of school age, these workers need training in developmental milestones and issues of children under 3 years of age.

Had our infant and toddler programs been in existence when Shirley was 16, they would have enabled us to engage with Shirley when she was first pregnant and work with her in the first 3 years of her child's life. In all likelihood, partnership with the Healthy Families home visitor assigned to support her first pregnancy and the first 3 years of Shirley's motherhood would have led to a radically different outcome for Shirley and the subsequent children she might choose to have. At a minimum, earlier intervention with Shirley and her children would have prevented or ameliorated the suffering that her first three children are living out today.

Nesting Families in a System of Care

Figure 16-2 illustrates how our initial vision of a single outreach worker grew into a network of teams within interlocking spheres of care that can encompass the needs of fragile families, beginning before birth. This system of care is designed to support children and families across a broad range of problems, including those at high levels of risk, acuity, and chronicity. The child and family are at the center of therapeutic wraparound because their voices and needs drive the unique blend of services and supports they receive. Spheres of care interlock both because in some cases they overlap (as, for example, in supporting the mental health needs of children in educational settings) and because linking systems of care through coordination and consensus is so essential. As parents find their own voice to tell their story to the team, a shared vision of the strengths, needs, and necessary therapeutic and community supports is created, along with consensual goals and clearly defined individual responsibilities. These elements are coordinated by the therapeutic network team, which is brought together on a regular basis by agency clinicians to ensure metasystemic communication. State agencies and local institutions are included on each family's therapeutic network team as key stakeholders whose level of consensus is critical for continuity of care.

What We Can Offer Shirley Now

Our partnerships with Shirley and so many others have given us the insight and motivation to transform and expand our clinical, community-based practice models and the Guidance Center. We now manage $8 million in human service resources, employ 160 staff, and directly serve more than 3,000 children and families. This includes the planning, purchasing, and oversight for services offered to selected families involved with our state child protective agency (Department of Social Services Family Based Services). Through a broad range of programs we influence the outcomes of many more lives through our extensive community-based consultations and universal early intervention developmental screenings in 25 child care centers throughout the Cambridge school system, psychoeducational parent groups, and numerous collaborative community-based projects.

Underpinnings of a System of Care

The system of care that evolved from our single outpatient clinic was able to grow because of five key elements. First, it was based on a firm philosophy of community-based work that included an understanding of the challenges facing families like Shirley's and a deepening commitment to core principles of wraparound care. This process grew out of a long-term process of facilitating change through training, active exchange of ideas, and consensus building.

The Guidance Center, Inc.
Mental Health Continuum

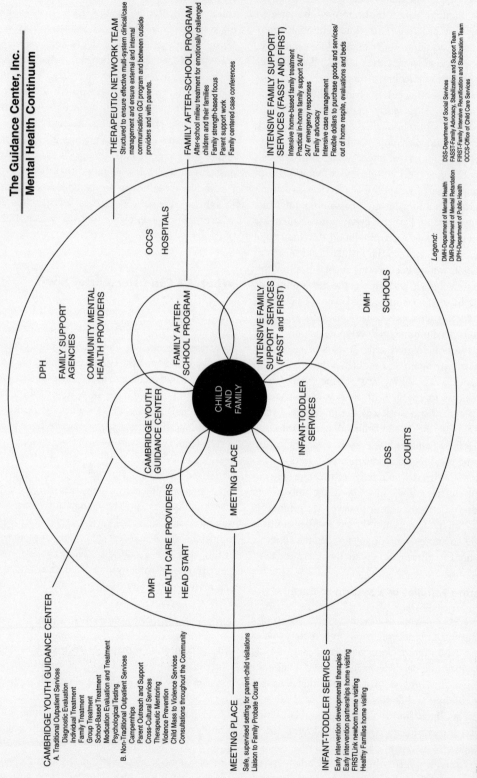

CAMBRIDGE YOUTH GUIDANCE CENTER
A. Traditional Outpatient Services
   Diagnostic Evaluation
   Individual Treatment
   Family Treatment
   Group Treatment
   School-Based Treatment
   Medication Evaluation and Treatment
   Psychological Testing
B. Non-Traditional Outpatient Services
   Campernhips
   Parent Outreach and Support
   Cross-Cultural Services
   Therapeutic Mentoring
   Violence Prevention
   Child Mass to Violence Services
   Consultations throughout the Community

MEETING PLACE
Safe, supervised setting for parent-child visitations
Liaison to Family Probate Courts

INFANT-TODDLER SERVICES
Early intervention developmental therapies
Early intervention partnerships home visiting
FIRSTLink newborn home visiting
Healthy Families home visiting

THERAPEUTIC NETWORK TEAM
Structured to ensure effective multi-system clinical/case
management and ensure external and internal
communication GCI program and between outside
providers and with parents.

FAMILY AFTER-SCHOOL PROGRAM
After-school milieu treatment for emotionally challenged
children and their families
Family strength-based focus
Parent support work
Family centered case conferences

INTENSIVE FAMILY SUPPORT
SERVICES (FASST AND FIRST)
Intensive home-based family treatment
Practical in-home family support 24/7
24/7 emergency responses
Family advocacy
Intensive case management
Flexible dollars to purchase goods and services/
out of home respite, evaluations and beds

Legend:
DMH-Department of Mental Health
DMR-Department of Mental Retardation
DPH-Department of Public Health

DSS-Department of Social Services
FASST-Family Advocacy, Stabilization and Support Team
FIRST-Family Intensive Reunification and Stabilization Team
OCCS-Office of Child Care Services

Figure 16.2. The Guidance Center, Inc. Mental Health Continuum

Second, our continuum grew because over time we were able to demonstrate an advanced knowledge of best practices, and we took advantage of every opportunity to implement it in our communities. Third, in addition to embracing best practices such as infant-toddler assessment and intervention, infant mental health (emphasizing the parent-child relationship), systemic family intervention, and wraparound principles of care, we have also sought to push the envelope. This has involved urging clinicians, researchers, payers, and lawmakers to recognize the value of testing models that have not yet been proved. After all, our first experiment in outreach had not been proved, and now we are able to develop even better models, backed by experience and data with and shaped by the knowledge of parents like Sylvia, who have partnered with us.

Fourth, we were able to maintain a high level of accountability by taking a leadership role in using empirical methods to describe the characteristics and needs of the families we serve and the outcomes they were able to achieve while with us. Rather than attempting to "prove efficacy" through impractical and expensive experimental designs, our research and presentations have focused on accurately describing the different challenges facing families we work with, and in identifying and quantifying key areas of family functioning in which positive change can happen (Lyman, Ayers, Siegel, Alvarez de Toledo, & Mikula, 2001). This has required committing the time of senior agency professionals with a range of skills in clinical practice and research methodology to design and implement a practical outcomes paradigm.

Fifth, we have consistently demonstrated our commitment to community partnership by actively seeking productive collaborations and creating opportunities to advocate at every level of local, state, and national government, and to seek private foundations, and local donors for ongoing improvements to our community's system of care. This, too, has involved the dedication of considerable time in coming together with other providers and payers to develop a shared vision of what a system of care should look like.

Finally, we have had the support of a board of directors that has shared our vision and realizes what an opportunity the Guidance Center has to have a profound impact on the quality of life for the children and families in our communities. This

consensus has resulted both from educating the board about the essentials of systems of care and from clearly demonstrating to it, through our outcomes work, the reach and effectiveness of our services.

System of Care Principles

This system of care is built around the following core operating principles that we have adapted from established principles of wraparound care (Stroul & Friedman, 1986): (1) Services for children and families need to be nested in a system of care with deep roots in the community. This rootedness includes the capacity of long-term relationships such as the one Shirley still has with Peggy, to preserve continuity of care. (2) Assessments of families must be strengths-based and metasystemic, determining every possible resource both within the family and within the family's community support system and network of providers. (3) The system must be consumer driven and have an inherent respect for the cultural identity of families and for their capacity to create their own solutions. (4) The continuum and its service models must have the elasticity to flexibly provide the most suitable service delivery models, including duration of service, and funding sources and to adjust multiple services according to the changing needs of different family members. (5) Flexibility must also include the capacity for urgent intervention for families with a familiar team at any time of day or night.

Model design, as well as ongoing accountability for implementation, must also be driven by empirical descriptions of population needs, as well as quantitative measurement of service access and outcomes. This can be done in a small agency such as the Guidance Center (Lyman et al., 2001) and does not necessarily require the negotiation involved in pooling funds across state agencies, such as one finds in many statewide wraparound systems. Our job will become infinitely easier as our state health and human service agencies, schools, and private funders continue to make progress in embracing the core principles and using them to guide the work they support, which might indeed result in the creation of true community-based systems of care across the state.[7]

Perhaps most important, operationalizing these principles rests on nurturing a flexibility in the thinking of clinical staff, who have often been trained in highly defined, often office-based therapies such as cognitive-behavioral, object relations, or a host of other theories and techniques. Though these approaches are highly valuable, it is important that clinicians be supported enough to accept the risks involved in accepting practical, community-based supports for families as critical elements of their interventions. To do this, it is absolutely essential that clinicians and family support workers be given systematized opportunities to receive training and consult with each other. This helps them to maintain awareness of the many community-based choices available and to hear other workers' experiences of what combinations of support and intervention have worked best for different types of families.

Accountability Through Outcomes

Our outcomes initiative enables us to be accountable to our stakeholders. State funders such as the Departments of Mental Health and Social Services need to know whom they are serving, what they are paying for, and how well it works, especially as they draw their monetary lines in the sand in tight financial times or make their case for funding to the legislature. They need more than just anecdotal descriptions of families like Shirley's. The social policy implications of this work are extremely significant. The capacity for profiling service populations tends to elude most state agencies, and hence social policy is created without sufficient information. Each state agency has a mandate to focus only on its own part of the elephant, so to speak, whereas community providers tend to be exposed to the whole animal, or at least most of it. Because we blend funding streams to craft wraparound services for families, hard data give us a chance to provide a "voice from the trenches" in the public policy debate about what seriously emotionally disturbed children and families need. In this capacity we can be a strong catalyst in bringing service to practice and practice to service.

Outcomes work is critical because it allows us to describe in quantitative terms the challenges faced by families like Shirley's. This provides critical information both to improve our services and to convince payers to fund them. Our work has resulted in demographic analysis that captures conventional family data, as well as a risk-factor matrix targeting both troubled children and their caregivers. By using functional assessments such as the Child and Adolescent Functional Assessment Scale (Hodges & Wong, 1996) and the Child Behavior Checklist (Achenbach, 1991) in combination with structured case disposition data, we are able to quantify outcomes. This is helpful to line staff, who are able to take a scientific look at whether or not progress is being made in their intervention, and to see that they are part of an organization that really is making a difference.

It is possible to do this outcomes work in a small agency such as ours by including outcomes measurement as one of the performance specifications for state contracts. By exploring software linkages between our outcomes database and our billing system, we are now able to tie together client demographics with outcomes, service duration, and cost to describe the effectiveness of different types of services with different types of families. Being able to profile families empirically has been a key component in determining family and community needs as we designed our service array. We are not able to conduct follow-up studies of the extent to which treatment gains are maintained over time. In part this is because payer-driven services are mandated to take care of serious family problems quickly in "brief" interventions, leaving little room either for prevention services or for follow-up work to determine how well families sustain treatment gains.

The Service Array Today

The core goal of our service array is to serve children of all ages and their families in our area, by addressing a broad range of challenges to healthy development at all levels of community-based service intensity. We intend to partner with parents and children and our community colleagues over time to support the growth of strong families. Our funding consists of multiple federal, state, and local contracts, third-party insurance payments, and an increasingly aggressive fund-raising program. In every case we attempt to blend our funds to create or enhance cutting-edge models of care that are uniquely tailored to fit family needs. Table 16-1 illustrates our Guidance Center continuum as it exists today.

Table 16-1. Programs at a Glance

	Cambridge/ Somerville Early Intervention (CSEI)	Families of Cambridge and Somerville (FOCAS)	Cambridge Head Start Day Care (CHSDC)	Cambridge Youth Guidance Ctr (CYGC)	Family Advocacy, Stabilization & Support Team (FASST)	Family-Based Services-DSS Lead Agency	Family After-School Program (FASP)	Temporary Care Services (TCS)	Meeting Place (MP)
Clients	Birth–3 years	Pre-birth–3 years	3–5	3–22	6–19	Birth–18 years	6–13	3–22	All ages
Services	Support and education for children at risk for developmental delays, and their parents	Pregnancy and parenting support to first-time adolescent parents age 19 and under	Preschool education, day care, and parent support	School, community, and clinic-based multicultural mental health and domestic violence	Intensive intervention for families, children, and adolescents at risk for hospitalization or	Manage $1.3MM of DSS services for families in Cambridge, Somerville and neighboring	Therapeutic after-school program for emotionally-challenged children and their families	Coordinate and provide respite for families of special needs children and young adults	Safe, supervised setting for parent-child visitation
Program headquarters	61 Medford St., Somerville	61 Medford St.	432 Columbia St., Cambridge	5 Sacramento St., Cambridge	1679 Mass Ave, Cambridge	1679 Mass Ave	1680 Mass Ave, Cambridge	5 Sacramento St.	5 Sacramento St.
Budget*	$1.8MM	$178K	$1.5MM	$1.2MM	$484K	$100K	$288K	$190K	$137K
Funding Sources	DPH, Insurance, Medicaid, CDBG, UW, Donors	DPH	Feds, DOE, City Contracts, OCCS	DMH, DSS, Medicaid, Insurance, UW, Donors, CDBG	DMH	DSS	DMH, DSS, Donors, United Way	DMR, Donors	Donors, DSS
Staff	44	5	47	16	5	2	6	7	4

*Budget figures are for FY 2000
DPH = Department of Public Health, CDBG = Community Development Block Grant, DOE = Dept. of Education, DMH = Dept. of Mental Health, DSS = Dept. of Social Services, DMR = Dept. of Mental Retardation, UW = United Way, OCCS = Office of Child Care Services
Note: Head Start is a program of Center, Inc. operated under a management contract with the Guidance Center, Inc.

Weaving Services for Families

Shirley, by telling her own story, has given us a rich picture, at some times tragic and at other times hopeful, of her fragility and resilience, of her fear and courage, of her disappointments as a parent and her wish to be a better grandparent. We have attempted to capture how our integrated service continuum has evolved with the intention of supporting the needs of families like Shirley's and others who seek support with their challenging tasks as parents.

We continue to look for opportunities to grow, always in adherence to our core vision of community-based services. These opportunities include the further development of expertise in the assessment and treatment of preschool age children and their families, after-school programming for troubled adolescents, and enhanced trauma services for victims of abuse. As we seek to further develop our system of care, we continue to use proven outcomes data along with narratives of our work with Shirley's and other families to influence public policy. Consistent themes of our advocacy work are that we must continue to press for innovative practices (both proven best practices and untested ones such as our outreach model once was) that shore up and integrate community-based services, to intervene early and provide the broadest possible range of supports to families like Shirley's.

We hope that we never again will hear the question, Where were you when I needed you? from a parent who has lived in Cambridge or Somerville for his or her children's formative years. By the time we found Shirley, her three oldest children, 16, 15, 13, were beyond the therapeutic reach of the Guidance Center. "I didn't have enough to give my oldest kids," Shirley sighs with regret. We were too late to partner with Shirley so she could have been a more present and effective parent for all her children. Thankfully, an enduring partnership has been formed with Shirley and a number of her children, and we will be there for their children if needed. We trust that together we have learned lessons that will enable us to listen to parents, children, and our community colleagues as we continuously refine the weave of our family-centered, community-based system of care.

Notes

1. This coauthorship represents the diverse talent and respectful partnerships that must exist at the heart of implementing the ambitious, shared vision of dynamic change told in this chapter.

2. Robert Reid, a child psychiatrist, was the first director of the Cambridge Mental Health Association (CMHA) and Cambridge Guidance Center. In 1968 his vision and leadership resulted in the creation of the Cambridge Somerville Mental Health and Retardation Center. The CMHA and Cambridge Guidance Center became the child mental health component of the center for the Cambridge community.

3. This was Susan C. Ayers, LICSW, current executive director and coauthor of this chapter.

4. A staff member's doctoral thesis had created this mentoring model and named it "companion tutor" because the traditionally trained staff did not believe that anything having to do with volunteers without graduate clinical training should connote that it was "therapeutic."

5. Peggy Worrall is now coordinator of outreach services at the Guidance Center.

6. Descriptive research on this model has been presented at local and statewide conferences, as well as at the 14th Annual Research Conference in Children's Mental Health in 2001 in Tampa, Florida.

7. Massachusetts has undertaken a process of assessment and reorganization of its state systems in relation to the systems of care principles. It is in its earliest stages, yet we want to be hopeful for positive outcomes.

References

Achenbach, T. C. (1991). *Manual for Child Behavior Checklist/ 4-18 and 1991 Profile*. Burlington: University of Vermont, Department of Psychiatry.

Ayers, C., & Colman, J. (1987). *Parents: The critical yet overlooked component of effective inpatient/ group care child treatment*. Paper presented at the Albert Trieschman Center conference, Boston, Massachusetts.

Bickman, L. (1996). Implications of a children's mental health managed care demonstration project. *Journal of Mental Health Administration, 23*, 107–117.

Bruns, E., Burchard, J., & Yoe, J. (1995). Evaluating the Vermont system of care: Outcomes associated with community-based wraparound services. *Journal of Child and Family Studies, 4*, 321–339.

Glasscote, R., Fishman, M., & Sonis, M. (1972). *Children and mental health centers*. Washington, DC:

Joint Information Service of the American Psychiatric Association and the National Association for Mental Health.

Hernandez, M., & Goldman, S. (1996). A local approach to system development: Ventura County, California. In B. A. Stroul (Ed.), *Children's mental health: Creating systems of care in a changing society* (pp. 177–196). Baltimore: Brookes.

Hodges, K., & Wong, M. (1996). Psychometric characteristics of a multi-dimensional measure to assess impairment: The Child and Adolescent Functional Assessment Scale. *Journal of Child and Family Studies, 5,* 445–467.

Joint Commission on the Mental Health of Children. (1969). *Crisis in child mental health.* New York: Harper and Row.

Knitzer, J. (1982). *Unclaimed children: The failure of public responsibility to children and adolescents in need of mental health services.* Washington, DC: Children's Defense Fund.

Lyman, D., Ayers, S., Siegel, R., Alvarez de Toledo B., & Mikula, J. (2001). How to be little and still think big: Creating a grass roots, evidence-based system of care. In C. Newman, C. Liberton, K. Kutash, & R. Friedman (Eds.), *A system of care for children's mental health: Expanding the research base* (pp. 49–58). Tampa: Research and Training Center for Children's Mental Health, University of South Florida.

President's Commission on Mental Health. (1978). *Report of the sub-task panel on infants, children and adolescents.* Washington, DC: Author.

Stroul, B. A. (1996). *Children's mental health: Creating systems of care in a changing society.* Baltimore: Brookes.

Stroul, B. A. (2002). *Systems of care: A framework for system reform in children's mental health.* Washington, DC: Georgetown University Child Development Center.

Stroul, B. A., & Friedman, R. M. (1986). *A system of care for seriously emotionally disturbed children and youth.* Washington, DC: CASSP Technical Assistance Center, Georgetown University Child Development Center.

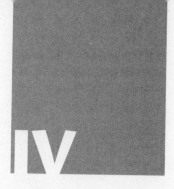

IV

Practice Examples

Martha Morrison Dore, Nancy Feldman,
and Amy Winnick Gelles

Family of Friends
Creating a Supportive Day Care Community to Prevent Child Abuse and Neglect

According to the oft-quoted African proverb, "It takes a village to raise a child." It also takes a village or, in contemporary society, a community to support parents to raise their children. Research studies have demonstrated the importance of community in the child-rearing process. One notable early study by Garbarino and Sherman (1980) illustrates this finding well. These researchers selected two low-income Chicago neighborhoods with similar sociodemographic characteristics, one with higher than average rates of reported child abuse and neglect, and the other with unusually low rates. They then examined differences in the two communities to determine what factors separated the high-incidence community from the low-incidence one. They found that in the low-incidence community, neighbors knew one another. Although economically deprived, the low-incidence community was quite stable, with little housing turnover. People looked out for one another, and for one another's children. When a family was in trouble, whether from loss of a job or a parent's emotional difficulties, neighbors were available to step in and provide needed support to the family.

Conversely, in the neighborhood with a high incidence of child maltreatment, there was a great deal of housing turnover, leaving neighbors unfamiliar with, and suspicious of, one another. Families were isolated behind locked doors, with few supportive resources to call on when trouble occurred.

Beginning in the mid-1980s, crack cocaine use became epidemic in the kind of low-income urban communities studied by Garbarino and Sherman, infecting many families in their prime childbearing and child-rearing years. Since the crack epidemic began, research has found deterioration in perceptions of community support in communities at low and moderate risk of child maltreatment, such that residents no longer perceive neighbors as a potential source of support during hard times (Coulton, 1996). Respondents in Coulton's study of Cleveland neighborhoods with low, moderate, and high risk of child maltreatment reported a significant change in the parenting capacities of individuals in these communities. Concern was expressed that children, even as young as 4 or 5 years of age, were unsupervised and allowed to wander the neighborhood at will. If a neighbor objected to a child's public behavior, the child's parent would often take the child's side, and there was a strong likelihood of retaliation by the parent or child, unlike years past, when neighbors frequently served as surrogate parents when children were outside the home, monitoring and correcting misbehavior. This changed perception of the role and involvement of neighbors has contributed to increased isolation of families and distrust of others in the community, according to Coulton (1996).

Other community-level factors that influence parenting and impact rates of child abuse and neglect have been examined as well. In his study of low-income Philadelphia neighborhoods, Furstenberg (1993) found that parents in violence-prone public housing projects isolated themselves and their children within their own homes. Their relationships with neighbors were guarded and suspicious. Even when there were neighborhood resources such as community centers that offered safe haven and activities for children, parents were reluctant to allow their children to participate, thus precluding the kinds of interpersonal relationships that could offer both children and their parents support in their daily lives. As in the Garbarino and Sherman study cited earlier, Furstenberg contrasted the experience of families in public housing projects to those of families in poor but stable neighborhoods with high levels of home ownership and strong kinship networks. In the latter communities, parents took a more active role in ensuring that appropriate community services were available for their children. Neighbor-to-neighbor relationships were characterized by mutual trust and interdependence, and neighbors fulfilled a surrogate parenting role for children outside their homes.

The finding that community social support mediates child abuse appears to hold true across cultures as well. Gracia and Musito (2003) recently reported the findings of a study comparing relationships between community social support and child maltreatment in communities in Spain and Columbia. In both cultures, maltreating parents were found to be less integrated into their communities, demonstrating lower levels of participation in community social activities and less use of formal and informal services than parents who had not maltreated their children.

In addition to studying the supports various communities offer for effective parenting, recent research has looked at community norms regarding various aspects of the parenting role. For example, community expectations with regard to corporal punishment may determine whether or not there is implicit permission for physical means of managing children's behavior. In neighborhoods where interpersonal violence is common, there may be more acceptance of physical aggression as an appropriate way of controlling the behavior of others, including young children (Lynch & Cicchetti, 1998).

In the face of community stressors such as the absence of employment and educational opportunities, inadequate and unstable housing, and few or no recreational outlets, reliance on aggressive methods of child management may quickly escalate into child abuse. A recent study that looked at the contribution of community structural factors including impoverishment, child care burden (number of children per adult caregiver), and instability (housing turnover within the community) to child maltreatment found that, on a measure of individuals' child abuse potential, there were few differences between residents of neighborhoods with low child maltreatment rates and those with high rates as measured by substantiated reports to the public child welfare agency (Coulton, Korbin, & Su, 1999). However, actual rates of child maltreatment varied considerably among the 20 neighborhoods studied and were closely correlated with the three community structural factors of impoverishment, child care burden, and instability. Coulton and her colleagues concluded that, while attitudes and beliefs about child rearing shown to correlate highly with child abuse may be pervasive among parents across all types of neighborhoods and communities, such attitudes are much more likely to turn into abusive parental behavior when other community-level stressors are present.

Another way in which community may interact with parenting to contribute to child abuse and neglect is through the psychological effects of living in an unsupportive, even hostile environment. Parents who must raise their children in neighborhoods permeated with violence and fear, and which lack even rudimentary resources for supporting child development such as adequate day care, community centers, libraries, or viable playgrounds, may be at greatly increased risk for depression and other mental health problems, as well as for drug and alcohol abuse (Cicchetti & Lynch, 1993; Klebanov, Brooks-Gunn, & Duncan, 1994). Both substance abuse and mental disorders, particularly depression, have been shown to be associated with increased risk of problems in parenting, including child neglect and abuse (Dore, 1993; Dore, Doris, & Wright, 1995).

As empirical evidence grows for the impact of community factors on parenting behaviors, there is increased interest in community-based interventions that can address those factors that contribute to maladaptive parenting, resulting in child abuse and neglect (McFarland & Fanton, 1997; Wilson & Melton, 2002). Such interventions must be designed to replace negative community factors such as widespread acceptance of aggressive child management strategies, including corporal punishment and verbal abuse, the social and emotional isolation of families with young children, and the lack of family-supportive community resources. In other words, they must replace unsupportive and detrimental communities with communities that create a climate that supports positive parenting and nurtures both parents and their children. The program discussed in this chapter, Family of Friends, represents one such effort to create an alternative, supportive, and nurturing community in collaboration with parents of preschool-aged children as a means of preventing child abuse and neglect.

Background

The Family of Friends project was developed by staff of the Boys and Girls Harbor, a large, multiservice voluntary community agency whose main site is located in the Spanish Harlem neighborhood of New York City. Family of Friends was designed to address agency concerns over the inadequate parenting skills and knowledge demonstrated by some parents whose children participated in the Harbor's three day care programs. There was also concern that some of these children exhibited behaviors indicative of possible maltreatment in their homes. Harbor staff applied for and received a grant from the National Committee on Child Abuse and Neglect, then located in the federal Department of Health and Human Services, Agency for Children, Youth and Families. This 3-year, $270,000 grant enabled Harbor staff to implement and evaluate the Family of Friends intervention model they had designed. The overall goal of the project, as defined by the grant-making agency, was to reduce the risk of child abuse and neglect among families residing in communities with high rates of substantiated cases of child maltreatment.

The underlying philosophy of Family of Friends draws on the concept of primary preven-

tion, a process of developing and strengthening compensatory or protective factors rather than directly addressing those community-level factors that increase child maltreatment risk. According to the primary prevention model, while it may not be possible, with limited resources, to adequately address community violence, poverty, inadequate education, unemployment, and other risk factors, it is possible to assist families and children in acquiring skills and developing competencies that enable them to better manage such risks. This intervention model is a strengths-based approach, which incorporates findings from the literature on resilience in the face of potentially overwhelming risk. This literature recognizes the importance of interpersonal support and connectedness in overcoming threats to positive psychosocial functioning.

The Family of Friends intervention model is also based on ecological systems theory, which holds that the risk of child abuse and neglect can be reduced by making the communities in which families function more supportive and responsive to families' needs (Garbarino, 1992; McFarland & Fanton, 1997; Shonkoff & Phillips, 2000). To this end, the intervention was designed to enhance three day care communities serving parents and children in East and Central Harlem, areas of New York City that statistically reflect factors that place children living there at increased risk of abuse and neglect. These factors include a high proportion of female-headed households, high rates of poverty and unemployment, high rates of community and domestic violence, and high rates of substance use and abuse.

Research on the etiology of child abuse and neglect offers a number of findings that informed the clinical components of the Family of Friends intervention model. Of particular importance were studies demonstrating that social isolation and inadequate social supports are significant contributing factors to the maltreatment of children (Bishop & Leadbeater, 1999; Coohey, 2001; DePanfilis & Zuravin, 1999, 2002; Kotch, Browne, Ringwalt, Dufort, & Ruina, 1997). Social supports, including relationships with neighbors and others in one's community, serve a variety of functions for parents in their parenting role, including buffering stress, providing models for appropriate parenting behavior, enhancing access to resources, services, and information, and providing emotional support. As noted earlier in this chapter, research has found that parents in low-income neighborhoods marked by community violence are constrained in the avenues available to them for developing supportive neighborhood networks because of the dangerous, often unpredictable nature of the neighborhoods themselves.

Research on stress and coping suggests that individuals with low educational attainment (less than a high school diploma) who live in high-stress communities such as those served by the Harbor day care centers may possess limited strategies for coping with the multiple stressors in their lives (Chapman, 2001). Numerous studies have examined the relationships between stress, coping strategies, and parenting dynamics (Hien & Honeyman, 2000; Levy-Shiff, Dimitrovsky, Shulman, & Har-Even, 1998; Tien, Sandler, & Zautra, 2000). The stresses associated with single parenthood, in particular, have been the object of extensive study. It appears that environmental stresses have less impact on the psychosocial development of children when parents are able to draw on active cognitive and behavioral coping strategies that moderate the effects of stressful life events on parenting practices (Holloway & Machida, 1991; Levy-Shiff et al., 1998; Tien et al., 2000). Mothers who are depressed, using drugs, or previously found to be maltreating their children have been found to employ fewer active coping strategies when dealing with the stresses of daily living (Hall, Gurley, Sachs, & Kryscio, 1991; Hien & Honeyman, 2000; Shipman & Zeman, 2001). Thus, these mothers are less able to modulate the negative effects of their own distress on their parenting. In the case of substance-abusing mothers, this often results in increased use of highly aggressive child management strategies (Hien & Honeyman, 2000), while in depressed mothers high aggression alternates with high passivity and emotional withdrawal (Hall et al., 1991). Both of these parenting practices are associated with child maltreatment risk and poor psychosocial outcomes for children.

Parents in stressful life circumstances may lack access to information regarding normative child development and behaviors, and on how to manage children other than by using aversive methods such as verbal abuse and corporal punishment (Cunningham & Zayas, 2002; Tamis-Lemonda, Shannon, & Spellman, 2002). Several studies of low-income parents' knowledge of child development appear to bear this out (Benasich & Brooks-Gunn,

1996; Maloney, 2000; Tamis-Lemonda et al., 2002). A study by Benasich and Brooks-Gunn (1996) found a significant association between a mother's understanding of child development at the time of the child's birth and the child's developmental outcomes at 12 months of age. In another study, of the relationship between low-income fathers' knowledge of child development and their potential for child abuse as determined by the Child Abuse Potential Inventory (Milner, 1994), there was a small but significant relationship between these two factors (Maloney, 2000). Similar to effective strategies for coping with stressful life events, knowledge of normative child development may act on parenting practices in such a way as to mediate risk factors for child maltreatment such as low educational attainment, poverty, and single parenthood.

Intervention Model

Family of Friends integrates these multiple research strands regarding factors that interact to result in child abuse and neglect: (1) social isolation and inadequate social supports; (2) inadequate strategies for coping with stress; (3) inadequate understanding of normative child development; and (4) lack of a full repertoire of child management techniques. These research strands are embedded in an intervention model designed to create a community context that supports parents' development in their parenting role. The intervention model contains several components designed to work together to enhance the overall experience of families and children in relation to the day care center and to create a sense of community within each center that provides social and emotional support to parents struggling to sustain their families and meet the emotional and developmental needs of their children.

Components of the Family of Friends model may be grouped together under three broad distal, or outcome, goals: (1) decrease potential for child maltreatment and increase capacity for positive parenting in families attending each day care center; (2) enhance collaboration of professionals, including day care staff, center social workers, and community allies, in supporting families; and (3) build the capacity of the day care community, including parents, staff, and administrators, to offer support and guidance to its members. More immediate, or proximal, program goals include the following:

- Increase parents' opportunities for giving and receiving social support;
- Increase parents' capacities for coping with stress;
- Increase opportunities for parent-teacher collaboration;
- Increase parents' overall sense of agency; and
- Increase parents' and teachers' knowledge of child development and strategies for managing child behavior

Chat Groups for Parents

The program elements designed to achieve these proximal goals included a variety of interventions that contributed to a sense of shared community in the three day care centers. One of these interventions, ongoing chat groups with parents that met at each center several times a week, morning and afternoon, allowed parents to drop in at their convenience to engage with other parents in discussions of child-rearing issues and challenges. These chat groups were scheduled and led by a master's-level social worker assigned to each center. Topics for discussion were suggested by parents and ranged from toilet training a toddler and managing bedtime resistance, to helping preschoolers prepare for kindergarten entry. A significant effort initially was put into recruiting parents for the chat groups. This was done in a variety of ways, according to the organizational structure and participating population of each day care center. One successful method, in addition to sending home the usual notices pinned to children's coats, was to have a table set up with coffee and doughnuts just inside the center's door, so that parents who were dropping off children could receive information about the chat groups as they stopped to pick up an early morning snack. To facilitate chat group involvement of working parents, arrangements were made to serve a simple evening meal at the evening groups and to provide child care during the group's meeting time. Initially, local restaurants and delicatessens donated food for the evening meals; eventually, the parents themselves organized potluck suppers to feed the attendees.

At one of the day care sites, where space was

not a premium, the center administration allowed the Family of Friends program to take over a small, unused room, which could accommodate the chat group meetings. Parents took responsibility for decorating the space, including donating paint, a coffee maker, pictures for the walls, and plants. A shelf of books, magazines, and pamphlets on various aspects of parenting and family life added to the usefulness of the space. In addition to housing the chat groups, the room served as a drop-in center for parents waiting to pick up their children or to meet with a teacher.

In addition to the center social worker, a parent support worker, selected from the center's parent population by the social worker, was an invaluable resource in contacting and recruiting interested parents for the chat groups. The parent support worker was especially effective in reaching out to parents who might not otherwise participate in a group experience but who were identified by center staff as potentially benefiting from the opportunity to engage with and gain support from other parents. These were often, though not always, parents whose children exhibited symptoms thought to indicate possible maltreatment and whose group participation could serve as a mechanism for bridging the chasm between home and school settings often found in low-income communities. Program personnel hoped particularly to engage parents of children whose behavior was problematic in the classroom, either because of high levels of aggression against peers or because of withdrawal and failure to engage with day care center staff or other children. Extra efforts were made to reach out to those parents through phone calls and one-on-one in-person invitations.

Over time, the chat groups became established and built a regular constituency, which was both positive and occasionally problematic because it made it more difficult for newcomers to join in. Having professional leadership of the groups was helpful in this regard; the social worker was able to support the entry of each newcomer into the groups and facilitate that process in a way that might not have occurred so smoothly in a purely self-help model.

As the chat groups became more stable and cohesive, parents shared openly their concerns over difficulties in parenting their children. For example, in one discussion, parents agreed that a particular frustration was giving a child repeated directives, only to have the child ignore them. Several parents in the group admitted that they would become enraged and hit their children at this point. This discussion provided a rich opportunity for the social worker to explore with the parents present how they issue directives to their children, why the children might "tune them out," and what some options for more successful interactions might be. They also discussed alternative disciplinary strategies to spanking or hitting a child and examined together how these strategies are carried out. "Teaching moments" such as this one allowed the social worker to explore potentially abusive attitudes and practices with parents and to continually educate them regarding more effective parenting strategies.

An interesting aspect to the chat groups' development was the subtle shift that took place over time from focusing almost exclusively on problems and concerns in parenting to addressing problems and concerns in other aspects of parents' lives. Depending on the day care site, many of the parents who attended the chat groups were single mothers struggling to balance the demands of parenthood with working outside the home. Employment-related issues, as well as other concerns in daily living, increasingly became the focus of group discussions. The social workers found themselves taking on case management functions for parents in the groups, linking them with resources in the community, locating job training programs, exploring housing options, providing information on how to obtain an order of protection against an abusive boyfriend, providing support during a protective services investigation, and counseling parents one-to-one on a myriad of personal concerns.

In one chat group, a young single mother, Ella W., attended regularly but rarely spoke in the group. After some weeks, she hesitantly approached the parent support worker after the group and asked if she could talk with her privately. Ms. W. tearfully revealed that she was in jeopardy of being evicted from her apartment because of differences with her landlord. She asked the parent support worker if she could accompany her to housing court the following day for an eviction hearing, sharing that she had no family or friends she could ask for support. While traveling to the hearing together, the family support worker learned that Ms. W. was 3 months behind in her rent. She had moved into the apartment from a

homeless shelter, where she had lived with her daughter for 2.5 years. Her family refused to help her because of her ongoing relationship with her daughter's father, who had abused her in the past. He had promised to pay child support that would have helped cover the rent, but he had not followed through. With support from the worker, Ms. W. was able to negotiate an agreement with the landlord to repay the overdue rent. Ms. W. was also helped to file a claim for back child support from her daughter's father, which resulted in restoration of regular payments to the family. In the months after these events, the classroom staff in the day care center noticed that Ms. W's 3-year-old daughter, who had previously exhibited serious behavior problems such as hitting, biting, and scratching her classmates, had become less aggressive toward her peers and more compliant with the teacher's directives.

The Parent Academy: A Self-Help Approach

Another interesting outcome of the chat groups was the development by parents at one of the day care sites of the Parent Academy concept that became part of the program model. The Parent Academy utilized parents of children in the day care center as peer educators on topics identified by center parents as of interest to them. Topics developed for workshop presentations by parents as part of the Parent Academy included behavior management of children, nutrition, building a child's self-esteem, stress management, and parents as role models. When parent expertise was not available on a particular topic, parents, in collaboration with the center social worker, identified a community expert to conduct the workshop. Topics delivered by outside speakers included financial planning, community advocacy (presented by the local councilman), and identification of child abuse. The Parent Academy allowed many parents to contribute substantially to the day care community, thereby increasing their sense of agency, as well as offering opportunities for both giving and receiving social support, two of the proximal goals of the Family of Friends project.

One intent of the Family of Friends intervention model was that parents would eventually assume responsibility for leading the chat groups and organizing the Parent Academy as a way of furthering the development of a sense of agency and ensuring the continuance of the program once funding ended. The mechanism for developing a coterie of parents who could take on this responsibility was the Peer Parents certification process. Parents could become certified as Peer Parents through completion of a progression of activities designed to develop their skills as program facilitators and managers. Beginning with attendance at chat groups and Parent Academy presentations, parents would progress to planning the Saturday family outings that were part of the Family of Friends model, and then to demonstrating their knowledge regarding various aspects of child development and child management through facilitating chat group discussions. Parents who met all the certification criteria received special recognition and certification as Peer Parents, who were qualified to take on responsibility for managing some aspect of the Family of Friends program. A special ceremony was held twice a year to honor those who had completed the Peer Parent certification process.

The Saturday Club

In addition to the chat groups, educational workshops, Parent Academy, and Peer Parent certification as strategies for decreasing parents' isolation and increasing their social networks, supports, and overall sense of agency, the Saturday Club was established to bring families together in more relaxed circumstances than the hustle and bustle of weekday life, to give parents some respite from sole and constant child care, and to provide parents with opportunities to engage in pleasurable activities with their children. The Saturday Club outings provided an opportunity for less competent parents to observe how more skilled parents interacted with their children, as well as giving parents a chance to socialize informally with one another. The Saturday field trips were also organized to expose parents and children to aspects of New York City that they might not otherwise see and to educate parents regarding low-cost or free activities that they could participate in with their children. As noted previously, although initial planning of these outings was carried out by program staff, the Parent Academy certification criteria called for parents to assume responsibility for planning these events.

This component of the Family of Friends program addressed several proximal goals, including increasing opportunities for giving and receiving social support, increasing parents' capacities for coping with stress, increasing parents' overall sense of agency, and developing a supportive environment for families.

Collaboration With Day Care Staff

An important element in the Family of Friends intervention model was the role of the daycare center staff—teachers and administrators—in the program's implementation. Although the on-site social worker and parent support worker were actively involved in the program's development, the collaboration of day care center staff in creating an environment to support and nurture families was essential. The active partnership of center staff was sought in a variety of ways. Because the Family of Friends project was initiated through the Harbor's mental health unit, the program staff was able to offer classroom observation and consultation to teachers regarding children identified as having behavioral or emotional difficulties. Family of Friends social workers and social work interns were an ongoing presence in each of the day care centers, participating in the daily routines of the classrooms, and sharing their expertise in early child development and developmental psychopathology with day care staff. They also provided educational opportunities for staff regarding the etiology and impact of child maltreatment, as well as information on management of children traumatized by abuse and violence in the home and community.

Over time, the presence of Family of Friends staff in the centers enabled teachers and administrative personnel to utilize them constructively as a sounding board for ideas on how to better approach and work with parents whose children were exhibiting classroom difficulties. Parent-teacher relationships had been strained in many instances, with parents feeling judged and their competence questioned by teachers, and teachers feeling that parents were unconcerned about problems their children displayed in the classroom. Some teachers, many of whom had, themselves, overcome obstacles and struggled to complete their education and training, had difficulty empathizing with the difficulties faced by center parents, particularly if they believed the parents were not trying hard enough to address their situation. As teachers were able to express these frustrations in discussions with the Family of Friends staff and gain ideas about how to better manage the children's difficult classroom behavior, they seemed to become more tolerant of parents and better able to engage them in working collaboratively to address behavior problems.

Occasionally teachers themselves appeared to lack knowledge and skills regarding appropriate child management strategies. One social work intern observed a teacher grow impatient with a new child in the classroom who was frightened and weeping during her first day at the center. The intern attempted to model a more nurturing, comforting approach than the impatient, rejecting stance of the teacher toward the child. Eventually, the intern's strategy worked, and the little girl stopped crying and joined in a storytelling activity. The intern noticed that, over the next few days, whenever the child became tearful and began to withdraw from the group, the day care teacher made an extra effort to engage her in activities that reassured her and diverted her attention from her feelings of fear and sadness.

As the teachers observed the engagement of many of the most distant parents with the Family of Friends staff in the chat groups, the Parent Academy workshops, and the Saturday Club, they began to extend themselves in community development activities. One volunteered to babysit with the children of parents who attended an evening chat group; others pitched in to help Family of Friends staff members arrange a potluck supper or volunteered to accompany families on a Saturday Club outing. In turn, parents, particularly those who sought certification as Peer Parents, volunteered to help out as teachers' aides a few hours each week. Each of these activities contributed to a lessening of the distance between parents and teachers, home and school, and facilitated the building of a community that supported and nurtured families in their child-rearing function.

Evaluation of the Family of Friends Program

Evaluation of the Family of Friends program was based on a developmental intervention research paradigm that identifies sequential stages and a recursive process in the development, implementa-

tion, and evaluation of innovative program models (Bailey-Dempsey & Reid, 1996; Patton, 1997; Peterson & Bell-Dolan, 1995; Rothman & Thomas, 1994). According to Patton (1997), a developmental approach to program evaluation involves a collaborative partnership between agency staff and researchers to design, implement, test, and revise new approaches in a "long-term, ongoing process of continuous improvement, adaptation, and intentional change" (p. 105). The developmental evaluation paradigm recognizes the realities of implementing social programs in field settings in that theoretical models, when implemented, are shaped and reshaped by their organizational and environmental settings in ways that cannot be foreseen. These influences become apparent only after the program has been implemented. The developmental approach calls for an ongoing evaluation process that provides continual feedback to those implementing the program regarding its effectiveness in meeting program objectives (Rossi, Freeman, & Lipsey, 1999).

The first three stages of this five-stage developmental evaluation paradigm call for intensive preparation for intervention development and include problem analysis and feasibility assessment, knowledge acquisition, and knowledge synthesis. These activities were carried out by Harbor staff in preparation for submitting their proposal for the Family of Friends program to the National Center on Child Abuse and Neglect.

The fourth stage of the research paradigm, the design phase, includes identifying measurable outcome objectives, selecting appropriate data collection instruments and planning the data collection process, designing participant recruitment strategies and ensuring human subjects protection, and developing procedural elements (structure of the intervention, a curriculum or manual) of the prototype intervention. It was at this stage that collaboration between researchers and Harbor staff was essential. Based on the work of stages 1 through 3, the evaluators aided key staff members in clarifying program goals and objectives and stating these in measurable terms. The goal of the Family of Friends program was to create a nurturing, supportive community for families in each of three Harbor-run day care centers as a way of preventing child abuse and neglect. It was hoped that creating such a community would carry out the following objectives: reduce social isolation, enlarge social networks, increase capacity for stress management, enhance knowledge of normative child development and effective child management practices, increase parents' sense of agency, and enhance parent-teacher collaboration.

Evaluation Design

To determine whether the Family of Friends program achieved its goal and objectives, data on the variables of interest (social isolation, social networks, stress management, child management practices, and parent-teacher collaboration) were collected from parents and, regarding parent-teacher collaboration, from teachers as well, prior to implementation of the Family of Friends program in each of the three day care centers in this project. These data formed a baseline against which to assess similar data collected after parents had participated in Family of Friends. The second round of data collection at each program site occurred approximately 9 months after the first, allowing sufficient time for the effects of program participation to be experienced by parents and teachers. As the program was implemented sequentially in the three sites, baseline or time$_1$ data in sites 2 and 3 could serve as comparison data for the outcomes in the program implemented previously.

In addition to data on program outcomes described earlier, information on the implementation of the Family of Friends model was collected as well. As noted by Bickman, Rog, and Hedrick (1998), conducting community-based research often involves multiple levels of analysis. While we were interested in the effects of the Family of Friends program model on individual participants, it was also important to understand the various organizational environments in which the program was being implemented and how these environments influenced the process of model implementation and, consequently, outcomes for participants. The Family of Friends program was designed to supplement the ongoing work of the day care centers. Understanding how each center functioned in its primary activity of providing day care to families with preschool-aged children, as well as its history, administrative structure, physical plant, staff composition, and shared views on parent-teacher collaboration, was essential to an analysis of the

implementation and impact of the Family of Friends program. As we were to discover, the three day care sites each had very different organizational dynamics, which significantly influenced how Family of Friends operated in each center.

Data Collection

Data were collected from parents and day care staff using structured interview schedules designed to capture information on the variables of concern. Embedded in the interview schedule for parents were two brief standardized assessment instruments, one on parenting stress and the other on social supports. Parents were interviewed by telephone for 15 to 20 minutes at two points in time, just prior to the introduction of the Family of Friends program in the day care center their child attended, and 9 months after program implementation. Day care center administrators and teaching staff were interviewed at these two points in time as well; however, these interviews were conducted in person at the day care center sites.

Data on organizational dynamics and on the implementation of the Family of Friends program in each site were gathered using multiple methods as advocated by Rossi et al. (1999). Interviews with day care center administrators and teaching staff, parents, and Family of Friends program staff were a rich source of information, as were social workers' written narratives of the chat groups and other program activities. Finally, social workers' and parent support workers' observations of relationships within the centers and experiences in the day care settings also served to enrich understanding of the organizational context for the Family of Friends program.

Human Subjects Considerations

To ensure that parent and staff participation in the data collection interviews was strictly voluntary, a number of steps were taken to obtain informed consent. In each day care site, the center administrator took initial responsibility for contacting parents regarding their willingness to participate in the program evaluation. Notices were sent home with the children describing the Family of Friends program and the evaluation process. These notices contained information on possible negative and beneficial effects of participation in the evaluation, the evaluation design, requirements of participants, and the mechanics of giving informed consent as required by federal research funding agencies. Parents were assured that there would be no negative consequences for refusing to take part in the Family of Friends evaluation. They could still participate in the program and receive other services as usual from the day care center. Parents who were willing to participate in the evaluation were asked to indicate on the form the best time to telephone them at home. Names of parents who returned a signed form to the day care center were compiled by each center administrator and passed along to the program evaluators. These parents were then called by the evaluators to set up a time for a telephone interview lasting approximately 15 to 20 minutes.

Rates of parent participation in the Family of Friends evaluation varied somewhat by day care site, averaging overall slightly less than half of all enrolled families. Demographic data analyzed by site revealed that the site with the highest levels of income and education had the highest rate of participation, while the site with the lowest average income and most children per family had the lowest. Family participation in the evaluation also reflected the ability and commitment of the center directors to the project. Again, the center with the most able and committed director also had the highest rate of participation by families, while the center with the lowest participation had a director who struggled to provide leadership to the center community.

For the follow-up telephone interviews with those parents who had been interviewed 9 months earlier, notices were sent home with the children informing parents that someone would be contacting them unless they indicated they did not wish to be interviewed a second time. A mechanism was established whereby parents could call and leave a message on an answering machine along with their name asking that they not be called again. Only one parent refused a second interview, so that the rate of participation in the follow-up data collection was similar to that of the initial interview.

Informed consent from day care center staff to being interviewed for the evaluation was obtained by the evaluators who conducted the interviews. Interviews with teachers and administrators were scheduled ahead of time, and at the beginning of each interview, the evaluator conducting the interview reviewed the consent form with the staff member. The staff consent form, like the form for parents, contained each of the elements required by the federal government to ensure protection of human subjects.

If the staff person agreed to participate in the interview, he or she would sign the form, and the interview would proceed. If the staff member refused to participate, the interview was terminated at that point. Like parents, teachers and administrators were reassured that there would be no negative consequences to them for refusing to participate in evaluating the Family of Friends program. Most day care personnel were willing to be interviewed, but there were a few refusals to participate in the evaluation, mostly because of confidentiality concerns despite written assurances that all material from the interviews would be kept strictly confidential and not disclosed to center administrators or Harbor personnel. Concerns about confidentiality spoke more to the dynamics of the day care centers than to personal issues, as will be discussed in the next section.

Findings

Overall, most evaluation participants were female (84%), and most worked outside the home (84%). About 38% of respondents were single heads of household, 34% were married, 10% were separated or divorced, 3% were widowed, and 15% lived with an unmarried partner. Family income across the three centers averaged $20,000 per year. The average age of participants in the evaluation was 26 years. Educational levels of parents were quite varied, with about 40% having at least some postsecondary education. Participating families had an average of slightly under two children, with the greatest number of families having just one child. About half of the families had only preschool-aged children, while the other half also had school-aged children and/or adolescents. Most respondents reported that all their children were currently living in the home (89%). Racially, families in the study were predominantly African American (76%), though there were a large number of Latino families at site 3.

Analyses of descriptive data on families in the study revealed interesting differences across program sites. In the first site, a freestanding day care center located in a blighted area of central Harlem, parents tended to be younger than in the other two centers, with 30% of parents less than 25 years old, as compared with 10% and 0% in this age range in sites 2 and 3. Parents in the first site also had less education; 33% had not graduated from high school, as compared with 10% and 14% in this category in the other two sites. One explanation for this discrepancy may be that the first day care site drew a number of African immigrant families living in the surrounding neighborhood who may have lacked educational opportunities in their home countries.

The day care center designated here as site 2 was located in a large public housing project on the Upper West Side of Manhattan, not far from Columbia University and near Harlem's main economic thoroughfare. This site had the most two-parent families, the most high school graduates, and the highest income levels of the three sites. Only 35% of families at this site had incomes of $20,000 or less, whereas at site 1, 53% and at site 3, 72% of families had incomes at this level. In addition to the lowest incomes, families at site 3 had more children, an average of 2.8 as opposed to 1.9 per family at the other two sites.

Findings on the variables relating to stresses experienced by parents suggested that, for most respondents, the three main sources of stress in their lives were finances, work, and parenting. Parents at site 3, in particular, reported experiencing high levels of stress in these three areas. Site 3 respondents also reported that their relationships with spouses, partners, and other family members were sources of stress for them, but respondents in the other two sites did not. When asked what was stressful about parenting, all respondents indicated that they felt they had too little time to do everything they needed to do for their children and that they had a hard time juggling multiple roles. Single parents specifically mentioned the difficulties inherent in single parenting. Forty percent of respondents at sites 1 and 3 indicated that their children often got on their nerves, and all respondents remarked on the amount of patience needed to be a parent.

With regard to sources of support, 75% of all respondents reported they were in contact with family or friends either daily or a several times a week. Most families indicated feeling that they could turn to family members or friends for emo-

tional support. Similar numbers could rely on the same sources for financial aid or advice in the case of an emergency. On the other hand, far fewer respondents reported that they were in frequent contact with other parents like themselves. About a quarter rarely or never had contact with other parents of young children, including parents at the day care center. A little more than one third agreed that they could consult with day care staff regarding concerns about their child. Close to half of the respondents said they seldom or never speak to their neighbors. These findings, like those in studies mentioned previously, suggest the difficulty parents experience in expanding their social networks in challenging urban communities. Again, there were notable differences on all the social support indicators between parents at the second day care site and parents at the other two sites, all in a direction favoring more resources and supports for site 2 families.

These site differences in family characteristics, sources of stress, and perceptions of social support are important in understanding the differential responses to the Family of Friends program by families in each day care center, as well as differences in parent-teacher relationships and in overall center dynamics. For example, the site 2 center, which served a somewhat better-educated, higher-income group of families, was clearly different from the others in its level of organization, its administrative leadership, its engagement of families, and the receptiveness of the day care community to the Family of Friends program. The director of this program was a dynamic woman who ruled her domain with an iron fist in a velvet glove. She had been director for a number of years and was a beloved figure in the community. The facility was clean, bright, and welcoming to families. Children's artwork covered the walls, and the friendliness of teachers and staff was noteworthy. Although the director initially was suspicious of the Family of Friends evaluation staff, having observed the negative effects of previous academic research projects on her staff and program participants, once she was assured of the benign intentions of the evaluators, she wholeheartedly supported the Family of Friends program and its evaluation. She was instrumental in encouraging families' participation in both the program and the evaluation. As a result, this site had the highest percentage of family participation in Family of Friends of any of the three day care centers.

Both site 1 and site 3 were beset with internal issues that impacted the implementation of the Family of Friends intervention to some extent. The first day care site had been taken over by the Harbor organization shortly before the implementation of Family of Friends; it had previously been run under the auspices of a for-profit day care agency. Many of the teachers and some administrators were holdovers from the previous ownership and were anxious about the change. Longtime teachers were concerned that the Harbor, located across town, might not respond quickly enough to the program's needs, noting the lack of teaching materials, supplies, and new curriculum initiatives.

Although the Harbor had put its own director in place when it took over this center, the administrator who was second in command had been with the day care center for many years and had prior relationships with many teachers and families. These circumstances made it somewhat difficult for the new director to assert his authority and created divided loyalties for some teachers and parents. Fortunately, the social worker who was employed by the Harbor to initiate the Family of Friends program in site 1 was an extremely able, engaging individual who was able to build relationships with families and center staff despite their struggles over the changes that were taking place in the center. In what turned out to be an extremely fortuitous move, the social worker hired the mother of a child in that center to be the Family of Friends parent support worker. The parent support worker was a woman from the community who had many positive relationships with families in the center and was able to engage even the most suspicious and fearful parents. She was highly energetic and willing to do whatever it took to address the problems and needs of families that affected their ability to parent. Because she was from the community, she understood the parents' struggles and was not viewed as part of an administrative elite. Her practical good sense and capacity to relate to a wide variety of parents were instrumental to the success of the Family of Friends program in site 1.

Despite the struggles of the staff and administration in the first site with the changes in center auspices, the Family of Friends program was quite successful in its implementation there, though it did get off to a slow start because of the initial reluctance of families to become involved. By the time of the follow-up interview 9 months after the program had begun, half of the families had participated in one or more aspects of the Family of Friends program such as chat groups, evening potluck suppers, Saturday Club outings, or Parent Academy workshops. Several of the fathers took active leadership roles in developing the Parent Academy, which, as noted earlier, was created by and for parents.

The last day care center to implement the Family of Friends program was site 3, located within the Harbor building itself. This center was also experiencing some internal struggles within and among staff. There were also ongoing concerns about negative perceptions of parents among the teaching staff and of teachers by parents. Many of the teachers, when interviewed at $time_1$ (T_1), indicated feeling that the center administrator was not providing strong leadership; she, in turn, felt disrespected by the staff, who often went over her head to the Harbor administration with their complaints. Much of the work of the Family of Friends social worker at this site was aimed at facilitating relationships among staff and attempting to enhance their interactions with parents, in addition to implementing programs for parents. The social worker tried to establish chat groups for teachers and to involve teaching staff in the Parent Academy workshops.

Despite these efforts, however, at the $time_2$ (T_2) interviews, there were few changes in the way staff viewed one another, the site director, or families' parenting skills. Their perceptions of the Family of Friends program at T_2 were that it was helpful to parents by increasing their participation in the day care center and giving them opportunities to support one another. Some classroom teachers reported seeing significant changes in children whose parents were involved in Family of Friends. According to one teacher, "We saw a dramatic difference in how the kids reacted and participated when their parents were in the [chat] group." This teacher gave the example of a child who was being raised by his grandmother. The child, who cried a lot and fought with other children in the classroom, changed dramatically when his grandmother began helping out in the class.

The parent support worker at the third day care site reflected in a T_2 interview on her experiences in helping to establish the Family of Friends program there. She noted that there was a core group of very engaged parents who consistently participated in the evening chat groups and the Saturday Club activities. This core group was supplemented by other parents who came and went. She felt that those parents who did participate in Family of Friends activities benefited greatly in that they learned to improve their relationships with classroom teachers, whom they had often treated as glorified babysitters in the past. She observed that site 3 had been the most difficult center in which to implement the Family of Friends program because of friction among staff and administration. She believed that some sense of community had been created, but that real implementation of the model would take much longer than 9 months or a year.

The T_2 telephone interviews with parents in the three program sites found that about half of the respondents were familiar with the Family of Friends program. Of those who knew about and had participated in the program, 60% had observed changes in the day care community since the program's inception. The same percentage had seen changes in other parents who participated in the Family of Friends program. Far fewer reported seeing changes in the day care center staff (22%) or in the children who attended the center (30%) since the beginning of Family of Friends. Agreement with the statement that parents can consult with day care staff with concerns about their child did not change significantly from T_1 to T_2, although there was a small shift toward positive agreement with the statement that families can participate in activities sponsored by the day care. There were larger increases in the percentages of parents who reported talking to other parents in the day care center on a daily basis (52% at T_1; 64% at T_2) and who knew other parents well enough to call them on the telephone (48% at T_1; 59% at T_2).

With regard to the sources of stress variables, the only observed reduction was in the stress related to coping with daily problems. Before the Family of Friends program was implemented, 42% of respondents found coping with daily problems to be very or somewhat stressful; afterward, 32% did so. Although there is no way of knowing from these data whether participation in the Family of Friends program was associated with this reduction, teaching coping skills as well as providing additional sources of social support were components of the program designed to help parents better manage the stresses of daily living.

There were significant reductions in the stress associated with parenting, according to the evaluation findings. The percentage of respondents reporting that their children often got on their nerves fell from 29% to 13.6% between the T_1 and T_2 interviews. Similarly, those who reported often feeling that children make too many demands fell from 23% to 9% over that time. While parents reported that these two conditions were still true sometimes, this positive change in frequency of irritation suggests that parents who participated in Family of Friends activities were feeling somewhat less stressed by the demands of parenting.

Conclusion

Family of Friends is an innovative program model designed to be implemented in day care centers and other preschool programs to create nurturing and supportive communities among participating families to ameliorate factors associated with child abuse and neglect. Its focus is based on the primary prevention concept of building capacity of parents to cope with the factors in their lives that present risks to adequate parenting. It draws on research on the etiology of child maltreatment in identifying a set of conditions that contribute to the incidence of child abuse and neglect. These conditions include social isolation and impoverished social networks, inadequate strategies for coping with stress, deficits in knowledge of child development and child management, and lack of opportunity to feel efficacious in daily life. Objectives of the Family of Friends program were to ameliorate these conditions, thereby preventing child maltreatment, through creation of a caring, supportive community for families of children in three day care centers, each with its own unique characteristics.

Implementation of the Family of Friends program model took place over a 3-year span in three separate day care centers that served predominantly African American and Latino families in three different Harlem neighborhoods. Evaluation of the implementation process found that organizational dynamics in each site, as well as demographic and other characteristics of the families served, significantly affected program implementation. It was necessary for program staff to adapt the intervention model to differing internal dynamics in each center, as well as to the needs of parent populations that differed overall by age, education, and income levels. While the basic program structure remained the same, how the various elements of the program were received and implemented differed a great deal by site. As the program was implemented sequentially over a period of 3 years, there was opportunity to use a developmental evaluation design to inform the development of the program as it was implemented in sites 2 and 3, based on earlier observations.

In each of the three day care centers, there was a group of parents, representing slightly less than half of enrolled families, who responded well to the various components of the Family of Friends program model. Some parents in each site participated in the chat groups, others were involved in the Parent Academy workshops, others enrolled in the Peer Parent certification process, and still others participated in the Saturday Club outings. Many parents participated in multiple aspects of the program.

In each location, the Family of Friends program staff—social workers and parent support worker—found it necessary initially to actively reach out to parents, using a variety of strategies to engage them in the program. They also frequently found themselves in the role of liaison between teachers and parents, and teachers and center administrators, working to create bridges between these various groups. The importance of having a highly trained, master's-level social worker at each site quickly became clear, given the difficult personal problems and issues with which some parents struggled. The parent support worker also played a key role in implementing the program because of her knowledge of the communities and her ability to connect with other parents like herself.

Program outcomes for Family of Friends were evaluated using a quasi-experimental design of collecting data before and after intervention. Sequential implementation of the program allowed for use of baseline data at sites 2 and 3 as control group (no treatment) data for outcome findings for sites 1 and 2. Data were collected through multiple methods, including telephone and in-person interviews with parents and day care staff, analyses of process recordings and other written narratives by program staff, and direct observations of organizational dynamics.

Analyses of postintervention (T_2) data indicated that parents who participated in the Family of Friends program activities demonstrated changes in their assessments of the stresses of parenthood and their capacities for coping with these stresses. They also indicated some increases in their social networks and sources of support in relation to the day care centers. Day care staff members observed changes in the level of parent involvement in the day care center activities and identified increased parent involvement as a factor in improved classroom behavior of some children in their care. However, center staff did not experience changes in the internal conflicts among staff and between staff and administrators within the day care centers.

A significant limitation of the Family of Friends experience was the 3-year time frame set by the program's funding. While the intention of the program from the beginning was to develop a parent base in each day care center that could sustain the program after the funding ended and the program's professional staff had to leave, establishing this parent base required ongoing effort and vigilance over an extended period. This was particularly a limitation in the third site, where internal difficulties greatly affected the program staff's ability to engage all the necessary constituencies in building a supportive, nurturing community with and for families. The parent support worker expressed the frustrations of all Family of Friends participants in site 3 in stating that they had just begun a process that had to end before it could be fully realized. Individual stories, however, indicated that the impact of the program was substantial for many families despite its ending too soon.

Acknowledgments

The authors would like to thank the many individuals who made the Family of Friends program possible. These, of course, include all of the parents and daycare center staff members who contributed their time and energies to program activities. They also include: Elsa Morse, grant writer for the Boys and Girls Harbor who contributed so much to the development and funding of the program model; the directors of the three daycare centers who generously supported the program and its evaluation, Rory Scott, Willisten Moore, and Zanaida Ramirez; Bernadette Wallace, Director of Harbor Preschool Programs; and the social workers and family support worker, Nadine Campbell Hauser, Pierre

Dolciney, Gail Murray, and Peter O'Neill, who were so instrumental in implementing the Family of Friends program.

References

Bailey-Dempsey, C., & Reid, W. J. (1996). Intervention design and development: A case study. *Research on Social Work Practice, 6*, 208–228.

Benasich, A. A., & Brooks-Gunn, J. (1996). Maternal attitudes and knowledge of child-rearing: Associations with family and child outcomes. *Child Development, 67*, 1186–1205.

Bickman, L., Rog, D. J., & Hedrick, T. E. (1998). Applied research design: A practical approach. In L. Bickman & D. J. Rog (Eds.), *Handbook of applied social research methods* (pp. 5–38). Thousand Oaks, CA: Sage.

Bishop, S. J., & Leadbeater, B. J. (1999). Maternal social support patterns and child maltreatment: Comparison of maltreating and nonmaltreating mothers. *American Journal of Orthopsychiatry, 69*, 172–181.

Chapman, P. L. (2001). *Maternal parenting and maternal psychosocial adjustment: Testing a structural model to explain adaptive social behavior of low-income three year olds*. Unpublished doctoral dissertation, Florida State University, Tallahassee.

Cicchetti, D., & Lynch, M. (1993). Toward an ecological/transactional model of community violence and child maltreatment: Consequences for children's development. *Psychiatry, 56*, 96–118.

Coohey, C. (2001). The relationship between familism and child maltreatment in Latino and Anglo families. *Child Maltreatment, 6*, 130–142.

Coulton, C. C. (1996). Effects of neighborhoods on families and children: Implications for services. In A. J. Kahn & S. B. Kamerman (Eds.), *Children and their families in big cities* (pp. 87–120). New York: Cross-National Studies Research Program, Columbia University School of Social Work.

Coulton, C. C., Korbin, J. E., & Su, M. (1999). Neighborhoods and child maltreatment: A multilevel study. *Child Abuse and Neglect, 23*, 1019–1040.

Cunningham, M., & Zayas, L. H. (2002). Reducing depression in pregnancy: Designing multimodal interventions. *Social Work, 47*, 114–123.

DePanfilis, D., & Zuravin, S. J. (1999). Predicting child maltreatment recurrences during treatment. *Child Abuse and Neglect, 23*, 729–743.

DePanfilis, D., & Zuravin, S. J. (2002). The effect of services on the recurrence of child maltreatment. *Child Abuse and Neglect, 26*, 187–205.

Dore, M. M. (1993). Family preservation and poor families: When "homebuilding" is not enough. *Families in Society, 74*, 545–556.

Dore, M. M., Doris, J., & Wright, P. (1995). Identifying substance abuse in maltreating families: A child welfare challenge. *Child Abuse and Neglect, 19*, 531–543.

Furstenberg, F. F. (1993). How families manage risk and opportunity in dangerous neighborhoods. In W. J. Wilson (Ed.), *Sociology and the public agenda* (pp. 231–258). Newbury Park, CA: Sage.

Garbarino, J. (Ed.). (1992). *Children and families in the social environment* (2nd ed.). New York: Aldine de Gruyter.

Garbarino, J., & Sherman, D. (1980). High-risk neighborhoods and high-risk families: The human ecology of child maltreatment. *Child Development, 51*, 188–198.

Gracia, E., & Musito, G. (2003). Social isolation from communities and child maltreatment: A cross-cultural comparison. *Child Abuse and Neglect, 27*, 153–168.

Hall, L. A., Gurley, D. N., Sachs, B., & Kryscio, R. (1991). Psychosocial predictors of maternal depressive symptoms, parenting attitudes, and child behavior in single-parent families. *Nursing Research, 40*, 214–220.

Hien, D., & Honeyman, T. (2000). A closer look at the drug abuse-maternal aggression link. *Journal of Interpersonal Violence, 15*, 503–522.

Holloway, S. D., & Machida, S. (1991). Child-rearing effectiveness of divorced mothers: Relationship to coping strategies and social support. *Journal of Divorce and Remarriage, 14*, 179–201.

Klebanov, P. K., Brooks-Gunn, J., & Duncan, G. J. (1994). Does neighborhood and family poverty affect mothers' parenting, mental health, and social support? *Journal of Marriage and the Family, 56*, 441–455.

Kotch, J. B., Browne, D. C., Ringwalt, C. L., Dufort, V., & Ruina, E. (1997). Stress, social support, and substantiated maltreatment in the second and third years of life. *Child Abuse and Neglect, 21*, 1025–1037.

Levy-Shiff, R., Dimitrovsky, L., Shulman, S., & Har-Even, D. (1998). Cognitive appraisals, coping strategies, and support resources as correlates of parenting and infant development. *Developmental Psychology, 34*, 1417–1427.

Lynch, M., & Cicchetti, D. (1998). An ecological-transactional analysis of children and contexts: The longitudinal interplay among child maltreatment, community violence, and children's symptomatology. *Development and Psychopathology, 10*, 235–257.

Maloney, J. M. (2000). *A study of the relationship be-*

tween empathy, social interest, knowledge of child development, and the potential for child maltreatment in fathers. Unpublished doctoral dissertation, Kent State University, Kent, Ohio.

McFarland, R. B., & Fanton, J. (1997). Moving towards utopia: Prevention of child abuse. *Journal of Psychohistory, 24,* 320–331.

Milner, J. (1994). Assessing physical child abuse risk: The child-abuse potential inventory. *Clinical Psychology Review, 14,* 547–583.

Patton, M. Q. (1997). *Utilization-focused evaluation* (3rd ed.). Thousand Oaks, CA: Sage.

Peterson, L., & Bell-Dolan, D. (1995). Treatment outcome research in child psychology: Realistic coping with the "Ten Commandments of Methodology." *Journal of Clinical Child Psychology, 24,* 149–162.

Rossi, P. H., Freeman, H. E., & Lipsey, M. W. (1999). *Evaluation: A systematic approach* (6th ed.). Thousand Oaks, CA: Sage.

Rothman, J., & Thomas, E. J. (Eds.). (1994). *Intervention research.* New York: Haworth.

Shipman, K. L., & Zeman, J. (2001). Socialization of children's emotional regulation in mother-child dyads: A developmental psychopathology perspective. *Development and Psychopathology, 13,* 317–336.

Shonkoff, J. P., & Phillips, D. A. (2000). *From neurons to neighborhoods.* Washington, DC: National Academy Press.

Tamis-Lemonda, C. S., Shannon, J., & Spellman, M. (2002). Low-income adolescent mothers' knowledge about domains of child development. *Infant Mental Health Journal, 23*(1–2), 88–103.

Tien, J-Y., Sandler, I. N., & Zautra, A. J. (2000). Stressful life events, psychological distress, coping, and parenting of divorced mothers: A longitudinal study. *Journal of Family Psychology, 14*(1), 27–41.

Wilson, K. K., & Melton, G. B. (2002). Exemplary neighborhood-based programs for child protection. In G. B. Melton and R. A. Thompson (Eds.), *Toward a child-centered, neighborhood-based child protection system* (pp. 197–213). Westport, CT: Praeger/Greenwood.

18

Chris Warren-Adamson and Anita Lightburn

Developing a Community-Based Model for Integrated Family Center Practice

This chapter describes integrated family center practice that offers protection, nurturance, and avenues for development for parents and their children. We write at a time when many, despairing of contemporary practices for at-risk children and families, are turning to explore new visions about developing child-centered communities in the United Kingdom (Local Government Association, 2002) and systems of care in the United States (Stroul, 1996). Our focus is the integrated family center (or family resource center) as a community-based single-site system of care, which arguably has an important role in the development of safe communities and new visions for children's services. As an alternative to existing child welfare services, they address fragmentation, defensive practice, and the disconnection from community that are serious problems in protective services. As stable community-based programs, integrated family centers provide a therapeutic milieu with a complex array of services to meet child welfare's primary goal—child well-being and family support. These integrated centers have the advantage of being a community, a place to belong to that grows with the family.

We particularly want to convey our belief in the family center's synergy created through the

multidimensional relationships, with staff working collaboratively with each other and with parents. This makes it possible for family centers to be a nurturing life force, a robust, complex community of care, able to respond to those at greatest risk, in need of more than traditional services offer. These centers are catalysts for professional and community knowledge. As witnesses to the vibrancy of this particular genre of family support, we are hopeful that this community-based approach will increasingly become an alternative to traditional mental health and child welfare services. At-risk families need access to reliable support, ongoing relationships, and the opportunity to be part of a community with a strong culture of care, a safe haven for those in need of protection.

Our focus throughout this chapter will be on lessons learned from our experience with family centers in the United Kingdom and the United States. We appreciate the difference national context means, and while we continue to gain insight from our differences, we also are taken with similar themes and concerns that have been variously described in different countries (Cannan & Warren, 1997; Warren-Adamson, 2001).[1] Internationally, we have observed wonderful cultural variation but with similar responsive characteristics. With this global perspective in mind, we have drawn from our individual experience, weaving together the common threads to offer a way of thinking about how families change in these comprehensive programs. Collaborating across national boundaries has stretched our thinking as we have sought to encapsulate the rich veins of practice theory and research in a model of practice for integrated family centers. We hope that advances in research methods will help us demonstrate the effectiveness of this comprehensive system of care that has been frequently described in case studies.

Defining Integrated Family Center Practice

We start by defining integrated family center programs, connecting recent developments to their evolution in the United Kingdom and the potential evident in a description of family center practice, in a UK family center. We consider the community ecology of this center and then move on to review the needs of high-risk families, the role of clinical services, and the potential of the family center to buffer risk and increase protection. A brief review of supportive research follows, pointing to important components of family center practice. We highlight in particular the importance of the center milieu that has a definable culture of care that distinguishes integrated family centers from other family support services, such as home-based family preservation. We share our thinking about the center as a developmental system, drawing useful concepts from developmental theorists and developmental science that contributes to a theory of change based on the tradition that values theory for the development and evaluation of integrated family centers. Our translation of theory into practice follows with a guide for working in this nontraditional setting, illustrated by a case example that shows how it is possible to provide early intervention to keep a family together, working responsibly with the mandate to protect children at risk for abuse and neglect.

Integrating the Protective Mandate With Family Support

Our starting point is the integrated family center or family resource center that has been given serious

attention over the last decade (Batchelor, Gould, & Wright, 1999; Hess, McGowan, & Botsko, 2000; Janchill, 1979; Lightburn & Kemp, 1994; Warren-Adamson, 2002). As a single-site resource, centers have a varied history of success in providing a continuum of services with good outcomes for fragile families (Comer & Fraser, 1998; Halpern, 1999; Seitz, 1990). The following overview highlights some of their more distinguishing characteristics. While family centers are friendly, open-door places, where parents can walk in without referrals and be welcomed to join in center programs, they are also places that engage in protective work with parents who are mandated to receive help because their children are at risk for abuse or neglect. These centers are unique because they frequently manage to integrate child protective work with a host of other therapeutic, educational, and supportive services. This integrative work requires patience, understanding, and a positive disposition toward all parents, communicating the belief in their ability to act in their children's best interest. The knowledge and skills of professionals shape services with developmental and mental health principles so that centers can both provide protection and support the special tandem development of parent and child (Germain, 1991). We are impressed with the center's therapeutic milieu that can function as a developmental system for all involved.

For center programs, there can be an inherent challenge in the "integration" of mandated protection and a focus on development. Staff need to recognize the different agendas that parents have (whether expressed or unspoken). While many have to master the challenges of mandated requirements to prove they are competent parents, others want to meet basic needs and find their way out of poverty. Others seek friendship and guidance in raising children in impoverished and/or dangerous neighborhoods. For staff there is the challenge of meeting parents' personal needs while balancing the needs of the whole community that require different approaches. There is both an art and a science to making it all work, with a good measure of humor and excellent management! The comprehensive programs offered in many centers make it possible to meet multiple social and mental health needs, which also incorporate community-building and empowerment approaches, reinforcing parents' strengths and their role as important advocates for safer communities (Batchelor et al., 1999; Feikema,

Segalavich, & Jefferies, 1997; Garbarino, 1986; Warren, 1997).

The Mission of Family Centers

The mission of a family center gives specific direction, with shared values influencing practice, such as commitments to prevention and early intervention. Family centers are located in, and are responsible to, neighborhoods and communities. Their mission reflects local needs and traditions that are shaped by leadership, the availability of professional staff, and partnerships with neighborhood helpers. The overarching mission of integrated family centers is to provide comprehensive services to support children's development and ensure their protection by helping families through crises, providing therapeutic and developmental support. This is achieved through parents, children, young people, grandparents, friends, and carers (an interdisciplinary group of helpers) coming together in community. In other words, families are defined widely, and they are joined by neighbors in a place where they can mutually benefit.

Location of Family Centers

In the United Kingdom and the United States, we are talking about family resource centers that are located in buildings with a range of activities operating under different auspices, for example, community centers, faith-based agencies, early childhood programs, schools, or a housing development. They are situated in neighborhood places. They represent a mix of the formal (individual, group, and family therapy, case management, and education), the informal (e.g., mentoring, after-school programs, recreation, and outreach) and are varied combinations of grassroots and professional collaborations. For example, a family support center in the United States or United Kingdom can be linked to early intervention programs, such as Head Start, Sure Start, and day care. These centers can be in a community center or in a full-service school, as in the United States. As might be expected, access to a range of services matters. Colocated services in centers enable families to make significant progress toward their goals. When there are limits to a facility's space for colocating services, good coordination and links with community resources become essential.

Historical Roots

Integrated family centers share many aspects of the older settlement movement (Cannan & Warren, 1997), with the important role of supporting low-income families and their children. The premise widely shared was that there should be neighborhood support for those who are disadvantaged by poverty, immigration, displacement, unstable communities, and personal misfortune. The more recent family center tradition in the United Kingdom, emerging in the late 1970s, was a response to a changing welfare state, and specifically the impact of change upon voluntary child care organizations that had invested in institutional care, for example, residential nurseries and homes. As well as a moral selling point, the family center also had an important professional, psychological implication, meaning the acceptance of the interconnectedness between child, parent, wider family, and community. Family work, family therapy, and community work could be developed in such settings. The Church of England Children's Society (now Children's Society) was at the forefront of these developments (Phelan, 1983). With the appointment of social workers and community workers, the context of the parent and child was the focus of helping with a mix of interventions, from the individual to the collective. Warren's survey of centers in 1990 recorded some 352 centers in England and Wales. It was a period of growth for family centers in both the United Kingdom and the United States.

Describing the Integrated Family Center: Program and Practice

We turn now to program description with our case study, which brings to life the complex world of practice in a UK center, beginning with a staff group's expression of center activities: counseling; play therapy; child behavioral programming; providing information; initiating and running expressive and instrumental groups (support, education, skill, action, community, therapy); providing recreational sessions; doing eco-maps and genograms; running crèches; offering behavioral and systemic family sessions; energizing depressed people; cooling down angry people; setting up and participating in music and arts; negotiating in groups; being a team person; changing nappies and general layette;

establishing routes to formal education and training; cooking and teaching cooking; working with the neighborhood; developing complex analysis; recruiting and supporting sessional staff; negotiating; staffing user meetings; planning; making judgments; writing reports well; appearing in court and giving evidence; liaising with professionals; developing projects; getting angry about issues and doing something about it; planning sessions; groups; outings; partying; pantomimes; driving the bus, sticking to your principles, especially against violence and racism; taking care of the physical side of the center; teaching formally and informally; encouraging; sticking around; being parental; facilitating; supervising and being supervised; negotiating, running, and receiving staff training; blowing the whistle on families; judging danger; getting cooperation, especially when the going gets tough; understanding depth as well as surface; using the law; keeping up to date; supporting weeping people; weeping and being supported; having people dependent on you; developing a network of professional allies; telling people off; breaking the worst of news; running angry or crazy neighborhood meetings; controlling the petty cash and toilet rolls; managing and explaining contact; explaining the difference between psychotherapy and psychoanalytic counseling; running a rummage sale; booking in a group; filling in at the after-school club; giving talks; doing courses; handling misuse of power, oppression, dirty tricks, damage, and theft; getting your timing right; negotiating; liaising with antagonistic professionals; explaining the one-way mirror; being imaginative; giggling; keeping the kitchen clean; being reliable; attending to health and safety; observing children and knowing about development; talking to visitors; explaining to skeptical managers that all this is really social work, this really is core business.

Many of these activities happen in one day. It is in your face, and you must remain at the same time empathic, nonjudgmental, suitably distant, and containing. So that is how it feels. It is a rich mixture of a professional domain and a mirroring of some of the complexity of family life. Such a domain can also be represented in a more conventional, programmatic way. Figure 18-1 depicts an account of this UK center, based in a converted school in a run-down urban neighborhood and operated by the local authority.

The Family Center Ecology

The family resource center works in and with the ecosystem in a dynamic, ever-changing way that responds to family needs from primary/early intervention that is preventive to tertiary intervention (based on the public health model). This family center has a robust interwoven web of services, programs, and opportunities for children and their parents envisioned in Bronfenbrenner's (1979) notion of human ecology usefully conceptualized as the microsystem, mesosystem, and exosystem. Accessible and friendly, centers are connected to a range of supports and important protective mechanisms, families are able to become involved in preventive programs that educate and offer balance to their lives, as well as support the development of family relationships and maximize means for nurturing and keeping children safe.

Let us focus first on the inner world of the center with the UK example presented in figure 18-1 that includes play therapy, counseling, information, and informal advice, as well as a teenage mothers group, parent and child games, and day programs. Here direct goals include assessment and behavioral change in the parent and child's personal world (the microsystem). Direct outcomes claimed would include "better parenting." Individual practices share the same agenda, for example, counseling or play therapy, and you can add couples work, family therapy, and the occasional specific behavioral program. This could be termed secondary and tertiary prevention. Users are most likely to be referred to the center. The fathers' group may be for men who do not directly care for their children and are looking for direction in their role as "absent fathers." The crèche support makes it possible for parents to take time out both informally and formally to participate in programs or to work.

Parents can also have active roles in helping with critical services in the center. The crèche also provides work for some parents and supports other center services and activities in the community such as adult education. The drama group and the painting groups are directly recreational, and indirectly they are expressive—they support their members, develop social skills, and create friendships. For lonely, isolated mothers this offers invaluable means for developing relationships.

Increasingly, centers are venues for family

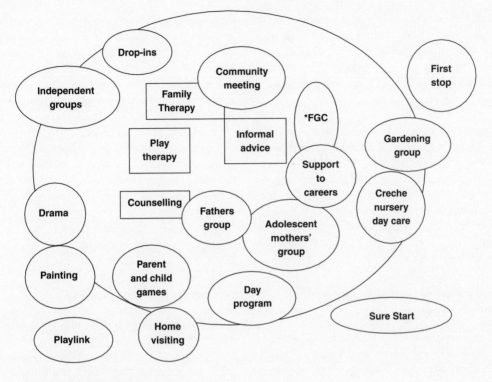

*Family Group Conferencing

Figure 18.1. The Integrated Family Center—A UK Example

group conferences (Burford & Hudson, 2000). This New Zealand innovation fits the style of the center—outcomes are often capacity building for parents, helping them plan and connect with resources, such as making a new decision for the care of their children with relatives or a friends network, to which the center is well placed to give its support.

Groups in the exosystem (the system beyond the family—school, social services, and local policies) have different relationships to the center. The center, by virtue of its early preventive stance and flexible and effective practice, may be asked to manage Surestart and Playlink, universal early intervention projects that may be based in the center or may work collaboratively with the center. Independent groups describe, first, the range of separate organizations that use the premises of the center and on which the center has indirect influence. It is argued that they ensure full use of the space, represent in their constitution a broad front to the world of early intervention, and offer the possibility

of connections, a network for participants in the family center.

Drop-in and community mornings occupy a position between systems. They are a link between the inner world of the center and the broader community. They are not just about a link with the neighborhood but represent stepping over the threshold informally to connect parents to important others. In Cigno's (1988) evaluation of this type of project, parents highly valued this type connection because it engaged them in an informal way on their own terms. Another informal means for engagement is the gardening group, where parents learn about soil technology and eating proper greens and gain support in the process by working with others.

First Stop, in the exosystem described earlier, is an example of a project promoting neighborhood development (Fletcher & Romano, 2001), where the center, because of its combined skills and knowledge, is able to broaden its scope and activities. This is a particularly valued role of the center, promoting awareness and action among local residents about child safety and protection. First Stop, which was developed in Brighton, England, promotes parent groups work in schools and includes information through publications and presence at community events.

This is the ecology of one family center that suggests the multiplicity of ways parents join activities, work with staff, and are linked to their neighborhood. However, grasping the real life of the center takes imagination, to see all of the comings and goings, the nonverbal expressions of encouragement and recognition, the weary staff changing gears once again to calm down a worried mother, and a group leader searching for a chair so a new parent has a place to sit.

Integration of Clinical Knowledge and Services

Clinical services build capacity in family centers to help children and parents who experience depression or post–traumatic stress disorder or who struggle with substance abuse or its effects. Clinically trained staff bring a developmental perspective that is useful in helping staff understand parents' competition with their children for attention and their emotional struggles with their own parents for not meeting their needs as they were growing up. Mental health needs are normalized as the need to learn to cope in a supportive home away from home, without the stigma associated with clinics and hospitals. Concerted efforts are made to form strong working partnerships with parents that emphasize their competence. Family life is best respected with strength-based approaches that work with the cultural heritage and traditions that contribute to a family's resilience (Berg & Kelly, 2000; MacAdoo, 1999; Saleebey, 2002; Walsh, 1998). There is a unique opportunity to blend clinical work with more informal helping. In particular situations this means weaving clinical knowledge of developmental needs into group work and activities that nurtures maturing relationships. For example, it is often the case that parents, because of lifelong disappointments, are in need of developing trust and support that involves testing and railing against those who are trying to help. In such situations there is the need for flexible responses that work to hold disappointment, anger, and frustration until

calm returns and there is strength to deal with the problems that provoked this response. This work necessarily occurs in multiple places, in mutual aid and community groups and individual therapy, and during activities, even standing in doorways, and resembles the holding or facilitating environment described by development theorists (Shuttleworth, 1989; Winnicott, 1960, 1990). Clinical services are also available through referrals, consultation, and on-site services that respond to individual and group needs. Our experience supports the findings of Batchelor and colleagues (1999) that consumers want a service model that bridges intensive therapeutic services and user-organized drop-in services.

Services for High-Risk Families

Integrated family centers are for all families; in fact, they work because families with different levels of need and resources participate. However, it is still helpful to remember the challenges that high-risk families bring. Parents often seek stability and care for themselves, as it is likely that many of them have experienced inconsistent parenting and still have unmet developmental needs. Many are victims of abuse and have lived chaotic lives, in and out of relationships. The added burden of living in poverty, frequently in disorganized communities, can mean that their survival needs are paramount. In need of support, they may have considerable difficulty receiving it. Trust does not come easily, and yet they live with hope that they will step out of loneliness and find belonging. Anger, alienation, frustration, and depression make initial connections in groups with other parents difficult. Problems are solved through cycles of crises. Substance abuse and domestic violence can further complicate their living situations as they try to provide nurturing homes for their children. Parents are also casualties of environments with multiple risk factors (such as marital discord, poverty, overcrowding, parental criminality, and maternal psychiatric disorder) that have been shown to lead to the development of psychiatric disorders later in life (Rutter, 1979). Too many parents have traveled down this road and are struggling with a heavy weight of problems. These challenges mean that concerted efforts in outreach and engagement are important in creating the relational bridge essential to bring families into center programs.

While accumulated risks make coping with everyday challenges difficult, parents' personal assets and strengths, and those assets in their networks and community, can be drawn upon to make it possible for them to parent and grow. Waller's (2001) synthesis of findings in resilience research is encouraging in this regard, where risk can be balanced with protective factors, as "a given risk/protective factor can have a 'ripple effect,' leading to further risk or protection" (p. 293). Involvement in a family center can provide the protective factors needed to cope with life's adversity. In essence, the family center experience offers a protective "ripple effect," a buffer and an organizing influence. Parents often come to family centers with a "negative sense of community," the psychological sense that has been used to describe single mothers' withdrawal from participating in community (Brodsky, 1996, p. 347). Over time, mothers' engagement in the life of the family center can mean that they will develop a new sense of community where they pool their strengths with others like themselves (Bowen, Bowen, & Cook, 2000). Their survival skills are valued, as they are challenged to learn new ways of protecting themselves and their children.

Research Points to the Potential of Integrated Centers

The integrated family center is one of the success stories in family and community work of the past 20 years. While there is limited research comparing integrated family support interventions (comprehensive programs) to other family support initiatives, such as family preservation programs and parenting education and support, a growing research base suggests the effectiveness of particular elements of such programs that are across a range of outcomes, not least of which is the protection and development of well-being of children and their families (Comer & Fraser, 1998). We highlight some of these findings because they underscore the efficacy of a range of activities that are integral in comprehensive programs in integrated family centers. We will draw on this research because it supports the theory of change we propose later in this chapter.

Comprehensive Programs Increase Protective Factors

Primary prevention is an important orientation for program development in family centers. Therefore, the risk and protective factor paradigm is particularly useful to consider, as research has shown that there is a positive relationship between increased protective factors (such as support, attachment, positive peer relationships, social skills, and quality educational programs) that decreases the probability of negative outcomes because of accumulated risk factors. For parents and children known to be at risk, the family center's comprehensive programs can provide the protective factors to increase their ability to cope with the stressors in their lives. The importance of this type of comprehensive program is underscored by the conclusions drawn from Durlak's (1998) review of 1,200 prevention outcome studies that shows that multilevel programs have obtained the most impressive results, In his view, "If risk exists at multiple levels and if multiple risk factors have multiplicative rather than additive effects, . . . the multilevel prevention programs are more likely to be successful than single level interventions" (p. 515). There is also evidence that intense programs produce stronger outcomes (Durlak & Wells, 1997; Hess et al., 2000; Layzer & Goodson, 2001; Nelson, Landsman, & Deutelbaum, 1990; Whipple & Wilson, 1996), and that positive effect sizes on various outcomes are a function of program characteristics, such as staffing intensity, with effects doubled with best practices (Layzer & Goodson, 2001). This evidence supports our experience that parents who participate in family centers benefit significantly from well-developed and well-staffed comprehensive programs.

Important Components for Family Center Programs

The recent U.S. National Evaluation of Family Support Programs provided a meta-analysis of 665 studies, describing the effectiveness of a variety of family support initiatives (Layzer & Goodson, 2001). We draw attention to a number of these researchers' findings, which suggest specific directions for practice. First there is an important lesson that needs to be understood regarding the positive relationship between a parent's own development and his or her child's development. Studies indicated that emphasis on parents' own development has been shown to correlate with children's social and emotional development and family cohesion (Berry, Cash, & Hoge, 1998; Blank, 2000; Comer & Fraser, 1998; Hess et al., 2000; Joseph et al., 2001). Other studies show that education and support led to significant improvements in parents' knowledge of mental health services and perceptions of self efficacy (Bickman, Heflinger, Northrup, Sonnichsen, & Schilling, 1998) and in reducing symptoms of depression and anxiety in mothers (Ireys, Divet, & Sakawa, 2002; Silver, Ireys, Bauman, & Stein, 1997; Whipple & Wilson, 1996). Therefore, programs that fit parents' needs and capabilities, including psychosocial education, will be an important staple of the family center. Added supports, such as child care, that enable parents to attend are also critical to positive outcomes (Dore & Lee, 1999).

Case Studies Describe What Works for Parents

Case studies also provide important descriptive program analysis that includes pre-post outcome evaluations. These studies show that ready access to services, outreach, user-friendly approaches, and integrated services colocated on-site overcome major obstacles with flexible services that are responsive to families at points of crisis. There are consistent reports that these services are highly valued by parents (Hess et al., 2000; Joseph et al., 2001; Lightburn & Kemp, 1994; Smith, 1992; Warren-Adamson, 2002; Wigfall & Moss, 2001).

Increasing Participation and Outcomes

The complex picture supported by layers of thick description demonstrates how centers contribute to family and child well-being, particularly with respect to engagement and participation (Hess et al., 2000; Lightburn, 1994; Warren-Adamson, 2001). And as Bond and Halpern (1986) have noted from reviewing family support program evaluations, there are signal signs of impact that are important to consider. For example, in a case study completed by the second author, family participation over an 18-month period was facilitated through ongoing negotiations by program staff that made it possible for these parents to complete their education and

work programs that were desired program outcomes (Lightburn, 1994). Lessons learned about the factors that mediated participation included the instrumental role center staff played in negotiations with different program providers, creating understanding of the realities of parents' lives, and interpreting parents' behavior as a product of their personal situations, not a lack of motivation. This made it possible to work out flexible schedules so parents could make it to their required programs. Without staff intervention, 20% of parents would have failed to reach their goals.

A second example involved center staff successfully advocating for the inclusion of parents to become part of the center team. This flexible, creative solution solved the problem caused by reduced funding that would have limited parents' participation in the center because it was no longer possible to support the salaries of staff to provide services for them. Parents saw themselves coming to the center program during the rest of their child's early years; they could not accept that this was their last year in the program. After much conferring with each other and staff, they decided to volunteer to mentor and support new parents at the beginning of the next year, as center members. In this way staff could continue to support them in their new role as mentors, and they could join in many of the activities for the whole community. Both of these examples show how center staff have a central role in mediating outcomes through their informal support and flexible roles that enhanced parents' engagement and completion of their specific program goals.

Translating Lessons Learned Into a Model for Integrated Family Center Practice

This section introduces ways of conceptualizing integrated family support practice. First we consider the importance of the center milieu that has a definable culture of care, which shapes participation and the development of community that both influences and protects children and family life. This milieu can also be productively thought of as a developmental system for parents, children, and center staff. Drawing useful concepts from developmental theorists and developmental science, we

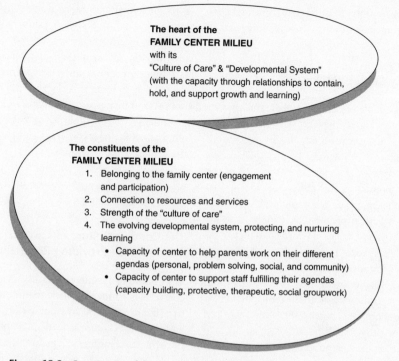

Figure 18.2. Constituents of the Family Center Milieu

describe how containment and a holding environment are part of a responsive developmental system that is similar to a family's nurturance. We will briefly elaborate on these concepts, describing how they contribute to the work of the center and, ultimately, the hoped-for outcomes such as child and family well-being, and protecting attachment bonds. Our goal is to map a more dynamic and inclusive guide for practice and research.

In summary, the components of the integrated family center model are as follows:

- The integrated family center milieu;
- The culture of care and the safe haven it provides;
- The developmental system of the integrated family center that contains, holds, and nurtures and provides opportunity for learning;
- The varied pathways to learning that promote development and change and build capacity for center parents and staff.

The heart of the center milieu, with its culture of care, is presented in figure 18-2, which shows the relationships of the milieu as the primary source

of support that makes it possible for the center to (1) protect and support parents and children; (2) nurture the learning of everyone in the center; (3) develop the capacity of the center to help parents work on their different agendas; and (4) support staff to meet their varied responsibilities in working with parents and building capacity in the center. We have used the term "agenda" for both parents and staff as a way to capture the different purposes that focus the work of parents and staff. Later in this chapter we will discuss these different agendas, conceptualizing the way staff and parents work together. As figure 18-2 shows, the constituents are parts of the whole, and as interrelated processes they influence parents' participation and strength of connection to the center, and ultimately their success in working on their different agendas (such as protecting their children, developing competence in life skills, and benefiting from mutual aid groups with other parents). In a similar way the developmental system and culture of care of the center milieu support staff so that they can also grow and be effective in their work. What follows is a more detailed look at how we understand the constituents and then how the developmental center milieu contributes to the whole of family center practice.

The Family Center's Milieu

As the UK example presented earlier in this chapter shows, family centers involve a way of living, and in doing so they provide a milieu that offers more than traditional clinic-based therapeutic approaches. Synergy, or "more than the sum of the parts," aptly describes this milieu that is a special interwoven social fabric, a community of care that transforms the way people live. Parents describe how their lives have been transformed as they manage to achieve goals they could barely imagine before they became part of the family center community (Lightburn 1994; Warren-Adamson, 2002). In an anthropological sense this milieu is a social invention (Bohannan, 1995), an organized system of care that blends resources (financial, professional, and personal) and builds capacity in staff and participants to meet families' diverse needs. Leadership (some combination of professional and grassroots) assists the community to develop a milieu where staff and parents can fulfill their responsibilities to each other. The milieu is the sum of all who participate in the center.

Integrated centers have been described by parents as "their family," a chosen family that is connected to the broader community of the neighborhood and beyond. This is the family that for many is missing, with whom they experience a normal round of life, with supports from survival basics to sharing information and managing daily upset. Recreation can be as important as a group that works on problem-solving skills. Outings and playgroups are part of the same whole that includes challenging learning situations. The integrated family center is a therapeutic milieu as it offers many healing experiences that are part of the community experience, in addition to supporting individual and family therapy. The power of the milieu to provide more than an individual therapeutic relationship is central, echoing the more-than-the-sum-of-the-parts synergy that flexes and responds in creative ways to meet individual and group needs.

The center milieu is also a developmental system that changes and grows with all who belong to the community. In many ways it is useful to think of the center as a learning organization that changes

through formal and informal relationships, evolving in natural ways and through community meetings, where staff and parents work together on program development, evaluating services, and determining guidelines for participation. Therefore, the focus of helping is also about developing community and being part of community, so that it is possible for the community to help a parent or child, a family, or a particular group of parents in the center. The professionals' role is to both help individual parents and children with the community milieu and work with the milieu so that it grows into a resource for all.

The Center's Culture of Care: A Safe Haven Providing Protection

The culture of a family center, like that of a school, contributes to the life of the participants in ways that culture shapes communication, experience, and identity. Culture is evident in the strength of the center community's shared values. Parents refer to this culture as their "safe haven," reflecting the power of the culture to protect and provide reason for attachment and belonging. This culture of care is in significant contrast to the culture of neglect and abuse many families know, where isolation, loneliness, anxiety, and fear rob children and parents of love and nurturance (Bowen, Bowen, & Ware, 2002; Duncan & Brooks-Gunn, 1999; Knitzer, 2000; Schwab-Stone et al., 1995; Warren-Adamson, 2002). Parents have described the ethos of this culture as the family that will not rob them, set them up and disappoint, take advantage of their children, or go away (Lightburn, 2002). Care in this culture means recognizing and attending to risk and abuse rather than tolerating or denying dangerous situations until it is too late. Protection is a serious matter, and the role of mandated supervision of children is part of this culture that draws authority from the larger community. It is a culture that supports development and growth through lively reciprocity that is typical of family life when it works well. Above all, it is a culture that affirms life and, where necessary, honors the need for respite. So while the family center can be experienced as chaotic, as described earlier in this chapter, it is the chaos of people colliding in the intensity of negotiating and working on relationships and problem solving, experiencing crisis in an environment that offers solutions, that is family centered and invested in keeping families together. It is also a culture where family and children are valued and celebrated, and in this regard center life celebrates achievements, holidays, and transitions, with rituals that reinforce belonging and enjoyment in community life (Lightburn & Kemp, 1994; Warren-Adamson, 2002).

Protection is a dynamic cultural phenomenon that involves the affirmative life force of the center in action. Protection for children and parents is evidence of the culture of care working. Earlier we described synergy as all the parts of the center working together. This synergy can also be thought of as correlated constraints, a way of conceptualizing positive factors that constrain the negative impact from accumulated risks. Drawn from the field of developmental science, correlated constraints are a way of explaining how the family center culture works to promote protection and, according to Farmer and Farmer (2001), increases the likelihood of positive outcomes. Correlated constraints are a result of the culture of care that is communicated in the way the center community works and mediates accumulated risk for parents and children.

The change process depends on promoting this positive culture that supports dependence and interdependence in staff and peer relationships. Therefore, the time given to supporting the culture of care will be an investment that increases protective factors that help parents cope. This suggests that it is necessary to focus on community building as a central means for helping. It is not enough to offer casework or case management, which primarily focuses on developing problem-solving skills and resource management, or that works on changing parents' internal world. We share Farmer and Farmer's (2001) concern that positive outcomes should represent more than changed behavior. Rather, meaningful outcomes should reflect a true understanding of developmental processes that would necessarily include measuring the positive correlated constraints and how they support change and development. After all, it is the quality of relationships and the actions of a community that make it possible to bear life's most distressing and hurtful experiences. To this end, center staff work to maintain positive norms such as mutual aid, hope, kindness, and positive expectation that there are solutions to violence and that there is continuity in relationships. Practitioners also need to promote guidelines that hold center life together,

through encouraging civic responsibility that benefits everyone.

The Integrated Family Center Community as a Developmental System

In our initial description of family centers, we suggested that it is useful to consider the integrated family center community as a developmental system. Our previous discussion has described how the center's culture is integral in the work of the developmental system as it protects and nurtures families. The center as a developmental system has a number of distinguishing functions. First, a developmental system works over time, and centers help families most effectively when they are involved with center programs and staff over extended periods of time. From our experience, family engagement can begin when children are very young and may involve the family throughout childhood and adolescence. The possibility for a family to have a long-term connection with the family center enables parents to be involved in relationships as they are able, creating the possibility of developing strong bonds that are necessary for healing and promoting mental health. As Garbarino (1995) reminds us, "time is wealth" (p. 102), and parents who have not received adequate nurturing will benefit from having time invested in their development. Time is one of the more important developmental resources available to families. Time is afforded to parents because of the family center's open structure, programming that provides long-term membership, and the varied ways parents can participate in the center that in effect provide ongoing "relational time." A developmental system also works implicitly through belonging and strong connections. When families become part of the family center community, they become anchored, part of a chosen family. They in effect join this special developmental system that supports attachment and bonds that make it possible to gain autonomy to manage life outside the center. For many this means that they are able to renew their conception of family and pass this new tradition of family on to the next generation. From the family center's perspective, we are also mindful of the time needed for the family center system to develop so that it can effectively meet parent and staff needs and respond to neighborhood concerns. In summary, family centers invest time in ways that ensure that both parents can grow because relationships are nurtured, and that the center's organization develops in ways that are responsive to all who participate.

A number of other relevant concepts drawn from developmental traditions further describe how the center's developmental system works for mothers and fathers. These are the familiar concepts of containment and support, which are functions of the relational holding environment (Shuttleworth, 1989; Winnicott, 1960, 1990). Also of import is the developmental process of mastering life's curriculum that involves transformative learning, recognition, and celebration of achievements (Kegan, 1998). Each of these dynamic processes is briefly elaborated on as guides for practice to be shaped to fit parents' different needs, starting places, abilities, and personal agendas.

Containment and the Holding Environment

An emerging message from parents is that such centers offer "containment" to them and their neighborhoods (Warren-Adamson, 2001). Containment in this sense implies a safe haven, which is possible because of the strength of the culture of care that makes it possible to weather charged emotions and challenging demands for attention. It is a holding environment that also supports and challenges parents to grow, as they develop new ways of thinking and gain confidence and skills. The notion of containment comes from object relations theory (Shuttleworth, 1989) and the capacity of the parent figure to "hold" and "manage" the projected emotion of those being cared for. This behavior is said to reproduce itself over the life span, especially in times of stress (Winnicott, 1960, 1990). For the parent, or in this case the center staff, it implies understanding and being with parents, providing unconditional love, empathy, and challenge, and in all it creates an energy that motivates.

Containment refers to boundaries that create physical and emotional safety, management of disorganizing experiences, and opportunities for reorganization. When parents are in crisis, the containment provided by the family center can be a mainstay until internal and external resources are available to stabilize and promote new means for coping. The quality relationships that instill trust and are reliable and durable, are the type of relationships that also need to stretch flexibly in order to handle emotional and physical stressors. As one

parent reflected, "I tested and tested you as I was so angry, I never expected you to let me come back. I kicked at you, and yet you let me return. Now my children have a different future." Acceptance communicated through attunement and empathy is woven throughout the stable relationships of the center, where parents are known and respected for their strengths, potential, and uniqueness. Staff recognizes parents' effort to manage the challenges in their lives. In the case of the mother just quoted, participation in the center enabled her to complete high school and cope with the demands of six children, while living on a marginal income and struggling with frequent patches of paranoia (schizophrenia; Lightburn, 1994).

A strong commitment to families affords an emotional connection with parents that can communicate understanding when they are not yet able to grasp what is wrong, or how their lives can change. The integrated family center milieu contains as it holds and engages parents in their own developmental process. This in turn enables parents to be more responsive to their own children, mirroring the support they have received. The family center's developmental system works for both parents and children, strengthening attachment through the dynamic process of containment and holding experienced in center relationships.

Mastering Life's Curriculum

Most parents seek support in managing their complicated lives. The notion of mastering life's curriculum is drawn from the work of developmental psychologist Robert Kegan (1998), who illuminates how this implicit curriculum nonetheless must be mastered by men and women for them to be good parents, partners, friends, workers and employees, and active citizens. Creating opportunities to master life's curriculum can be a primary focus for center programming. Mastering the implicit "life curriculum" is a continued challenge that is intensified when conditions of living are complicated by factors such as poverty, low incomes, single parenthood, domestic violence, and chronic illness. And while it is important to offer parent education programs, it is also a worthy investment to provide educational opportunities to help parents master life's implicit curriculum. Parents need help identifying what they need to learn and how this best can happen (for an expanded discussion of how to develop an educational approach within a clinical frame, see Lightburn & Black, 2001). As noted earlier, research has supported this focus, as parents' investment and achievements in their own development are correlated with their child's positive development (Layzer & Goodson, 2001). Golding (2000) has also shown that when parents learn in a community-based program that meets their multiple needs, they become more competent in managing their children's serious behavior problems. It is fortunate that the center's developmental system, which provides understanding and nurturing relationships to help discouraged parents keep going, further facilitates their personal development in educational programs. As parents become more resilient, they more readily understand their children's needs and are more able to manage crises.

The Many Pathways to Learning in Family Centers

Psychosocial education, transformative learning, and being part of a learning organization are key pathways that can revitalize learning in the family center. All these approaches benefit from using group process to support learning. Research indicates that collaborative learning in support groups is particularly valuable for parents (Berry et al., 1998; Golding, 2000; Ireys et al., 2002). This is not surprising, as parents are relieved to discover other parents share their experiences. They need to speak about the stress that is overwhelming because they do not have required information and skills, and they have not been exposed to different ways of thinking, helping them to develop their own voice.

Psychosocial Education

Psychosocial education or psychoeducation increases psychosocial understanding with information that is directly useful and connects with parents' experience. This pathway focuses on life experiences and draws on personal and interpersonal issues such as understanding and managing intimate relationships, managing aggression and conflict in families, coping with substance use and abusers, and successful parenting. The intent of psychosocial education is to help parents gain understanding and skill with the social and psychological realities of life, thereby increasing their self-esteem and self-worth. Adult education offers many resources that will support shaping and facilitating

different types of learning programs (Merriam & Clark, 1991). Therefore, achieving an educational goal, such as developing parents' competence in behavior management, would be dependent on parental understanding of child development, as well as interpersonal dynamics between themselves and their child.

A Learning Organization Approach That Builds Family Center Capacity

Earlier we suggested that the family center could benefit from being a learning organization. Drawing from Peter Senge's (2000) approach, which emphasizes the interdependence of all parts of the center, participants would share in a commitment to work together on the changes needed, starting with developing a vision of the center's future. Based on collaborative learning principles, parent, children, staff, therapists, and volunteers learn with and from each other as they shape the focus for learning in community meetings, program development, and evaluation. There is a unique opportunity to draw on the bank of knowledge that honors what parents and staff already know about child development, rearing children, and living in loving relationships and in their neighborhoods. The learning organization approach emphasizes sharing knowledge and creating an openness to new ideas. Professional knowledge is not privileged over other knowledge, and enacting this perspective helps parents to respect what they know and can do, and can result in their challenging each other so that new ways of coping emerge that strengthen the center's culture.

A case in point involves a center where parents were most concerned about their children's safety after school. They learned to work as part of the team in the center's organizational review, which resulted in refocused priorities and the development of supervised after-school activities at the center. Through enacting new roles, parents strengthened the mutual aid and the center's culture of care (Warren-Adamson, 2001). At the same time, such action strengthened parents' sense of efficacy in protecting their children.

Capacity Building

A similar approach drawn from community development is the tradition of capacity building that increases knowledge and skill of staff and parents. This is a strength-based approach that benefits from an integration of best practices in community development (building capacity) and draws on clinical knowledge to prepare nonprofessionals and parents to join in the center's work. The approach has a long tradition in the trainer model and development of nonprofessionals, mentors, tutors, parent advocates, and outreach workers. Respecting the knowledge and skill of parents, it provides ways to formalize their tacit knowledge. For example, with more specialized training and support, parents can become teacher's aides and mentors of other parents. As mentors, parents become an invaluable resource for other parents, helping stressed parents keep their families together through strategic support and advocacy.

Transformative Learning and Empowerment

Empowerment practice respects parents' goals and ability to take charge of their lives that enables them to more effectively advocate for and influence change in their families and communities. Transformative and experiential learning are well-developed, dynamic approaches in adult education that support empowerment practice. Empowerment depends on a critical learning process that involves dialogue, respecting each parent's knowledge and way of knowing. With roots in Freire's (1985) pedagogy of the oppressed and the politics of liberation, transformative learning involves challenging what is known and how it is known.

There are an increasing number of well-developed road maps and examples of transformative learning linked with adult development and activism. Transformative learning benefits from a collaborative approach to examine life experiences, challenge personal and social beliefs, and to gain a critical perspective that can lead to new ways of understanding and acting (Daloz, 1992; Heron & Reason, 2001; Mezirow & Associates, 2000; Parsons, 1991; Vella, 1995). For parents involved in workshops or groups focused on mastering the implicit life curriculum, this can mean learning how to cope with racism and sexism, or power relationships in critical institutions, such as schools, hospitals, and the workplace. Transformative learning results in a change of consciousness that is the foundation for new ways of acting and relating, which ultimately transform parents' powerlessness in the face of these challenges so that they can voice their concerns and negotiate successfully for themselves.

Taking Stock and Pointing to a Theory of Change for Family Centers

Thus far we have endeavored to present a description of the integrated family center, especially its holistic quality, and how it is part of community ecology. We regard family centers as a community that functions like a developmental system, where families grow with the community. Families belong to the center community. They have a history and identify with this special culture of care that is experienced in sharp contrast to the culture of poverty, neglect, and abuse that most high-risk families know too well. We have emphasized the importance of the synergy in these centers, a phenomenon where the sum is more than the parts, similar to the notion of correlated constraints, where protective factors are developed to buffer risk for parents and children. Primary prevention and early intervention are part of the center's mission, as they provide comprehensive services to meet a wide range of needs. Parents see the family center as their safe haven, a place of protection that also may involve mandated attendance to ensure protection for their children. The developmental system of the center can be a holding environment to respond to parents' developmental needs, even as they stretch to master life's implicit curriculum. A range of approaches to learning have been identified that are synchronous with the goals of empowerment and capacity building that help parents increase competence and grow. In sum, we have described how family centers are powerful social inventions that have the capacity to transform the way families live.

Developing a Theory of Change

We are now at the point of proposing a theory of change for families in integrated centers, revisiting the material presented earlier, and continuing our attempts to unravel complexity, describing how transformation happens. A theory of change (Chaskin, 2002) helps us to understand desired outcomes, what we need to know, and actions we need to take to promote child and family well-being, and inevitably humbles us in our quest for certainty in our interventions. A lack of a theory of change has been an enduring problem for family support program practice, despite the fact that different models of intervention have been proposed over time.

The theory of change illustrated in figure 18-3 details the contextual resources that are critical to supporting change for families. We have set out major goals that focus the work of integrated family centers, and while these can vary, we believe that it will always be important to include the goal of building a family center community milieu so that it is possible to provide a comprehensive program that is not just a set of services but rather a community, a developmental system that changes in response to participants' needs.

Our theory emphasizes a focus on nurturing both parent and child development because this tandem focus makes sense and is reinforced by research, as discussed earlier. A responsive developmental system (such as the center milieu) nurtures development in the way parents are supported and challenged and are allowed to start and stop in their personal work. Mastery is possible because of the opportunities to work on getting things right, and that happens best when parents have long-term involvement in a program where there is appreciation for their abilities and recognition of the stresses in their lives, where support makes the difference to their success. When families are involved with protective services and are working toward reunification with their children who have been placed in foster care, the center has an important role in facilitating visiting and developing supports, such as a parent mentor, to make the transition to home work.

We have described a range of possible outcomes based on a family's involvement in a center that offers both a supportive developmental system and specific opportunities for therapeutic help and pathways to learning. These outcomes include child and parent well-being, child and family development, and protection of attachment bonds that reduce the need for child placement.

An important proximal outcome of the work of the family center is the developmental capacity of the center itself to support parents and staff to achieve the longer-term outcomes of parent and child development and well-being. It is expected that the developmental capacity of the center is directly related to the development of the center, that is, one contributes to the other. The success in building the center milieu will be critical to all outcomes, as the developmental system (which includes the culture of care activities such as containment, holding, and learning) provides protection that increases the likelihood of positive outcomes

for parents and children. In effect, building capacity results in the necessary change in the family center, and increasing flexibility that supports engagement and participation.

The theory of change proposes that protection comes from providing a safe haven and culture of care that facilitates attachments and containment within the milieu. This enables families to participate for an extended period of time during their children's early years and sustains them when stressors are overwhelming and their personal resources are scarce. Families experience this domain of supportive activity, which goes beyond the known effects of specific interventions and has been identified and struggled with by colleagues over time as social and informal support (Tracy & Whittaker, 1987) to account for this hard-to-know world of change.

Provision of a comprehensive program also increases protective factors that can buffer risk (such as opportunities for mentors and positive peer relationships, and opportunities to participate in the program). Integral to such a comprehensive program is synergy, where the sum is more than the parts. This synergy is the creative ability of the center milieu that enables all to deal with risk.

Enhancing the developmental system (the therapeutic milieu of the center) is also a means for developing correlated constraints that increases protective factors for the participants. The developmental system also provides valuable support and learning (psychosocial education, transformative and collective learning) that contribute to families' competence in managing the challenges of parenting, relationships, and work.

In summary, this comprehensive, multilevel approach is most appropriate for families and children at risk, where poverty, low income, lone parenting, substance abuse, and domestic violence challenge coping and create cycles of disadvantage that can be broken through the protection offered in this unique developmental system.

A Model for Practice

In this section we will shift our focus to consider the actual work of centers from the parent perspective and the professional perspective. Earlier we introduced the notion of the parent "agenda" and the professional "agenda" as a way to conceptualize the purpose of each and how these different agendas represent parent and staff's collaborative work.

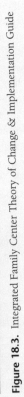

Figure 18.3. Integrated Family Center Theory of Change & Implementation Guide

To facilitate development, protection, and collective efficacy, it is useful to have a model of practice to guide helping activities. Our thinking draws on an organizing framework developed by David Howe (1987) in which theories of intervention are reorganized according to an epistemological grid embracing theories of knowledge and theories of action.[2]

The Parents' Agenda

We propose understanding an individual parent's needs as an agenda that brings him or her to the center to join other parents, find resources, learn, and work on a wide range of goals. Although parents come for many reasons, and have unspoken and unrecognized needs, we think it is helpful to group the range of possible needs and motivation into four different agendas as guides for service development, as presented in figure 18-4.

From our experience, one agenda usually leads to the development of other interests and hence new agendas. A parent will also develop the ability to work on other agendas; for example, it can take time to feel confident enough to join a group or an educational program. A parent's agenda reflects unexpressed and expressed needs. A number of factors influence engaging parents to work on their agenda, such as how the mission of the family center is communicated, the way parents perceive the mission, how able parents are to communicate their needs, and the responsiveness of center staff to parents' priorities and to helping parents identify unexpressed needs. It also depends on parents' ability to work on their agenda. For example, if the center's mission focuses on the protective mandate and requires participation in parenting classes, then regardless of the parents' agenda to meet their personal needs for belonging and support services, they of necessity will make the protection (problem-solving) agenda their priority. However, their success in working on this problem-solving agenda would be furthered if their personal agenda for support was addressed first, or even concurrently. For example, a parent's overwhelming stress caused by family disruption or by threats of his or her child being placed in foster care can be mitigated with personal support that then makes it possible for

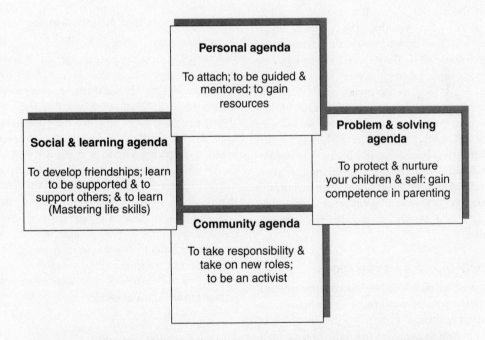

These four agendas conceptualize different ways parents engage and work in Family Centers. Often the work on one agenda overlaps or leads to the work on another. Work on one agenda is determined by both a parent's priorities and the priorities of the center determined by protective mandates to ensure the safety of children.

Figure 18.4. Parent Agendas

him or her to want to engage in learning to be a more competent parent.

Parents' Personal Agenda

In figure 18-4, the parent's personal agenda is represented as central to all the others because of the needs of most parents: to attach, to be guided and mentored, and to gain resources. The personal agenda is both conscious and practical: to gain resources for themselves and their children, such as housing, food, clothing, education, and day care, and to meet unspoken needs for a relationship with someone who is able to understand how hard it is to trust and be consistent. Usually, parents who are isolated, with few supports or models to learn from, want someone to help with direction. Very quickly, centers learned that families need to develop relationships over time, to attach and reattach, to be guided, mentored, and in many cases to experience qualities of parenting, which they themselves had missed.

Parents' Problem-Solving Agenda

Many centers begin with parents' problem-solving agenda when families are referred because of concern about child rearing that soon evolves into work on other agendas. The problem-solving agenda includes learning how to protect and do the best for oneself and one's children, and gaining competence in parenting. Others may dictate this agenda, so that attendance may be compulsory if parents are to maintain or regain custody of their children. Parents are engaged in problem solving with staff to develop plans that will be best for their children. It is hoped that this plan involves maintaining attachment bonds and keeping the family together. However, it is also important to deal with the realities of parents' lives and assist them in making the best decision considering their circumstances.

Parents' Social and Learning Agenda

The need for friendships and social relationships is central to parents' social and learning agenda. Basically, parents seek friendship with other parents; this can include an unspoken need to be supported, to find mutual aid that involves learning to receive help from and give help to others. They also need to experience respite, have fun, and gain balance through relationships with others. Parents' learning agenda can start with needed help with parenting and broaden to include mastering life's implicit curriculum, including understanding and coping with interpersonal relationships, preparing for work, managing budgets and household affairs, and dealing with substance abuse in the family and community.

Parents' Community Agenda

Parents are drawn by other parents' example to be more actively involved in center life and in their community. At first this may start with being a supportive participant in center community meetings; later it may evolve into active work on behalf of the center, joining with other parents in community organizing activities. It can also involve learning to take responsibility in the family center, through different informal and formal roles that support community life. Informal roles include working on projects in the center, such as developing recreational activities for families. Formal roles can mean becoming part of the center staff as parent aides in day care programs or as parent mentors to support parents who need outreach, coaching, and additional help at home.

The Interrelationship of Parents' Agendas

As can be readily imagined, over time parents will be involved in all of the possible agendas. It is also important to recognize that parents need time to be involved in one agenda and then to consider working on another. Figure 18-5 describes the ways these agenda also interact, so that it is possible, for example, for work on the social and learning agenda to prepare parents to be engaged in working on the community agenda. We believe that just as a synergy exists between all the parts of the center that results in the sum being more than the parts, so it can be with parents' experience as they are involved in working on multiple agendas; the sum, or outcome, from their work on multiple agendas is greater than reaching each agenda's goals. Success in one area increases success in another, as reinforcing and transformative.

The Professional Agenda

Program and practice in the center need to anticipate and respond to parents' different agendas. From the practitioners' perspective, their profes-

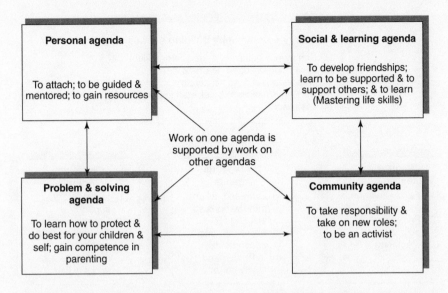

The Parent Agenda model shows the interaction among the different agendas. Although one agenda may begin as the primary focus, other agendas develop over time. Parents' work in meeting their goals in one agenda will influence their work in other agendas.

Figure 18.5. Parent Agendas Interactive Model

sional agenda would include responding to parents' personal priorities and needs, including their need for therapy, with added responsibilities for protection of the child and parent, and capacity building that is critical to the development of the center milieu and to professional collaboration and effectiveness. Figure 18-6 describes the professional agenda, with capacity in community building as central to all other work, which includes the regulatory-protective agenda, the therapeutic, and the community agenda.

The Capacity and Community Building Agenda

The community agenda involves developing capacity in the center milieu and facilitating parents' involvement in the broader community. Building capacity in the center requires building a team that includes parents as part of the service team, supporting teamwork, coordinating the entire center's services to promote integration, and supporting staff through supervision and training. Community development activities are focused on helping parents become part of the center milieu, as cocreators of the culture of care responsible for the vibrancy of center life. Collective learning that supports a learning organization approach reinforces parents' investment in and contribution to center programs.

Community organizing approaches also develop connections between the center and its neighborhood and enhance the center's role in community change. Many centers seek to connect with the local community development agenda. For example, centers increasingly are drawn to Boushel's (1994)[3] schema as a framework for developing child-safe communities (Jones & Ely, 2001).

The Therapeutic Agenda

The therapeutic/counseling and alliance-building agenda accounts for the basics of interpersonal relationships, the conventional one-to-one therapeutic relationship, and the way in which key workers signpost and facilitate the families' route in and around the center. It provides the foundation for connection and containment, with anchoring relationships that are sustaining because they provide continuity. Assessment and decisions about therapeutic approaches to meet need are developed with parents as partners in the helping process. Family and individual therapy are provided as needed, including referrals for substance abuse treatment.

Regulatory-Protective Agenda

The regulatory agenda accounts explicitly for protective work, where change is a requirement for safe

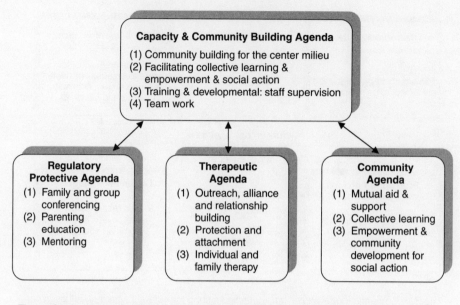

Figure 18.6. Professional Agenda Model

children; contemporary approaches include parent education programs, family work, play therapy, physical health intervention, cognitive-behavioral training, and assessment. This is where work intersects with the child welfare system, and the family center has a role in collaborating with parents and protective systems to make sure that a child's well-being is ensured. Ongoing work can include planning and transitional support for reunification if a child is in out-of-home placement. In situations of domestic violence, the professional agenda will also include work with parents to ensure their safety.

Community Agenda:
Group Work and Education

The community agenda embraces a broad range of therapeutic, mutual aid, and support groups, collective learning and action groups, and recreation. There is the unique mandate to build community, one where mutual aid brings support and a foundation for individual and group efficacy. At the same time, collective learning is important to building community capacity, as discussed earlier in this chapter.

How It All Comes Together

We conclude with a case example that describes the journey of a parent in a UK family center who, after 3.5 years, has continued to be an important part of center life. The brief introduction to her experience captures how this model helps describe the focus for work and, more important, how the family center became the community that helped her keep her children and regain a sense of worth after long years of abuse.

Case Example From a UK Integrated Family Center

Annette was referred to the center by her social worker. Her two children, ages 5 and 9, are listed on the "at-risk" register. The concern is neglect. Annette's partner, and the children's father, has left the home after a long period of violence toward Annette. His children are regular witnesses to his unpredictable outburst of anger and abuse. Annette acknowledges she has great difficulty in controlling, caring for, and expressing emotion to her children. Their behavior is very challenging at home and at school. Annette agrees to attend the parenting program at the center and is introduced to the center by her health visitor, with whom she has a trusting relationship. This took time, but good collaboration between the center and social work health practitioner resulted in Annette becoming engaged in the center.

Annette began her time in the center with a mixed agenda that included her personal needs, but foremost in her mind was the problem-solving agenda: she wanted to keep her children. Her health visitor would have introduced other possibilities, although she was unsure Annette would absorb them at this time. She was too beaten down and hopeless about her situation. The professional agenda concerned Annette's immediate need to keep her children (rooted in the protection agenda), yet her team was mindful of how important work on other agendas would help Annette develop the support and experience she needed as a valued community member. Her problem-solving agenda led to a full program that involved a behavioral plan, observed play, a one-way mirror and earpiece for Annette so she could receive coaching, and sustained encouragement and firm advice. Because Annette came to the center for these different services, she also began to participate in the center's activities, such as rituals, celebrations, and outings, had meals with other parents, and received needed resources.

Over the next months, Annette began to act like she belonged, dropping in when she did not have appointment to talk with other parents and staff. She was becoming part of the family center community. Initially, she expressed needs that she came to understand as part of her personal agenda; she needed to work with an individual therapist on her relationships with abusive men. After 8 months, as courage and confidence developed, with challenge from work on the required protective agenda (nagging, nudging, and support to do something to break through her tendency to isolate), there emerged a collaborative sense that a social and learning agenda could now make sense for her. In the next 10 months, in three different support groups (a survivors group, a cooking group, and an art group), Annette reports significant change in her behavior and the way she feels. She ascribes such change to the support that enables her to continue through the many tears (struggling with challenges that demanded new things of her), working through old hurts, and encounters with fear and lack of confidence in her ability to cope, not least of which was the ups and downs of keeping to the agreed program.

Opportunities to engage differently in the center and elsewhere—*the community agenda*—are encountered by Annette in explicit and implicit ways. Peers show her possibilities, and staff (part mindful of the center's several agendas) give signposts as to where she could make a real contribution. This experience results in Annette engaging in other activities, and over time she becomes a support worker and encourager to new parents contemplating the program. What was so important for Annette was being held and accepted through the connections in the center while she lived through the pushes and pulling away, not getting too close to staff. This all was part of her growth, as well as acting out projections on center staff, rejecting them before they could reject her, all painful reenactments of her early history of repeated loss. Now that a different culture of care accepts her and recognizes her reactions, she learns that the center staff will not abandon her when she needs to dramatically move away from them. They have not forgotten or rejected her; they recognize her struggle, and that she is worthy of their care. When she is ready, they accept her back to continue her work. In sum this meant that Annette has had more than a therapist, more than a coach for parenting, more than mutual aid from a group of survivors like herself, more than opportunities to participate in the center. She belongs to a caring center, with a culture that invited her belonging, encouraged her attachment and enabled her dependence on others, and worked with her to make sure she completed the work that she had begun. Through all this, Annette developed a multifaceted sense of self (participant, parent, friend, helper, and contributor) from her many roles in the community. The center has also gained an important resource and provides a stronger caring culture for other parents because Annette is part of the team.

Conclusion

We have argued that the integrated center is a system of care that integrates services that have been fragmented, bringing the mental health and child welfare services together to develop well-being in families and children. The integrated family center as a social invention provides a milieu that has a strong culture of care that offers an alternative developmental system to families who are isolated, who struggle without resources, and who face unimaginable challenges in the face of violence, poverty, and mental illness.

We believe that there is accruing evidence that centers are a resource that can be an effective alternative to child welfare as we know it, where the focus is on placement and foster care rather than prevention. Instead, we believe that it is possible to support families so that they are able to have continued connections to their children, supporting attachment, protection, and development. Comprehensive community-based programs such as integrated family centers are unique because of their therapeutic milieu and their capacity-building function, which are important to the development of parents, staff, and their communities.

We have proposed a theory of change for family support practice as a step in explaining how these centers contribute to a host of important outcomes and as a guide for practice and evaluation. Our practice model emphasizes the possible agendas of parents and professionals, suggesting the synergy possible from work on multiple agendas that significantly influence positive outcomes. We believe the integrated family center provides protection and acts as a buffer for the accumulated risks that impede development for children and their parents because the center truly is more than the sum of it parts. This is a major reason parents tell us that family centers work for them and for their children, and are "beacons" in their communities.

Notes

1. These texts identify centers in Greece, France, the United States, the United Kingdom, Canada, Germany, Ireland, and Scandinavian countries.

2. The grid is based on two continuums, first between subjective knowledge and objective knowledge, and second, ideas of society and change.

3. Boushel gives us an illuminating framework with which to develop protective environments for children, based on the value attached to children; the status of women and their careers; the social connectedness of children; the extent and quality of the available protective safety nets.

References

Batchelor, J., Gould, N., & Wright, J. (1999). Family centers: A focus for the children in need debate. *Children and Family Social Work, 4*, 197–208.

Berg, I. K., & Kelly, S. (2000). *Building solutions in child protective services*. New York: Norton.

Berry, M., Cash, S. J., & Hoge, L. A. (1998). Creating community through psychoeducational groups in family preservation work. *Families in Society: The Journal of Contemporary Human Services, 79*, 15–24.

Bickman, L., Heflinger, C. A., Northrup, D., Sonnichsen, S., & Schilling, S. (1998). Long-term outcomes to family caregiver empowerment. *Journal of Child and Family Studies, 7*, 269–282.

Blank, S. (2000). *Good works: Highlights of a study on the Center for Family Life*. Baltimore: Annie E. Casey Foundation Press.

Bohannan, P. (1995). *How culture works*. New York: Free Press.

Bond, J., & Halpern, R. (1986) The cross-project evaluation of the Child Survival/Fair Start Initiative: A case study of action research. In H. Weiss & F. Jacobs (Eds.), *Evaluating family programs* (pp. 347–370). Hawthorne, NY: Aldine de Gruyter.

Boushel, M. (1994). The protective environment of children: Towards a framework for anti-oppressive, cross-cultural and cross-national understanding. *British Journal of Social Work, 24*, 173–190.

Bowen, N., Bowen, G., & Cook, P. (2000). Neighborhood characteristics and supportive parenting among single mothers. *Families, Crime and Criminal Justice, 2*, 183–206.

Bowen, N., Bowen, G., & Ware, W. (2002). Neighborhood social disorganization, families, and the educational behavior of adolescents. *Journal of Adolescent Research, 17*, 468–490.

Brodsky, A. (1996). Resilient single mothers in risky neighborhoods: Negative psychological sense of community. *Journal of Community Psychology, 24*, 347–363.

Bronfenbrenner, U. (1979). *The ecology of human development: Experiments by nature and design*. Cambridge, MA: Harvard University Press.

Burford, G., & Hudson, J. (Eds.). (2000). *Family group conferencing*. New York: Aldine de Gruyter.

Cannan, C., & Warren, C. (Eds.). (1997). *Social action with children and their families: A community development approach*. London: Routledge.

Chaskin, R. (2002). The evaluation of "community building": Measuring the social effects of community-based practice. In T. Vecchiato, A. Maluccio, & C. Canali (Eds.), *Client and program* perspectives on outcome evaluation in child and family services: A cross-national perspective (pp. 28–47). New York: Aldine de Gruyter.

Cigno, K. (1988). Consumer views of a family center drop-in. British Journal of Social Work, 18(4), 33–38.

Comer, E. W., & Fraser, M. W. (1998). Evaluation of six family-support programs: Are they effective? Families in Society, 79, 134–148.

Daloz, L. (1992). Effective teaching and mentoring: Realizing the transformational power of adult learning experiences. San Francisco: Jossey-Bass.

Dore, M. M., & Lee, J. M. (1999). The role of parent training with abusive and neglectful parents. Family Relations: Interdisciplinary Journal of Applied Family Studies, 48, 313–325.

Duncan, G. J., & Brooks-Gunn, J. (1999). Consequences of growing up poor. New York: Russell Sage Foundation.

Durlak, J. (1998). Common risk and protective factors in successful prevention programs. American Journal of Orthopsychiatry, 68, 511–520.

Durlak, J., & Wells, A. (1997). Primary prevention mental health programs for children and adolescents: A meta-analytic review. American Journal of Community Psychology, 25, 115–152.

Farmer, T., & Farmer, E. (2001). Developmental science, systems of care, and prevention of emotional and behavioral problems in youth. American Journal of Orthopsychiatry, 71, 171–181.

Feikema, R., Segalavich, J., & Jefferies, S. (1997). From child development to community development: One agency's journey. Families in Society, 78(20), 185–195.

Fletcher, T., & Romano, M. (2001). Justice, child protection and family centers. In C. Warren-Adamson (Ed.), Family centers and their international role in social action (pp. 105–126). Aldershot, UK: Ashgate.

Freire, P. (1985). The politics of education, culture, power and liberation. Basingstoke, UK: Macmillan.

Garbarino, J. (1986). Where does social support fit into optimizing human development and prevention of dysfunction? British Journal of Social Work, 16, 23–27.

Garbarino, J. (1995). Raising children in a socially toxic environment. San Francisco: Jossey-Bass.

Germain, C. (1991). Human behavior in the social environment. New York: Columbia University Press.

Golding, K. (2000). Parent management training as an intervention to promote adequate parenting. Clinical Child Psychology and Psychiatry, 5, 357–371.

Halpern, R. (1999). Fragile families. New York: Columbia University Press.

Heron, J., & Reason, P. (2001). The practice of co-operative inquiry: Research "with" rather than "on" people. In P. Reason & H. Bardbury (Eds.), Handbook of action research: Participation, enquiry and practice (pp. 179–188). London: Sage.

Hess, P., McGowan, B., & Botsko, M. (2000). A preventive services program model for preserving and supporting families over time. Child Welfare, 79, 227–265.

Howe, D. (1987). Introduction to social work theory. Aldershot, UK: Ashgate.

Ireys, H., Divet, K., & Sakawa, D. (2002). Family support and education. In B. Burns & K. Hoagwood (Eds.), Community treatment for youth: Evidence-based interventions for severe emotional and behavioral disorders (pp. 154–176). New York: Oxford University Press.

Janchill, Sister M. (1979). People cannot go it alone. In C. Germain (Ed.), Social work practice (pp. 74–106). New York: Columbia University Press.

Jones, E., & Ely, D. (2001). Justice, child protection and family centres—Part 1 (Inside). In C. Warren-Adamson (Ed.), Family centres and their international role in social action: Social work as informal education (pp. 192–104). Aldershot, UK: Ashgate.

Joseph, R., Friedman, R., Gutierrez-Mayka, M., Sengova, J., Uzzell, D., & Hernandez, M.C.R. (2001). Final comprehensive report: Evaluation findings and lessons learned from the Annie E. Casey Mental Health Initiative for Urban Children. Tampa: University of South Florida, Louis de la Parte Florida Mental Health Institute, Department of Child Studies.

Kegan, R. (1998). The mental demands of modern life: In over our heads. Cambridge, MA: Harvard University Press.

Knitzer, J. (2000). Promoting resilience: Helping young children and parents affected by substance abuse, domestic violence and depression in the context of welfare reform. New York: National Center for Children in Poverty.

Layzer, J., & Goodson, B. (2001). National evaluation of family support programs. Cambridge, MA: ABT Associates.

Lightburn, A. (1994). Hall Neighborhood House family support program demonstration, 1990-1993: Final evaluation for the Office of Head Start (Administration of Children, Youth and Families, Health and Human Services). New York: Author.

Lightburn, A. (2002). Family service centers: Lessons learned from national and local evaluations. In T. Vecchiato, A. Maluccio, & C. Canali (Eds.), Client and program perspectives on outcome evaluation in child and family services: A cross-national perspective (pp. 153–173). New York: Aldine de Gruyter.

Lightburn, A., & Black, R. (2001). The client as

learner and the clinician as teacher: Working with an educational lens. *Smith Studies in Social Work, 72*, 15–33.

Lightburn, A., & Kemp, S. (1994). Family support programs: Opportunities for community-based practice. *Families in Society: The Journal of Contemporary Social Services, 75*, 16–26.

Local Government Association. (2002). *Serving children well: A new vision for children's services*. London: LGA Publications, the Local Government Association, Local Government House.

MacAdoo, H. (1999). African-American families: Strengths and realities. In H. McCubbin, E. Thompson, A. Thompson, & J. Futrell (Eds.), *Resiliency in African-American families* (pp. 17–30). Thousand Oaks, CA: Sage.

Merriam, S., & Clark, M. (1991). *Lifelines: Patterns of work, love and learning in adulthood*. San Francisco: Jossey-Bass.

Mezirow, J., & Associates. (2000). *Learning as transformation: Critical perspectives on a theory in progress*. San Francisco: Jossey-Bass.

Nelson, K., Landsman, M., & Deutelbaum, W. (1990). Three models of family-centered prevention services. *Child Welfare, 69*, 3–29.

Parsons, R. (1991). Empowerment: Purpose and practice principle in social work. *Social Work with Groups, 14*(2), 7–21.

Phelan, J. (1983). *Family centers: A study*. London: Children's Society.

Rutter, M. (1979). Protective factors in children's response to stress and disadvantage. In M. Kent & J. Rolf (Eds.), *Primary prevention of psychopathology: Social competence in children* (Vol. 3, pp. 49–74). Hanover, NH: University of New England Press.

Saleebey, D. (Ed.). (2002). *The strengths perspective in social work practice*. Boston: Allyn and Bacon.

Schwab-Stone, M., Ayers, T., Kasprow, W., Voyce, C. Barone, C. Shriver, T., & Weissberg, R. (1995). No safe haven: A study of violence exposure in an urban community. *Journal of the American Academy of Child and Adolescent Psychiatry, 34*, 1343–1352.

Seitz, V. (1990). Intervention programs for impoverished children: A comparison of education and family support models. *Annual of Child Development, 7*, 73–103.

Senge, P. (2000). *Schools that learn: A fifth discipline fieldbook for educators, parents and everyone who cares about education*. New York: Doubleday.

Shuttleworth, J. (1989). Psychoanalytic theory and infant development. In L. Miller, M. L. Rustin, M. Rustin, & M. Shuttleworth (Eds.), *Closely observed infants* (pp. 22–51). London: Duckworth.

Silver, E., Ireys, H., Bauman, L., & Stein, R. (1997). Psychological outcomes of a support intervention for mothers of children with ongoing health conditions: The Parent-to-Parent Network. *Journal of Community Psychology, 25*, 249–264.

Smith, T. (1992). *Family centers and bringing up young children*. London: HMSO.

Stroul, B. (Ed.). (1996). *Children's mental health*. Baltimore: Brookes.

Tracy, E., & Whittaker, J. (1987). The evidence base for social support interventions in child and family practice: Emerging issues for research and practice. *Children and Youth Services Review, 9*, 249–270.

Vella, J. (1995). *Training through dialogue: Promoting effective learning and change with adults*. San Francisco: Jossey-Bass.

Waller, M. (2001). Resilience in ecosystemic context: Evolution of the concept. *American Journal of Orthopsychiatry, 71*, 290–297.

Walsh, F. (1998). *Strengthening family resilience*. New York: Guilford.

Warren, C. (1997). Family support and the journey to empowerment. In C. Cannan & C. Warren (Eds.), *Social action with children and their families: A community development approach* (pp. 103–123). London: Routledge.

Warren-Adamson, C. (Ed.). (2001). *Family centers and their international role in social action*. Aldershot, UK: Ashgate.

Warren-Adamson, C. (2002). Applying a parenting scale in family resource centers: Challenges and lessons. In T. Vecchiato, A. Maluccio, & C. Canali (Eds.), *Client and program perspectives on outcome evaluation in child and family services: A cross-national perspective* (pp. 120–134). New York: Aldine de Gruyter.

Whipple, W., & Wilson, S. (1996). Evaluation of a parent education and support program for families at risk of physical child abuse. *Families in Society: The Journal of Contemporary Human Services*, April, 227–239.

Wigfall, V., & Moss, P. (2001). *More than the sum of its parts: A study of multi-agency childcare network*. London: National Children's Bureau.

Winnicott, D. W. (1960). The theory of parent-infant relationship. *International Journal of Psychoanalysis, 41*, 585–595.

Winnicott, D. (1990). *The maturational process in the facilitating environment*. London: Karnac.

19

Sandra Gossart-Walker and Robert A. Murphy

Children and HIV

A Model of Home-Based Mental Health Treatment

The human immunodeficiency virus and acquired immune deficiency syndrome (HIV/AIDS) has become a potent disease that affects not only infected individuals but also entire families and communities. A growing number of children are directly affected by HIV/AIDS in their immediate families in the United States who are not necessarily infected with the virus (Dane & Levine, 1994; Geballe, Gruendel, & Andiman, 1995; Michaels & Levine, 1992; Murphy, Forsyth, & Adnopoz, 2002). Children affected by HIV disease and AIDS not only face multiple challenges beyond those of the disease but also can present notable challenges to their families and to mental health professionals. Children with HIV/AIDS in their families often lose one or both parents, as well as multiple other family members, to the disease. The inconsistency and diminished availability of adult caregivers due to the disease and its associated complications can impair children's ability to master developmental milestones and build appropriate coping skills. With each loss, they are often confronted with the prospect of further losses. For many HIV-affected children losses to AIDS only add to other losses associated with violence, poverty, and substance abuse. These children must then face the many developmentally ex-

pectable hurdles of childhood with the added burden and commotion AIDS creates in their families.

Despite the multiple mental health issues of HIV-affected children and their families, few resources are available to adequately address their needs (Burr & Lewis, 2000; Gerwirtz & Gossart-Walker, 2000). Those services that are available for affected families often focus on patients' medical and concrete support needs and terminate upon their death. Available services often focus on the case management needs of the patients and often cease upon the patient's death, leaving little, if any, support for the children and their new caregivers. These services end at the time of death because of funding constraints; as a result, the family may lose its housing, food subsidies, case management, and other supportive services, all of which may have been supported through AIDS-specific funding.

The dire toll of HIV disease often compromises families' ability to utilize available mental health care. Traditional modalities of office- and clinic-based care may be ill suited to families who must contend with HIV/AIDS. Obstacles such as transportation, overwhelming and chaotic family life, and feelings of stigma, as well as the disease itself, prevent some families from seeking mental health and supportive services for their children. In light of these obstacles to traditional service utilization, the Yale Child Study Center, through its Program for HIV-Affected Children and Families, has developed a community-based approach to the mental health care of children and families beset by HIV/AIDS. This chapter will explore the unique opportunities inherent in providing mental health care to HIV-infected and HIV-affected children using nontraditional techniques. The chapter will begin by briefly providing a history of HIV-affected children on a national level, followed by a detailed discussion of the Program for HIV-Affected Children and Families, including the issues faced by these children and their families. Two case vignettes will illustrate the need and challenges of home-based work with HIV-affected children.

HIV-Affected Children in the United States

AIDS was first identified by the Centers for Disease Control in the United States in 1981 among gay men in California and New York (Centers for Disease Control [CDC], 2000). Once the disease was identified as an epidemic, the focus was on its contagion, epidemiology, and medical treatment. Early in the epidemic and throughout the 1980s, social service and mental health interventions focused solely on the infected individuals, most often adults. During the mid-1980s, attention turned to babies born to HIV-infected women, about a quarter of whom would develop AIDS within the first year or more of life. The focus remained, however, on their medical treatment as individuals, not as family members within a community. In the public realm, there continued to be concern about contagion; the epidemic was thought to center only on marginalized populations. There was strong and sustained advocacy among the gay community for better treatment and services; however, the voices of children were missing. In rare instances when the general population thought about AIDS and children, they thought of AIDS babies, often hearing stories of their abandonment in hospitals or their early deaths (Stein, 1998). Although tragic, the exclusive focus on their plight obscured the broader segment of youth whose lives were being devastated by HIV/AIDS in their families.

In 1992, more than 10 years after the first case of AIDS was identified in the United State, David Michaels and Carol Levine identified the overwhelming numbers of children who had been and were expected to be orphaned to the disease (Michaels & Levine, 1992). They estimated that between 72,000 and 125,000 children and adolescents would become motherless due to AIDS (Michaels & Levine, 1992). In addition, women, typically of childbearing age, were comprising a growing percentage of AIDS cases reported in the United States, especially in large urban settings (CDC, 2001). The percentage of women diagnosed with AIDS increased from 8% in the 1980s to 22% in 2000 (CDC, 2001). Most of these women's children were not infected themselves but faced the loss of their parent(s) and would need alternate care. The needs of these children were tremendous; however, interventions were either lacking or not delivered in ways that children and their families could access or use sufficiently (Burr & Lewis, 2000).

In 1999, the National Pediatric and Family HIV Resource Center at the University of Medicine and Dentistry of New Jersey studied HIV-infected mothers to identify the health and social service needs of families, describe model projects that were successfully meeting those needs, and characterize unmet needs that required program or policy responses. In their summary report, Burr and Lewis (2000) stated that families affected by HIV frequently are challenged by the difficulty of coordinating each family member's health care. Furthermore, services that are specific to family members with HIV disease are unlikely to be appropriate for those children who are uninfected. For example, women often receive health care or case management services in agencies that primarily serve adults. Within these service models the needs of children and other family members are not considered or addressed. For the children of HIV-infected parents of particular concern is the serious underutilization of important child services. The complexity involved in accessing multiple systems presents a substantial barrier to securing adequate medical and psychiatric care. Health care providers working with HIV-positive women exacerbate their problems when they fail to recognize the roles and responsibilities of active parenting and fail to offer appropriate support services. For example, Roth, Siegel, and Black (1994) noted that HIV disease may decrease a parent's ability to provide a secure holding environment that fosters optimal child development and psychosocial adaptation. Despite advances in HIV treatment that have dramatically changed the course of the illness, families continue to experience a "roller coaster" effect of treatments that may yield promising results in terms of mortality and quality of life, yet may also fail to alleviate episodes of illness and stressors associated with a chronic and life-endangering illness.

Adolescents and young adults now constitute the majority of new incidences of HIV infection, unlike earlier years when prenatal and perinatal HIV transmission accounted for the majority of infected children. Rates of infection among this age cohort now exceed those of any other age-group (UNAIDS, 2000). The widely lauded decrease in infections among younger children and adults in the United States has not been evident among youth (CDC, 1998), for whom the epidemic is marked by higher prevalence among young women than among men, due to rates of sexual contact with older males. Among young men with HIV infection, homosexual transmission accounts for the single largest risk group. The advent of new antiretroviral therapies appears to have spurred a resurgence of unsafe sexual practices among gay youth (UNAIDS, 2000). Additional risk factors contributing to the alarming rates of HIV infection among teens and young adults include an exponential increase in diagnoses of sexually transmitted diseases (STDs), thought to be a preceding marker for possible HIV infection due to high rates of unsafe sexual practices. In addition to direct transmission via intravenous (IV) drug use, other forms of substance abuse lower inhibitions and impair judgment skills needed to make sound decisions about safer sex practices. Despite their heightened risk, youth may also be relatively more amenable to altering their sexual practices than are older adults, who may be less flexible (Murphy et al., 2002).

The Scope of Mental Health Problems Among HIV-Affected Youth

Youth diagnosed with psychiatric disorders may engage in a range of behaviors that heighten their risk for contracting HIV (Brown, Danovsky, Lourie, DiClemente, & Ponton, 1997). Those diagnosed with conduct disorder or a depressive disorder engage in higher rates of substance abuse, including IV drug abuse, and unprotected sexual activity, including prostitution (Stiffman, Dore, Earls, & Cunningham, 1992). Their characteristic pessimistic outlook may interfere with their ability to apply the information they have received to alter their high-risk behaviors (Brown et al., 1997). Children with disorders marked by problems with impulse control may be at greater risk for infection due to their multiple risk behaviors (Booth & Zhang, 1997). For example, adolescents with diagnoses of conduct disorder or attention deficit/hyperactivity disorder (ADHD) abuse substances at higher levels, engage in sexual activity with a greater number of partners, and more frequently contract STDs relative to nondisordered youth. Even among runaway and homeless adolescents, who are much more likely than most adolescents to engage in high-risk sexual activity and injecting drug use, those with a comorbid diagnosis of conduct disorder are still more likely to have engaged in an exchange of sexual activity in return for money or drugs and to have had unprotected sex with multiple partners. A diagnosis of conduct disorder increased the likelihood of injecting drug use by more than a 2:1 margin (odds ratio [OR] = 2.28) and the likelihood of exchanging sex for drugs or money by almost a 3:1 margin (OR = 2.82). Similarly, adolescents who knew someone infected with HIV were also at greater risk for drug injection (OR = 1.40) or sexual exchange (OR = 1.29) (Brown et al., 1997). Despite an absence of detailed estimates, seroprevalence rates in excess of the 0.2% to 2.2% rates among adolescents of indeterminate psychiatric status are likely, as has been the case for psychiatrically compromised adults, where prevalence rates have ranged from 5.5% to 14%, suggesting that psychiatric symptomatology increases the likelihood of engaging in activities that pose particular risks for HIV infection.

Developmental Perspectives on HIV/AIDS

Interventions for children infected with or affected by HIV disease require a comprehensive, developmentally informed approach to their complex psychological and social needs and those of their families (Murphy et al., 2002). As with their overall cognitive development and capacity for logical reasoning, children's understanding of HIV and AIDS can be expected to follow a predictable sequence. Preschool and early school-age children explain AIDS in terms of events that occur together in time or location but which may actually have little relation to one another. In effect, young children overgeneralize causal relationships where they may not be warranted, for example, inferring that a parent's illness is a result of their own misbehavior. At this age, children also may recognize that symptoms are the result of an underlying illness, but they probably cannot explain the etiology of HIV as a virus that is contracted in specific ways. With development, the causation of AIDS can be described as a sequential process related to certain types of behavior, for example, sexual activity, blood exposure, or drug use. Typically, these explanations may provide school-age children with a factually accurate account of how HIV/AIDS may be contracted, yet the explanation remains based on a series of events culminating in illness, with little understanding of broader contexts or individual behaviors that contribute. The final stage of understanding is based on the expanded capacity for abstract reasoning that accompanies adolescence, and youth become able to describe the origins of HIV/AIDS in terms of its underlying disease etiology (Walsh & Bibace, 1991).

Infants and Toddlers

The quality of attachment between infant and caregiver sets the stage for later development and influences how children progress in terms of their sense of self, their capacity for relationships with others, and their emotional resilience. Preoccupation with the medical and psychological demands of coping with HIV disease may deplete families of the energy and psychological resources available to attend to early aspects of normative childhood development. While most caregivers remain able to provide for their infant's basic needs, for others, HIV may interfere with the establishment of a predictable and reciprocal pattern of interaction between caregiver and their infected and/or affected babies, resulting in episodic and irregular dyadic engagement.

The expectable acts of defiance and desires for separation that mark toddlerhood may heighten unconscious fears of loss and permanent separation for affected children. The anger and defiance of the toddler represent developmentally appropriate and necessary assertions of autonomy and distinctness

from a parent or primary caregiver (Mayes & Cohen, 1993). Infected, symptomatic young children may require an enhanced degree of caretaking and protection that may constrict the expression of their normal drives toward the external world, while affected children may find their symptomatic caregivers unable to withstand their developmentally appropriate challenges.

Early Childhood and Preschool Years

In this phase of development, imaginative play, which is intimately connected to language and cognitive development, represents a primary means for integrating internal thoughts and feelings with external experiences (Marans & Cohen, 1996). The play of a child affected by HIV might involve repeated scenarios related to illness or loss, even though the same child might never be able to verbalize these concerns. Although children may gradually be able to understand basic facts about HIV illness and death, their ideas will likely remain concrete and specific to their life experiences. Metaphors about death may engender greater confusion, as young children are unable to abstract basic concepts that death represents a final end to life.

When HIV becomes involved at this stage of development, emotional conflicts involving the simultaneous experience of loving and rivalrous or aggressive feelings may become especially threatening and upsetting. Parents with HIV/AIDS may be too psychologically and physically fragile for a child to express these concerns freely. The egocentric orientation of this stage may potentiate feelings of guilt and responsibility, as children may assume that their actions have caused their parent's illness. Independence and engagement with peers and a broader social world may be experienced as a rejection of the already fragile caregiver. Unable to negotiate the competing developmental tasks involving loyalty and closeness to caregivers and a desire for greater independence and autonomy, some children may find themselves compromised in their ability to negotiate this expectable developmental step.

School-Age Children

As school-age children turn increasingly toward accomplishments in the broader realms of school and friendships, they must rely on a relatively distinct sense of self that is still dependent on their primary caregivers. Children who have been unable to resolve conflicted feelings about their medically compromised parents may remain tied to them in a manner that precludes their developmentally appropriate ventures into the world of peers and school. Mastery of basic logical principles allows a child to infer cause-and-effect relationships, devise alternate solutions to problems, and comprehend reciprocal relationships, advances that may be invaluable as children attempt to understand their own illness or that of a parent. Language serves a regulatory as well as a communicative function; a child who can put words to his or her feelings is able to refrain from acting on those feelings and acquires greater mastery over his or her experiences.

Adolescents

While most adolescents strive to loosen the ties of childhood dependency by substituting intimate and romantic relationships with peers, those who must contend with personal or familial HIV may be hampered in efforts toward individuation and the formation of an independent sense of self. Expected rule transgressions and rebellions against parental rules also become fraught with danger, real and imagined, about the potential consequences of their emerging sexuality and the strength of their angry, hostile, or defiant feelings. Adolescents contend with their desire for adult sexuality and relationships in the context of the potential for HIV infection. Out of their own discomfort, they may be unlikely to approach parents with these concerns, especially if these relationships are already marked by conflict, dispute, or unexpressed concerns about HIV disease. While avoidance of HIV-related topics may reduce immediate feelings of discomfort and prolong a wish to protect teenagers through extending a protected childhood, adolescents continue to engage in sexual activity at ever-younger ages. Initial sexual encounters among teens are rarely planned, decreasing the likelihood of their using birth control or engaging in sexual practices aimed at reducing the chances of HIV transmission, thereby heightening the risk for HIV and other STDs and limiting attention to issues of risk amelioration (Brown et al., 1997; Hein, Dell, Futterman, Rotheram-Borus, & Shaffer, 1995).

High-Risk Adolescents

Adolescents have been cited as a high-risk group for HIV infection and AIDS. However, the relationship between knowledge about HIV/AIDS and risk behavior remains unclear, with investigators reporting contradictory results about whether or not adolescents apply knowledge of HIV to their actions. For example, Rotheram-Borus, Draimin, Reid, & Murphy (1997) noted an increase in high-risk behavior among adolescents who had been informed of their parents' HIV infection. Clinicians in the Yale program have observed similar situations in which affected teens engage in multiple instances of unprotected sexual activity, suggesting that denial may be a predominant mechanism by which adolescents cope with the complex emotional sequelae of HIV infection in themselves or loved ones. Detachment and avoidance of emotion provide defenses against the overwhelming anxiety related to a history and future defined by the specter of loss. Among some HIV-affected youth, reenactment of the very behaviors that led their parents to contract the AIDS virus may represent a developmentally appropriate desire to feel invulnerable, along with a desperate effort to control overwhelming anxiety among youth who confront their own sexual drives in the context of HIV. Thus, adolescence in general involves a period of risk taking that can heighten the probability of HIV infection. Youth from high-risk backgrounds characterized by familial HIV, socioeconomic adversity, and psychosocial and psychiatric difficulties may be still more likely to be exposed to or contract HIV, as these multiple factors represent an exponential increase in risk.

Despite predictions of a rising incidence of HIV infection among adolescents, appropriate prevention efforts and clinical responses have often been lacking (Kalichman, 2000). Prevention curricula using a psychoeducation and problem-solving approach to sexual and other risk behaviors have demonstrated a range of positive outcomes in general school and community settings, including increased condom use during intercourse, decreased high-risk (unprotected) sexual behavior, decreased sexual activity with multiple partners, increased age at time of first intercourse, and increased discussion of sexual practices between parents and children (Jemmott, Jemmott, & Fong, 1992; Lefkowitz, Sigman, & Au, 2000; Main et al., 1994; St. Lawrence et al., 1995). The extent to which primary preventive approaches may generalize to high-risk, psychiatrically impaired, or juvenile delinquent cohorts outside of these mainstream settings remains untested (Schoeberlein, Woolston, & Brett, 2000; Schonfeld, 2000). Those at greatest risk for contracting HIV/AIDS tend to be the same adolescents whose isolation from traditional health and mental health treatment systems complicates or primary and secondary prevention efforts.

Loss and Stigma

A child faced with HIV/AIDS in his or her family is often unable to express anger and rage toward the ill or dying caregiver. They may fear that their anger will hasten their parent's death and make the child the responsible agent of the death. Though feeling certain that their ill parent will die, children cannot predict with certainty the nature, shape, and potential impact of the events that will precede this loss. Thus, they are left with an ever-present sense of doom that colors the ways in which they interpret and make sense out of their experience. Children must then repress their rage and keep feelings tightly contained, with limited scope of expression. Children do not understand what these powerful feelings mean. Some children may act out that rage toward themselves and others in destructive ways. Very often, when acting out and malicious behavior is occurring in the home, families are already emotionally depleted and are unable to connect the behavior to the rage and sadness about illnesses and deaths. It is possible for children and their "problem" behavior to become the targets for the family's anger and hence perpetuate the behavior.

HIV disease can also impact the parent's caregiver role. Fatigue and medication side effects can make it difficult to handle everyday parenting tasks and make coping with children's emotional or behavioral problems seem beyond their personal resources. Infected parents often need access to support and parental guidance to learn effective ways to manage children at home while they are ill. It is also important for them to have appropriate referrals and advocacy for in-home help. It is our experience that fears of stigma and issues of privacy may compel families to prohibit children from openly discussing the disease, despite the gradual deterioration in health status. Children cannot help

but observe what is happening. They are forbidden to talk to adults about their observations, and without adults' direct explanation they have no clear way to express their worries and concerns and are left alone with their fears.

Long before the AIDS epidemic, Erving Goffman defined stigma as "an attribute that is deeply discrediting" (1963, p. 3). This definition captures the feelings many families experience with AIDS. We have found, however, that AIDS becomes a stigma attached not only to the infected individual but also to those associated with him or her. The illness becomes a secret that is often guarded carefully by families (Nagler, Adnopoz & Forsyth, 1995). The circle of the stigma expands from the infected person, attaching itself to those closely associated with him or her, especially family. For many families, the issue of AIDS becomes a toxic family secret (Boyd-Franklin, 1989). Fearing their children will be ostracized by playmates, and by playmates' parents, parents struggle to keep the "secret" to "protect" their children from the same dilemmas they face (Gossart-Walker & Moss, 1998).

The staff of the program is well aware of the stigma felt by the families they serve. The teams often approach families with careful explanations of the services offered and a firm commitment to protecting families' privacy. With each form to be completed and each referral made, the team repeatedly assures the families of their confidentiality. They assure the families that they will not disclose information within their family and neighborhood or to other professionals without explicit permission. With the disclosure of HIV status to other family members, including children, the teams work at the pace the family finds comfortable. Outside pressures to disclose are discussed and explored, but the team never insists on disclosure.

Permanency Planning

All children need a sense of stability and permanence to support development. Most parents want their children to grow up in environments that are stable and safe. However, HIV-infected and HIV-affected children are prone to experience unstable and unpredictable relationships, accompanied by multiple disruptions in placements with the emotional distress that follows numerous losses and an uncertain future. The inconsistency and frequent unavailability of infected adult caregivers due not only to the course of the illness but also to the comorbidity of socioeconomic stressors, substance abuse, and mental illness can heighten the risk of out-of-family placement for these children.

Parents may approach their potential death with untested assumptions about their children's future welfare, for example, assuming that a relative or older sibling will take custody of younger children. Children who lose a parent to AIDS typically remain in the care of relatives, yet siblings are separated in more than 50% of cases (Draimin, 1995) at a time where the continuity of their relationships is especially crucial. In effect, parental loss becomes exacerbated through separations from remaining family members.

Despite adversity and trepidation about their own foreshortened lives, many parents are able to consider potential permanency plans that will sustain sibling and family relationships. For example, in a study of 151 HIV-infected parents and their 171 adolescent children (Rotheram-Borus et al., 1997), almost three quarters of the teens had been told of their parent's HIV diagnosis, and a slightly larger percentage of parents (81% of mothers and 75% of fathers) had developed formal or informal custody plans for their children. Virtually all the parents who made a permanency plan consulted the potential guardian, and almost all the plans were agreed to by the chosen guardian. Among both the disclosing and nondisclosing parents, however, legal custody arrangements were rare, occurring in less than one quarter of cases in which there existed some form of permanency arrangement. The high rates of permanency planning and their communication to affected children are encouraging, as they indicate that many parents are able to address their children's needs in a planful and thoughtful manner. The relative lack of legally sanctioned custody arrangements raises greater concern because during a period of grief, arrangements based on verbal agreements may be jeopardized.

Bereavement

In Worden's (1991) work on grief and loss he outlines circumstances that may lead to abnormal grief reactions. These circumstances are all too familiar in HIV-affected families, including those with chil-

dren. He states that in experiencing multiple losses the sheer volume of people to be grieved can be overwhelming. He also adds that social factors can lead to complicated mourning because "grief is really a social process and is best dealt with in a social setting where people can support and reinforce each other in their reactions to the loss" (p. 69). He adds that if the loss is unspeakable or socially negated, or if there is an absence of a social support network, one can expect that complicated grief reactions may occur. All these circumstances are present with children affected by HIV/AIDS. Bereaved children appear to be at increased risk for psychological trauma if support from primary caretakers is limited. Social support also decreases as children are shuffled among adult caregivers, often losing contact with their neighborhoods, schools, and other social institutions. Thus, children's needs go unmet for nurturing, consistent, and predictable relationships that can further their capacity to tolerate and adapt to painful life experiences in the wake of HIV/AIDS (Gossart-Walker & Moss, 1998).

Through work with the infected parents and extended family members, clinicians and family support workers guide families through the complex and often frightening issues of planning for and moving toward the transfer of guardianship that the parent's illness eventually necessitates. Because such transitions are difficult and taxing for both children and caregivers, follow-up services and support groups are offered to the newly identified guardians, as well as the biological parents. Legal advocacy is provided to families in conjunction with the Yale Law Clinic and Legal AIDS Network of Connecticut.

Disclosure and Secrecy

The stigma associated with AIDS may prevent open discussion and true expression of concern and worry, hampering appropriate developmental trajectories. Often, families are not open to discussing the HIV status of their members with their children (Armistead & Forehand, 1995; Armistead et al., 1999; Armistead, Tannenbaum, Forehand, Morse, & Morse, 2001; Faithful, 1997; Hackl, Sonlai, Kelly, & Kalichman, 1997). The psychological issues of affected children and families remain closely tied to the issue of secrecy and stigma that prevent open communication between children and their caregivers. As a result, many children are not told of their parent's and/or other family member's HIV infection (Nagler et al., 1995). Responses to stigma prevent many families from getting their needs met; for example, a mother with AIDS may not tell anyone at her child's school about her illness. The child may be having difficulty at school because of his inability to concentrate due to his worries about his mother. The school mislabels the child, and he is directed toward behavioral consequences, whereas providing the opportunity for the child to call home twice per day may have diminished the negative behavior.

Due to the lack of open communication about the disease, children will often develop fantasies about family secrets. Fantasies often can loom large and be dire, engendering a sense of shame and isolation. Children can sense the prohibition and shame attached to expressions about the illness and respond to their parents' unrecognized communication of their own fears about discrimination, rejection, and abandonment. Frequently, in their desire to be "good" and to protect their fragile adult caregivers, children will not confront or ask about the secret, thus continuing the cycle of silence. Children are burdened by this powerful secret (Gossart-Walker & Moss, 1998).

Some children are aware of a secret within their families but are unable to name it. We have termed this as "naming vs. knowing" (Nagler et al., 1995), when children have been denied the name or even permission to know the name for the illness that they already recognize. Naming the illness permits a child to organize his or her ideas, fears, and feelings. However, many, if not most, caregivers worry about giving the name to their children. Using this conceptualization of the difference between "knowing" and "naming" has allowed us to work with parents and children in ways that we think are less assertive and confrontational than solely focusing on the issues of disclosure. With this strategy, we can try to help parents come to terms with what they believe their children already know, and to work with them about how to give their children the language with which to talk about the illness and their fears. In our work, we have learned that when children are able to develop a language for the disease that so devastates their families and alters their universe, they are no longer compelled to

act out their fears and their rage through maladaptive behaviors.

Community Approaches to Service Provision

Children and families who are most vulnerable to the deleterious effects of HIV/AIDS may also lack access to sufficient mental health care. For many disadvantaged families, access to adequate mental health care is already limited by restrictive criteria for obtaining health insurance and utilizing benefits within an existing managed care plan. Families who also contend with the chronic and acute effects of HIV-related illness in addition to poverty, social disadvantage, and individual and family psychopathology may be further hindered in their efforts to access traditional clinic- or office-based services when they are available. In essence, those with the greatest need may receive the least care. In response to these concerns, there has been a proliferation of community-based services where mental health care is provided in homes, schools, and community settings, with an emphasis on stabilization of individual and family psychopathology, collaboration with other community providers, and attention to the psychological needs of children affected by HIV/AIDS (Aber, Jones, Brown, Chaudry, & Samples, 1998; Boyd-Franklin & Bry, 2000; Bor & du Plessis, 1997; Burr & Lewis, 2000; Family Health Project Research Group, 1998; Gewirtz & Gossart-Walker, 2000; Murphy et al., 2002; Pilowsky, Wissow, & Hutton, 2000; Rotheram-Borus, Lee, Gwadz, & Draimin, 2001; Schonfeld, 2000; Woolston, Berkowitz, Schaefer, & Adnopoz, 1998).

The services offered by the Program for HIV-Affected Children and Families at the Yale Child Study Center are designed to meet the complex needs of children and families who are attempting to cope with HIV/AIDS and the related issues of loss, separation, and impending death. We have found that home-based family therapy and support, as well as community-based groups and home-based individual psychotherapy, are uniquely effective in addressing the mental health needs of children directly impacted by HIV/AIDS in their families. Because of the medical, psychological, and social complications of AIDS, families often require that services be provided in nontraditional ways.

The clinicians in the Program for HIV-Affected Children and Families recognize that while families may be willing to bring their children in to treatment, there are many obstacles to doing so, such as balancing multiple appointments for multiple family members and caregivers. By moving services into the home, we have been able to meet children's needs directly and avoid the problems of failed or missed appointments and other barriers to accessing mental health services in traditional settings. Within the home setting, children can receive psychiatric evaluation, psychological and developmental assessment and testing, and psychosocial evaluation in addition to psychotherapy. Because the therapeutic environment is selected on the basis of what is most appropriate to the specific child, individual therapy may be provided in the home or in a public place (e.g., school); when appropriate, the child may be transported to the therapist's office.

Program for HIV-Affected Children and Families at the Yale Child Study Center

HIV infection is a disease that not only affects the identified patient but also has marked significance for those persons who are within the patient's family and social networks. Whether the infected person is a parent, sibling, or child, the effects of the disease ripple throughout the immediate and extended family. When parents are infected, children are affected, and the possibility of separation from and loss of parents or other family members can have profound influence on intellectual, behavioral, and psychological development. When children themselves are infected, they must contend with their own physical illness, as well as with possible disruptions and disturbances in all other areas of their lives. Without direct early intervention, both affected and infected children are at risk for adverse, potentially devastating psychological effects.

Families affected by HIV/AIDS who may be poor, minority, isolated from community support, and struggling with substance abuse and/or mental illness (Geballe et al., 1995; Stein, 1998) may be those who are least able to use traditional mental health resources. Although they may need and desire intensive services, they may be unable to access

such services because of psychosocial stressors, medical symptomatology, conflicting priorities across multiple care systems, and lack of transportation. The Program for HIV-Affected Children and Families at the Yale Child Study Center attempts to overcome obstacles to care by providing mental health services directly in the homes and communities of children and their families (Gewirtz & Gossart-Walker, 2000).

The program is designed to follow families throughout the course of the illness and well after the death of the infected family member(s). Assistance is provided for children through their difficult transition period following the loss of their parent or caregiver, supporting them through the grieving process. Clinical staff assist affected children and families to express and resolve the practical, as well as psychological, problems related to an HIV diagnosis that often complicate and impede the process to obtain appropriate long-term custodial care for children. Goals are met through the provision of services most accessible to the client. Therefore, staff meet with children and their families in their own homes and in community settings such as schools, hospitals, and clinics.

Since its establishment in 1989, the Program for HIV-Affected Children and Families has mirrored the national needs of HIV-affected families (Adnopoz, Forsyth, & Nagler, 1994). Its initial focus was on the medical needs of HIV-infected infants and children, providing in-home support to assure medical compliance in an effort to prevent the children from being removed from their parents' care. Within 2 years the program expanded to include permanency planning with HIV-infected parents and supporting alternate caregiving arrangements. By the fifth year, a formal mental health intervention was established to provide services to HIV-infected and affected children in their homes and communities. The most recent expansion has included staff dedicated toward adolescents and youth who are HIV infected, affected, or at high risk for contracting the virus.

A master's-level social worker and a doctoral-level child psychologist coordinate the program, which includes master's-level social workers and family therapists (i.e., MSW and MFT) and family support workers. In addition, the program serves as a community training site for predoctoral psychology fellows, MSW interns, and BSW students.

Family support workers are nondegreed para-professionals who are recruited with a sensitivity to the cultural and ethnic backgrounds of the communities in which families reside. These workers bring with them experience in successful parenting in difficult circumstances, experience in negotiating social service systems, connections and credibility with the community, and a strong sense of affiliation with their clients.

The family support worker is an integral part of the team with the clinician. The clinical team initially meets with the family to assess their needs. As plans and goals are established, the clinical team may divide the work between its members. Often the family support worker will provide direct intervention with the parent, providing parent guidance, case management, and support, and the clinician will lead family therapy sessions, evaluate the children, and provide liaison with the schools. At times the family support worker provides the bridge between the formal clinical intervention and the family, interpreting the services in a way that the family can understand and accept. Because New Haven is a small city, some family support workers are personally familiar with the families in the program. Issues of professional boundaries are discussed in supervision and among the teams. The boundaries are made explicit to the families as well. For example, a family support worker may say, "Our children are in the same classroom, however, any information that I learn from you will not be shared with others outside our team, and any information I learn about you through our community will be kept private unless you would like me to share that with our team." With open communication, among the family support worker, the families, and the team, appropriate professional boundaries can be maintained. Families will often test the limits of the boundaries. With good supervision and team support, the family support worker will be comfortable in establishing and preserving boundaries.

The program currently provides home-based intervention with HIV-infected and HIV-affected children and adolescents, their parents, and alternate caregivers. A comprehensive range of child-oriented and family-focused mental health and supportive services includes the following:

- Home-based family therapy;
- Home-based individual child psychotherapy;
- Psychological evaluations (based in home, office, or community);
- Psychiatric consultations (based in home, office, or community);
- Support groups for HIV-affected children;
- Support groups for caregivers of infected and affected children;
- Life skills development group for infected and affected adolescents;
- Clinically informed case management;
- Collaboration and coordinated service planning with HIV-related and other agencies providing psychosocial services.

Philosophy of Intervention

The simple introduction of a child and/or parent to a mental health professional is most often insufficient to ensure successful treatment. Instead, an active outreach process consisting of home visits, follow-up phone calls after canceled and/or failed appointments, and arrangements for transportation to clinic-based appointments are a necessary process of forming a therapeutic alliance. This type of approach demands a high level of case coordination, comprehensive service linkage, and an integrated system of referral, all of which strengthen the capacity of individual agencies and programs to provide effective service, and improves the accessibility, availability, and appropriateness of the care received by children and families. Mental health services provide us a timely way, instead of waiting for crises to erupt, to help HIV-infected and HIV-affected children and their families cope with the trauma of HIV infection, prevent out-of-family placements, and mitigate the emergence of more serious psychopathology.

Each service provided by the Program for HIV-Affected Children and Families enables families to work through the psychological and emotional issues related to an HIV diagnosis that often complicate and impede their ability to obtain appropriate medical care for both children and adults. The program assists families to plan for alternate caregiving during periods of acute parental illness. In the event of death, plans enable children to avoid out-of-family placements at the critical times when they most need to be with adults they know and trust. The flexibility of the program enables families to receive services that are most appropriate at any given point in time, makes it possible for families to determine their own course of intervention, and assures that services remain in place for as long as necessary. Thus a family may receive services at varying levels of intensity that can include individual and family modalities provided in a range of settings and in consultation with a variety of providers (i.e., school professionals, child protective service workers, juvenile justice and law enforcement personnel, and medical providers). For example, over the course of an extended treatment, interventions might focus on practical life skills and problem solving, psychiatric symptoms secondary to HIV illness, coordination of service providers, or compliance with complicated medication regimens.

Using a team approach, clinicians and family support workers provide home-based clinical evaluation and intensive intervention to maintain HIV-infected and HIV-affected children safely within their families, prevent the disruption of the child's ties to primary caregivers, reduce the child's distress, and avert unnecessary placements. Upon accepting a referral, the clinical team begins the lengthy process of engagement that is often necessary to support the entry into treatment by HIV-infected and HIV-affected persons. This process includes home visitation, outreach, and building a relationship with the caregiver(s) to facilitate their comfort and willingness to allow the child to engage in therapy. This essential engagement process requires the expenditure of significant time, which can vary from days to months, and requires considerable clinical skill and understanding, as well as close coordination with the referring agency, to ensure that the children and families whom they identify as needing service actually enter the system. The clinical team must be respectful of families' hesitance and resistance to intervention. The approach to engagement must be at their pace. Often, the team must prove their motivation for engagement rather than the traditional reversal of the client proving his or her motivation for treatment.

Despite the intensity of the work, the staff within the Program for HIV-Affected Children and Families are able to balance the needs of a large number of children and families by creating flexible, individualized plans for each person involved in the program. Interventions are calibrated to meet the needs over time of the individual family in a flexible and useful manner. In some periods the intensity of our intervention is increased in re-sponse to particular crises, often occasioned by an impending or actual loss. For example, clinical teams have accompanied children to hospitals, providing direct support and intervention at times of greatest need. Similarly, in some periods a weekly or biweekly scheduled session is sufficient to support the children and families. This offers needed maintenance and often prevents reemergence of serious symptoms, averting problems before they disrupt fragile family systems.

Most challenging to this type of work is building the trust of resistant families. Repeated failed home visits are frustrating for the clinical team. The teams are often confronted by families who state by phone that they will be available, when the team arrives 20 minutes later, no one answers the door. This same scenario also provides the most valuable aspect of the work. As the team engages the family and earns their trust, the door (literally) opens and treatment begins. Once this occurs, the families will use the clinical team to explore their overwhelming concerns about their children, their illness, and potential death, often for the first time. Once the trust has been established, the clinical team can set into place services that will enhance the families' lives, including better housing, adequate food, and more appropriate academic placements.

Coordination With Other Providers

Due to the nature of the illness, few, if any families, enter or continue with our program without the active involvement of other providers. At the very least, HIV medical specialists are integral to the treatment. In the absence of specialized medical care or sufficient medical compliance, early interventions encourage and support a positive connection between the HIV-infected individual and medical providers. The program staff may broker this relationship to ensure appropriate care. While the focal point of the Program for HIV-Affected Children and Families may be the children, both infected and affected, the clinicians in the program develop positive working relationships with the children's HIV-infected parents and/or caregivers. Through this relationship, issues of parenting, illness, and stigma can be addressed. We have often seen that parents will attend to their children's health care needs before their own. The clinicians therefore are very mindful of the work that needs to be done to help a parent access health care.

Through a partnership with the parents, and with their ongoing collaboration with health care providers, clinicians are able to link the two together. Clinicians often find that reluctant HIV-infected parents are more willing to obtain their own health care if they are provided adequate support. Therefore, clinicians can provide a supportive ride to the clinic, can wait for the client in the waiting room, or can meet with the health care provider along with the client.

Emma was 3 years old when her parents' medical provider phoned the program for a consultation. He expressed worry because both parents were very ill, yet they refused any type of services. Over the next 2 years, [the social worker] spoke with the medical team periodically. She provided information on normative child development and language that they could use with the parents to offer guidance as they continued to refuse intervention for their daughter. When Emma was 5, her mother was critically ill in the intensive care unit and was resuscitated twice. Emma's father asked for assistance with his daughter; specifically, he wanted his daughter to have a person to talk to about her fears. The extended family refused, remembering that Emma's mother was emphatic about Emma seeing a therapist. A home visit was arranged with the father that included his in-laws and Emma. The service was explained, and they were encouraged to think about the needs of Emma. The family then "tested" [the social worker], leaving her alone with Emma but observing from another room ([the social worker] was unaware at the time that she was being observed). They then agreed to treatment with certain restrictions: [the social worker] could not tell Emma of her parents' ill health or use the words "dying," "dead," or "AIDS." Individual therapy was begun, once per week at either her father's or her grandparents' home. Emma often played spelling games as she tried to understand the secrets in her life. Family therapy sessions were impromptu, [the social worker] meeting with whomever was around during home visits. This successfully included the grandfather, whom all the other family members stated would not become involved. In fact, he requested scheduled family sessions periodically. Another team member met with the mother separately per her request. Emma's therapist also met with the mother at a nursing home to alleviate the mother's worries that the ther-

apist was disclosing too much. The team worked closely with the family and the medical providers through the deaths of both parents. They attended both funerals. They assisted in drawing up guardianship plans. Emma was able to make a smooth transition to her grandparents' home. At the time of this writing, she was doing well at school, and her grandparents were struggling, as they should, in their dual roles as grandparents and parents.

Other essential collaborations occur with AIDS-specific case managers, housing advocates, substance abuse treaters, child protective service workers, educators, and other mental health providers. Formal relationships have been established to ensure active and continuing discussions between program staff and community-based AIDS case managers and a local housing support agency. These relationships enhance case coordination and diminish duplication of services. Most important, these collaborations enhance the opportunities for the families to secure adequate housing, food, utilities, and other basic needs that are necessary prerequisites to mental health interventions. In addition, the clinical staff of the program support and teach case managers and housing advocates about family dynamics and child development, at times interpreting the behaviors displayed by the children and families to ensure that continued services are provided. For example, at times of intense stress and fear of death, some parents may lash out at their service providers. Through careful understanding, and a supportive team approach, the parent will not be discharged from a program but will be provided more individualized intervention.

The team is also involved with other aspects of the family members' lives and community network. The team will join the family at graduations and celebrations, when clinically appropriate. The team will set boundaries when invited to more intimate occasions such as baby showers but will supply cameras and film to document the celebrations. With the family's permission, the team will go to funerals. Again, at the funeral, professional boundaries are set. Often the family may want the team to become more intimately involved, such as sitting with the family at the service, but we find it important to maintain boundaries. Therefore, the team will often attend the funeral service but not attend the burial or a family reception that follows. While paying respects to the family, the team communicates that this is an important time for the family to be together, and that the team is available to them, but at a distance.

In addition to these collaborations, the team is active in the policy aspects of HIV/AIDS. Members of the program are on the board or are participants in a number of policymaking groups throughout the state. We encourage and support our clients to become involved as consumer advocates as well. Therefore, we will provide transportation or companionship to ensure their comfortable participation.

Supervision

Many of the children in our program have additional needs or limitations, such as mental retardation, psychiatric disturbance, or serious developmental delay, that require specialized interventions appropriate to their cognitive level and sensitive to the HIV issues in their families. These considerations make it necessary, even for otherwise well-trained mental health professionals, to be particularly knowledgeable about the disease and its sequelae when engaged in treating affected clients.

Clinicians who are confronted with difficult material—unexpected crises, maladaptive behavior such as aggression, and reports of deaths of caregivers and children—must be not only flexible and creative but also attuned to subtle nuances and aware of complex developmental and psychological factors. To continue to respond effectively and compassionately to these concerns, clinicians benefit from an ongoing, multidisciplinary forum that supports acquiring and honing the development of knowledge, therapeutic skills, and techniques. Essential to effective service provision is the range of knowledge that comes from a multidisciplinary team, with its multiple visions and ideas. We provide clinicians and family support workers with ongoing training and supervision that are uniquely specialized to HIV disease and specific to work with children. All program staff have access to multiple training opportunities through the Yale Child Study Center and through the AIDS training seminars offered by a number of entities throughout the state. Weekly individual supervision meetings, weekly conferences on group dynamics, and weekly multidisciplinary rounds provide the clinical support, feedback, and knowledge necessary to maintain our standards of intervention.

Evaluation and Program Sustainability

Reports by the Institute of Medicine (2000) and the Office of National AIDS Policy (Office of National AIDS Policy and the White House, 2000) highlight worrisome developments in the HIV/AIDS epidemic that require a coordinated national and international effort toward prevention of new infection and provision of care to those who are already infected. A comprehensive strategy to ameliorate the effects of HIV disease on children and adolescents should arise from such a concerted, national strategy focusing on both prevention of new HIV infection and treatment provision to HIV-positive and HIV-affected youth. Research will be needed to evaluate the transportability of prevention programs from school and clinic settings to community settings where youth at greatest risk are likely to be found, for example, juvenile justice and psychiatric settings and facilities. The availability of effective treatment for HIV disease does not, at present, portend a cure. Nonetheless, counseling and testing remain crucial ingredients in a public health approach to HIV and service provision.

Given the myriad psychosocial stressors encountered by HIV-infected and HIV-affected children and youth, comprehensive and effective medical and mental health services remain crucial to the success of medical treatment and to the stability of child and family psychological and social functioning. Access to care must be extended to children, adolescents, and families who have traditionally existed at the margins of the health care delivery system. Psychiatric treatment must support children's well-being in the context of their families. Interventions need to focus on maintaining stability of caregiving relationships and safety through a comprehensive strategy that addresses the medical and mental health needs of individual children, supports family functioning, addresses permanency planning for infected and affected youth, and coordinates care among psychiatric, medical, and social service providers (Burr & Lewis, 2000; Casey Family Services, 1999; Murphy et al., 2002).

Service programs face significant challenges in developing and sustaining mental health services for HIV-affected children and youth. Concerns about funding, including reliance on grant support, with its typically limited duration, or health insurance reimbursement, with its medical necessity and utilization management criteria, leave programs with an insecure funding base to provide services to a population beset by both acute and chronic mental health problems. Social workers and other professionals who have dedicated their careers to providing service to HIV-affected children and youth may feel understandably defensive about growing demands for accountability and outcome data to justify productivity or funding. For many, this is an unwelcome and unfamiliar agenda that seems to interfere with the main focus of their work. From another perspective, collection and analysis of service and program data may be viewed as an integral component of learning from one's clinical experience and modifying one's approach based on its relative strengths and weaknesses. One approach to dissemination research emphasizes the use of descriptive data about programs and services in an effort to traverse the distance between research and practice. Providers and researchers together form and sustain a "learning community" (Rosenheck, 2001a, 2001b) focused on providing the highest-quality service possible to a population that is often underserved in terms of both the quantity and quality of interventions. In the Yale Child Study Center program, an ongoing evaluation is designed to clarify the psychiatric and social functioning of affected children and determine conditions that facilitate or impede the implementation of permanency plans for affected youth.

Case Vignette

The R. family was referred to the Program for HIV-Affected Children and Families by a hospital social worker. Both parents had AIDS and alternated inpatient hospitalizations over the past year. They had three young girls, all HIV negative. The program clinician made arrangements to meet the parents at their home. Over several weeks, she had difficulty reaching them at their home, although it was clear that someone was inside but not answering the door. The family did not have a telephone, so she left handwritten notes in their mailbox indicating her phone number and when she would return. She learned from the hospital social worker that both parents were very sick, and they had ar-

ranged a system so that one would always be home with the girls, while the other, whichever was sicker, would go to the hospital for treatment. The clinician finally met with the father while he was hospitalized. He stated he was most worried about the fate of his girls, worried that both he and his wife were near death and there was no one to take the girls. He stated that his wife was very angry and distrustful of social workers because she feared the girls would be taken away from them. The clinician attempted to meet with the mother at home. She was in fact angry and hostile but was willing to talk through the closed door of her bedroom. Over time, the clinician gained the trust of both parents. As she sat by their sickbeds, not repulsed by their disease, making an effort to display care for them and their children, they were more willing to share their concerns and begin to establish a permanency plan. The clinician was finally given permission to meet with the girls, ages 5 to 10. She quickly observed that one girl was developmentally delayed, one was described as difficult, and the oldest was parentified. The parentified behavior included making all the meals, disciplining the younger children, and speaking as if she were the adult in the home.

Over the next few months the clinician, along with colleagues on the treatment team, began to help the family identify relatives who might be willing to raise the children upon their parents' death. Extended family members were identified, and plans were drawn up. The clinician established herself as a partner with the parents, both verbally and nonverbally indicating that they were the experts on their children, and she was there to support them in their parenting.

After several assessment sessions, the clinical team decided that the girls should receive weekly sibling sessions that would address their combined worries about their parents and their future. The oldest child began individual therapy sessions because her school had identified her as having behavioral problems in class. The sibling sessions took place at home in their kitchen. The individual therapy sessions took place at the girls' school. Concerns about their parents' health were clearly evident in all sessions. The girls drew pictures of houses and played with dolls. They clearly were afraid not only of their parents' deaths but also of not having adults to care for them. The primary clinician continued to work with the parents, focusing not only on the emotional support they needed but also on exploring all possibilities within the family and community for the girls. She sat silently during their sessions as the parents' conditions worsened. She was bearing witness to the family story.

During this process, other immediate but concrete issues were identified. The girls had chronic problems with lice. The school was frustrated with the lack of care the parents were able to provide in this area. The team consulted the local health department to assist in eradicating the lice from the girls' apartment. Financial assistance was obtained from various agencies. The treatment team remained in close communication with both parents' medical teams, including the visiting nurse and hospital social worker, to coordinate care and be prepared to intervene as their health declined. This was crucial upon the mother's death. The program team was available to assist the father in telling the girls. The mother died 9 months after the beginning of the intervention. Her husband died shortly afterward. The team continued to meet with the girls, now at their alternate caregiver's home. The team also worked closely with the school, providing consultation to the teachers and the principal on how to deal with the grieving girls, and support to the teachers who felt much sorrow about the girls' suffering.

The team continued to work with the girls, providing sibling and individual therapy, and attempted to provide support to the alternate caregivers. Unfortunately, the caregivers changed their minds about taking the girls within months of them moving in. The program team worked closely and intensively with the child protection agency to ensure that the girls were placed together. With the assistance of the school, they also continued in the same school through the end of the school year. The girls were placed in a foster home, which resulted in a failed adoption (this family changed its mind as well). At the time of this writing, the girls are now in a new "pre-adoptive" home. They have been there 1 year, but this new set of parents is having some questions. The team continues to work closely with the girls and all other service providers to attempt to establish a permanent plan. Issues of abandonment are clearly at the forefront for the girls. They lost their biological family, then the adoptive family, and now maybe another family. As they get older, the possibility of a permanent family will diminish. And, unfortunately, it is the paid staff of the Program for HIV-Affected Children and Families who has become the holder of their history; it is the program that knew their parents, knew their neighborhood and schools, and followed them from home to home. It is the program team that has kept them connected to their community.

From the beginning of treatment, a memory book was created by the program staff and the girls. While the staff did not anticipate the multiple transitions, the memory books have been useful to document not only the bad times (deaths, losses of families), but also the good (awards at school).

Although this is not a successful case of the Program for HIV-Affected Children and Families, it does illustrate the frustrations associated with this disease. Without home-based intervention, the parents would have never been able to make use of mental health or supportive services. Without these services, there is a good chance that the child protection agency may have removed the children before their parents' deaths and have separated the girls. Through the respectful and thoughtful engagement process, both parents were able to die peacefully, knowing that they had resolved their anger and connected with their children. Through intensive intervention, which includes everyone in the children's lives, they have been able to locate older half siblings, who, while not able to raise the girls, have become an important part of their lives.

References

Aber, L., Jones, S., Brown, J., Chaudry, N., & Samples, F. (1998). Resolving conflict creatively: Evaluating the developmental effects of a school-based violence prevention program in neighborhood and classroom context. *Development and Psychopathology, 10*, 187–213.

Adnopoz, J., Forsyth, B., & Nagler, S. (1994). Psychiatric aspects of HIV infection and AIDS on the family. *Child and Adolescent Psychiatric Clinics of North America, 3*, 543–555.

Armistead, L., & Forehand, R. (1995). For whom the bell tolls: Parenting decisions and challenges faced by mothers who are HIV seropositive. *Clinical Psychology: Science and Practice, 2*, 239–250.

Armistead, L., Summers, P., Forehand, R., Morse, P., Morse, E., & Clark, L. (1999). Understanding of HIV/AIDS among children of HIV-infected mothers: Implications for prevention, disclosure and bereavement. *Children's Health Care, 28,* 277–295.

Armistead, L., Tannenbaum, L., Forehand, R., Morse, E., & Morse, P. (2001). Disclosing HIV Status: Are mothers telling their children? *Journal of Pediatric Psychology, 26,* 11–20.

Booth, R., & Zhang, Y. (1997). Conduct disorder and HIV risk behaviors among runaway and homeless adolescents. *Drug and Alcohol Dependence, 48,* 69–76.

Bor, R., & du Plessis, P. (1997). The impact of HIV/AIDS on families: An overview of recent research. *Families, Systems, and Health, 15,* 413–427.

Boyd-Franklin, N. (1989). *Black families in therapy: A multisystems approach.* New York: Guilford.

Boyd-Franklin, N., & Bry, B. (2000) *Reaching out in family therapy: Home-based, school and community interventions.* New York: Guilford.

Brown, L., Danovsky, M., Lourie, K., DiClemente, R., & Ponton, L. (1997). Adolescents with psychiatric disorders and the risk of HIV. *Journal of the American Academy of Child and Adolescent Psychiatry, 36,* 1609–1617.

Burr, C. K., & Lewis, S. (2000). *Making the invisible visible: Services for families living with HIV infections and their affected children.* National Pediatric and Family HIV Resource Center, University of Medicine and Dentistry of New Jersey, Newark.

Casey Family Services. (1999). *Planning children's futures: Meeting the needs of children, adolescents and families affected by HIV.* Shelton, CT: Author.

Centers for Disease Control. (1998). Young people at risk: Epidemic shifts further toward young women and minorities. *CDC Update,* pp. 1–2.

Centers for Disease Control. (2000). U.S. HIV and AIDS cases reported through December 1999. *HIV/AIDS Surveillance Report, 11*(21), 5–6.

Centers for Disease Control. (2001). *Morbidity and Mortality Weekly Report, 50*(21), 2.

Dane, B., & Levine, C. (1994). *AIDS and the new orphans.* Westport, CT: Auburn House.

Draimin, B. (1995). A second family? Custody and placement decisions. In S. Geballe, J. Gruendel, & W. Andiman (Eds.), *Forgotten children of the AIDS epidemic* (pp. 125–139). New Haven, CT: Yale University Press.

Faithful, J. (1997). HIV positive and AIDS-infected women: Challenges and difficulties of mothering. *American Journal of Orthopsychiatry, 67,* 144–151.

Family Health Project Research Group. (1998). The Family Health Project: A multidisciplinary longitudinal investigation of children whose mothers are HIV infected. *Clinical Psychology Review, 18,* 839–856.

Geballe, S., Gruendel, J., & Andiman, W. (Eds.).

(1995). *Forgotten children of the AIDS epidemic.* New Haven, CT: Yale University Press.

Gewirtz, A., & Gossart-Walker, S. (2000). Home-based treatment for children and families affected by HIV/AIDS: Dealing with stigma, secrecy, disclosure and loss. *Psychiatric Clinics of North America, 9,* 313–330.

Goffman, E. (1963). *Stigma: Notes on the management of spoiled identity.* Englewood Cliffs, NJ: Prentice Hall.

Gossart-Walker, S., & Moss, N. (1998). Support groups for HIV-affected children. *Journal of Child and Adolescent Group Therapy, 8,* 55–69.

Hackl, K., Sonlai, A., Kelly, J., & Kalichman, S. (1997). Women living with HIV/AIDS: The dual challenge of being a patient and a caregiver. *Health and Social Work, 22,* 53–62.

Hein, K., Dell, R., Futterman, D., Rotheram-Borus, M. J., & Shaffer, N. (1995). Comparison of HIV+ and HIV− adolescents: Risk factors and psychological determinates. *Pediatrics, 95,* 96–104.

Institute of Medicine. (2000). *No time to lose: Getting more from HIV prevention.* Washington, DC: National Academy Press.

Jemmott, J., Jemmott, L., & Fong, G. (1992). Reductions in HIV risk-associated sexual behaviors among black male adolescents: Effects of an AIDS prevention intervention. *American Journal of Public Health, 82,* 372–377.

Kalichman, S. (2000). HIV transmission risk behaviors of men and women living with HIV-AIDS: Prevalence, predictors, and emerging clinical interventions. *Clinical Psychology: Science and Practice, 7,* 32–47.

Lefkowitz, E., Sigman, M., & Au, T. K. (2000). Helping mothers discuss sexuality and AIDS with adolescents. *Child Development, 71,* 1383–1394.

Main, D., Iverson, D., Mcgloin, J., Banspach, S., Collins, J., Rugg, D., & Kolbe, L. (1994). Preventing HIV infection among adolescents: Evaluation of a school-based education program. *Preventive Medicine, 23,* 409–417.

Marans, S., & Cohen, D. (1996). Child psychoanalytic theories of development. In M. Lewis (Ed.), *Child and adolescent psychiatry: A comprehensive textbook* (pp. 156–170). Baltimore: Williams and Wilkins.

Mayes, L., & Cohen, D. (1993). The social matrix of aggression: Enactments and representations of loving and hating in the first years of life. *Psychoanalytic Study of the Child, 48,* 145–169.

Michaels, D., & Levine, C. (1992). Estimates of the number of motherless youth orphaned by AIDS in the United States. *Journal of the American Medical Association, 268,* 3456–3461.

Murphy, R. A., Forsyth, B.W.C., & Adnopoz, J.

(2002). Neurobiological and psychosocial sequelae of HIV disease in children and adolescents. In M. Lewis (Ed.), *Comprehensive textbook of child and adolescent psychiatry*. Baltimore: Williams and Wilkins.

Nagler, S., Adnopoz, J., & Forsyth, B. (1995). Uncertainty, stigma and secrecy: Psychological aspects of AIDS for children and adolescents. In S. Geballe, J. Gruendel & W. Andiman (Eds.), *Forgotten children of the AIDS epidemic*. New Haven, CT: Yale University Press.

Office of National AIDS Policy and the White House. (2000). *Youth and HIV/AIDS 2000: A new American agenda*. Washington, DC: Author.

Pilowsky, D., Wissow, L., & Hutton, N. (2000). Children affected by HIV: Clinical experience and research findings. *Psychiatric Clinics of North America, 9*, 451–464.

Rosenheck, R. (2001a). Organizational process: A missing link between research and practice. *Psychiatric Services, 52*, 1607–1612.

Rosenheck, R. (2001b). Stages in the implementation of innovative clinical programs in complex organizations. *Journal of Nervous and Mental Diseases, 189*, 812–821.

Roth, J., Siegel, R., & Black, S. (1994). Identifying the mental health needs of children living in families with AIDS or HIV infections. *Community Mental Health Journal, 30*, 581–593.

Rotheram-Borus, M. J., Draimin, B., Reid, H., & Murphy, D. (1997). The impact of illness disclosure and custody plans on adolescents whose parents live with AIDS. *AIDS, 11*, 1159–1164.

Rotheram-Borus, M. J., Lee, M., Gwadz, M., & Draimin, B. (2001). An intervention for parents with AIDS and their adolescent children. *American Journal of Public Health, 91*, 1294–1302.

Schoeberlein, D., Woolston, J., & Brett, J. (2000). School-based HIV prevention: A promising model. *Psychiatric Clinics of North America, 9*, 389–406.

Schonfeld, D. (2000). Teaching young children about HIV and AIDS. *Psychiatric Clinics of North America, 9*, 375–388.

Stein, T. (1998). *The social welfare of women and children with HIV and AIDS*. New York: Oxford University Press.

Stiffman, A., Dore, P., Earls, F., & Cunningham, R. (1992). The influence of mental health problems on AIDS-related risk behaviors in young adults. *Journal of Nervous and Mental Diseases, 180*, 314–320.

St. Lawrence, J., Brasfield, T., Jefferson, K., Alleyne, E., O'Bannon, R., & Shirley, A. (1995). Cognitive-behavioral intervention to reduce African-American adolescents' risk for HIV infection. *Journal of Consulting and Clinical Psychology, 63*, 221–227.

UNAIDS. (2000, June). *Report on the global HIV/AIDS epidemic*.

Walsh, M. E., & Bibace, R. (1991). Children's conceptions of AIDS: A developmental analysis. *Journal of Pediatric Psychology, 16*, 273–285.

Woolston, J., Berkowitz, S., Schaefer, M., & Adnopoz, J. (1998). Intensive, integrated, in-home psychiatric services: The catalyst to enhancing outpatient intervention. *Child and Adolescent Psychiatric Clinics of North America, 7*, 615–633.

Worden, W. (1991). *Grief counseling and grief therapy: A handbook for the mental health practitioner*. New York: Springer.

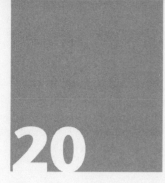

20

Phebe Sessions and Verba Fanolis

Partners for Success
10 Years of Collaboration Between a School for Social Work and an Urban Public School System

This chapter will present the work of Partners for Success (PfS), a collaborative project between Smith College School for Social Work (SSW) and an urban public school system of a midsize city in the Northeast. In a context of widespread experimentation in locating mental health services in the public schools, this program succeeded in achieving the goals of providing multisystemic mental health services consistent with system-of-care principles, while preparing social work interns for clinical and leadership roles in school-based mental health services. The services were provided through the placement of teams of social work interns in elementary schools (four full-time interns in each of two schools for 35 hours per week over the course of an 8-month field placement) with on-site supervision, supported by a training program from the SSW.

In this chapter, we will describe the impetus for the project, the initial negotiations between the two partners, the agreed-upon goals, the initial stages of entry and engagement, a lengthy period of stability and expansion, the clinical model that evolved over time, evaluative studies of the degree of satisfaction experienced by different stakeholders, and the process of adjustment to recent financial crisis in the schools, with reduction in the scope of the program, coupled with integration into the structure of the school system. We will supplement our story by integrating discussions of important issues from the literature about school-based mental health practice, as well as with case examples of our work.

Impetus for the Project

Our project began in the early 1990s at the instigation of both the public school system and the SSW. The school system was embarking on a period of major reform with a new superintendent who was determined to set high standards for achievement in this urban school system, which had undergone a demographic shift toward a greater concentration of low-income children and families of color. He sought a collaboration with the SSW with the hope of infusing the youthful energy of interns and the mental health and social service expertise of social work into the schools as a part of his reforms. The faculty of the SSW, in turn, had been searching for ways to enhance our ability to prepare graduates for practice with at-risk children and families in community-based settings. They were also formulating as part of the school's mission a commitment to becoming an antiracist institution, which involved examining all its programs to consider how they could be enhanced to more proactively address problems of racism. One of the concerns uncovered in this examination was that many child- and family-serving social agencies were insufficiently serving the changing population of the area, particularly children and families of color. As a result, our interns were not receiving sufficient preparation for effective practice with these populations. With reform occurring in a nearby school system, the SSW became interested in a partnership in which excellent service and excellent training could support each other.

Both professions, education and mental health, were responding with concern at that time to several disturbing trends affecting American children, including evidence from epidemiological studies of emotional and behavioral disorders of a rise in diagnosable conditions in children; increase in child poverty and greater knowledge of its deleterious effects; increased exposure of children to violence in families, schools, and neighborhoods; cultural mismatches between professionals in both education and mental health, with the children and families they serve due to changing demographics; increased pressure on schools to be accountable for equitable outcomes for all children, without sufficient resources to ensure these outcomes; and lack of increase in the capacity of child mental health services to cope with these changes.

Rates of Emotional and Behavioral Disturbance

One concern centered on the rising rates of psychiatric symptomatology among American children and the effects of such symptoms on the ability of children to succeed in school and develop into emotionally and vocationally successful adults. Achenbach, Domenci, and Rescorla (2003), in a review of reports of emotional and behavioral disturbance in children by parents and teachers from 1973 to the present, revealed that rates had increased dramatically from 1973 through 1993 when we initiated our program; rates of increase from 1993 to 2003 have slowed but remain unacceptably high, with approximately 20% of American children showing the symptoms of a *DSM-IV* emotional or behavioral disorder (Center for Mental Health in Schools at UCLA, 2003b). Though the prevalence of disturbance has increased, the avail-

ability of specialized resources for effective interventions has not improved enough to address these needs. Studies by Jane Knitzer (1982) and special commissions to examine the state of children's mental health (U.S. Department of Public Health, 2000) have revealed serious gaps in the quantity and quality of care, especially for children with serious emotional disturbance and for children in socially disadvantaged environments (Lourie, 2003). Recent studies in fact indicate that children with severe emotional disturbance are less likely to receive specialized mental health care than are children with milder disturbance (Harrison, McKay, & Bannon, 2004).

Increased Poverty Among Children and Recognition of Its Effects

During the 1980s, the rate of poverty among American children rose substantially. Reviews of studies examining the effects of poverty document higher rates of impairment among low-income children due to a concentration of risk factors and fewer protective factors in their lives (Evans, 2004; Linver, Fuligni, Hernandez, & Brooks-Gunn, 2004; Luthar, 1999). Evans (2004) reports that more than 50% of low-income families have three or more risk factors, whereas 60% of non-low-income families experience no more than one risk factor. Access to comprehensive mental health services is severely limited by variables of social class, race, and severity of symptoms. A majority of mental health services (about 75%), especially those that are available to disenfranchised populations, are provided through the public schools (Stroul, 1996). Without such services, many low-income children who might benefit substantially from them are diverted into juvenile justice and child welfare systems. These frequently overburdened public bureaucracies are often not sufficiently prepared to address mental health needs, contributing to the greater likelihood that low-income children, particularly children of color, will have their mental health symptoms managed with restraint and punishment.

Concerns About Violence in Schools, Families, and Neighborhoods

Similarly, the substantial rise in the exposure of American children to violence at home, in their schools, and in their neighborhoods throughout the 1980s and well into the 1990s alarmed all child-serving professions. Osofsky (1997) and Garbarino (1999) documented the rise in exposure to violence and commission of violent acts by children, as well as the deeply troubling consequences of violence for children's well-being. Though most children who are exposed to violence do not develop symptoms of post–traumatic stress disorder, many do suffer neurodevelopmental effects from chronic hyperarousal of the sympathetic nervous system during and after these events (Perry, 1997). It is also clear that exposure to violence increases anxiety, behavior disorders, difficulties in concentration, depression, problems with sleep, and difficulties in trusting social institutions as providers of nurturance and protection. Pynoos, Steinberg, and Goenjian (1996) have found that exposure to trauma has its most severe effects on the child's cognitive schema about moral authority in his or her social world. All these effects profoundly influence children's readiness to show up in a classroom able to attend to cognitive learning.

Cultural Mismatches Between Professionals and the Children and Families They Serve

The racial and ethnic composition of the U.S. population has been changing markedly, particularly among younger families. According to Pumariega (2003), youth of color currently constitute 30% of the under-18 population, with their percentage expected to rise to 40% by 2020 and to surpass 50% by 2030. Despite these changes in demographics and the stated goals of multicultural competence, both education and mental health have been slow to adapt teaching and clinical practice methods. They also have been timid about addressing the historical legacy and current dynamics of racism as they affect their professions. Professor of education Sonia Nieto (1996, 1999) notes that there continues to be what she calls a "hidden curriculum" of unintentional messages, which contradict school policies of equity, leading to children of color receiving "watered-down" curricula, less experimental teaching, lower expectations for achievement, and greater likelihood of being tracked into poor achievement levels. Nieto also expresses concern about the relative absence of talk about cultural difference in schools, leaving many social and inter-

personal issues and tensions unaddressed. Like some African American educators and scholars (Ferguson, 2000; Hale, 1994), Nieto (1999) observes that many low-income students of color may come to view education as a process of "deculturalization," which they feel they should resist:

> Because schools have traditionally perceived their role as that of an assimilating agent, the isolation and rejection that come hand in hand with immigration and colonization have simply been [brought through] the schoolhouse door. Curriculum and pedagogy, rather than using the lived experiences of students as a foundation, have been based on what can be described as an alien and imposed reality. The rich experiences of millions of our students, and their parents, grandparents, and neighbors, have been kept strangely quiet. . . . No child should have to make the painful choice between family and school and what inevitably becomes the choice between belonging and succeeding. (p. 3)

Pressure on Schools for Accountability

Public schools have been under increased pressure, through both legislation and public policy, to provide education for children with a wide range of disabilities, including those challenged by emotional and behavioral disorders, in the most normative settings possible. Meeting the standards for special education services requires cross-disciplinary planning meetings of many participants providing these supportive services. At the same time, schools are also required to demonstrate that they are producing equitable outcomes for children despite substantial differences between socially advantaged and disadvantaged children in the "cultural capital" that has been available to them. With schools receiving widely disparate amounts of financial support through local taxation, socially advantaged children are more readily prepared for success, and less socially advantaged children for obstacles to success. Yet schools in less privileged communities are currently threatened with punitive measures if their children cannot perform successfully on standardized tests of achievement. To cope with these competing mandates and enhance the likelihood of academic success, public schools have needed more support from other child-serving disciplines.

Restrictions of Insurance in Mental Health Settings and Effectiveness of School-Based Mental Health Practice

Mental health clinicians have encountered increasing obstacles in the provision of multisystemic interventions for children and families. Recent implementation of fee-for-service contracts means that clinicians are often paid only for direct service interviews with child and/or family, depending on the policies of particular third-party payers. They are often not paid for no-show appointments or for collaborative meetings with other professionals to coordinate services. These policies have led clinicians to avoid outreach to clients with complex psychosocial needs requiring a lot of advocacy and interagency coordination. Since effective child mental health services are most dependent on these activities in socially disenfranchised communities, there has been an active search by service providers and planners for alternatives. Locating mental health services in the public schools helps with the problems of access to children in need and collaborative work with teachers. Furthermore, research into the effectiveness of school-based mental health services indicates that outcomes are at least equivalent and with some populations superior to those delivered in a clinical setting (Armbruster & Lichtman, 1999).

Initial Negotiations

In the initial meetings between the SSW and the administrators of the school system, common ground was immediately established around shared interests in the work of Peter Senge and Paolo Freire. With *The Fifth Discipline* (Senge, 1990) displayed prominently on his desk, the superintendent began to describe his interests in reforming the school system around Senge's principles for changing organizations, including school systems, by developing a "learning organization" that enhances the effectiveness of all participants. The principles that guide a learning organization include developing a shared vision for change, support for teamwork, a systemic perspective on the interdependence of all parts of a system, active questioning of fixed models that interfere with receptivity to new ideas, and a constructionist orientation that emphasizes our responsibility for generating the future we desire (Senge, 2000). These principles resonate deeply with the priorities of social work. The interest and respect for these principles and goals to guide both education and mental health created a dynamic foundation to our collaboration.

Other administrators in the school system were actively trying to use the critical pedagogical ideas of Paolo Freire to instigate reform (Senge, 2000). Freire emphasized the need to draw upon learners' own experiences in their education to achieve literacy, so that they are not simply recipients of abstracted knowledge systems but are actively engaged in cocreating knowledge through the sharing of their own indigenous wisdom based on life experience. A critical perspective on the "banking concept" of education, which conceives of teaching as putting expert knowledge into an empty receptacle, recognizes instead the value of multiple sources of knowledge. Though Freirian ideas have been more influential in education than in mental health, they do have corollaries in social constructionist, empowerment models in mental health practice, which focus on eliciting clients' strengths and ensuring client self determination in shaping the direction of therapy (Gutierrez, Parsons, & Cox, 1998).

The priorities for the project from the school administrators included the following:

1. Mental health services that were sensitive to and respectful of the educational mission of the public schools;
2. Full integration of the project into the ongoing life of the schools;
3. Extensive family outreach and positive engagement of families in their child's education; and
4. Cultural competence in the program, which integrated knowledge of the cultural traditions of students and families.

School administrators were familiar with different models of collaborative programs, including "school-linked services," in which child mental health professionals from agencies in the community provided services on-site in the schools. The school system also had placed adjustment and guidance counselors in every school, and each school had access to part-time school psychologists. The goal of the schools in seeking this collaboration with the SSW was not to displace these traditional school-based professionals or to eliminate mental health services from the local agencies. Administrators were interested in having the project provide services that were complementary to what they were already offering, with a particular focus on work with children who would not otherwise have access to intensive work, integration of a mental health perspective into the life of the school, and outreach to families and community.

One concern that had to be addressed in this initial negotiation was a legacy of conflict between the school system and some institutions of higher education in the area. School administrators were concerned that previous affiliations with universities had led to substantial research projects in the schools. Though this research contributed to knowledge development in the field of education, it had failed to make a lasting impact on the resources of the school system itself. Therefore, they wanted some guarantee that knowledge generation would be balanced by a long-term commitment to bring enduring resources and add value to the schools.

Additional priorities of the SSW were to balance excellent service with excellent training. We felt that could best be achieved through a concentration of resources in a limited number of schools. Sizable teams would promote team learning and enable delivery of a full range of intensive services that could be flexibly designed to respond to the needs of individual children and families. They would ensure that the project would have the capacity to provide multisystemic interventions and that it could maximize the infusion of mental health knowledge into the life of the school. We also wanted to be located in schools with a high level of psychosocial need, with principals and counseling staff who would actively collaborate with the program. We understood that the SSW teams would be providing many hours of service in the schools, and to make the project work, we were requesting many hours of collaborative time from intensely busy professionals. We also understood that to respond to their requests for full integration of teams in the schools, we would have much to learn about the mission, values, structure, and procedures of public education.

Goals and Structure

Out of this period of negotiation, the partners achieved agreement on the following goals:

1. Delivery of mental health services that addressed problems at multiple systemic levels, including those of the individual child, family, school community, and neighborhood;
2. Training of social work interns with support of on-site supervisors and a training program through the SSW to ensure infusion of current "best practices";
3. Management of program through integration of feedback from evaluative studies and collaborative participation of multiple stakeholders in the public schools and SSW;
4. Partnership that brought resources to the public schools from SSW of multicultural competence and responsiveness, knowledge base about the effects of trauma on children and families, capacity for bridging the gulf between school, families, and communities and that, in turn, brought resources from the public schools to SSW about the integration of mental health and the professional priorities of education.

The structure of the program varied over the course of 10 years but has generally included the following elements:

1. A program director and a supervisor to provide on-site training in two central-city elementary schools with between 600 and 800 students;
2. Two teams of four full-time social work interns who worked for 35 hours per week on 8-month field placements;
3. Weekly training sessions in individual, family, group, and community practice provided by SSW faculty;
4. Consultation regarding cross-cultural issues in practice from cultural consultants;
5. Twice-yearly meetings with public school administrators;
6. Weekly meetings with principals and guidance and adjustment counselors;
7. Evaluative studies every 3 years with an outside evaluator;
8. Service provision, including crisis intervention, individual and family assessment and

counseling, groups for parents and for children, family outreach, advocacy, and engagement in the life of the school, intensive and ongoing collaboration with teachers, both within and outside of the classroom, and psychoeducational presentations to enhance capacity for children, families, and school professionals;

9. From 3 to 5 hours of service by each of the social work participants in the program, including the director, in a community after-school program, providing a bridge between school and community and contributing mental health resources to community workers;

10. Dissemination of information about the program through conferences, curriculum development, and a follow-up study on the professional activities of the graduates of the program.

Entry and Engagement

The project represented a significant increase in person power for the two elementary schools we joined and was enthusiastically received from the beginning. The SSW team were pleased with their welcome into the school community and the access they had to work with children and families in a nonstigmatizing setting. For many low-income families, seeking "mental health" services carries the burden of stigma of possible "craziness" and a damaged identity. The specialized language and procedures of formal mental health clinics can seem remote from everyday pressing concerns for families. While families and children may have little understanding of how "therapy" might be useful, they do have a greater understanding of "counseling" in the context of an educational setting. Locating mental health services in the schools did indeed eliminate many of the problems of access. Children quickly learned to use the resource of a team of social workers committed to helping them in times of trouble, and few families refused an offer of engagement with the project. The emphasis on building relationships carefully and empathically with everyone in the system was continuously upheld by the project director and supervisors, modeling these skills for interns. Nevertheless, our social work teams and the school-based professionals underwent serious growing pains of mutual adjust-

ment. Adjustment issues for the SSW team included the following:

1. Learning about and understanding the host profession of education;
2. Developing relationships with school-based professionals in a range of roles;
3. Developing a structure for services that honors the knowledge base and represents the priorities of both professions; and
4. Dealing with the specific issues that frequently create friction between mental health workers and educators in the schools, including issues of confidentiality, privacy, space, time for crisis response, and time for community engagement.

Understanding the Host Profession

Though the supervisors and some interns had previous experience in school-based settings, our goals of full integration into the school community demanded that we become much more knowledgeable about public education: its mission and public mandates, current controversies and challenges, issues facing the local school system, and the methods and procedures of the particular schools in which the project was located.

Education in this country is a hotly contested political issue, since schools have a significant role in providing and managing social and vocational opportunities for the next generation. Americans may agree about the central importance of education in civic life, with every president in recent history assuming the mantle of "the education president," but they have strong disagreements about how schools should be structured, managed, financed, and evaluated. Widely debated topics of bilingual education, the role of standardized testing, rights to inclusion of children in mainstream classrooms who have a range of physical, emotional, and behavioral challenges, effectiveness of violence- and drug-prevention programs, inequity in resources available to school boards in low-income communities that are largely dependent on local taxes, school choice through vouchers or charter schools, as well as the advisability of integrating mental health and social service resources in the schools, powerfully shape educational practices (Allen-Meares, 2004; Center for Mental Health in Schools at UCLA, 2004). Though social work as a profession educates practitioners to be knowledgeable about, and advocate for, significant policy issues, practitioners in mental health settings often experience greater insulation from public debate than do educators. While there have been important federal commissions to advise and plan for mental health policy, these debates take place at a much more subdued level of exposure. For mental health professionals to enter into the world of public education is to become swiftly immersed in the public controversies affecting education and their very real effects on institutions and the people they serve. Our social work teams needed ongoing training opportunities to understand the systemic effects of these public issues.

The mission of education is to prepare children and youth for contributing social roles through the acquisition of the knowledge and skills in school that will enable them to perform these roles. Emotional health and competence in children are contributing factors in the achievement of this mission, but it is not the primary mission of education to promote them. For mental health practitioners to be relevant in the school setting, they need to understand how their efforts to promote emotional health contribute to the primary educational goal of knowledge and skill development. Emotional and behavioral problems have increasingly been conceptualized in the school-based mental health practice literature as "barriers to learning" (Center for Mental Health in Schools at UCLA, 2003a). Schools sanction the involvement of mental health practitioners because of their ability to remove such barriers, allowing learning to occur. Mental health professionals, however, tend to view the achievement of emotional health and reduction in symptoms of emotional and behavioral disorders as ends in themselves. These differences in primary goals set up sources of strain between the professions if they are not understood and, to some extent, harmonized.

Relationships With School-Based Professionals

When polarized, school professionals see themselves as supporting a classroom and community of learners; mental health professionals see themselves as dealing with a caseload of individual children and families. School professionals often see mental health professionals as "naive" when they advocate for greater empathy for the individual child in the classroom, and they believe that mental health workers do not understand the effect of the child's behavior on the learning environment. They often believe that mental health workers can easily be manipulated by children in a one-to-one therapeutic relationship, and that they underestimate children's aggression and responsibility. Mental health professionals often see school professionals as overly zealous in discipline or critical feedback, undermining their efforts to engage the child positively in the learning activities of the classroom. They often advocate that school professionals consider the individual circumstances of the child, respond empathically, and/or set up elaborate behavioral reinforcement systems. The power of a therapeutic relationship is indeed fueled by empathy, consideration of the complexity of the individual circumstance, and analysis of the functions of particular behaviors. Consequently, mental health professionals often use the expertise of their own professions to advise school professionals to approach children as though they were in a therapeutic environment. However, this advice may fall on deaf ears because it runs into conflict with the responsibility of the teacher to the classroom as a whole, and the methods of the teaching profession.

In our entry into the public schools, we quickly encountered such misunderstandings between our clinical team and school professionals. To put it bluntly, many interns were seriously distressed that some of the teachers were "too mean." An oft-repeated incident occurred when an intern arrived in a classroom at the appointed hour for a student and a teacher announced to the class: "You've come to pick up José for counseling? That's great. He's been terrible today, hasn't he, boys and girls?" Teachers, in turn, felt that the interns sometimes were "too soft" and, their favorite term, "naive." Consolidation of pejorative images around adjectives like "mean" and "naive" can undermine effective collaboration between the two professions.

In the initial stages of the project, leadership by the on-site supervisors was critical in preventing this kind of polarization. Supervisors modeled for interns how to enter classrooms and truly listen to teachers' concerns. In a hierarchical system, teachers tended to feel "equal" to the supervisors but not to the interns. Efforts by the interns to provide "expert" advice were not welcomed. The major lesson from this period was the importance of care in the negotiation of collaborative relationships. Too much "expertise" from the mental health team was sometimes experienced as intrusive and undermining of the school professionals' understanding of their own roles. Too little "expertise" would quickly lead to concern about valuable time being wasted. The sensitive and effective negotiation of these relationships was critical to the later stabilization and success of the project.

Development of a Structure for Services

The school social work literature lists as roles for social workers in schools: consultant, clinical interventionist, enabler and facilitator, collaborator, educator, mediator, advocate, diversity specialist, manager, case manager and broker, community interventionist, and policy initiator and developer (Franklin, 2004). We certainly found that effective practice in the schools does indeed require implementation of all these roles. Their multiplicity, however, is daunting, particularly for social workers who, as in most schools, are alone in their school and must manage their roles without much access to other social workers. As we entered into our partnership with the public schools, we were confronted with the need to develop a strategic plan for service delivery, allocating specific amounts of time and resources to these diverse roles.

The pace of activity in schools is intense, fueled by youthful energy and relatively frequent crises. School professionals had no difficulty generating ideas about how the intern teams could be useful. The presence and active involvement of adults in monitoring and protecting children during transitional times, such as coming to and leaving school, lunchtime, moving between classes, during outside trips, and at recess, is a critical need in schools. Research into violence in schools shows that most violent incidents occur not in the classroom but in these transitional spaces (Astor, Benbenishty, Pitcher, & Meyer, 2004). Consequently, children are most fearful of bullying and other forms of aggression during these times. To be a fully engaged participant in the school community, each team member was required to contribute at least an hour each day to these supportive activities. This was not always a popular requirement among the interns,

some of whom resented having to perform what they considered to be "nonprofessional" roles. However, their work in the school community earned them visibility, relationships, and respect. They soon learned that these activities were also exceptional and unique opportunities for making effective interventions in the lives of troubled children.

Case Example

A young male intern from a military background had been concerned about his field placement assignment to an elementary school. He feared that he lacked both the sensitivity and the interest to be useful in his work with children. He was assigned to work with a 7-year-old Puerto Rican boy who was showing signs of significant depression. Ramon was living in a multigenerational all-female household, since his father had been imprisoned several years earlier with a lengthy sentence. The father's crime and imprisonment were a source of shame for the family, so his name was seldom mentioned. The intern was beginning to understand through his work with Ramon individually and with the family how significant the loss of the father was to Ramon, when a critical incident occurred while the intern was on lunch duty. A group of classmates were teasing a tearful Ramon about his lack of a father and called to the intern to settle the dispute. "Hey, mister! Ramon says you're his father. But he don't have no father. Are you his father?" The intern felt momentarily paralyzed by the challenge to respond helpfully in such a public setting. But his response was heartfelt and created a turning point in Ramon's ability to function in the classroom and his own level of interest and confidence in working in the school setting. He said, "I would be very proud to be Ramon's father." This response transformed the certain humiliation and defeat for Ramon into victory, with the valuable and truthful affirmation of his worthiness as a son.

School professionals were also more than happy to recruit an intern in the halls to come help with a crisis of student behavior in a classroom. Without structure, reactivity to crisis could have consumed most of the time available to the team. Project supervisors assumed leadership in working out protocols with assistant principals and student support staff for making decisions about crisis intervention. To avoid redundancy, promote clarity, and provide structure, a decision-making tree was developed for crisis response, which centralized authority in school staff and the project supervisors. While interns did provide crisis intervention services, the amount of time committed to this role was centrally managed.

Similarly, assignment of cases for more intensive work required centralized planning. It was important to the project that we serve as a kind of "safety net" in the spectrum of counseling and mental health services. Any children whose families would accept and follow through on a referral to an appropriate outside agency were referred. Work with children whose principal needs involved straightforward educational assessment and planning continued to be done by guidance and pupil adjustment counselors. Our project was concerned to identify, in collaboration with the counselors, those children whose learning was compromised by emotional and behavioral disorders and who would not, for a variety of reasons, have access to mental health services in any other way. There was, unfortunately, no shortage of referrals. At first, most referrals involved children with behavioral problems whose aggression in the classroom prompted frequent trips to the assistant principal's office. Identification of children who had suffered from trauma, leading to various kinds of internalizing disorders, required outreach to teachers to help them recognize these kinds of symptoms.

Other Adjustment Issues for Mental Health Professionals

Mental health professionals working in the public schools frequently encounter difficulties in establishing what many consider "basic necessities" for practice: privacy, confidentiality, space, and regularities in scheduling. "Office space" for our project ranged from converted supply closets to corners in the library or cafeteria, to real offices with four walls, some of which were specifically renovated for our project. Our teams were very creative in making what initially appeared to be marginal space into warm, stimulating environments for professionals and for children. Scouring for games, toys, decorative items, furniture, and books at tag sales, as well as soliciting the support of local businesses, became regular autumn events. Though these activities sometimes stimulated concern among interns about "nonprofessional" roles, they in fact

contributed significantly to team building. Interns, like other school-based professionals, also learned that the structure of "the office" is not the critical variable in creating a "facilitating environment" in which careful and compassionate attention to the present reality of a child enables growth and development to occur.

Scheduling and use of time are also challenging for mental health professionals in the school setting. With greater demands for accountability in performance on standardized tests and requirements for "time on learning," schools have become increasingly cautious about releasing children from classroom instruction for supportive services. Recognizing these constraints, our project worked diligently to balance the need for regularly scheduled appointments so that interns could follow through with children consistently, and the need to work around important instructional periods. Children also sometimes did not want to interrupt their completion of an important educational activity. Because we had made an initial agreement with the school administration to respect the priorities and mission of education, we felt it was important to respond flexibly with scheduling. Teachers, in addition, were very pleased that the intern team would be present during all school hours. Many expressed the opinion that most mental health professionals do not begin work until 9:00 A.M. Embedded in that assumption are feelings about the relative degree of professional autonomy and privilege that many teachers believe that mental health professionals enjoy.

Privacy in the school setting is challenging for mental health professionals to achieve. They assume that a closed door sets a boundary for privacy. School-based professionals tend to assume instead that they are operating within a community of interdependent people, and that in a fast-paced environment, accessibility is a high priority. During the early stages of the project, the intern team was regularly distressed by the degree of what they regarded as intrusions. Much thought and conversation across disciplinary lines went into establishing some boundaries with different kinds of signs on doors that would protect the ability of clinicians to work with some degree of privacy.

Similarly, confidentiality is understood very differently by educators and mental health professionals. The project kept records on our work that were separate from the school records available to all personnel within the school. An important skill for the interns to develop was the ability to communicate with teachers, providing useful feedback about their work with children and families without disclosing personal details that were not critical for the educational purposes of the teacher's work with the child. Family circumstances are particularly sensitive issues. Many families did not want "their business" known widely in the school. Families especially wanted to retain confidentiality about paternity, mental and physical illnesses, illegal activities, imprisonment, or substance abuse of family members. School professionals often feel that mental health professionals withhold feedback about what takes place in private offices. When a child is taken out of a classroom for an intervention and then returned, sometimes in a state of emotional upset, teachers understandably have questions about what has occurred. Successful collaboration in such circumstances relies on a legacy of good relationship and communication, as well as the skills of distilling what of the child's context is relevant for the teacher to be able to do her job, while honoring mental health professionals' ethical obligations to confidentiality with clients. Teachers also need to be reassured that clinicians will make every effort to help the child reestablish emotional equilibrium and preparedness to learn before returning to the classroom.

Stability and Expansion

After a period of adjustment of the schools and SSW to each other, the program settled into a reliable structure of service provision. However, as we grew more knowledgeable about each other, opportunities arose for prioritizing other ways of thinking and kinds of intervention. Sources of change included feedback from the intern teams, collaborative meetings with school administrators, ongoing discussions with the multiple participants in the school communities, and developments in the field of school-based mental health practice. In this section, we will examine some of these changes as they evolved in the areas of work with individual children, work with families, work with groups, crisis work, collaborative and psychoeducational work, and work in community.

Work With Individual Children

Children of elementary school age are referred for counseling in schools because of presenting problems that interfere with learning, including behavioral and academic problems, attentional problems, hyperactivity, impulsive and aggressive behavior, poor peer relationships, social withdrawal, or excessive anxiety (Davies, 1999). School-based professionals have a wealth of understanding of child development and the pathways to emotional and behavioral disorders to inform them about how to intervene successfully with these problems, especially when a problem is focused and self-contained. Referral to specialized mental health services in schools becomes particularly significant when these presenting problems are nested in a complex web of neurological, psychological, and/or social challenges, requiring interventions on multiple levels. In a public health framework, this occurs when there are multiple risk factors and relatively few protective factors (Hoagwood & Johnson, 2003; Hunter, 2003; Weist, 2003). Multiple risk factors often occur in highly stressed families who, for a variety of reasons, do not follow through with referrals to outside social agencies.

Our project welcomed referrals in these complex situations because we had the person power to deal with the multiple layers of intervention that they required. During the first few years of the project, a high percentage of our work focused on individual and group work with children. It was what could most easily be accommodated within the school setting. Over time, the demand for effectiveness led us out into ever-widening circles of social influence, into the ecology of the problem, so that the balance of interventions shifted. However, the project ensured that interns were grounded in a knowledge base for understanding, assessing, engaging, and helpfully interacting with children. For many years, interns received training from a Winnicottian consultant about play as a vehicle for entering into the subjective world of the child. The "squiggle game," in which intern and child cocreate a visual image and narrative about it, based on their sequential elaborations after an initial mark on a paper, became a staple skill for assessment and intervention. The squiggle game had the virtue of richly engaging the child's imagination, promoting meaningful interaction between intern and child, and being highly transportable in a school setting where continuity of office space could not always be assured. It helped interns become less dependent on words and cognition as the exclusive route to understanding children. Play techniques were extremely useful in helping children express their thoughts and fears and the meaning of significant relationships; many important issues about relationships could be effectively addressed through this medium.

However, exclusive reliance on psychodynamic methods was insufficient for the school-based setting. Cognitive-behavioral interventions have the most direct applicability within schools because of their consonance with how educators think and practice. In addition, they have the most confirmation from research into their effectiveness in an era in which evidence-based practice methods are of increasing importance (Fonagy, Target, Cottrell, Phillips, & Kurtz, 2002; Hoagwood, 2000). Observing children in classrooms helps clinicians understand the contexts in which particular behaviors emerge and the functions that particular behaviors serve. Talking with children about their behaviors helps clinicians understand the interpretive frameworks that children are applying to themselves and others. Children can then be helped to challenge or distance themselves from core negative beliefs about self and others, which interfere with social, emotional, and cognitive skills, and to develop behavioral alternatives.

Over time, the interest in cognitive-behavioral interventions evolved into attention to narrative therapy models. Narrative therapy texts provide richly detailed examples of the importance of helping children to "externalize" the problem, recognizing the problem as a dynamic external force exerting unwelcome influence over the child's life (Smith & Nylund, 1997; Winslade & Cheshire, 1997). With the inclusion of a narrative therapy consultant, interns enthusiastically embraced this way of thinking and set of skills, and the tenor of trainings became more playful. Children seemed to be particularly pleased with the "narrative turn." Using narrative methods, they began imagining the problem as an energized opponent, helping to relieve them of identification with the problem as an inherent part of their personality. The opponent could be named, visualized, and described, and his tricks and strategies analyzed (White, 1995). Dealing with such a skilled opponent requires strategies

for counteracting its influence, leading to the child's recognition of his or her own capacities. The child can be helped to identify those times, "sparkling moments," when he or she is more empowered than the crafty but outmaneuvered opponent; the recognition of these incidents marks the beginning of a "preferred identity" that the child can choose to move toward. The child can be helped to identify his or her resources, both internally and in relationship, for supporting these choices and strengthening a preferred way of being. Like psychodynamic methods, narrative methods utilize and enhance imaginative play, which draws naturally on children's resources and ways of knowing. Unlike more interpretive psychodynamic traditions, narrative methods are problem-solving, present-oriented, and strengths-based approaches, making them more consistent with the preferred ways of addressing problems within educational settings.

Work With Families

This school system had recognized the value of positive engagement with families, and most schools had Comer-inspired site-based management teams for involving parents in management decisions (Corbin, this volume). Nevertheless, despite good intentions, tension between school-based professionals and families was palpable. Based on her studies of the parent-teacher conference, Sara Lawrence-Lightfoot (2003) has eloquently described the experience of insecurity and dread with which many families approach interactions with school-based professionals. She draws from the metaphor of "ghosts from the nursery," developed by infant researcher Selma Fraiberg, to describe the effects of a legacy of trauma and poorly developed attachment on people throughout their lives, and discusses the problem of "ghosts from the classroom" for both families and school-based professionals:

> Even when the rhetoric and policies of the school seem to support parental engagement and participation, many parents feel as if they are trespassing when they cross the threshold of the school, as if they are treading on territory where they don't belong. This makes them feel ill at ease, off-balance, and often defensive. Other parents—particularly those who speak a different language, who are poor, or who them-

selves were school dropouts—feel excluded by an institutional bureaucracy that seems opaque and unwelcoming, hard to understand and difficult to navigate. And they feel demeaned by a subtle message that they are inadequate parents who have not prepared their children to succeed in school. (p. 230)

For many families in low-income communities, the "ghosts" of previous school failure, experience of racism and social class prejudice, and brittle hope for a different outcome for their children, tempered by expectation of repetition of the past, haunt the current interactions. For mental health clinicians in the schools, the first phone call to families, who are generally highly stressed in multiple domains of life, is fraught with peril. Mental health professions have their own legacy of "blame-filled" discourse about parents, especially those in low-income communities, which clinicians have acquired both through their professional education and through internalization of prevalent social attitudes. In addition, their empathic responses to the pain of children who have been treated with insensitivity and/or abuse make it challenging to extend themselves empathically and respectfully to families who have contributed to such pain, or been unable to protect their children from it. Interns were helped to develop skills in outreach to families through the following:

1. The acquisition of a "strengths perspective" (DeJong & Miller, 1998);
2. Training for cultural competence to recognize the sources of resilience in groups different from their own (Boyd-Franklin, 2003; Canino & Spurlock, 1994; Falicov, 1998; Koss-Chioino & Vargas, 1999);
3. An ecosystemic perspective on the effects of multiple sources of stress on families (Allen-Meares, 2004; Boyd-Franklin, 2003; Falicov, 1998);
4. Pragmatic recognition of "what works" to enhance family capacity to protect and support children (Center for Mental Health in Schools at UCLA, 1999; Dupper, 2002; Fonagy et al., 2002; Murphy, 1999); and
5. Training and supervision for the development of specific skills in engagement of families who may have no reason to trust in the beneficence of "the friendly caller" from the school

(Boyd-Franklin & Bry, 2000; Dupper, 2002; Madsen, 1999).

Specifically, interns were helped to learn this knowledge base and set of skills through supervision and training, which included role-playing in family therapy theory and skills, and presentations of cases to cultural consultants. Family therapy has a long history of elaborating the therapeutic implications of systems theory, understanding the complex interactions, reciprocal influences, and feedback loops of different components of a social system. Structural family therapy has a successful legacy of practice in inner-city low-income neighborhoods. Interns were helped to use its framework for assessment, analyzing patterns in families of alliances and coalitions, hierarchies of authority, and subsystem boundaries and applying intervention strategies of engagement and pragmatic action for change (Aponte, 1995; Boyd-Franklin & Bry, 2000).

However, application of the structural model, like the psychodynamic model, had to be modified for the school setting. Few families viewed themselves as mental health clients in their work with interns. Instead, they were assumed to be, and experienced themselves as, collaborators in planning for and implementing strategies to help children succeed in school. Much change could be leveraged through the relationship between clinician and family when this more collaborative stance was assumed. The most well-researched model for practice with families who have behaviorally disordered children and teens, the multisystemic therapy model, is grounded in a collaborative stance, with goals that express the priorities of the family for change (Cunningham & Henggeler, 1999). Like the multisystemic therapy researchers and practitioners, we also felt that sensitive negotiation of the engagement process was critical to success. This required flexibility in time and place of meetings with families, with much work consequently taking place in the home. Interns expressed concern at the beginning of field placements about home visiting because of both safety issues and the challenge of listening with "multidirectional partiality" to multiple voices and usefully structuring a meeting of potentially argumentative family members. Role-playing family meetings was of some, though insufficient, assistance. Modeling by supervisors was more helpful. Most useful was the pairing of interns for home visits early in the year so that each intern had another perspective, which could be brought to bear to understand complex and intense interactions. Direct observation of others' work has been a critical feature of family therapy training since its beginnings in the 1960s. The team structure of these field placements allowed this kind of observation and shared participation to occur, enabling interns to overcome initial apprehensions about engaging families.

As with the individual work, over time, the project became very interested in the evolving narrative therapy models of practice. The narrative therapy developed by Michael White and colleagues has moved beyond a narrow focus on clinical interventions with individuals and families to be much more concerned about community integration and development (White, 1995). The "reauthoring" of clients' lives facilitated by narrative therapy actively helps people to expand their social connections and meaningful involvement with others in ways that help them consolidate construction of a preferred identity. Often this involves becoming engaged with networks of people who have wrestled with similar challenges and the mutual sharing of strategies that empower the gift giver as well as the receiver. Annual international conferences on narrative therapy and community work are providing profoundly different models of collaboration, transcending the dichotomy between professional "helpers" and "help seekers." While PfS never developed formal reflecting teams or coalitions of mutual aid and advocacy, as are commonly practiced in narrative therapy, our team structure kept the clinical work open to ongoing feedback from others. A case example of the use of narrative therapy methods in the project is presented in the chapter by Mary Olson (this volume).

The presentation of clinical work for the input of cultural consultants who could deepen the interns' understanding of cultural context was significant. Early in the academic year, trainings focused on cultivating an awareness of culture as central to identity development. Sue and Sue (2003) have cited several components of awareness for cultural competence that clinicians need to cultivate, including sensitivity to one's own cultural heritage; respect for differences based on sociodemographic variables; awareness of bias toward people of color; and recognition of when referral of a client due to cultural mismatch may be in order. In addition,

clinicians need to gain knowledge in several areas for cultural competence, including specific information about particular groups; dynamics of marginalization of groups in this society; limitations of particular models of practice cross-culturally; and institutional barriers that prevent diverse clients from using mental health services. Finally, on the level of skills, they recommend use of a wide variety of verbal and nonverbal responses; ability to understand and respond to different communication styles; advocacy within institutions on behalf of clients; anticipation of the impact of one's own limitations on the clients; and environmental interventions.

In our schools, 80% of the student population, as well as both school principals but few teachers, were of African American or Latino heritage. Our training program provided ongoing knowledge and skill development through the inclusion of cultural consultants with expertise for practice with African American and Latino families and children. They reviewed cases and advised about interventions in the classrooms and school communities. Work with the case of Amy and her family, which follows, utilized this training.

Referral and Presenting Problem

Amy is a 7-year-old girl in the second grade who lives at home with her biological mother, stepfather, 10-year-old sister, 8-year-old brother, and 5-year-old half brother. Amy was referred to PfS because of her refusal to speak in school since she first entered the school in kindergarten. The school had attempted different interventions, including psychological testing and work with a speech pathologist. When these efforts did not lead to speech in the classroom, Amy's second-grade teacher referred her to the PfS project. She was concerned that Amy's reading ability could not be evaluated without her willingness to read aloud.

Family Background

Amy's family, including her mother, two older siblings, and Amy, moved to the United States from the Dominican Republic when Amy was 4 months old. Amy's mother had left an abusive husband to come to the United States. After arrival here, she sought treatment for significant symptoms of depression. She soon became romantically involved with Amy's stepfather, who quickly developed positive relationships with Amy and her older siblings, as well as a new child. Shortly before Amy began school, her stepfather was diagnosed with a chronic degenerative illness. Though the children know that he is ill, the parents have not shared with them the specific diagnosis. The family is involved with a Pentecostal church, and they attend services several times a week, finding much support in this community. Their primary language is Spanish, which is the language most frequently spoken at home by everyone but Amy. Amy generally speaks English at home and at church. She is being taught in an English-speaking classroom. She will speak neither Spanish nor English in school.

Amy in School

Amy is described by her teacher as a cooperative, quietly engaged student who appears from her written work to be learning at a second-grade level. All three of her siblings attend the same school; the older two siblings are protective of Amy, seek her out during the day, and communicate with school personnel on her behalf. Amy occasionally whispers to her siblings, but she speaks to no one else in the school. Amy's siblings are known for their sociability and extroverted personalities. Amy has acquired the identity throughout the school as "the girl who won't talk." In individual sessions, Amy drew many pictures of human faces, which she promptly scribbled over.

Interventions

The PfS intern actively pursued information about the cultural context that might help her provide more effective interventions. She learned that "selective mutism" occurs with much greater frequency among bilingual/bicultural children. Additional historical and social variables, which appear to contribute to this problem, include a history of surgery to the mouth, family secrets, and early life trauma. Amy and her family had undergone severe stress during the period of immigration to the United States, and Amy had required minor surgery to her mouth during infancy. Although the family had made many successful adaptations to life in the United States, they were threatened with the impact of the deteriorating health of a nurturing and economically contributing stepfather. Neither the stresses nor the resilience experienced by this family could be fully understood without a larger framework of knowledge about the "journeys of migration and adaptation" experienced more generally by Latino families (Falicov, 1998) and the stresses on children entering into American schools with complex demands on identity development (Nieto, 1996). Cohesion and protection for the family were significant issues, which were both internal and external to the life of this particular family. With the flexibility of the PfS program, we were able to work with Amy individually around issues of self-expression through play in weekly meetings, with Amy and her siblings around issues of protection and autonomy in biweekly meetings, and with the family as a whole in monthly home visits to support the parents' leadership around these issues. The school continued to be impatient for speech from Amy. However, direct efforts to induce speech through discipline or behavioral rewards had failed. Intensive, culturally informed work with Amy and her family helped to provide a protective bridge between contexts for Amy, which eventually led to speech, greatly reduced anxiety, and school achievement.

Work With Groups

Group work in schools is an important modality for helping children to develop social skills and is highly valued by schools. In the early years of the project, we relied exclusively on the referrals we received from school-based professionals to form the groups. Teachers were most interested in "anger management" groups for acting-out boys. The project soon discovered that concentrating boys with various kinds of oppositional and aggressive behaviors in the same group contributed to spiraling, out-of-control behavior, leading in one memorable incident to group members' hurling verbal abuse out the windows to a dismayed school community during the boarding of buses at the end of the day. We sought ongoing consultation on children's groups through the training program, which enabled us to become much more skillful in design and implementation of a group program. Over time, it became clear that groups were needed around times of transition, for social skill development, and for interventions to help children cope with particular psychosocial stressors. At all times, each intern was expected to be co-leading at least two groups of either short- or longer-term duration.

"Transition" groups were developed to help children with entry into the first grade and with preparation for middle school. The first-grade groups evolved out of the teachers' concerns that many of their children had not been involved in any kind of preschool experience and were therefore not equipped with the social and behavioral skills that would enable them to function in a classroom. Our intern team both observed ongoing classes and broke the classes into small groups of children to assess and teach social skills. When particularly poorly prepared children were identified, we were able to continue with them in small groups to help them to catch up with their classmates. Over the course of several years, we developed our own protocol with relevant psychoeducational materials for the conduct of these groups. Children with more challenging social and emotional difficulties could also be identified through this process early in their school careers and followed in "booster sessions" through the second grade or provided with more intensive individualized services.

Fifth- and sixth-grade groups were devised around different themes to help with the transition to middle school or junior high. In our schools, children were beginning to feel some of the pressures of sexualizing relationships and recruitment into gang activities during these years. They experienced conflicted feelings about leaving the relatively protected environment of elementary school and entering into larger school environments with greater demands for maturity and greater temptations for diverging from the path of maturity. Some girls' groups were developed as a result of particular conflicts between coalitions of girls, with the intention of undermining bullying dynamics. Girl groups addressed body image issues through the use of photography, and emerging sexuality and relationship issues through psychoeducational approaches. Boy groups similarly addressed gender-based challenges about images of maleness and paths to success. Both girl and boy groups addressed expectations for the higher academic demands of the next stage of schooling.

"Lunch bunches" were social skills groups for children with poorly developed interpersonal skills that isolated them from other children. They allowed interns to provide such insightful, on-the-spot feedback as "If you stick baloney on your forehead during lunch, no one is going to want to sit next to you."

Groups were often formed around particular shared experiences, such as death in the family and foster care. Losing a parent or sibling through death is a more common experience for children in low-income communities than for children in more privileged communities, through higher rates of chronic disease and violence. The loss and bereavement groups helped children to feel less alone in their experiences and to benefit from the coping strategies of other group members. Foster care can also be an intensely isolating experience for children; all too frequently children would come to school with green trash bags filled with their belongings with the expectation that the child welfare worker would transport them from school to a new home. Interns initially were horrified at the apparent lack of careful attention to processing the meaning of these transitions for children. As the project evolved, they became more impressed with how supportive elementary schools are for children with highly disrupted lives. Some of the necessary support could be provided in the school context with crisis work, groups for children in foster care, and greater coordination with child welfare workers. Supportive groups helped children to cope more effectively with these painful situations and develop coherent narratives for severely disrupted lives (Murphy, Pynoos, & James, 1997; Williams, Fanolis, & Schamess, 2001).

Crisis Work

Intervention in crises occurs because of disruptions in the classroom leading to the removal of a particular child, crises in the families of children, violent or tragic events that affect the local school community, or national crises that trouble everyone. The person power of the intern team enabled us to assist regularly with the crises experienced by individual children (Fanolis, 2001). Local tragedies, such as the accidental shooting death of one child by another, led us to help with in-class discussions to honor the life of the deceased, help children express feelings of loss, and reassure children of their safety. The shootings at Columbine High School in April 1999 were a national crisis with reverberating effects for children all over the country. Our teams were asked to lead discussions in every classroom following this tragedy. These discussions were profoundly shaped by the developmental needs and cognitive capacities of the children. Older children tended to be preoccupied with and even traumatized by particular visual images, especially of a teen jumping out a window onto a car. Younger children were frightened that the shooters could be, and some thought probably were, present in their school. Neither the distance between Colorado and the East Coast nor the reality of the deaths of the shooters was reassuring to the younger children at their level of cognitive development. Some children were distressed that the shooters were not in jail, feeling that this form of justice was more protective than death. Children needed the concrete reassurance of the protective measures already available in their school from the adults they knew, in the context of relationships they could trust, before they could let go of their anxiety.

On a policy level, the program director worked with the school administration to develop the crisis plan for the school district, incorporating mental health principles to cope with the multiple forms of crisis that schools increasingly have to be prepared to implement. Her background as the director of a project at a child guidance clinic working with families who had experienced murder or other forms of violent death was invaluable. In addition, one of the interns wrote a master's thesis on school-based crisis plans that was utilized by the school administration.

Collaborative and Psychoeducational Work

The evolutionary changes in the collaborative relationships between the project and the teaching staff were dramatic. Polarities between the "mean" teachers and the "naive" interns gave way to more universal appreciation of each other's professional competence. For the interns, this was facilitated by the involvement of Smith College Department of Education consultants who, early in the training year, prepared interns with compelling descriptions of the job of teaching. Some of this material emerged from their involvement in the program developed by Parker Palmer (1997) to replenish the vitality of teachers. Because of concerns about the numbers of teachers who leave the profession during their first 5 years (estimated to be 50%), and the amount of "burnout" experienced by disillusioned, formerly idealistic teachers, Palmer has developed a program of ongoing training and support that integrates a spiritual perspective on the meaning of teaching with specific strategies for renewal and development of capacity. Informed by this perspective, Smith Department of Education profes-

sors helped the intern team to know how to talk to teachers in a way that elicits and develops capacity, while recognizing the sources of stress in the extremely important but highly contested roles that they perform.

Teachers, in turn, instead of complaining about the interns' naïveté, began to recognize the value of helping interns gain the skills in classroom participation and collaboration that were required. After several successful years of the project, they knew that the interns would become contributors to the well-being of their individual students and their classrooms, and they increasingly thought of themselves as cotrainers of the interns at the beginning of each year. Each cohort of interns profited from the legacy of goodwill and success generated by the previous group, leading to enhanced ability to collaborate on every level.

Work in Community

Over time, the "bridging" or networking function of the intern team, working within the school community and on the boundaries between family and school, and school and community, was greatly enhanced. Initially, Smith SSW had offered to contribute training opportunities for school-based professionals on topics such as trauma identification and intervention, behavior management, and depression and anxiety in children. Teachers responded positively to these trainings but expressed concern that single trainings were not nearly as useful to them in their on-the-ground work as the development of collaborative relationships over time. Their responses are quite consistent with studies which show that brief trainings do not have much influence on professional behavior (McGinty, Diamond, Brown, & McCammon, 2003). We concluded that there is no shortcut around time-intensive relationship development and "being there" when "stuff" happens. This lesson was driven home during the third year of the project, when a flood in one of our schools led to the physical relocation of the school community. A "school" had to be immediately created out of a vacant, lifeless office building. Everyone rolled up their sleeves and, disregarding professional status, contributed to solving whatever was the most pressing problem at the moment. The intern team took particular responsibility for contributing to the creation of a "school library." This involved soliciting contributions in the community and carrying endless numbers of books for the school librarian to catalog. While these tasks did not appear on the surface to be the skills the interns were paying tuition to acquire, in fact, it was an extremely valuable lesson in crisis response and community building. Within a couple of weeks, a barren space was transformed into a child-welcoming, brightly decorated, organized learning environment. The intern team was never again experienced as "marginal," and the relationships that were forged during the performance of these "nonprofessional" roles enabled the professional collaborations to occur.

Five years into the project, we decided to take a further step out into the community through the development of a collaborative partnership with a community agency that focused on youth development programs in a low-income, African American community. In this agency, 85% of the children served and 100% of the professional and nonprofessional staff were African American. The few Caucasian youth who came to the agency were drawn from the suburbs into the inner-city by the desire to improve their basketball skills with players who could help them. They did not bring resources into the program. In her review of the development of this partnership, the agency director shared what had been her serious reservations about how a team of mostly white social workers from Smith College would "fit in" and be useful to their program. The racial identity of "whiteness," the "child removal" reputation of social work, and the social privilege of Smith College were all seen as potential sources of conflict and mutual rejection. Interns who had grown up in or had extensive experience in low-income communities of color quickly found meaningful roles. For those interns without this social experience, entry was more challenging but facilitated by the team structure of the project, which enabled the give-and-take of experiences and assets among team members. Open discussion of the meaning of the problematic identities of whiteness, privilege, and power, not particularly welcome in the school setting, was extremely useful in the community setting. Flexibility in roles, modeled by the PfS director, enabled different kinds of participation to occur, including tutoring in the after-school program, collaboration with community workers to support children with challenging emotional and behavioral problems, and social skill-building interventions for children known in

the school settings who needed to be supported in after-school activities. Some interns with particular skills in dance, yoga, and drumming formed groups to help children with these activities. The drumming group was received with particular enthusiasm. The teams came to be embraced as "our interns."

Evaluation

PfS has undergone three evaluative studies in the past 10 years. In addition, there has been one follow-up study of graduates of PfS, examining the influence of the program on their professional choices. In the most recent and thorough study (Corwin, 2000), administrators, school adjustment counselors, and teachers were asked to evaluate the project in terms of its contributions to school health climate, meeting the social, emotional, behavioral, and academic needs of children, quality of collaboration, quality of feedback and follow-through, advocacy and mediation for children, and culturally sensitive interactions with students and parents. The project received particularly high evaluative feedback on the level of integration of the team into all aspects of the school community and the quality of services. The project was favorably compared to other kinds of mental health collaborative models, with clinicians only providing direct services to children. Despite very positive ratings and feedback about the relevance of our services, school personnel emphasized that even more orientation of the intern teams for the institutional realities and priorities of public schools would be useful. School personnel also seek more diversity in the intern teams in gender, race, and ethnicity. In addition, feedback from PfS graduates indicates that a high percentage (67%) remained in school-based practice, addressing a critical need for mental health professionals prepared to practice from a system-of-care set of principles (McGinty et al., 2003).

Financial Pressures and Redirection of the Project

Financial support for the project came through blended funding streams from the public schools, Smith SSW, and the contributions of local and national foundations, particularly the General Mills Foundation. Every year, there were issues to be negotiated among partners in the funding of the program. Both Smith and the public schools wanted to see the program put on a solid foundation with permanent integration into the structure of the public school system. The public school administration believed that this would be most effectively accomplished by having Partners for Success take responsibility for developing preschool mental health services for the city, with the positions of project director and supervisor fully funded by the school system. Smith SSW would continue to provide interns, training, and technical support for the pursuit of outside funding to study and evaluate the effectiveness of the interventions.

The school system's request was motivated by pragmatic concerns to find a permanent "home" for the project without the continuing perils of obtaining "soft money" to support a successful, albeit ongoing, project and by their need to respond to the increasing concerns about the emotional and developmental vulnerability of many of the children they were seeing in their expanding preschool programs. The field of infant and early childhood mental health has been undergoing enormous development in recent years, and the importance of early identification and intervention into emotional and behavioral problems recognized (Knitzer, 1996a, 1996b). Two years ago, PfS began adapting its model and working in two preschool sites. Interns were assigned to work in specific classrooms for several hours a day to learn about developmental issues in preschool-aged children, identification of particularly vulnerable children, curriculum and teaching methods for preschoolers, and social skills development in the classroom. A violence-prevention curriculum for preschoolers was introduced to teachers, parents, and children. Skill development for emotional and behavioral competence is a critical mental health need in the preschool population, and this highly developed curriculum was enthusiastically received. The project also was persuaded by evidence that enhancing parents' skills in positive emotional engagement and stimulation of their children's abilities was significant in social and emotional development and school readiness. We incorporated training in filial therapy, which coaches and supports parents in stimulating and emotionally responsive play with their children, into our project. Initial responses to this model of in-class involvement and assessment by interns, a curriculum for social skill development, and a clinical intervention that helps parents guide the psychosocial development of their own children were very positive.

However, enthusiasm for this important and promising work soon encountered an unmovable constraint: extreme financial hardship for the public school system and recognition of the need for fiscal restraint in the SSW as well. The school system was challenged to maintain its existing programs with dramatic cuts in professional staff and could not support the preschool expansion it so much desired. The suddenness and severity of this crisis led to the suspension of the PfS program because of the inability to fund the supervisory positions. Supervisors for the PfS project have recently been given full-time positions within the school system but have not been assigned to preschool services. The program director of PfS has been selected by the school department to participate in a program to prepare her for a leadership role in the system. As this chapter goes to press, decisions about any next step in continuation and/or transformation of the project are yet to be made by the partners.

In Conclusion

In rethinking what allowed this program to flourish for 10 years, we come back to where we started: our ability to build upon Senge's (1990) ideas about learning organizations. The school system and the SSW shared a particular vision for enhancing emotional and behavioral health of schoolchildren and their families through intensive and flexible interventions at multiple systemic levels with sizable teams of mental health professionals in training. We learned about and shared principles of collaboration based on respect for each other's professional needs and priorities. We allowed our models of practice to evolve over time with input from experience, feedback from our partners and participants, and the changing base of knowledge that was available to us. We emphasized practice and learning for practice rather than the study of practice. Responding to the needs of the children, families, and school community as we became more deeply familiar with them, we were able to mount a program that was comprehensive in the scope of its services, integrated into the ongoing life of the schools, built upon principles of early intervention as well as intervention for children at high risk of chronicity, influential in changing some aspects of school climate, and successful in preparing future generations of school-based clinicians for a diversity of roles in socially stressed urban school systems.

References

Achenbach, T., Dumenci, L., & Rescorla, L. (2003). Are American children's problems still getting worse? A 23-year comparison. *Journal of Abnormal Child Psychology, 31*, 1–11.

Allen-Meares, P. (2004). *Social work services in schools* (4th ed.). Needham Heights, MA: Allyn and Bacon.

Aponte, H. (1995). *Bread and spirit*. New York: Norton.

Armbruster, P., & Lichtman, J. (1999). Are school-based mental health services effective: Evidence from 36 inner-city schools. *Community Mental Health Journal, 35*, 493–504.

Astor, R., Benbenishty, R., Pitcher, R., & Meyer, H. (2004). Bullying and peer victimization in schools. In P. Allen-Meares & M. Fraser (Eds.), *Intervention with children and adolescents: An interdisciplinary approach* (pp. 417–449). Boston: Allyn and Bacon.

Boyd-Franklin, N. (2003). *Black families in therapy* (2nd ed.). New York: Guilford.

Boyd-Franklin, N., & Bry, B. (2000). *Reaching out in family therapy: Home-based, school and community interventions*. New York: Guilford.

Canino, I., & Spurlock, J. (1994). *Culturally diverse children and adolescents*. New York: Guilford.

Center for Mental Health in Schools at UCLA. (1999). *An introductory packet on social and interpersonal problems related to school aged youth*. Los Angeles: Author.

Center for Mental Health in Schools at UCLA. (2003a). *Addressing barriers to learning: A comprehensive approach to mental health in schools*. Los Angeles: Author.

Center for Mental Health in Schools at UCLA. (2003b). *Youngsters' mental health and psychosocial problems: What are the data?* Los Angeles: Author.

Center for Mental Health in Schools at UCLA. (2004). *Mental health of children and youth and the role of public health professionals*. Los Angeles: Author.

Corwin, M. (2000). *Evaluation of Partners for Success*. Unpublished manuscript.

Cunningham, P., & Henggeler, S. (1999). Engaging multiproblem families in treatment: Lessons learned throughout the development of multisystemic therapy. *Family Process, 38*, 265–281.

Davies, D. (1999). *Child development: A practitioner's guide*. New York: Guilford.

DeJong, P., & Miller, S. (1998). How to interview for client strengths. In E. Freeman, C. Franklin, R. Fong, G. Shaffer, & E. Timberlake (Eds.), *Multisystem skills and interventions in school social work practice* (pp. 5–16). Washington, DC: NASW Press.

Dupper, D. (2002). *School social work: Skills and intervention for effective practice*. Hoboken, NJ: Wiley.

Evans, G. (2004). The environment of childhood poverty. *American Psychologist, 59*, 77–92.

Falicov, C. (1998). *Latino families in therapy: A guide to multicultural practice*. New York: Guilford.

Fanolis, V. (2001). The use of crisis teams in response to violent or critical incidents in schools. *Smith Studies in Social Work, 71*, 271–278.

Ferguson, A. (2000). *Bad boys: Public schools in the making of black masculinity*. Ann Arbor: University of Michigan Press.

Fonagy, P., Target, M., Cottrell, D., Phillips, J., & Kurtz, Z. (2002). *What works for whom? A critical review of treatments for children and adolescents*. New York: Guilford.

Franklin, C. (2004). The delivery of school social work services. In P. Allen-Meares (Ed.), *Social work services in schools* (4th ed., pp. 295–327). Needham Heights, MA: Allyn and Bacon.

Garbarino, J. (1999). *Lost boys: Why our sons turn violent and how we can save them*. New York: Free Press.

Gutierrez, L., Parsons, R., & Cox, E. (1998). *Empowerment in social work practice*. Pacific Grove, CA: Brooks/Cole.

Hale, J. (1994). *Unbank the fire: Visions for the education of African American children*. Baltimore: Johns Hopkins University Press.

Harrison, M., McKay, M., & Bannon, W. (2004). Inner-city child mental health service use: The real question is why youth and families do not use services. *Community Mental Health Journal 40*, 119–131.

Hoagwood, K. (2000). State of the evidence on school-based mental health services—NIMH perspectives. *Emotional and Behavioral Disorders in Youth, 1*, 13–15.

Hoagwood, K., & Johnson, J. (2003). School psychology: A public health framework: I: From evidence-based practice to evidence-based policies. *Journal of School Psychology, 41*, 3–21.

Hunter, L. (2003). School psychology: A public health framework: III: Managing disruptive behavior in schools. *Journal of School Psychology, 41*, 39–59.

Knitzer, J. (1982). *Unclaimed children: The failure of public responsibility to children and adolescents in need of mental health services*. Washington, DC: Children's Defense Fund.

Knitzer, J. (1996a). Meeting the mental health needs of young children and their families. In B. Stroul (Ed.), *Children's mental health: Creating systems of care in a changing society* (pp. 553–573). Baltimore: Brookes.

Knitzer, J. (1996b). The role of education in systems of care. In B. Stroul (Ed.), *Children's mental health: Creating systems of care in a changing society* (pp. 197–215). Baltimore: Brookes.

Koss-Chioino, J., & Vargas, L. (1999). *Working with Latino youth: Culture, development and context*. San Francisco: Jossey-Bass.

Lawrence-Lightfoot, S. (2003). *The essential conversation: What parents and teachers can learn from each other*. New York: Random House.

Linver, M., Fuligni, A., Hernandez, M., & Brooks-Gunn, J. (2004). Poverty and child development: Promising interventions. In P. Allen-Meares & M. Fraser (Eds.), *Intervention with children and adolescents: An interdisciplinary approach* (pp. 106–130). Boston: Allyn and Bacon.

Lourie, I. (2003). The history of child community mental health. In A. Pumariega & N. Winters (Eds.), *Handbook of child and adolescent systems of care* (pp. 1–17). San Francisco: Jossey-Bass.

Luthar, S. (1999). *Poverty and children's adjustment*. Thousand Oaks, CA: Sage.

Madsen, W. (1999). *Collaborative therapy with multistressed families*. New York: Guilford.

McGinty, K., Diamond, J., Brown, M., & McCammon, S. (2003). Training of child and adolescent psychiatrists and child mental health professionals for systems of care. In A. Pumariega & N. Winters (Eds.), *Handbook of child and adolescent systems of care* (pp. 487–509). San Francisco: Jossey-Bass.

Murphy, J. (1999). Common factors of school based change. In M. Hubble, B. Duncan, & S. Miller (Eds.), *The heart and soul of change: What works in therapy* (pp. 361–386). Washington, DC: APA Press.

Murphy, L., Pynoos, R., & James, C. B. (1997). The trauma/grief-focused group psychotherapy module of an elementary school-based violence prevention/intervention program. In J. Osofsky (Ed.), *Children in a violent society* (pp. 223–256). New York: Guilford.

Nieto, S. (1996). *Affirming diversity: Sociopolitical context of multicultural education* (2nd ed.). New York: Longman.

Nieto, S. (1999). *The light in their eyes: Creating multicultural learning communities*. New York: Teachers College Press.

Osofsky, J. (1997). *Children in a violent society*. New York: Guilford.

Palmer, P. (1997). *The courage to teach: Exploring the inner landscape of a teacher's life*. San Francisco: Jossey-Bass.

Perry, B. (1997). Incubated in terror: Neurodevelopmental factors in the "cycle of violence." In J. Osofsky (Ed.), *Children in a violent society* (pp. 124–150). New York: Guilford.

Pumariega, A. (2003). Cultural competence in systems of care for children's mental health. In A. Pumariega & N. Winters (Eds.), *Handbook of child and adolescent systems of care* (pp. 82–107). San Francisco: Jossey-Bass.

Pynoos, R., Steinberg, A., & Goenjian, A. (1996). Traumatic stress in childhood and adolescence: Recent developments and current controversies. In B. van der Kolk, A. McFarlane, & L. Weisaeth (Eds.), *Traumatic stress: The effects of overwhelming experience on mind, body, and society* (pp. 331–359). New York: Guilford.

Senge, P. (1990). *The fifth discipline: The art and practice of the learning organization*. New York: Doubleday.

Senge, P. (2000). *Schools that learn: A fifth discipline fieldbook for educators, parents, and everyone who cares about education*. New York: Doubleday.

Smith, C., & Nylund, D. (1997). *Narrative therapies with children and adolescents*. New York: Guilford.

Stroul, B. (1996). *Children's mental health: Creating systems of care in a changing society*. Baltimore: Paul Brookes.

Sue, D. W., & Sue, D. (2003). *Counseling the culturally diverse: Theory and practice* (4th ed.). New York: Wiley.

U.S. Department of Public Health. (2000). *Report of the Surgeon General's Conference on Children's Mental Health: A national action agenda*. Washington, DC: Author.

Weist, M. (2003). Challenges and opportunities in moving towards a public health approach in school mental health. *Journal of School Psychology, 41*, 77–82.

White, M. (1995). *Reauthoring lives*. Adelaide, South Australia: Dulwich Centre Publications.

Williams, S., Fanolis, V., & Schamess, G. (2001). Adapting the Pynoos school-based group therapy model for use with foster children: Theoretical and process considerations. *Journal of Child and Adolescent Group Therapy, 11*, 57–76.

Winslade, J., & Cheshire, A. (1997). School counseling in narrative mode. In G. Monk, J. Winslade, K. Crocket, & D. Epston (Eds.), *Narrative therapy in practice* (pp. 215–233). San Francisco: Jossey-Bass.

21

Joanne Corbin

School-Based Clinical Practice and School Reform

Application of Clinical Social Work to the School Development Program

School settings offer a wealth of opportunities for social workers to learn, practice, and enhance their social work knowledge and skills. Clinical practice in schools has generally focused on providing services to individual students related to behavioral, social, and academic issues, often involving collaboration with parents, caregivers, and teaching staff. Clinical social work practice may also involve group sessions with students around behavioral and social interaction issues. Working with site-based decision-making teams, taking an active role in leadership activities, or engaging in school reform are areas that generally have not been attended to by social workers. This chapter will look at the role of social work in the context of school leadership and systemic reform through the involvement of one school reform program. Recommendations will be offered to support those desiring to work in this manner.

Scope of Social Work Practice in Schools

Few studies provide good estimates of the number of social workers working in schools. One study looked at the number of support staff in public elementary and secondary schools in the United States and found approximately 1.3 million support staff working with the approximately 50 million students (National Center for Education Statistics, 2001).[1] Social workers are included in this overall figure but are not recorded separately. Torres (1996), in a study of 57 American educational jurisdictions, found that 34 of these jurisdictions indicated having 9,337 social workers employed. The average was 274 per jurisdiction, and 62% of the responding jurisdictions reported fewer than the average. A study by Allen-Meares (1994) identified 11,285 names in a search of state associations in the United States that identified school social workers. Although a more precise number of social workers in schools is not available, this information does give a sense that there is an opportunity for social workers to be more active in influencing and creating change in the policies and decisions of schools and school districts, in addition to working with individual students, caregivers, and teachers.

One related lack of clarity about the nature of social work practice in schools is understanding the range of tasks that social workers perform in schools. An analysis of job descriptions reported in the Torres (1996) study found the following social work job-related activities: casework, liaison, assessment and testing, consultation, referral services, record keeping, truancy, advocacy, supervision, participation in professional development, in-service training, program planning, implementation and evaluation, and functioning as a team member of an interdisciplinary team. Allen-Meares (1994) found the following categorization of job dimensions of social workers in schools in order of importance as perceived by the social workers to be (1) administrative and professional tasks, (2) home-school liaison, (3) educational counseling with children, (4) facilitating and advocating families' use of community resources, and (5) leadership and policymaking. She also looked at the differentiation of mandated tasks such as home visits, referrals to community agencies, and working with individual students versus preferred tasks such as acting as an advocate with community agencies, helping change school-community relationships, and meeting with parents in groups. It is important to consider this aspect of mandated versus preferred because many social workers feel that it is important to attend to the mandated tasks before addressing the preferred tasks. Engaging in the work of decision making or leadership tends to be viewed as "not mandated"; therefore, it is not a priority and does not become a part of the work. In the Allen-Meares study, the area of leadership and policymaking was not viewed as a preferred task and was considered to be least important in the context of the job dimensions. If this area is not a mandated task and not a preferred task, there is little question as to why there is not much written on this topic. However, without involvement in the leadership and policymaking aspects of the school, social workers have no power, and their voices are not involved in decision making. This is antithetical to the mission of social work.

This area of leadership and policymaking is important because it relates to the application of clinical social work knowledge and skills to schools' site-based decision-making teams or central office administrative decision making. This systemic application of clinical social work is just as important, and perhaps more so, as the delivery of services to individual students. It may be more important because of the potential for systemic decisions and policies to affect many more students and families than individual-based services. Systemic decisions and policies also have a greater possibility of be-

coming institutionalized, that is, they become part of the operational system of the school or school district.

How Systems Impact Students

Schools are made up of various subgroups or systems that include students, teachers, custodians, cafeteria workers, security personnel, support staff, music/art/physical education teachers, caregivers, administrators, and others. Schools are also affected by other systems or groups outside of the school, such as the neighborhood and community, community resources such as health and mental health centers, businesses, colleges, the central office administration to which the school is accountable, and city and state policies and funding. When providing services to an individual student, we may not consider the interplay of all these systems, but they are always involved to a greater or lesser extent (see figure 21.1).

A student's disrespectful verbal behavior toward a teacher may result in the student being disciplined in some way, such as in-school suspension, detention, communication with caregivers, and so forth. It is necessary to consider that a student's behavior may not be solely about the individual student but may relate to the student's earlier negative interaction with classmates, difficult family situation, or perhaps a recent transfer from another school. Very often other staff within the school know about these related experiences; however, this information is not included when decisions are made about how to respond to the student. There often are many barriers that prevent this larger assessment of systems affecting an individual from being attended to, such as limited time, limited resources, and reluctance to incorporate this perspective regarding student behavior. Creating the time and appropriate structure for these wider discussions to occur can change the climate of the school community and encourage more sensitive responses to the situations of students within schools.

Using the social worker's clinical knowledge to better understand how students are affected by other students, teachers, school policies, curriculum, school district decisions, and sociocultural forces to create more appropriate student-level interventions is essential. As a social worker in a com-

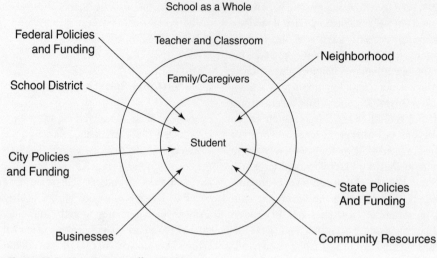

Figure 21.1. How Systems Affect Students

munity mental health agency, I supported individual students from outside the school structure, forming collaborative relationships with other social workers, counselors, or teachers within various schools. This work was focused on the needs of individual students. It was not until I began working with a school reform model and working with educators[2] that I understood the importance of a social work perspective in school-based decision making. The next section will describe this school reform program, the School Development Program[3] and will indicate the aspects of this program that connect to a social work perspective.

School Development Program Mission and Program Structure

Evaluation and assessment of the School Development Program (SDP) have been substantial and consistent since the 1980s. Studies on the SDP have documented increases in student achievement (Cauce, Comer, & Schwartz, 1987; Cook, Hunt, & Murphy, 1999; Haynes, 1994; Haynes, Comer, & Hamilton-Lee, 1988), school climate (Cook et al., 1999; Haynes et al., 1988), student self-concept (Haynes & Comer, 1990), and student behavior (Haynes, 1994; Haynes et al., 1988). In addition to these outcomes, research has also found increased parental involvement, reduced discipline problems, and increased agency as a school to effect change

(Noblit et al., 1997). A case study by Noblit, Malloy, and Malloy (2001) examined the effects of the SDP on five schools across the United States that were performing well when each decided to select the SDP as a reform model. The case study revealed an interesting aspect of the "value-added" (p. 110) provided by the SDP, meaning that some characteristic provided by the SDP enabled the schools to do better than their prior good performance. This characteristic was a sense of a collective agency:

> In each of these schools, the structures in place before the SDP were rather traditional. Traditional school structures isolate staff and students into classrooms and separate administration from instruction. The principal is then invested with the agency to act for the school as a whole. In the Comer Schools we studied, the SDP alters the traditional structure and creates opportunities for collective agency. Moreover, the schools then use this agency in the service of improving the schools. (p. 111)

A closer look will allow us to see what it is about the SDP that enabled schools to make these advancements. The SDP began in 1968 with Dr. James P. Comer and colleagues at the Yale Child Study Center in New Haven, Connecticut, working with two of the city's elementary schools, including the staff members, students, parents, and community members. At that time, a significant percentage of students were performing below grade level, students were viewed as unmotivated and disruptive, and parents and community members felt disenfranchised by the school. Parents, teachers, and students, in fact, the school community as a whole, were divided and viewed each other as unhelpful. Comer (1980) believed that to turn things around in these schools and to improve student achievement, all the stakeholders (parents, students, teachers, administrators, and involved community members) needed to have working relationships that could be used to support the students. Comer explains the hypothesis on which the SDP was created: "The application of social and behavioral science principles to every aspect of a school reform program will improve the climate of relationships among all involved and will facilitate significant academic and social growth of students" (p. 60). This passage gives evidence to the importance of a strong attention to child and adolescent development knowledge and subsequent ability to develop effective relationships.

How the SDP Works

Three major teams are created to enable this process to work: the school planning and management team (SPMT), the student and staff support team (SSST),[4] and the parent team (PT). The structure provided by these teams is a crucial factor in creating working relationships between the stakeholder groups. These teams enabled the school community to focus its energies. Additional elements of the SDP (three functions and three guiding principles) that will be discussed later allowed these energies to be used effectively to support the students.

The SPMT, the lead team, is composed of representative stakeholders in the school community. It makes decisions regarding the school program, policies, and practices. Although this team has representative membership, the meetings are open to anyone within the school community. The SSST is composed of the educators responsible for delivering student resources in the areas of cognitive, social, psychological, ethical, linguistic, and physical development. The SDP refers to these six areas as the six developmental pathways. The purpose of the SSST is to ensure the positive overall development of students within the school. The PT is designed to involve all parents of students in the

school in some way. The efforts of this team go beyond the traditional activities of parent-teacher organizations. Because Dr. Comer realized that parents and school staff tend to be alienated from one another, the PT must create linkages between the community and the school. Parents and community members must be involved in planning these efforts (Anson et al., 1991; Comer, Haynes, Joyner, & Ben-Avie, 1996).

The three major functions of these three SPMT-led teams are to develop a comprehensive school plan, to ensure that the professional development program of the school supports the actualization of the plan, and to make sure that the school has a way of evaluating and modifying it. The comprehensive school plan consists of goals and objectives for the academic, social development, and public relations or community involvement aspects of the school. The functions give the teams a purpose, helping to guide the efforts, rather than have the teams work in an undirected fashion.

The SDP operates under three guiding principles: no-fault, consensus decision making, and collaboration. These principles lay the ground rules for how teams function. No-fault pertains to team members not using judgmental or attacking language. When team members are attacked, they are less likely to be fully engaged as team members. Consensus decision making gives members the expectation that all viewpoints will be considered and not ignored, as is often the case with voting. This type of decision-making process builds a sense of inclusiveness among group members. Collaboration refers to individuals or subgroups avoiding the use of positions of power to muscle through decisions or stalemate the process (Comer et al., 1996).

In addition to the structures, the functions, and the guiding principles, the SDP demands that all the academic and psychosocial development activities, polices, or decisions that occur within this model are discussed, planned, implemented, and assessed within a developmental perspective, using the six developmental pathways as a framework and guide for decisions. Because schools consist of students with varying experiences along each of the six developmental pathways, schools can engage in wonderfully creative discussions about how best to attend to the learning needs of students. It is in this intersection of developmental understanding and academic planning that the training and preparation of social workers have the potential for exciting application in site-based decision making.

Training and Support

Educators attend the SDP's foundational training, which consists of two 1-week sessions designed to prepare them to be the key change agents for their school or district. The program also offers a 1-week session for principals to focus on their role as academic leaders in this implementation process. A separate week is geared to classroom-based teachers and support service staff to integrate child development principles into their practice. Another category of training addresses the academic areas of curriculum alignment, literacy, and teacher instructional dialogue.

To monitor and support district-level implementation of the model, an implementation coordinator from the SDP staff is assigned to work with a particular district. Additional consultation may be established if work on a specific curriculum area is needed. The implementation coordinator is responsible for assessing the district's needs, its capacity for change, and the abilities of the key district educators who will be managing the program in between the visits of the implementation coordinator. An emphasis of the SDP is on building the capacity of the district to do this program on its own from the very beginning. Being in this role of implementation coordinator for more than 10 years shaped my understanding of the relationship between clinical social work and school reform.

Relationships

The vision for how this program should support students and families is compatible with the social work belief in building relationships with those with whom you are working. This small phrase, "building relationships," does not come close to identifying the many different aspects that must be attended to to establish good, genuine relationships. For example, the membership of the various teams is determined; representative membership of the SPMT and PT is desired. The SSST may not be as inclusive due to the at times confidential nature of information being addressed. Establishing criteria of membership sends a clear message regarding the boundaries and scope of the work of the teams. The three teams allow these relationships to be

built around a common purpose. Each team identifies its expected outcomes. It is most important that the three teams communicate and plan their work in coordination with each other. The SDP does not just say that relationships are important; it identifies aspects that schools need to attend to in order to have effective relationships. In a similar fashion, social workers are prepared to attend to the many different aspects of building relationships with their clients.

One of the first interventions for SDP schools is to assess the school climate within the building, which indicates the ability and potential of individuals to work collaboratively. School climate consists of those elements within a school community that affect the development and maintenance of interpersonal relationships necessary to accomplish defined and agreed-upon tasks. It can also affect intrapersonal issues that might have an influence on achieving these tasks, such as an attitude or belief about the ability of all children to succeed in school. The elements of school climate that have been identified and researched by the School Development Program are academic focus, achievement motivation, caring and sensitivity, order and discipline, parent involvement, sharing and fairness, physical appearance and maintenance of the school, students' relationships with teachers, students' relationship with other students, and school-community relations (Haynes, Emmons, Ben-Avie, & Comer, 1996).

It is the responsibility of the school leadership to establish the norms of behavior needed to improve school climate. This does not just mean establishing a list of rules for students to abide by but understanding, as Dr. Comer has stated, that "in every interaction you are either building community, or breaking community" (Comer et al., 1996, p. 148). This statement puts *every* aspect of interaction within the school up for critical examination and provides a stringent standard for self-examination. The school leadership must model the desired interactions if the school community is to adopt the same norms (Comer et al., 1996).

A Social Worker Enters the Field of School Reform

After a number of years working with individuals, families, and groups in an outpatient mental health center, I explored working with the SDP, a national school reform program, with the goal of using my clinical training in a larger system. Early on, while training educators in the SDP, I realized that applying aspects of child and adolescent development theory to the micro-, meso-, and macrosystems of a school, which were second nature to me due to my social work background, was not a priority within the decision-making practices of schools. Decision making often occurred with little incorporation of the developmental needs of students. An illustration of this issue can be found in a discussion that occurred in one of the SDP training sessions on child and adolescent development. When the situation of quiet lunch periods was raised for discussion, we began by examining the reasons for schools instituting quiet lunch periods. The lack of a separate cafeteria in schools, the proximity to classes, and previous disruptive behavior were given as reasons for quiet lunch periods. We then used the six developmental pathways to consider how children were being affected by this decision and identified children's need for unstructured interactions, to release energy and tension, to problem solve, and to connect to others. We then related these developmental needs to how a quiet lunch and often no or little recess were not supportive of healthy development. Some teachers were surprised by these ideas, and others felt reaffirmed in their beliefs about the potential negative consequences on both children's development and school performance with quiet lunch periods. The developmental needs of students are often not taken into consideration when decisions, such as this one to institute quiet lunchrooms, are made; this example points to the tendency to treat problems as a management issue without considering the role of psychosocial development on decisions affecting students.

When conducting trainings on the Student and Staff Support Team (SSST) component of the model, I began to infuse child and adolescent development theory into the discussions that school staff was having. An SSST is a team in which educational specialists, counselors, social workers, and others meet to discuss and develop a plan for a student's difficulties related to academic or social behavior issues. Usually these teams discuss individual students one by one, looking at academic performance issues. It was important for me, as a social worker, to move educators beyond addressing the needs of one student to understand the developmental needs of all the students within the school, or all students who might be experiencing a similar situation as the one student being discussed. The educators would then practice applying this developmental understanding to the curricular and instructional goals of the school, resulting in a shift from the usual team discussion of student-level interventions to interventions involving students, caregivers, teachers, and the larger school community—systemic interventions.

Skills of the Social Worker

Franklin and Streeter (1995) identified five areas of expertise in which social workers are trained to bring to their work with schools: environmental assessment, mediation, goal attainment, resources assessment, and political action. These areas are necessary for social workers doing clinical work with the larger systems, such as schools and the school community. As I think back on the ways I have used my skills as a social worker implementing school reform, I find that these five areas of expertise accurately reflect the actual work. I will describe experiences for each of the three teams identified earlier and indicate which of the areas of expertise are being used.

Environmental Assessment

Introducing a systemic perspective to a team discussion or putting students' behavior within a developmental perspective can help broaden staff members' understanding of the system, as well as help in the creation of more effective but typically different from usual interventions. An example of needing to assess what was occurring at multiple levels of the school environment occurred during one school's SSST meeting. During this particular team discussion, a member raised the concern of students creating potentially dangerous situations in the halls during the change of classes. There was an increase in pushing and shoving to the point that someone could be injured. Other staff members agreed with this sense of potential danger, and the team began to discuss what teachers could do to decrease the level of activity during this transition time. At this point in the meeting, the team was focused on how to stop the students' dangerous behaviors. Suggestions included having teachers come out of their classrooms and be present in the halls during this time, with the thought that their presence, watchful eyes, and possible comments would be a deterrent to this behavior. The linear relationship between "acting-out students" and increased teacher presence as the solution was troubling to hear as a social worker, mainly due to the idea of teachers "controlling" students, which seems counter to the positive climate of a learning environment. Educational settings are ones in which school and community climate are essential building blocks for learning. Structure, consistency, and high expectations are important elements of that learning climate; control is not, and overemphasis on it has a negative effect on learning. During this discussion, I stated that earlier in the meeting the members had discussed their own feelings of insecurity from an administration standpoint. The principal of the school was experiencing a serious illness and had been absent for a length of time, and the educators and students did not know when the principal would return. I suggested that, rather than looking at the students' behavior in isolation, there might be a parallel process occurring between the educators and the students around the issue of uncertainty and insecurity resulting from the void of leadership and a sense of vulnerability around a medical issue. This began a discussion of how the students may be experiencing the same insecurity and vulnerability as the educators but be displaying it in a different way. Without my background in clinical social work to offer another perspective of the situation, it might have only been viewed as problematic behavior that required limit setting or restrictive intervention, and possibly disciplinary action for those students who continued with the pushing and shoving. Although no specific action was taken to address the uncertainty related to the principal's illness during this meeting, there was a softening in the tone of that discussion and consideration of the students' perspective. Changing a school's tendency to respond to situations as isolated individual acts versus connected to other situations and people, a moving toward a systemic perspective, takes time, and the first step of awareness is necessary even if a systemic intervention does not follow in the initial attempts. It is important to be able to take in all aspects of the community that might affect the current situation; without a good assessment, an appropriate intervention may not follow.

Mediation

The need for mediation is evident when individuals from various backgrounds and experiences begin to work together on such teams as those of the SDP. Site-based decision-making teams (the SPMT is an example) can provide a way for schools to identify the priorities for students' academic and social development needs in a given year. The importance of this is that site-based decision-making teams often are viewed as rubber-stamping entities or a way for a school to say it has parent or community involvement without really involving the parents or community in making decisions. A site-based decision-making team should be committed to bringing key issues of programming, curriculum, school-level policies, or even school climate issues to the table for discussion and input by all members. All decisions are made by consensus, so there is ample opportunity for discussion. As teams are learning to operate in a more collaborative way, it is sometimes difficult for members to stop thinking they are working on an issue alone. For example, an SPMT may struggle with the issue of how to increase parental involvement. This is a good topic because, although it may not be obvious to see why a school should spend time discussing parent involvement versus student achievement or student behavior, we know that without some manner of parent involvement, the issues of student achievement or behavior will never be adequately addressed.

A school's SPMT just beginning on this path may have various members talking about their individual efforts to increase parent involvement, because that was the way it was done in the past. There can be reluctance on the part of team members to have others involved in their work, or anxiety when they are asked to stop their particular activity to work with others to ensure another activity's success. Helping people see the benefits of working as a team and identifying common goals, and putting aside personal fears of not being totally in control or having to work with someone else, takes a skill and experience level that most social workers have. Many school teams fail to be effective because they cannot surmount this issue. School reform may direct schools to use teams, but it may not tell schools how to develop these teams. I had the opportunity to work with a reform model that included a process to which I could bring my social work skills. When I work with schools that are not using a reform model, I still have to use my group skills to bring individuals together around a task. No one is asking that I do this; I can identify the need or the missing relational element and make recommendations to address these issues. I think most social workers in schools find themselves in a similar situation and have to identify the need or the gap in the effective performance of teams and come up with strategies to address these needs. I believe that social workers need to initiate the implementation of these strategies because other educators within the school are not trained to identify and assess these types of interpersonal issues.

Goal Attainment

Goal attainment or goal identification can be seen in this example of a parent team experience of working with a group of teachers when one school's PT did not feel collaborative or on the same wavelength as the teachers. Parents, teachers, and school administrators expressed dissatisfaction with the working relationship between the PT and the school staff. I conducted a training session for parents and teachers of this school on the six developmental pathways. All participants were divided into groups of five or six members, with teachers and parents mixed within each group. Their task was to look at each of those six developmental pathways and determine what specific goals or characteristics they wanted their children/students to be able to develop or achieve within each pathway. There was much conversation, and as the groups presented their final list of goals on large pieces of newsprint to the entire group, they realized there were more similarities between the parents and teachers about what they wanted for their children than they expected. Parents and teachers came away with a sense that they had something in common, and this was a starting point for future discussions. My clinical experience in running groups and doing family therapy was extremely important in this situation because it allowed me to attend to the process of the relationships, such as getting people to see commonalities, and not just

attend to the task that needed to be accomplished, such as disseminating information. This was only one activity in a school year. It is important to recognize that without a continuous plan of nurturing and developing these relationships, the positive outcome of one activity will be short-lived.

Resources Assessment

Resources assessment consists of taking an inventory of the resources available within the school's community and determining how and when to engage the available resources, or how and when to offer school resources to community agencies. One principal I worked with did two things when she started in a new school. First, she walked the streets of the neighborhood and introduced herself to people at each store and business, no matter how large or small, including churches. No doubt she also introduced herself to neighborhood members whom she saw on a regular basis. She wanted to establish a relationship with the community from which her students were coming. She wanted the community to know her, and she wanted to know who she could call upon if a time or situation arose when she needed to enlist the community's resources. The second thing she did was to make an effort to call each parent to find out what interest or skill they could contribute to the school. This sounds overwhelming, but when she decided to create a school garden to help the students connect to the school and learn science, she knew which parents to call on. A good question to consider is, as social workers, are we thinking strategically about the relationships that we need to do our work to the fullest in school communities? Although this example involved a school principal, one can see that a social worker might easily be pictured in this role. As an aside, this principal had a daughter who became a social worker several years later.

Political Action

So far I have described teams within a school environment working in a more systemic way and with a developmental focus. Work with school districts can be equally effective as we try to support schools, school districts, boards of education, and teachers' unions to work toward the same goals for students. A school district I worked with for 2 years was implementing the SDP at the school level, and schools were seeing levels of application that varied widely. The district did not understand that there needed to be a commitment at its level to support the implementation in the individual schools. This commitment may require providing funding for schools to send staff members to training, working with a school around their team meetings (SPMT, SSST, or PT), or bringing in relevant staff development for areas of child development, instruction, or classroom management. These are good efforts and should be done. However, by observing all the schools involved, the district may come to understand the common barriers to effective implementation; rather than only attend to each school's problem, it may learn that a district-level structural change needs to occur.

While working with one school district that was implementing the SDP, I spent most of a year promoting monthly meetings to discuss the implementation process. One way to ensure that a district focuses on a program and takes responsibility for its success is to create a time for the central office to receive information about the program's progress, even if it is only a brief review or update. The district wanted to discuss more management-type topics during this meeting, such as budget issues, staffing issues, and decisions made by the state department of education or the school board. Although these were important and necessary issues to address, I knew that if the implementation of the SDP was not on the agenda in a significant way, its implementation would continue to vary widely from school to school, with no true investment by central office administrators. I planned my implementation visits to coincide with the district meetings as best I could and had a standing request for the SDP implementation to be a part of the agenda, asking that each principal discuss how his or her school used the three teams to advance its goals. By working in this way, the individual-level work of each school was highlighted in a central office forum, and principals had an opportunity to share successes with one another and to identify areas in which they could use some suggestions. This built a more collegial relationship among the principals, and it allowed the central office administrators to get an overall sense of the work and make some helpful suggestions. The entire district staff then knew what was happening with this particular program and knew how they could support

one another. Their comments to one another both during and after the meeting confirmed the importance of doing this. I heard comments such as, "We should do this at each meeting." One individual realized that this was what we had been trying to do all year. Without constant attention to this process and ensuring that members feel safe enough to share in this manner, or get the message that it is important to discuss implementation issues in this way, the central office system will no longer be supportive.

National School Reform

I have used the SDP as the focus for understanding the connection between social work and school reform, and the relationship between social work and the leadership and decision-making structures of schools and districts. The SDP is just one of many school reform models, and it is important that social work practice in schools is viewed within the changing landscape of the national school reform movement. Public education has been in a state of continuous reform since the report *A Nation at Risk* (National Commission for Excellence in Education, 1983), which focused on America's declining educational standards. Since that time, various programs have been designed to improve compartmentalized aspects of school functioning, such as social skills programs, reading programs, parent involvement programs, and so forth. In 1991, the New American Schools Development Corporation (NASDC), which was created by business leaders, funded innovative and "break-the-mold" educational ideas. The design teams that were established through NASDC were often existing school reform models or collaborative ventures between several existing educational models. For the most part these designs were to include parent involvement, community involvement, and staff development (McDonald et al., 1999; North Central Regional Educational Laboratory, 2002). The focus was to bring the compartmentalized models together to deliver a more comprehensive approach to school reform.

In 1994, Title I legislation was expanded to include funding for schoolwide or comprehensive initiatives (National Clearinghouse for Comprehensive School Reform, 2002). The interest in the NASDC design teams and individual schoolwide/

comprehensive initiatives grew, and in 1997 Congress passed the Obey-Porter Comprehensive School Reform Demonstration (CSRD) legislation that initially provided $145 million to state education agencies for incentive grants to school districts, on a competitive basis, for schools that elected to pursue comprehensive school reforms. In 1998, the initial funding year, 1,800 schools in 50 states received grants, in 1999, 2,800 schools received grants and in 2001, 5,300 schools received grants (*About CSR*, 2002). Individual schools received up to $50,000 per year for 3 years to implement a research-based, comprehensive school reform model. A major aspect of school reform was the decentralization of decision making from the district office to the individual school. The types of decisions that were decentralized varied from state to state, but increased involvement of school staff, parents, and community members on site-based decision-making teams was common.

Social Work and School Reform

School reform has left a legacy of increased site-based decision-making teams, more types of teams to address the prereferral to special education needs of students, parent and community involvement, and comprehensive educational programs. That is not to say that all these teams are effective, and some may actually exist in name only; the point is that there is an opportunity for someone who knows how these teams can be better used to support students. The names of the specific teams will differ from district to district, but these teams exist, and social workers need to be involved with them and know how to use them. These teams have opened new avenues for (1) improving relationships between and among the various systems within the school community, and (2) integrating child and adolescent development knowledge in more aspects of school decision making. Insufficient attention has been given to how to build productive relationships within the school community to support the students; this is a key area in which the training and skills of social work have much to contribute. Site-based decision-making teams, child study teams, student and staff support teams, and even crisis teams, commonplace in schools since school reform, have a responsibility to attend to the issues within a school that affect not only the

educational process but also the developmental process for students.

To play a more active role in school reform or education in general, social workers will need to consider the following areas: know the teams, understand your potential contribution to the team, help educators understand the connection between the individual clinical work that you do and the larger systemic impact that you can have, and, finally, increase your visibility within the school community through participation on decision-making teams.

Know the Teams

Social workers must know what teams exist in the school. First, there is usually some type of decision-making team identified by a name such as "leadership team," "site-based decision-making team," "local site council," "school committee," "management team," and "school planning and management team" (the SDP version). The team involves the principal as the lead decision maker in the school and typically handles curriculum, achievement, policy, and planning and budget issues, among others. Second, there are teams designated to address the educational or learning needs of students; most are familiar with the referral team for special education issues that is mandated by state law. Third, there are other teams sometimes known at prereferral teams, for example, child study teams, student support teams, care teams, and student and staff support teams (the SDP version). These teams are able to consider ways to improve a student's success in school before the student needs to be referred for special education services. Moreover, this level of team can look at the overall needs of all students, or students within a specific grade, classroom, or even coming from a particular neighborhood, to see if there needs to be a systemic intervention to support their needs. For example, a middle school I worked with received word that a local newspaper was going to publish pictures of all the teenagers who had been killed in the local community due to violence within the past year. The student and staff support team met immediately to discuss this new information and developed a plan of action for the homeroom teachers to address the newspaper story the first thing the next morning. The SSST members were available in case some students were distressed and/or reacted in response to the newspaper story. Under a very tight time schedule, this team was able to not just react to a potentially disruptive event but to develop a plan of response that probably helped the students and educators feel more secure emotionally.

Fourth, other teams that social workers need to consider working with are the parent or parent and teacher teams, such as PTAs, PTOs, booster clubs, and parent teams (the SDP version). These teams have a wonderful resource of parents and community members who may not be involved in the life of the school in as many ways as possible. Being able to mediate between teachers and parents about ways to improve or support the school can lead to more powerful networks of support and power for a school or principal who may not have power through the district's central administration. Fifth, there are also grade-level (elementary school) or department-level meetings (middle and high school). As teachers are planning lessons, knowledge of the social and cultural environments of the students or specific child development information can be brought in to improve the level of instruction. Finally, there are faculty meetings. Often these are administrative, but well-developed materials about a topic that can be passed out fairly quickly with brief commentary can go a long way toward increasing access to information about child and adolescent development and indicating an area where teachers can use you as a resource.

See a Place for Your Contribution

Regardless of whether you have knowledge or training in child or adolescent development, psychodynamically oriented therapies, systems-oriented therapies, group process, multicultural issues, or another area, as a social worker you have preparation in the five areas of expertise identified earlier and are able to apply your particular specialty to any of the previously mentioned teams. At this point there is no step-by-step guide on how to do this; however, it starts with being present on these teams and listening to the discussions. As you are listening, ask yourself, What is the main concern here? Is it an issue related to the students or an issue about the adults (teachers, administrators, parents)? Often the discussions in schools are not about the students; one thing everyone can do is to bring the discussions back to focus on how to improve the situation of

students. Next, you can think about whether the discussions and decisions related to the students take into consideration the multiple layers of the system. It is almost a setup to provide a detailed behavior modification plan for a student addressing his or her classroom behavior, when the student may not be getting appropriate nutrition in the morning before school starts.

Academic achievement, staff development, scheduling issues, budgeting, and so forth may not be considered to be the domain of the clinician, but they are. Consider the effects on students when the teaching staff changes curriculum, instruction goals, and objectives based on state or district mandates without thinking about the consequences on the established academic climate and student academic self-concepts. In one school, I listened as a teacher who had been a part of a school reform effort and really understood child development described changing the curriculum plan to meet the students' needs. This fifth-grade mathematics teacher recalled that at the beginning of a school year, the curriculum guide indicated that the students were to start with the multiplication of fractions. This teacher immediately discovered that most of the students did not know their multiplication tables. The teacher went against the district's written curriculum and started where the students were, which was to learn multiplication, something they were supposed to have mastered the previous year. After a few months, the students had caught up to where they should have been. Other teachers in the same grade began the year following the written curriculum, and several months down the road they found themselves wondering what to do because their students did not have the prerequisite knowledge and skills to handle the mathematical tasks. This may seem solely like an educational issue, but the effect on the self-esteem of the children and teachers and the impact on classroom climate and academic motivation demonstrate the interconnection between the academic program and the psychoemotional factors that affect academic achievement. This example illustrates that once the developmental discussions take hold within a school, the educators begin to "own" this developmental perspective and are able to integrate it into their daily work. Including clinical practitioners at the table for these types of discussions would make a substantial impact on the process and climate of education.

Understanding the Connection

Social workers can help educators understand the connection between individual-level situations and larger systemic situations. Winters and Gourdine (2000) discuss the importance of social workers being a part of the site-based teams and indicate that the school system may not recognize the importance of the social worker in this capacity, and therefore may not accept them in this role. Social workers not only should address the individual problems and crises that arise within a school but also must attend to the transactions between the various subsystems within schools that interfere with a student's ability to effectively engage in the educational process (Winters & Easton, 1983). Making the connection between individual-level issues and larger systemic issues occurs over a period of time, but it must be constantly attended to. In the following example, an incident in a training event was a reminder of the power of changed perspective and support of colleagues.

During this particular training session, my colleagues and I had been engaged in a weeklong series of sessions and activities focused on increasing understanding of the developmental, social, and cultural contexts of the children within schools, and the importance of connecting this understanding to the instructional practices. Typically 100 to 150 teachers from all over the United States attend such events, and they are placed in groups with teachers from other districts. At the end of the training, groups have an opportunity to display what they have learned and what they will take back to their respective schools. During one of these final sessions, one teacher described how she had reached an "understanding" with her students; if they don't hassle her, she won't hassle them. She explained that there were a few adolescents in the class who were particularly unruly, and this was her way of creating a classroom where she felt she could get some teaching accomplished without having as many disruptions. As this teacher relayed her experience the entire room was silent; many were nodding their heads in agreement. She continued by saying that as a result of using a developmental perspective and the discussions with the other educators in the room, she knew she had abandoned her responsibility to all her students. She made a promise in front of the entire room to go back and reconnect with each of her students, and received much support from the others in that room. Although this situation occurred after an intense weeklong training focused on development, a continued focus on child development applied to individuals and system-level responses in schools can have similar effects. Social workers can create opportunities for discussions among school staff that can result in this type of personal and professional transformation.

Increased Visibility

Streeter and Franklin (1993) indicate that with school reform, specifically because decision making is decentralized and staffing and budgeting decisions are closely related to the school's ability to meet educational objectives, social workers need to show how they impact this overall objective. It becomes essential that social workers within schools are able to document and quantify their effectiveness. This also means that the visibility and involvement of social workers in the larger planning aspects of schools must increase. Staff members within the school need to be informed about what social workers are doing with students, and they need to know how their work can support the clinical work being done and vice versa. Clinical work usually occurs in isolation, and the school staff generally does not know what a social worker does with a referred student. I frequently hear teachers say that they do not know what the social worker does or what a SSST does. When I try to build acceptance of the social worker by the school staff, it becomes important to continually educate the staff about what the social worker can and cannot do. If the social worker is invisible in a school, that individual's work may not be valued. This does not necessarily mean that clinical work is not valued but that the social worker will not be used as effectively as possible. If we follow Streeter and Franklin's conclusion, this invisibility may translate into fewer social work positions in the long term.

Conclusion

Social workers in schools have a heavy workload, assigned tasks that vary from state to state, and an enormous number of individual students in need. Thus, it is not without hesitation that I identify yet another area of work within schools that would benefit from incorporating clinical practice. Social workers' participation in schools in a more systemic way is important for the following reasons. First, when the larger systemic issues are focused on, there can be a decrease in the individual-level cases because the system is better situated to handle them. Second, team meetings that address such topics as budgets, curriculum, discipline, and collaborations with community resources are just as critical as the psychosocial needs of individual students, and time must be set aside for social workers to participate on these decision-making and policymaking teams. Third, site-based decision-making teams, prereferral teams, and parent teams all have varying degrees of impact on school budgets, staffing, educational programs, and the ways that resources are provided to students. Therefore, it is an optimal opportunity for the presence and participation of social work.

This type of work calls for an end of thinking about social work in school settings as occurring in a "host" agency. Although the business of education may be the focus in a school, true education does not occur without a solid foundation of effective relationships and an in-depth knowledge of the student body; by this I mean child and adolescent development knowledge. Therefore, social workers and educators must work hand in hand; if they do not, we will continue to see the declining conditions of education and educational communities.

The expanded application of clinical social work described in this chapter provides a lens for perceiving and understanding what is occurring beyond individual, isolated behaviors to affect change within the larger systems of the school. The core aspects of social work education and preparation make social workers extremely qualified to be involved in the establishment and ongoing work of the leadership and policymaking teams within schools. The theoretical perspective of social workers enables them to attend to the individual issues within the context of the larger systems issues. Social workers must be willing to step into this role and make a greater impact on the legacy of school reform.

Notes

1. The positions included in this figure are psychologists, social workers, attendance officers, and other support categories, such as data processing, health, building and equipment, bus drivers, and security and food service workers.

2. I use the term "educators" to include teachers, administrators, and nonteaching staff within a school.

3. Information about the School Development Program and districts implementing this reform model can be obtained online at http://info.med.yale.edu/Comer/.

4. The student and staff support team was initially named the mental health team. The change occurred in the early 1990s to ensure that the work of the team focused on holistic development, not mental health alone.

References

About CSR. Overview of the comprehensive school reform program (CSR). Available: http://www.ed.gov/offices/OESE/compreform/2pager.html. December 11, 2002.

Allen-Meares, P. (1994). Social work services in schools: A national study of entry-level tasks. Social Work, 39, 560–565.

Anson, A. R., Cook, T. D., Habib, F., Grady, M. K., Haynes, N., & Comer, J. P. (1991). The Comer School Development Program: A theoretical analysis. Urban Education, 26, 56–82.

Cauce, A. M., Comer, J. P., & Schwartz, D. (1987). Long-term effects of a systems-oriented school prevention program. American Journal of Orthopsychiatry, 57, 127–131.

Comer, J. P. (1980). School power: Implications of an intervention project. New York: Free Press.

Comer, J. P., Haynes, N. M., Joyner, E. T., & Ben-Avie, M. (1996). Rallying the whole village: The Comer process for reforming education. New York: Teachers College Press.

Cook, T. D., Hunt, H. D., & Murphy, R. F. (1999). Comer's School Development Program in Chicago: A theory-based evaluation. Evanston, IL: Northwestern University, Institute for Policy Research.

Franklin, C., & Streeter, C. L. (1995). School reform: Linking public schools with human services. Social Work, 40, 773–782.

Haynes, N. M. (1994). School Development Program. Research Monograph No. 1. New Haven, CT: Yale University Child Study Center School Development Program.

Haynes, N. M., & Comer, J. P. (1990). The effects of a school development program on self-concept. Yale Journal of Biology and Medicine, 63, 275–283.

Haynes, N. M., Comer, J. P., & Hamilton-Lee, M.

(1988). The School Development Program: A model for school improvement. *Journal of Negro Education, 57*, 11–21.

Haynes, N. M., Emmons, C. L., Ben-Avie, M., & Comer, J. P. (1996). *The school development program: Student, staff and parent school climate surveys.* New Haven, CT: Yale Child Study Center School Development Program.

McDonald, J. P., Hatch, T., Kirby, E., Aimes, N., Haynes, N. M., & Joyner, E. T. (1999). *School reform behind the scenes.* New York: Teachers College Press.

National Center for Education Statistics. (2001). *Statistics in brief: Public school student, staff and graduate counts by state, school year 1999–2000.* Retrieved July 18, 2003, from http://nces.ed.gov/pubs2001/2001326r.pdf

The National Clearinghouse for Comprehensive School Reform. *About CSR.* (2002). Available: http://www.goodschools.gwu.edu/about_csr/index.html. December 12, 2002.

National Commission for Excellence in Education. *A nation at risk* (1983). Online. Available: http://www.ed.gov/pubs/NatAtRisk/risk.html. December 11, 2002.

Noblit, G., Malloy, C., Malloy, W., Villenas, S., Groves, P., Jennings, M., Patterson, J., & Rayle, J. (1997). *Scaling up supportive environment: Case studies of successful Comer schools.* Chapel Hill: University of North Carolina Press.

Noblit, G., Malloy. W., & Malloy, C. (2001). *The kids got smarter: Case studies of successful Comer schools.* Creskill, NJ: Hampton Press.

North Central Regional Educational Laboratory (2002). *New American schools.* Available: http://www.ncrel.org/sdrs/areas/issues/students/atrisk/at6lk50a.htm. December 11, 2002.

Streeter, C. L., & Franklin, C. (1993). Site-based management in public education: Opportunities and challenges for school social workers. *Social Work in Education, 15*, 71–81.

Torres, S. (1996). The status of school social workers in America. *Social Work in Education, 18*, 8–18.

Winters, W. G., & Easton, F. (1983). *The practice of social work in schools: An ecological perspective.* New York: Free Press.

Winters, W. G., & Gourdine, R. M. (2000). School reform: A viable domain for school social work practice. In June G. Hopps & Robert Morris (Eds.), *Social work at the millennium: Critical reflections on the future of the profession* (pp. 138–159). New York: Free Press.

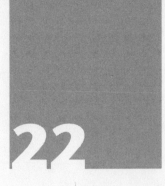

22

E. Martin Schotz, Ruth Grossman Dean,

and Jane Crosby

Social Work and the "Community of Concern" in an Urban American Public Elementary School

An Interim Report

Beginning Anew

In life, human beings are always beginning in the middle and moving backward and forward simultaneously. We begin in the middle of a world confronting us with problems, which are not of our own making. We must move forward in tackling these problems, while we move backward, attempting to more fully assimilate and understand our history and our human heritage (including the history of the problems) in order to be equal to life's challenges.

So it was approximately 4 years ago that a group of four clinicians (three social workers and a psychiatrist; in addition to the three authors of this chapter, Joe Sarra and various mental health interns have been part of the working team) in the family services clinic of a community health center came to form a children's services team and attempted to begin anew. This team had rather spontaneously emerged in the clinic, united by a desire to approach their work from a radical perspective. Each member of the team had received "traditional training" in his or her field. However, each had independently come to the conclusion that people's problems, which were traditionally seen as individual defects or the re-

sult of family problems, were, in a deeper sense, a reflection of the difficulty people and their families were having responding to the chaos and violence that dominated our society.

In speaking of "chaos and violence," we are not referring only to the most obvious manifestations, which one witnesses daily on the evening news. We refer as well to ruling forces in society that by their very nature pit people against each other in a daily struggle for survival—forces that foster vast disparities of wealth both within our own country and throughout the world, forces that obstruct people's efforts to secure meaningful employment along with access to high-quality health services, education, housing, recreation, arts, and a safe and healthy environment.

As soon as one begins to conceive of "social" and "psychological" problems within this framework, it becomes obvious that mental health workers, being products of the same system, are both a part of the problem and hopefully part of the solution. The mental health worker is a part of the problem in that he or she more often than not is a privileged "middleman" in the vast system of maldistribution. And the system surrounds the mental health worker with rationalizations that justify the problem and "blame the victim" (Ryan, 1976). To

336

the degree that workers cannot resist such ideas, they become extensions of the system of oppression. But how is one to resist? Where is one to find ideas that offer an alternative?

In pursuing its project, the team found two theoretical sources most helpful. Both are aspects of our heritage that have been marginalized in this day and age. One was the Christian prophetic tradition, as reflected in the writings of advocates of nonviolence such as Harriet Beecher Stowe (1852/1965, 1999; see also Hedrick, 1994), and the Catholic worker movement founded by Dorothy Day (1997) and Peter Maurin. The other tradition was to be found in the struggles for socialism and social democracy, a tradition of political activists and writers on the left such as Jane Addams (1960), W. E. B. DuBois (1970, 1971), David Gil (1996, 1998), Florence Kelley (1986), Jonathan Kozol (1992), Bertha Capen Reynolds (1951, 1991), Paul Robeson (1978), and William Ryan (1976). Ultimately, these traditions seemed to intertwine in the liberation theology of Latin America (Borge, 1987; Brockman, 1989; Friere, 1972; Gutierrez, 1996; Menchu, 1984) or in our country in the writings of Martin Luther King Jr. (1986). In referring to these writings, we only wish to indicate a few of the most immediate sources of guidance for us. Each member of the team has been influenced by a myriad of religious and political traditions and experiences.

As the work has progressed, more and more the team has come to see that we all need an alternative to the present social, economic, and political system. For our health, as well as the health of the people we seek to serve, we need to hasten into being that "community of concern," based on ideals as old as Christ's Gospels, and articulated in Martin Luther King Jr.'s last work, "Where Do We Go From Here: Chaos or Community" (1986).

In this regard it is worth recalling the "Credo" of Bertha Capen Reynolds, first published in *Social Work Today* in 1941. In this statement she affirms the possibility of understanding and "intelligently aligning oneself with the movement of social and economic forces" in the world and proposes that people have the strength to work together to change life conditions and achieve their goals and not goals set for them by others (1991, p. 186). In her view, the path to individual fulfillment is through joining with others who share the same purposes.

On Working With Social and Psychological Problems

Drawing on this literature of liberation and social justice, the team has developed its own credo:

1. We believe that problems of social injustice are at the core of social and psychological problems, and that all people want to belong, to be embraced, loved, respected, and celebrated for their struggles and successes.
2. We believe that an essential aspect of our work is making people aware of their rights and seeking to understand the forces in society that obstruct the full enjoyment of those rights.
3. We believe that when a person experiences him- or herself as being loved—embraced, celebrated, and cared for—the person naturally experiences a desire to give back the same.
4. We believe that an essential task of the social worker is to help develop the "community of concern," in which each person's difficulty is everyone's responsibility.
5. We believe that the "community of concern" is necessary to adequately respond to the individual's and the institution's need for social and psychological healing.
6. We believe there is an essential connection between working for and with an individual and working for and with institutions, and that each nurtures the other.
7. We believe that a creative use of community, institutional, group, and individual resources woven together in varying patterns and combinations constitutes the essence of community-based practice.
8. We believe that working to address the social problems of individuals or institutions is a long-term process and requires a long-term commitment. With this in mind, we encourage people to think in terms of a hundred-year plan.

In the narrative that follows, we hope to demonstrate how we put these principles into action.

Shifting the Frame

As an example of the shift in the team's approach to problems, we might cite the issue of "out-of-control" children. Without abandoning traditional knowledge about social and psychological problems, the team began to approach disturbing, disruptive, or "symptomatic" behavior differently. While it is well established within the framework of traditional psychoanalytic thought that "symptomatic" behavior is not simply a sign of pathology but is simultaneously an attempt on the part of the individual to cope, psychoanalytic theory does not locate the origin of the problem as well as the solution in the social order.

It is rather typical for children to be diagnosed as "out of control" and for clinicians to develop strategies aimed at getting them to control themselves better. However, the team felt that children who were labeled "out of control" were generally children whose behavior was problematic for the adults who were supposed to be in control of the situation. In other words, the children were disturbing. Instead of seeing the problem of the disturbing child as a case where greater self-control was needed, the team considered that the problem was with the self that the child was expressing. Instead of pressing the child to control an unhappy self, why not try to find ways of fostering a happier sense of self in the child? To do this the team needed to seek out positive resources for the child in the community—resources that would not approach the child with the bias that he or she was the problem.

Seeing the origins and solutions to the problem in the community, the team acknowledged that people who are subjects of violence and abuse tend to defend themselves in any way they can. A person's healthy response to abuse, violence, and oppression requires healthy social institutions that are prepared to identify with victims of oppression and support them in finding positive responses. The need for such care is not an alternative to but rather an addition to individual and family services. Thus, throughout the clinical process, the team is always attempting to connect the individual or family with supportive services that are part of the "community of concern," such as church groups, after-school programs, night schools, mentoring programs, arts programs, sports and recreation programs, and political organizations.

When we speak of connecting others and ourselves with a "community of concern," we understand that we are only speaking of such a com-

munity in its earliest stages, with its few components rather fragmented. Nevertheless, we believe it is important to conceive this community, for it is truly what we all deserve. This perspective calls on us to change ourselves, as well as the ways we see clients.

Search for a "Community of Concern"

From the outset, the team saw its foremost priority as beginning to connect itself with various institutions in the community, all of which in one way or another were seen as the seeds of a "community of concern." The institutions with which the team sought links were quite varied in size and focus. One program was the Paul Robeson Institute, a Saturday program led by African American men for African American boys, which aimed at helping the latter develop positive self-images. Another program was the Victory Generation Program of the Black Ministerial Alliance of Boston, a coalition of the city's African American churches, which had launched an ambitious program of developing 40 after-school programs for children across the city. There was the Earn-a-Bike program developed by an organization called Bikes Not Bombs, which held 8-week sessions in which children learned about the mechanics of a bicycle, and in the end built a bike that they could take home with them. There was a small law firm dedicated to working with parents to defend their children's rights in regard to education. There was a graduate school of social work, which placed social work interns with the team and sponsored the work of one of its faculty members with the team. And there was the primary focus of our work, a public elementary school located a couple of blocks from the clinic.

The Elementary School

In the following sections of this chapter, we report on the progress of various aspects of the team's work using a community practice approach in the public elementary school. Located in a large city in the northeastern United States, the school, which includes kindergarten through fifth grade, is housed in a low, rambling building that occupies a city block. It has an open plan, typical of school design in the 1970s, and a noisy atmosphere, with few rooms having walls that reach the ceiling. Classrooms are spread throughout the building, and many are located far from the main office. The section of the city in which the school is located is socially and economically diverse, but the majority of families whose children attend the school are low income and Hispanic. Out of a total student body of 778 students, 33% are officially classified as having "special needs" educationally, 40 % are bilingual, and 82% come from homes in which English is not the first language. Because children are bused to the school from neighborhoods all over the city, the school has only a limited connection to the surrounding neighborhood. Nonetheless, the principal has developed many strong relationships with local merchants, firemen, police, and downtown community leaders, who provide help of different sorts. For example, staff from one of the large "downtown" financial institutions have been volunteering a lunch hour a week to visit the school, eat lunch, and read with a student. Students, delighted with this opportunity, have been heard to say to one another on the appointed day, "I can't talk to you now, I have my 'power lunch.'"

For a number of years, members of the team ran a traditional mental health clinic in the school, providing individual and group psychotherapy to students. Over the past 4 years, the team has broadened its approach and, in alliance with the principal, has attempted to help the school develop a culture of nonviolence. The team's individual and group work with children and parents is billed through the mental health clinic; public and private grants cover the more broadly defined supportive services, and some small portion of team members' time is voluntary.

In the material that follows, examples of the team's work in the elementary school illustrate how it is attempting to put into practice the teachings of those who locate "social work" in communal and collaborative efforts. Although for purposes of organizing this writing, work with various groups in the school is discussed separately from work with individuals, these distinctions are relative. The team's work with individual administrators, teachers, parents, and students occurs simultaneously with work with groups in the school, and each provides a context and support for the other. The team also sees its work in the community outside the school as intimately connected with the work in the school. The relationships it has developed with various agencies become resources to draw on, as needed, to enrich the work in the school.

Some History

Prior to the arrival of a new principal in the fall of 1996, our elementary school had been seen as a large, unruly, and problem-filled place where academic achievement was low. The teachers and staff were often in conflict with one another. There was little sense of community, and collaborative efforts to address difficulties were limited.

Mrs. Hernandez, the school's new leader, is a tall, impressive, gregarious, and very bright Hispanic woman, who arrived full of energy. Before taking this new position, she had extensive experience as a teacher and had been head of bilingual education for the entire city. She came to the school deeply committed to raising academic standards and creating a new atmosphere for students, teachers, and parents. Perhaps symbolic of her energy and values was a large poster of César Chávez, the founder of the National Farm Workers Association, which she hung on the wall of her office.

At about the time Mrs. Hernandez was arriving, something had happened at our clinic. In 1995, Nelson Mandela's autobiography, *Long Walk to Freedom*, first appeared. In response, a member of the clinic, who would later become a member of our team, was so impressed with the book that he was moved to write an essay entitled "Confronting Violence in Our Schools With a Culture of Nonviolence" (Schotz, 1996). The essay attempted to use key concepts from Mandela's autobiography as a way of orienting oneself to clinical practice. At the heart of this analysis was the concept that violence was not merely physical assault or the threat of such but was anything that breached in any way the dignity or human rights of anyone. Mandela had eventually come to see the task as liberating whites as well as blacks, for as blacks were enslaved by apartheid, whites were enslaved by hate and fear.

Drawing on this insight, the essay offered a vision of all of us as trapped in a structurally violent system. The critical task was to help people find ways of working within the system without identifying themselves with the system and without adopting its values. Peace was seen not as the absence of open hostility but as the order that flows from social justice. The essay developed the values of "freedom," "equality," "justice," "discipline," "identification," "understanding," "respect," "patience," and "humility" as providing an orientation for clinical, educational, and administrative practices.

The members of the team who were working in the school reported that a new energy was emanating from the principal's office. It occurred to them that perhaps the new principal might be interested in the essay, and so they shared it with her. For the next few months they heard nothing about it. When they finally asked the principal about the essay, they learned that she had liked it quite a bit and was interested in discussing it with the team. Thus, a meeting was arranged.

At this meeting the team and Mrs. Hernandez found that they shared many ideas and values, and that the essay seemed to provide a conceptual basis for them to start collaborating on building a "culture of nonviolence" in the school. Mrs. Hernandez spoke of the range of pressures she experienced as principal. There were learning issues, standards, and testing. On an administrative level, she faced budget problems and budget cuts, union pressures, and many other issues. Then she talked about the frustration and tension in her relationship with the teachers, who were not always in accord with the changes she was trying to bring to the school.

Another concern was the lack of parental involvement in the school. Many of the students' families struggled with severe financial pressures, crowded living conditions, health problems, and violence in their neighborhoods and at times in their homes. A high percentage of the children and their families did not speak English. Many parents worked during the day and were unavailable to meet with teachers; others stayed away because they were afraid of institutions like the school. This was especially true of recent immigrants and parents unable to speak English. Some students lived in other parts of the city far away from the school, others had siblings to be cared for, or the parents had no easy means of transportation.

Then Mrs. Hernandez told the story of the "kindergarten from hell." As it turned out, often the children in the school with the most violent disruptive behavior were the youngest, the kindergartners. The previous year had seen a class that was so unruly it had been labeled by the staff as the "kindergarten from hell." Month after month, teachers and administrators had struggled with this group. Finally, toward the end of the school year, the "kids finally seemed to get it," and the class had become much better disciplined and well behaved. As the end of the year approached, the staff looked forward to a graduation ceremony, at which they would celebrate with the children and parents the great progress the class had made. Finally the day came, and as the kindergartners marched on the stage, dressed in their best clothes for their graduation, the ceremony was interrupted before it began as two parents got into a physical fight over a seat, only to be cheered on by other parents. The team members could not help but laugh with Mrs. Hernandez over the wild absurdity of this story. At the same time, the team was being educated as to the range and depth of some of the challenges it would face.

As the meeting drew to a close, Mrs. Hernandez suddenly exclaimed, "I know how I will use you—you will be my consultants." Mrs. Hernandez's suggestion seemed very much in line with the team's ideas. It was clear that everyone in this situation was suffering, including the principal. If she were to be able to successfully help her staff take better care of the students, she needed people who would offer her the support and understanding she deserved and was sorely lacking. This, then, was the first step in our collaboration. From that point on, the team has met regularly with the principal—sometimes monthly, sometimes more often as she felt the need.

Many initiatives have evolved from these meetings. In the material that follows, we discuss efforts with several groups—the teachers' support group, the discipline committee, and the Parent Alliance (La Alianza Para Padres). This is followed by a description of work with an individual student.

The Teacher's Support Group

The idea of a teachers' support group naturally flowed from the focus of developing a culture of nonviolence in the school community. From the earliest meeting, the principal indicated that such a group for the teachers was timely, as she had found herself quite beleaguered by their pressing needs and demands.

An announcement was made to the entire faculty that two social workers from the team would offer a weekly support group for all teachers who wanted to attend. At the outset, those teachers who came seemed quite overwhelmed and angry and directed a good deal of that anger at the principal. The team found itself in the middle of a seeming conflict between a principal who was frustrated with the resistance of teachers and teachers who were frustrated and angry at the demands they perceived the principal to be making.

The team's understanding of the nature of oppression in our society was critical to the way it approached this conflict. In our society, workers in the field of public education tend to be fragmented into different disciplines (e.g., teachers, clinicians, paraprofessionals, administrators). The ideology of the system encourages everyone to believe that if one does his or her job correctly, then he or she will be successful. This belief is inculcated at the same time that the social and material resources that are provided to public educational institutions are woefully inadequate. If one accepts this ideology, when failure comes, as it inevitably must, the question becomes, Who is to blame for the failure? In the case of a teacher, one could blame oneself, which would lead to guilt, shame, frustration, and feelings of being burned out. Or one could blame the children or families or the administration. No matter whom one chooses to blame, one is angry and frustrated, and a general climate of poor morale tends to develop. From their first meeting, the team members who led the teachers' support group were confronted with exactly such feelings.

After listening to the teachers, the team members began to offer a different perspective on their situation. Specifically, the team encouraged the teachers to realize that everyone in the school was a victim of violence—the teachers, the students, and the parents, as well as the administrative staff. Because the resources necessary to do the job were so inadequate, it was self-defeating to feel guilty about this or to blame oneself or others for the failures. Rather, the task was to come together and try to improve the situation collectively. Improving the situation did not necessarily mean that it would fulfill the ideal of what people truly deserved. As people are taught in 12-step recovery programs, progress, not perfection, needs to be the goal.

As a result of this approach, the teachers began to see that they had a responsibility to take care of themselves, as well as the students and the principal. The teachers began to have a greater sense of respect for themselves. Reciprocally, this same perspective was used in working with the principal, who was helped to appreciate the frustrations and needs of her staff while at the same time relinquishing the idea that it was reasonable for her to expect to be able to meet these needs. Even though she could not realistically hope to meet all their needs, she could make herself available in a way that might helpful. Thus, the principal was encouraged to set aside a couple of open hours a week when she would be available to any teachers who wanted to come and talk with her.

The combined work with the teachers and principal began to foster a new quality of relating. One example involved Mrs. Baldwin, a teacher who very much wanted Mrs. Hernandez's approval but had always found her intimidating. One day in a professional development workshop, Mrs. Hernandez was explaining a program to the teachers. Mrs. Baldwin did not understand the instructions, and upon asking for further explanation felt humiliated by the principal's reply. Mrs. Baldwin was extremely upset that Mrs. Hernandez considered her "dumb" for not understanding the first time. She went home, thought about it, and the next day went in to see Mrs. Hernandez. Mrs. Baldwin told her, "I wanted to let you know that when I asked a question in the workshop yesterday, your answer made me feel stupid!" The principal, who was quite surprised, apologized and emphatically stated that she did not intend to make anyone feel stupid and that she welcomed questions. They had an excellent exchange, and the principal thanked Mrs. Baldwin for the feedback.

Mrs. Baldwin, elated by the interchange, attended the teachers' support group a few days later and told the group what had happened. The group discussed Mrs. Baldwin's courageous encounter with Mrs. Hernandez as an excellent example of a teacher seeing herself as a peer of the principal and approaching the principal from a place of respect for herself as well as the other person. The principal was no longer the person on whom to place the blame out of a feeling of powerlessness and hopelessness but was rather a colleague among active, capable colleagues.

The Reemergence of the Discipline Committee

In the fall of 2000, two separate incidents in which teachers in other public schools in the city had been assaulted deeply affected members of the teachers' support group. In the first instance, the assault was by a high school student; in the second, the assault was by the parent of an elementary school student. Members began expressing a great deal of anger about the lack of physical security they felt in the school. Following some discussion of this within the team, it appeared to us that there was a real crisis among the teachers, and that the crisis was potentially an opportunity to take the concepts of nonviolence and the process of building a nonviolent culture to a new level. We decided to offer a consultation to the teachers from a team member who had not been working directly with the teachers' support group. Thus an additional early morning session, "Staying Safe at Work," was announced.

Twenty-five teachers and a vice principal attended this special session. The consultant opened the meeting with a general discussion of the ubiquitous nature of violence in our contemporary society, and the tendency we all have to adjust to this by denying our fears. He pointed out that this was a dangerous response because fear is a warning signal that something is wrong. Furthermore, from the team's point of view, teachers, like everyone else in the society, had a right to live and work free of the danger of violence from others. The fact that such a right could not be achieved at a particular moment in no way lessened the fact that it was a right, and that the violation of that right was itself a form of violence. The consultant reviewed with the group the notion that teachers' attending to their own safety was a precondition for being able to help the children do the same. With this in mind, he invited them to reflect on these ideas and to bring up specific situations in which they were feeling unsafe.

While various individual issues were brought up, all the teachers were concerned about the school's poorly working intercom system, which often did not allow them to be in contact with the administration immediately when an unsafe situation arose in the classroom. The teachers wanted the administration to do something about this problem, but how were they to press their concern? At this point the vice principal mentioned that, in the past, the school had an official discipline committee, made up of interested teachers and some administrators, that was supposed to address issues such as this. Unfortunately, the committee had been dormant for some time. Following a discussion with the consultant, the administration decided to reconstitute the committee, and several of the teachers and the vice principal committed themselves to attending the bimonthly meetings. It is worth noting that the teachers were not nearly as unanimous in the decision to reconstitute the discipline committee as they were in their articulation of the problem. Some expressed the feeling "We've been here before. Nothing will come of this." Such sentiments alerted the team to the importance that the committee not fail this time around. As a result, the team decided that, if the committee members approved, it would assign one of its members to attend the discipline committee as a consultant. Thus, in addition to the weekly teachers' support group, there now was a bimonthly discipline committee meeting.

For the first several months the discipline committee set about tackling problems of security in the school. One by one, the committee worked on a number of safety concerns. For example, inadequate screening of persons entering the building through the main entrance was addressed. In regard to the intercom system, following discussion with the principal, the discipline committee decided to petition the superintendent of schools. Describing the safety concerns associated with the antiquated nature of the current system, they requested a new intercom system for the school. Every teacher in the school signed the petition and, as the year came to a close, the petition was sent with the principal's approval to the superintendent.

Much to the teachers' amazement and joy, when they returned to school at the end of the summer, they found electricians installing a brand-new intercom system. This success was a great boost to the morale of the new discipline committee as it began its second year. Having dealt with the most immediate and obvious issues of building security, the committee now began to turn to the much more complex issue of discipline problems that were arising in the classrooms.

At this point the team's consultant to the discipline committee offered some of the team's thinking in regard to the problem. Specifically, the consultant pointed out that the word "discipline" is linked etymologically to "disciple," and that being disciplined as an individual involves having positive role models that one wishes to emulate. From this perspective, discipline is not something adults do to children but is something that adults convey to children by being disciplined themselves. The relevance of these concepts emerged in the second year of the discipline committee's work as the group began to share different notions of what children and teachers really needed in order to develop discipline in the classroom. Some teachers saw the problem as a simple one, which could be remedied by having rules and enforcing them. But not all teachers agreed. Thus conflicts arose in the committee, and the teachers in the group had to learn how to listen to each other, respect each other, and, most difficult of all, be open when one honestly disagreed. The emergence of these values in the group was slow and difficult, but as spring approached, there was a definite shift in the way the group was working together.

It was at this point that the committee began to consider offering itself as a resource to other teachers in the school who were having "discipline problems" with students. Acknowledging that working differently with a child often means changing oneself, the committee decided to test its capacity to consult by first consulting with its own members. It was with some humor and courage that the first brave souls began to bring some of their concerns to their fellow committee members. Each painstaking step was important in the gradual process of creating a committee that would be a safe place where teachers could look at themselves, as well as at the problems the students were having—a committee that might be a lever for nonviolent change in the school community.

From the point of view of the team, this process in the discipline committee was an embodiment of its idea of a "nonviolent" or "nonviolating" community—one in which people speak up when they witness what they believe is a violation of one person or group by another. To do this respectfully but clearly and with a sense of doing unto others what you would want them to do unto you was the essence of nonviolence as the team defined it.

The Parent Alliance (La Alianza Para Padres)

From the outset of our work at the school, there had been a recognition that working with parents and helping them become more engaged in the school would be an important component of a nonviolent culture. Thus, from our earliest meetings with Mrs. Hernandez, the issue of how to reach parents was discussed. Everyone agreed that we hoped to help parents feel more at home in the school and increase their capacity to make their homes institutions of learning. This was a wonderful idea, but how were we to realize it practically?

We returned to the idea, often mentioned by Mrs. Hernandez, that the kindergartners were the "biggest" behavior problems in the school. Many were attending school for the first time and often were the first member of their family to matriculate in the Boston public school system. The parents of most kindergartners were invisible at the school for all the reasons already mentioned.

From the team's perspective, the behavior problems of the kindergartners reflected problems of discipline in the homes from which they were coming. A key concept for our team involved the notion of disciplined parenting as a reflective art. As indicated earlier, the stress needed to be on "conveying discipline to children" as opposed to "disciplining them." If parents want to convey discipline to their children, they must develop their capacity to be disciplined parents. But what is a "disciplined parent"? One way of thinking about this is that a disciplined parent is one who is able to take parenting seriously as a discipline. And like in any discipline, be it law, medicine, art, or others, developing oneself involves an ongoing process of practice and both formal and informal study. There is conversation with others who are practicing the discipline. There is an awareness that a discipline is an infinite process with a history, a process that one never fully masters but which is interesting, challenging, and an outlet for creative, loving energies.

Based on these ideas, the decision was made to

begin a series of monthly meetings with the parents of the kindergartners by starting the Parent Alliance (La Alianza Para Padres) and to involve as many parents of kindergarten children as possible. Then, in subsequent years, the parents of the incoming kindergarten class would be invited to join, so that eventually parents from all grades in the school would be included. After the first year, the team decided that each month there would be an evening meeting, as well as one in the morning, to increase accessibility. Typically, each session lasts for 2 hours, with an hour of structured discussion or activity, and an hour of free discussion. All sessions are bilingual.

In the third year of the alliance meetings (2002–2003), the morning sessions have included opportunities for parents to observe their children's classrooms, thereby increasing their involvement in their children's learning. The principal prepares the parents to observe particular aspects of the classroom related to the subject being discussed by the alliance that month. For example, when the focus was "Reading to Your Child," parents were encouraged to observe the ways that reading was taught in their children's classes. Following the observation, parents had the opportunity to discuss and increase their understanding of what they had observed. For many parents, these were their first experiences of their children's classrooms in progress.

In the second, more unstructured part of the meeting, topics discussed ranged from strategies teachers are using to teach math or literacy to ways of managing children's demands, to how to cope with their own and their children's reactions to events such as 9/11 or the war in Iraq. One month, the activity involved learning how to organize a study corner at home. In the unstructured hour, led by members of the team, parents have an opportunity to express their concerns in a more free-flowing discussion. Parents share solutions with each other, as well as problems, giving and getting helpful advice and support. In this way parents recognize their own and other parents' strengths and learn new strategies to try out. Sometimes problems are identified at meetings that enable the team to reach out to children and families in need of further help.

For the first 2 years, the parenting program developed slowly. Despite a monthly newsletter reminding parents about meetings, and some calls from teachers and team members, turnout was variable and low. A core of about seven parents came regularly, with some new parents attending each meeting. Although parents almost always reported that the meeting had been helpful, they did not necessarily return.

In reviewing the alliance, the team and the principal concluded that the it needed a full-time staff person in the school whose main responsibility would be outreach to parents. This conclusion flowed naturally from our recognition that part of our task was to develop sufficient resources to be able to achieve our goals. While unable to establish a full-time position, the principal was able to create a new half-time position; in addition, the clinic applied for and received a small grant that allowed one member of our team to be reimbursed for increased hours on this project.

The team member began by identifying parent assistants in each classroom who receive a small stipend for their work of reaching out to other parents by calling them before meetings and encouraging them to come. Parents who attend four or more meetings receive certificates honoring their participation. As a result of these efforts, attendance increased dramatically. One hundred and three parents have attended at least one meeting in the alliance's third year, with more than 50% attending two or more meetings. The team hopes to eventually develop a system that will enable parents to play a larger role in the organization of the alliance and in setting its agenda. This will be an indication that we are achieving one of our goals of helping parents feel more at home in the school.

Having outlined our work with various groups in the school, we now turn to an example of work with an individual.

Tackling a Runner

Walter Sanchez began meeting with a member of our counseling team, Ms. Jane Crosby, 3 years ago, shortly after the murder of his mother's boyfriend, a man he referred to as "Dad." At the time, he was in the second grade. When Ms. Crosby first went to Walter's class, she found him sitting apart from everyone else at his own table in the back of the room, looking sad and angry. His teacher explained that he was refusing to do any work and oscillated between being extremely defiant and having crying spells. Because he was mean, none of the other children liked him. The teacher felt frustrated and blamed Mrs. Sanchez, who came to the school infrequently. When she did, she chastised Walter in front of other students and the teacher.

In contrast, in the initial counseling sessions, Ms. Crosby found Walter to be fun-loving and intelligent. He related easily and loved to play games and draw. Though guarded about his home life and his emotions, his drawings about the murder of "Dad" revealed some of his fantasies and questions about it. After 6 months of working together, Ms. Crosby felt that she had a good relationship with Walter. Gradually he began to show signs of being happier in school.

Concomitantly, Ms. Crosby met occasionally with Mrs. Sanchez and offered her support regarding the violent loss of her boyfriend. Like Walter, his mother was also emotionally guarded. She acknowledged her own anger, but it was difficult for her to express or examine her feelings.

In the midst of this fragile beginning, Mrs. Sanchez had a very negative experience with the school. On one occasion Walter was so out of control that the school called the BEST Team (the city's emergency response team for mental health–related emergencies) and summoned his mother. During the evaluation process, a member of the BEST Team told Mrs. Sanchez that her son could be arrested for his behavior. This comment infuriated Mrs. Sanchez, who abruptly left the school with her son. For many months afterward, Ms. Crosby and Mrs. Sanchez talked on the phone, trying to come to some understanding of what had happened. However, the incident seemed only to substantiate the mother's negative view of the school.

Thus far, a traditional approach had been taken in the work with Walter and his mother. Ms. Crosby worked on building a trusting relationship through individual sessions with Walter. Using play and conversation, she tried to explore and better understand his fears and behavior. At this point, her attempts to engage Mrs. Sanchez in the treatment were largely unsuccessful.

When Walter returned as a third grader the following September, he had more energy, which propelled him toward two other "bad boys" in the class. Their combined behavior made it very hard for the teacher to maintain control. Sometimes Walter left the classroom and ran unattended around the school. When an administrator (who had been alerted by his teacher) caught him and set strong consequences for his behavior, he dissolved into fearful crying.

Walter continued his therapy sessions, but they did not seem to affect his classroom behavior. His mother remained angry, complaining at the number of phone calls she received from the school. She wanted the school to handle her son's problems without bothering her and indicated that she was at risk of losing her job if the interruptions from the school continued.

At this time, Walter was the topic of discussion at one of the team's meetings with Mrs. Hernandez. The team considered how Walter had become "a problem that needed fixing." This view of Walter was being enacted every day. Walter had no opportunity to feel good about school or himself as a member of the school community. The traditional approach was not working, and it was necessary to "shift the frame." Here was a child whose ways of expressing unhappiness were upsetting the adults around him. In keeping with its emphasis on fostering a happier sense of self in such a child, the team tried to find a context in which Walter's habit of running would be helpful and he would be appreciated for it. Mrs. Hernandez suggested that Walter might use his running ability to the benefit of physically handicapped children in gym class. She consulted the gym teacher and arranged for Ms. Crosby and Walter to visit the class.

The gym teacher turned out to be a flexible and lighthearted person. He had his hands full with Alexander, a feisty 7-year-old with a big smile. Every time he had a chance, Alexander would run to a wooden ladder attached to the wall and climb it. The gym teacher explained that it would be a big help if Walter could ensure Alexander's safety by preventing him from climbing the ladder. It was agreed that Walter would volunteer weekly in this gym class for special needs children.

The idea was a stunning success. Walter never tired of his assignment. Each time Alexander "ran," Walter laughed and patiently brought him back. Alexander loved Walter's attention. Whenever Walter arrived at the classroom, Alexander called out Walter's name, gave him a big smile, and ran over and took his hand. Gradually Walter and Alexander formed an alliance that went beyond the classroom. Walter told Ms. Crosby that he and Alexander rode the same school bus, and Walter looked out for his small friend there as well. They also played together on the playground during recess. By the end of the third grade, Walter definitely seemed to be a happier student who was enjoying some aspects of his school experience, even though he still had behavior problems.

Over the summer Ms. Crosby arranged for the health center to pay for Walter to attend a day camp outside the city with a beautiful lake and big playing fields. Walter loved the camp activities and the new friends he made there.

At the start of the fourth grade, Mrs. Hernandez placed Walter in a small, highly structured classroom where he was the most advanced student. His teacher, who was very nurturing, explained to him that the school's goal was for him to succeed in this small setting and then move to a regular classroom by the middle of the year. Walter's academic testing showed that he was working on grade level. In the small classroom, he was able to work through some of the tensions he had about school in the past. He was very secure with his classmates, and his teacher gave him ample support. Counseling sessions with Ms. Crosby continued. By this time, Walter had stopped leaving the classroom and roaming the halls. He was overcoming his fear of failure.

At midyear, according to plan, he was moved back to a regular classroom. His new teacher found him difficult to manage, especially during transitions. Walter regressed. He became withdrawn, but he did not run, and he participated actively in class. In therapy, he expressed the fear that his peers did not like him.

After some discussion between the team and the principal, Ms. Crosby suggested to Walter that he and she might approach the class together and ask if some of the children wanted to be his friends. Walter initially opposed the idea, but with her encouragement he eventually agreed. After obtaining the teacher's permission, Ms. Crosby and Walter met with the class. She explained that Walter was feeling lonely because he did not have any friends. "Were any members of the class interested in being friends with Walter?" she asked. To Walter's amazement, two hands immediately shot up, followed by the hands of almost every child in the class. Ms. Crosby chose the two children who had volunteered initially and, after obtaining their parents' consent, initiated weekly meetings of the Friends of Walter Club.

For a while the counseling sessions became club meetings structured around the idea of what it meant to be a friend of Walter's, and how he could be a friend in return. Ms. Crosby suggested that the two students could show their friendship by giving Walter insight into how his actions in the class affected other children. Walter could be a friend to the two students by listening carefully to what they were saying.

All three children attended each week with great enthusiasm. Walter's friends were thoughtful and direct with him, and he took their feedback seriously and showed that it mattered to him. They told him about their own troubles and struggles. One of the "friends," Mario, had great emotional courage and shared many personal things. This encouraged Walter to share his own struggles and thoughts more fully, and the children seemed to develop empathy toward one another. As the year progressed, Walter was able to settle into the regular classroom and do his work more consistently. He was more secure that he had a place there and was liked. When the team informed Mrs. Hernandez about the remarkable insights Mario had into Walter's behavior, she smiled and informed us that "our star co-therapist" had himself been transferred to the school the previous year because of disciplinary problems he had been having.

During the school year, Ms. Crosby stayed in touch with Walter's mother by phone. But despite many invitations to discuss Walter's progress, Mrs. Sanchez refused to meet with Ms. Crosby. Finally, in early spring, she agreed to a meeting, but at the appointed hour, she used her cell phone to inform Ms. Crosby that she was outside the school but could not find a parking space. Knowing that this might be a manifestation of Mrs. Sanchez's ambivalence about meeting, Ms. Crosby went outside and sat in the car for the hour-long session.

As the year progressed, Walter showed increasing openness in therapy, sharing difficulties he was experiencing at home. Toward the end of the year, in the midst of a behavior problem, Walter revealed that he was extremely afraid of his mother being called because she had been beating him over reports of his misconduct. It appeared that the ability of the school to create a positive environment for Walter had ultimately resulted in his having sufficient confidence in himself to assert his desire not to be abused. This in turn led to a new level of involvement and confrontation with Mrs. Sanchez. This information also aided the team's understanding of Walter's behavior. The knowledge that he had been experiencing physical abuse for a long time helped to explain his anxiety and fearfulness. His lack of discipline and meanness toward other children could also be seen as a possible mirror of his mother's treatment of him.

In response to Walter's disclosure, Ms. Crosby and the school filed a report of suspected abuse with the Department of Social Services and arranged a meeting with Mrs. Sanchez. When Walter's mother arrived for the meeting with Ms. Crosby, Mrs. Hernandez, and an assistant principal, she was extremely angry. Mrs. Hernandez began the meeting by reviewing what had happened and explaining why the report had been filed. In the midst of this discussion, as Mrs. Sanchez became even more furious, Ms. Crosby tried to intervene, feeling that by now they had developed a relationship that could withstand the confrontation. Speaking as calmly as possible, Ms. Crosby explained why she thought that striking Walter was very harmful. She said she felt confident that with help, his mother could find other ways to work with her son. Mrs. Sanchez's anger only increased in response to this intervention. She screamed that no one had a right to tell her how to raise her son, since she was the person putting clothes on his back and food on the table. Ms. Crosby persisted, saying that while she knew her to be a committed and caring mother, hitting her son was not permitted under the law. Mrs. Sanchez became increasingly furious and then suddenly burst into tears and started to leave the room. Mrs. Hernandez and the vice principal got up and guided her into the assistant principal's office. Once in a different office and without Ms. Crosby's presence, Walter's mother became calmer. In the course of discussing what had happened, she insisted that she no longer wanted Ms. Crosby to see her child, and that she would send a note to this effect the following day.

In processing the confrontation, the team was impressed with the level of honesty in the exchange between Ms. Crosby and Mrs. Sanchez, and saw this as an opportunity to help Walter's mother see that deep anger could be expressed without destroying a relationship. With the team's encouragement, Ms. Crosby called Walter's mother after a few days and expressed sorrow about her being upset. She asked the mother to allow her to continue her work with Walter for the few remaining weeks of school. To Ms. Crosby's surprise, Mrs. Sanchez was quite receptive and agreed to ongoing meetings and plans for Walter to attend camp that summer. Ms.

Crosby and Walter's mother met a few months later and shared the belief that this confrontation with anger was a turning point in their relationship.

The work with Walter and his mother exemplifies the team's focus on helping individuals experience themselves as respected and beloved members of a community. Over a period of several years, Ms. Crosby has been helping Walter and his mother develop connections with concerned administrators, teachers, and peers whom they might experience as the beginning of a "community of concern." The work required the creative use of institutional resources. It could not have occurred without the strong relationship that has gradually evolved between the team and the school. This relationship is also manifested in the work of the teachers' support group, discipline committee, and Parent Alliance. Each example is part of a long-term and ongoing commitment by all involved toward the goal of creating a culture of nonviolence in the school.

Conclusion

In this chapter we have reviewed the work of a community mental health team in an urban public elementary school. We have provided examples of the work with administrators, teachers, parents, and students. As the title of this chapter suggests, in recounting the work of our team over 4 years, we can only provide the reader with an early interim report. A great deal remains to be done. What has been accomplished is just a beginning. Over the next 5 to 10 years, with the principal's help, we hope to extend these concepts to build a schoolwide culture involving everyone—students, teachers, administrators, and parents.

To do this, the concepts we have elaborated here will need to manifest themselves in a more systematic fashion throughout the school. With this in mind, the principal and the team have been exploring an approach to building community pioneered by the North American Family Institute. Founded on principles of openness and democracy, this approach draws everyone in an institution into the development of a common mission, which is articulated in a system of values and norms that apply to everyone. In our school, the mission is building a community of concern in which "anyone's trouble is everyone's concern." The principal, having instituted major reforms in the literacy and math curricula, is now determined to engage in a process of reforming the moral culture of the school. Exactly what form these developments will take, if they are realized, is impossible to predict. Change such as we are discussing is subtle, slow, and incremental. At the present time, the discipline committee appears to be a group that might begin to play a major role in elaborating for teachers and students the concept of the school as a "community of concern." So, while maintaining and improving what we have been doing so far, this appears to be the next step in our process.

To be sure, the future of our efforts is extremely uncertain. Today, in addition to the enormous social forces that lie behind the problems we are attempting to confront, we must add a deteriorating economic situation in which fewer and fewer resources are being made available to our public schools as city and state budgets are subjected to massive cuts. Nevertheless, we have hope that our vision can be realized. In *The Human Side of School Change: Reform, Resistance, and the Real-life Problems of Innovation,* Robert Evans (1996) has written eloquently about the complexity, frustrations, and possibilities of school reform. Evans addresses himself to the issue of hope for change by reminding the reader of the words of Václav Havel, the poet and former president of Czechoslovakia, a man with some experience in the struggle for radical changes in the institutions of society:

Hope in this deep and powerful sense is not the same as joy when things are going well, or willingness to invest in enterprises that are obviously headed for early success, but rather an ability to work for something to succeed. Hope is definitely not the same thing as optimism. It is not the conviction that something will turn out well, but the certainty that something will make sense, regardless of how it turns out. It is this hope, above all, that gives us strength to live and to continually try new things. (Havel, in Evans, 1996, p. 298)

References

Addams, J. (1960). *Jane Addams: A centennial reader.* New York: Macmillan.

Borge, T. (1987). *Christianity and revolution: Tomas Borge's theology of life* (Andrew Reding, Ed. & Trans.). Maryknoll, NY: Orbis Books.

Brockman, J. R. (1989). *Romero: A life.* Maryknoll, NY: Orbis Books.

Day, D. (1997). *Loaves and fishes: The inspiring story of the Catholic worker movement.* Maryknoll, NY: Orbis Books.

DuBois, W.E.B. (1970). *W.E.B. Dubois speaks: Speeches and addresses 1920–1963* (Philip S. Foner, Ed.). New York: Pathfinder.

DuBois, W.E.B. (1971). *W.E.B. Dubois: A reader* (Andrew Paschal, Ed.) New York: Collier Books.

Evans, R. (1996). *The human side of school change: Reform, resistance, and the real-life problems of innovation.* San Francisco: Jossey-Bass.

Friere, P. (1972). *Pedagogy of the oppressed.* London: Penguin.

Gil, D. (1996). Preventing violence in a structurally violent society: Mission impossible. *American Journal of Orthopsychiatry, 66,* 77–84.

Gill, D. (1998). *Confronting injustice and oppression: Concepts and strategies for social workers.* New York: Columbia University Press.

Gutierrez, G. (1996). *Essential writings* (James B. Nicoloff, Ed.). Maryknoll, NY: Orbis Books.

Hedrick, J. D. (1994). *Harriet Beecher Stowe: A life.* New York: Oxford University Press.

Kelley, F. (1986). *Notes of sixty years: The autobiography of Florence Kelley.* Chicago: Kerr.

King, M. L., Jr. (1986). *A testament of hope: The essential writings of Martin Luther King, Jr.* (James M. Washington, Ed.). San Francisco: Harper and Row.

Kozol, J. (1992). *Savage inequalities: Children in America's schools.* New York: Harper Perennial.

Mandela, N. (1995). *Long walk to freedom.* Boston: Beacon.

Menchu, R. (1984). *I, Rigoberta Menchu: An Indian woman in Guatemala* (E. Burgos-Debray, Ed., & A. Wright, Trans.). London: Verso.

Reynolds, B. C. (1951). *Social work and social living: Explorations in philosophy and practice.* New York: Citadel Press.

Reynolds, B. C. (1991). *An uncharted journey.* Silver Springs, MD: NASW Press.

Robeson, P. (1978). *Here I stand.* Boston: Beacon.

Ryan, W. (1976). *Blaming the victim.* New York: Vintage.

Schotz, E. M. (1996). *Confronting violence in our schools with the culture of nonviolence.* Unpublished manuscript.

Stowe, H. B. (1965). *Uncle Tom's cabin.* New York: Harper Classics (original work published 1852).

Stowe, H. B. (1999). *The Oxford Harriet Beecher Stowe reader* (Joan Hedrick, Ed.). New York: Oxford University Press.

Ann Marie Glodich, Jon G. Allen, Jim Fultz,

George Thompson, Cindy Arnold-Whitney,

Cheri Varvil, and Chris Moody

23

School-Based Psychoeducational Groups on Trauma Designed to Decrease Reenactment

The extent of adolescents' exposure to violence has become a national concern. Either direct participation and victimization or witnessing violent events may lead to posttraumatic symptoms, as well as having a broader adverse impact on psychosocial development (Eth & Pynoos, 1985; Garbarino & Kostelny, 1997; Osofsky, 1997; Pelcovitz, Kaplan, DeRosa, Mandel, & Salzinger, 2000; Perry, 1997). Hence, communities must place a high priority on developing interventions that promise to decrease exposure to violence and reduce the associated potential for enduring psychosocial trauma.

Over the course of several years, we have been researching and refining psychoeducational interventions for adolescents exposed to violence and abuse. We first designed and implemented interventions with adolescents being treated in inpatient, residential, and outpatient programs. Although we started with the intention of teaching participants about the potential impact of trauma on their life and strengthening their coping skills (Allen, Kelly, & Glodich, 1997; Glodich, 2001), we gradually shifted our focus to patients' recurrent engagement in risk-taking behaviors. Risk-taking behavior is one of the most pernicious traumatic effects of exposure to violence because it exposes the individual to further violence. The most striking

example of this phenomenon is substance abuse, which increases risk of trauma exposure and subsequent development of post–traumatic stress disorder (PTSD; Giaconia et al., 2000). We concluded that it would be futile to endeavor to help adolescents with their posttraumatic symptoms when their impulsive, high-risk behavior continually placed them at risk for additional violence exposure and the associated trauma. Thus, we directed the adolescents' attention to the link between their past trauma and their current risk-taking behavior, employing the concept of reenactment (van der Kolk, 1989).

Plainly, there are multiple origins of impulsive, risk-taking behavior. Yet we found it helpful to encourage adolescents with a trauma history to understand their high-risk behavior in the context of propensity to re-create traumatic experiences through reenactment. Our approach follows Pynoos and colleagues' (Pynoos, 1993; Saltzman, Steinberg, Layne, Aisenberg, & Pynoos, 2001) view that adolescents may reenact their trauma by actively pursuing thrill seeking. Pynoos and Nader (1992) noted that teenagers are at particularly high risk of involvement in violent reenactments, given their ready access to alcohol, drugs, cars, and guns. Moreover, we are particularly concerned that repeated exposure to potentially traumatic events may sensitize the sympathetic nervous system and thereby systematically undermine resilience (Post, Weiss, Smith, Li, & McCann, 1997; Post, Weiss, & Smith, 1995). Specifically, in contrast to desensitization, where repeated exposure to a stressful situation leads to lessened fear and greater mastery, sensitization results in an increasingly reactive nervous system with repeated stress exposure. Repeated, extreme, uncontrollable stress is most likely to sensitize the nervous system, resulting in increased emotional reactivity over time.

Thus, on the basis of our early clinical experience in conducting psychoeducational groups for traumatized adolescents, we decided to focus specifically on averting further trauma exposure. Emphasizing the concept of reenactment, we engaged participants in understanding the relation between their trauma history and their high-risk behavior, and we supported their developing healthier ways of coping with emotional distress stemming from their trauma-related impairment in affect regulation. Concomitantly, we recognized the need to go beyond tertiary prevention in a clinical setting, at which point considerable psychosocial damage already has been done. Thus we extended the program into the public schools. School-community collaborations have been an essential means of providing support to children and adolescents in high-risk situations (Allen-Meares, Washington, & Welsch, 1996; Ceballo, 2000; Glodich, Allen, & Arnold, 2001; Saltzman et al., 2001; Scannapieco, 1994; Williams, Fanolis, & Schamess, 2001). Schools provide ready access to the population in need of service. Schools also provide a setting that can normalize trauma-related problems insofar as schools do not carry the stigma associated with mental health facilities (Herz, Goldberg, & Reis, 1984). Moreover, our psychoeducational approach is highly compatible with a setting wherein students are accustomed to classes and learning.

Over the course of several years, we have implemented, evaluated, and continually refined a protocol for psychoeducational intervention. The protocol aims to increase adolescents' awareness of the impact of trauma on their functioning, thereby setting the stage for helping them cope more effectively with stress—all in the service of diminishing the likelihood of reenactment and risk-taking behaviors. The school-based protocol has gone through several stages of development. We began by conducting two pilot groups that consisted of males and females ranging in age from 14 to 18. These pilot groups served to establish a milieu in the school conducive to the intervention, to develop procedures for implementation, to refine the inclusion and exclusion criteria, and to experiment with different aspects of the intervention. Then we conducted three studies of the effectiveness of the intervention, refining the protocol at each stage. First, we evaluated the effectiveness of an 8-session intervention and learned that an expansion of the protocol was indicated. Second, we conducted a 12-session intervention that also included more refined assessment techniques. Although clinical impressions suggested that this 12-session intervention was effective, the results of the quantitative assessments were disappointing and appeared insensitive to the impact of the intervention. Hence, we conducted a third study that included a qualitative evaluation of the 12-session protocol.

This chapter describes the current status of the protocol, its evolution through the process of evaluation, and its potential for wider applications in the community. First, we present the latest version of the protocol. Second, we trace the course of its evaluation, from a quantitative to a qualitative approach, the latter developed to better validate our clinical impressions. Third, we present a framework to conceptualize the role of this intervention in violence prevention. Finally, we spell out some of the implications for future community applications.

Intervention Protocol

Although the protocol focuses on minimizing further trauma exposure by highlighting awareness of reenactment and risk-taking behavior, a number of additional topics and themes are included to buttress this central agenda. Our guiding assumption throughout this work is that enhanced self-awareness plays a key role in self-regulation. The protocol draws attention to the potential damage trauma can do to self-worth (Allen, 2001; Harter, 1999; Janoff-Bulman, 1992) and endeavors to enhance self-worth, for example, through the encouragement of compassion for the self. In conjunction with damaged self-worth, many trauma survivors feel they are not deserving of care; they neglect themselves and put themselves at risk for harm.

Hence, to some degree, self-worth is a foundation for self-control, a theme the groups emphasize in the context of will, attention, and responsibility. Structured exercises enhance participants' awareness of the *feeling* of self-control. Yet, to provide containment for affective distress, self-regulation must be bolstered by social support (Allen, 2001). Hence, many of the interventions are intended to facilitate supportive interpersonal relationships. In conjunction with role-playing, a continual focus on compassion fosters participants' ability to take the perspective of others. A specific exercise to facilitate compassion is introduced early in the protocol, and each subsequent session concludes with this compassion exercise. Thus, the intervention is designed to help participants learn skills not only for emotional self-regulation but also for interpersonal negotiation in a climate of interest, openness, tolerance, and respect.

Participants

Participants for the intervention are referred by school counselors and social workers, based on the belief that they have been adversely affected by having experienced or witnessed violent events that were highly stressful and potentially traumatic. Such events include living in a high-crime area where community violence is a daily occurrence; being exposed to community violence; witnessing or participating in an attempted or actual drive-by shooting, or in an attempted or actual shooting or stabbing; rape; traumatic accidents; traumatic loss (sudden or violent death of parent, relative, or friend); or family violence (witnessing or experiencing physical, sexual, or emotional abuse).

Session Synopses

The psychoeducational intervention is relatively structured in two senses. First, the protocol provides a topical focus for each of the 12 sessions, although avoidance of reenactment is a broad topic that spans a number of sessions. Second, each session includes a discussion of didactic material pertaining to the topic, along with one or more tasks that promote active involvement in learning (e.g., coping skills). The protocol is described in more detail elsewhere (Glodich & Allen, 2000; Glodich, Allen, & Arnold, 2001), and the gist of each session is presented here. Several exercises have been adapted from Palmer (1997) and are summarized briefly here; readers are referred to Palmer for details.

Session 1

The co-leaders introduce the group by reviewing group norms (emphasizing confidentiality and mutual respect) and presenting the overall framework for the 12-week group. The leaders review situations in which adolescents may be exposed to violence in the community, the school, and the home. Potentially traumatic effects of exposure to violence are discussed, and the session focuses on the role of power differences in violence. Two tasks are included: (1) Participants are requested to write down a personal experience of violence or abuse and sources of strength that have helped them cope; and (2) the leaders use Kivel and Creighton's (1997) Power Chart to expand the adolescents' awareness of the contribution of societal contexts to violence, abuse, and trauma. The leaders also foster discussion about the consequences of having power and lacking power, with an eye toward understanding how violence can erupt both from power and from powerlessness.

Session 2

The session focuses on three posttraumatic phenomena: the fight-or-flight response, reexperiencing symptoms (e.g., flashbacks, nightmares), and reenactment. A discussion of the concept of "will" is introduced to foster self-awareness and a sense of self-control. Focusing on will promotes a sense of self-efficacy (Palmer, 1997) and has the advantage of being a familiar, everyday concept (e.g., as in "willpower"). Participants are encouraged to see how thoughts, feelings, and actions can be controlled by the will. Consistent with the literature on learned helplessness (Seligman, 1975), we describe how the experience of violence and trauma can have a debilitating effect on individuals' sense of ability to make their own choices, that is, their will. This session also introduces the significance of a compassionate attitude toward the self and others. Two tasks are included: (1) We employ a task adapted from James (1989), the violence-related Trauma Bag. Each bag contains a topic pertaining to reexperiencing, reenactment, and risk taking. Each participant examines the chosen topic and elects whether to talk about it or simply to read it aloud. The co-leaders participate by providing further information about the topics, emphasizing exercise of self-control. (2) Participants complete a Compassion Exercise (Palmer, 1997) that fosters empathy by asking individuals to think about persons they like and dislike in a way that draws attention to shared feelings and struggles. This exercise is repeated at the end of each subsequent session.

Session 3

The leaders focus on emotional abuse as a common example of a potentially traumatic experience that may undermine self-worth, play a role in miscommunication, elicit defensiveness, and contribute to self-destructive behavior. Discussion emphasizes how emotionally abused adolescents not only may become self-critical but also may seek out critical or emotionally abusive relationships in traumatic reenactments. The leaders explicate the goal of processing trauma in the context of containment provided by self-regulation and social support. The session includes three tasks: (1) Participants join in the Heart Exercise (Kivel & Creighton, 1997), which the leaders use to demonstrate that violence, reenactment, and risk taking can result from damaged self-worth associated with emotional abuse and miscommunication. Potential ways to overcome these patterns of miscommunication are discussed and further explored throughout the rest of the sessions. (2) To provide participants with a concrete experience of controlling their behavior by an exercise of will, the co-leaders explain and role-play the Acting as Aware Will Exercise (Palmer, 1997). Participants coach each other in this exercise.

Session 4

The leaders place the concept of reenactment in an explicit interpersonal context by explaining a set of roles integral to traumatic relationships. This discussion builds on the widely discussed roles of victim, perpetrator, rescuer, and witnessing bystander (Davies & Frawley, 1994; Gabbard & Wilkinson, 1994; Saakvitne, Gamble, Pearlman, & Lev, 2000; Twemlow, Sacco, & Williams, 1996). Further exploration of self-control through exercise of the will is incorporated into discussion of avoiding the victim role. Two tasks are included: (1) The leaders present a reenactment diagram (Allen, 2001) that illustrates a set of interconnecting and potentially traumatic roles, three active (rescuer, abuser, neglector) and three passive (rescued, victim, ne-

glected). The diagram also contrasts these traumatic relationships with a parallel set of ordinary interactions, three active (helping, hurting, ignoring) and three passive (helped, hurt, ignored). The diagram thus illustrates how ordinary interactions can trigger posttraumatic experiences and contribute to full-blown reenactments of trauma. Discussion focuses on identifying the roles and on determining coping strategies that are less likely to lead to further reenactment and trauma. Session 4 concentrates on the victim role, and the other roles are explored in session 5. One of the co-leaders models a victim role. The other co-leader asks the participants to attempt to talk the first co-leader out of the victim role. Participants are requested to pay particular attention to any feelings that arise while they are attempting to "change the victim." Invariably, feelings of helplessness and anger at the victim are evoked. Participants discuss how victims are scapegoated, how they are not able to "get their needs met" in this role, and how they may incur further violence. (2) Participants are asked to consider if the victim role can be brought under control of their will. To concretize this discussion, participants and co-leaders complete Palmer's (1997) the Will Rules All Exercise, demonstrating how deliberately changing thoughts and behaviors can induce positive emotional states.

Session 5

This session continues the discussion of traumatic interactions in terms of role relationships and applies the concepts of will and attention to self-control. The group discusses anger and guilt feelings in relation to self-blame and an excessive sense of responsibility for traumatic events. Elaborating on the prior session, two tasks are introduced: (1) The co-leaders model various relationship roles (being the abuser, rescuer, victim, neglecter, or helpless witness; feeling neglected). Participants are asked to pay particular attention to any feelings that arise while they are observing the role play. Then participants take turns modeling the various roles (including the victim role), while the others observe and note feelings that are evoked. To model an alternative strategy to traumatic interactions, the leaders introduce an additional role, the compassion role, which provides a means of defusing violence and avoiding reenactment, while also fostering awareness of others' mental states. (2) To illustrate the voluntary control of attention and its potential influence on mental states, participants complete the Behavior of Attention Exercise (Palmer, 1997). This exercise demonstrates self-control over attention (e.g., voluntarily shifting attention from the outer world to the inner world) and also helps participants appreciate how what they pay attention to affects their feelings.

Session 6

The session continues the use of role-playing to promote discussion of the role of will, voluntary attention, and compassion in defusing violence, as well as the various feelings evoked by enactment of trauma roles. Two tasks are included: (1) Participants develop and videotape a role-played situation that depicts a stressful or traumatic incident. They may use a situation from their personal experience or devise a situation based on a pertinent problem of interest to them. (2) The leaders work with the students to develop a second role play (not videotaped) that demonstrates ways of using the will, voluntary attention, and compassion to avoid further violence, reenactment, risk taking, and trauma exposure.

Session 7

The videotape created in session 6 serves as a springboard for further discussion of reenactment and contributors to risk taking. The task for the session entails reviewing the role-play videotape from the previous session. Specifically, participants identify perpetrator, victim, rescuer, witness-neglecter, and other roles. They discuss how individuals are drawn into these roles, how enacting them can contribute to reenactments of trauma, and how to avoid trauma. The videotape is erased at the end of the session.

Session 8

Participants discuss reenactment and trauma exposure in the high-risk situation of interactions with police officers. Two local police officers in street clothes join the co-leaders in conducting this session, emphasizing ways of defusing violence by increasing constructive communication and promoting positive interactions. The task for the session involves police officers conducting a role-play with the participants, demonstrating how to defuse violence in extremely tense situations. The Power Chart is brought into the discussion (see session 1). The co-leaders help facilitate the dialogue, reiter-

ating how participants may use voluntary attention and will to foster self-control in these potentially explosive situations.

Session 9

This session continues discussion of potentially problematic interactions with police officers, and the two local police officers attend the session in uniform. Participants engage in further discussion of how to increase communication and positive interactions between the police and the participants, and the task for the session entails role-playing positive interactions with police officers.

Session 10

This session fosters discussion of how fear, anger, self-hatred, guilt feelings, and externalization of blame can contribute to reenactment, risk taking, and violence. Discussion emphasizes the role of will in regulating actions, the importance of taking responsibility for one's actions, and the value of being open and honest with oneself and others. Two new tasks are introduced: (1) The Self-Deception Signals Exercise (Palmer, 1997) increases participants' awareness of the extent to which their own actions may be similar to the actions of others who have caused them emotional distress and pain. They learn how it can be easier to recognize troublesome behavior in others than in oneself. They are encouraged to identify their own contributions to current interpersonal conflicts. This exercise epitomizes a theme running throughout the groups: "Think before you act." (2) The next exercise, the Enlightened Justice Procedure (Palmer, 1999), further encourages compassion, self-responsibility, and restraint from potentially risky, damaging, and violent behaviors.

Session 11

This penultimate session serves to counteract participants' sense of hopelessness and helpless about their future. Several ways of avoiding reenactment in the long-range future are discussed: knowing oneself, being aware of emotional triggers, recognizing the potential traumatic impact of substance abuse and other risk-taking behavior, noting the warning signs of abusive relationships, and using one's will in the service of self-control and in making healthy choices. Participants are encouraged to articulate life goals and plans for how they will be able to achieve those goals. The group is organized around the task of generating a future family diagram (Glodich, 2001) that was adapted from Bowen's (Bowen, 1980) genogram. Individual participants volunteer to construct and draw on the blackboard a diagram of how they envision their future family. Co-leaders and other participants raise questions, and co-leaders interweave themes from previous sessions in the discussion. Intergenerational transmission of abuse and trauma is a prominent theme.

Session 12

The final session reviews what participants have learned, and the leaders reiterate the key themes of the group. Participants are also invited to provide feedback about the group, discussing aspects that were helpful and unhelpful. The task for the group entails participants rewriting the traumatic experience they described in the first session. They are encouraged to review differences, if any, between their first and second narratives.

Evaluation of Effectiveness

Three studies were designed to evaluate the effectiveness of the group. The first two studies included quantitative measures of effectiveness and involved wait-list control groups; on the basis of the results of the first study, the protocol was expanded and its assessment was refined. The core quantitative measures employed in studies 1 and 2 generally failed to reveal any significant positive impact of the intervention, notwithstanding facilitators' strong clinical impressions that many participants had derived substantial benefit from the groups. Hence, study 3 included a qualitative evaluation of the effectiveness of the expanded protocol.

Study 1

The initial study was based on an eight-session protocol developed after two pilot groups were conducted in the school. Details of the methods and results are presented elsewhere (Glodich, 1999) and will be summarized here.

Fifty adolescents attending an urban high school and ranging in age from 14 to 18 were randomly assigned to one of two intervention groups or a control group. We employed the Screen for Adolescent Exposure to Violence (Hastings & Kel-

ley, 1997) to assess frequency of violence exposure and to assess posttraumatic experiences, dissociation, and psychiatric symptoms. To assess attitudes toward risk-taking behavior, we employed the Adolescent Risk-Taking Instrument (Busen, 1991; Busen & Kouzekanani, 2000). We also developed the Trauma Knowledge and Insight questionnaire (Glodich & Allen, 2000) to assess the students' level of trauma knowledge before and after the group intervention. Finally, we included a feedback questionnaire in the post-group assessment to measure participants' satisfaction (i.e., participants rated the extent to which the intervention helped them, the extent of their learning, and the extent to which they liked the group).

Participants reported a high level of exposure to violence, as well as a high level of engagement in risk-taking behaviors. Yet they showed minimal symptoms of any kind. As anticipated, the intervention group participants showed a marked gain in knowledge about trauma and its effects, whereas the control group's knowledge remained essentially unchanged. Yet, despite significant learning, intervention participants showed no significant change in attitudes toward risk taking over the course of the group (i.e., pretest to posttest). Nonetheless, we found a significant positive correlation across all participants between extent of acquired knowledge about trauma and adaptiveness of attitudes toward risk-taking behaviors. Furthermore, overall, participants' satisfaction ratings indicated a highly positive response to the group: participants found the group helpful, felt they learned, and liked the group. We suspected that the limited effects of the group might have been associated with somewhat poor attendance coupled with a limited number of scheduled sessions. Hence, we expanded and elaborated the protocol for the second study.

Study 2

Design and Participants

Sixty-one participants comparable to those in study 1 completed study 2, meeting similar inclusion criteria. Half of the students were randomly assigned to one of three identical 12-week groups that were conducted over the course of a school semester, and the other half of the students were placed in a wait-list control group (the latter group receiving the intervention in the next semester). All students were assessed both before and after their participation in the groups on measures of violence exposure, risk-taking behavior, emotional responses, and knowledge about trauma-related phenomena. We refined the Trauma Knowledge and Insight questionnaire and retained the participant satisfaction questionnaire from Study 1, and we included more current measures of trauma-related phenomena being developed and tested by leading research groups. To measure trauma exposure, we employed the Things I Have Experienced measure, a 38-item scale developed by Pynoos and colleagues in the UCLA Trauma Services that includes items relating to exposure to violence, disasters, accidents, losses, deaths, and other forms of trauma. We also employed a parallel scale developed by this UCLA research group to assess a range of feelings experienced at the time of the most troubling trauma, as well as posttraumatic symptoms. To measure risk-taking behavior, we employed the questionnaire Things I Did in High School, developed by Garbarino and colleagues at the Cornell Family Life Development Center. This scale includes items pertaining to substance abuse, illegal behavior, sexual activity, aggression, self-destructive actions, and victimization.

As in study 1, participants in the intervention group demonstrated a substantial gain in knowledge about trauma (test scores of 21% correct at pretest versus 78% correct at posttest), along with expressing a high degree of satisfaction with the groups. Paralleling the students' satisfaction, the facilitators found participation in the groups highly gratifying, and all the facilitators stated an interest in continuing in the project. Despite participants' learning about trauma and feeling positively about the groups, the quantitative measures of exposure to trauma and loss, posttraumatic distress, and risk-taking behavior failed to demonstrate any significant impact of the intervention. Repeated measures multivariate analyses of variance comparing pretest and posttest scores did not approach significance on any of these measures (all p's $> .10$).

Working against positive findings, however, was a high level of attrition and a low rate of attendance. In addition, the leaders had reason to believe that some students may have minimized their problematic behavior on the questionnaires prior to participating, and that they were more honest and open after participating. Hence, we speculate that some students may have had higher scores on problematic behavior owing to an increase in openness

from pretest to posttest. Moreover, given that students are generally inundated with tests and questionnaires, it is possible that they did not complete them carefully. Abundant clinical impressions of students' active participation and seeming benefit from the group (e.g., in their reporting avoiding violent situations and increased reaching out to counselors for help) suggested that the quantitative measures failed to capture the main benefits of the intervention, and that the measurements needed to be refined in future applications.

It was imperative that efforts to investigate the impact and effectiveness of the intervention continue, particularly in light of the mixed findings from the first two studies. In an effort to strengthen the evaluation, the leaders conducted focus groups involving all the facilitators in the high schools, as well as the police officers who had participated. The focus groups were intended to guide the development of a more qualitative assessment of the impact of the intervention. Specifically, the focus group members engaged in three tasks: (1) elucidating leaders' clinical impressions of the nature of the positive impact of the intervention; (2) developing interview questions that might elicit information from future participants bearing on the hypothesized positive effects; and (3) role-playing structured interviews of participants and critiquing the interviews.

Study 3

Design and Participants

Study 3 employed the same criteria for inclusion as the first two studies. Participants were 44 students ranging in age from 14 to 18 who were attending one of two local urban high schools. Four time-limited groups of 12 one-hour sessions were conducted over the course of an academic year in two urban high schools. Study 3 did not include a control group, given that the core outcome measure was a semistructured interview about the impact of the group, and this measure would not have been appropriate for members of a control group.

Measures

The measures for the participants included the Trauma Knowledge and Insight questionnaire, along with the interviews. As noted earlier, the outcome interview was designed on the basis of input from facilitators of previous groups who participated in focus groups in which the perceived benefits of group participation were discussed. All intervention group participants were seen in a pre-group interview, which asked about trauma-related problems and goals for the group. The post-group interview addressed several questions: Did the group make a difference, and if so, in what way? Was the participant aware of any problems being connected to trauma? Did the participant use his or her will to make better choices or good decisions? Did the participant actively avoid exposure to violence and trauma? Did the participant employ coping skills to deal with emotional reactivity and reenactment? Using these questions as a prompt, interviewers were asked to probe for specific examples that would provide evidence of a perceived benefit (e.g., if a participant indicated that she had learned to avoid fights, she would be asked to give a specific example of when and how she did so). At the end of the interview, participants were asked if they had any idea of how the group might be helpful to others they know. Interviewers were group facilitators who made detailed notes regarding participants' responses on the interview form.

Upon completion of the first round of interviews, the authors held a series of meetings to develop a coding scheme based on a content analysis of interviewers' notes. We conceptualized the content of the responses in three broad domains: Awareness and Will, Coping, and Relationships. In addition, we divided each of the three broad domains into subdomains, each defined by a set of exemplars. We designed this coding scheme such that we could tabulate the percentage of participants giving responses indicative of benefit within each subdomain.

Specifically, we broke down the interview content within each of the three domains as follows: (1) In the Awareness and Will (Insight) domain, we coded (a) *self-awareness* (e.g., awareness of the impact of trauma history and its connection to present behavior; awareness of how material learned in the group related to the self; and awareness of the influence of the group on the self-concept); and (b) awareness of *will* (e.g., awareness of thinking before acting; awareness of making choices and decisions; and having a sense of responsibility for actions). (2) In the Coping domain, we sought evidence for (a) *trauma avoidance* (e.g., being alert to avoid harm or danger; extricating oneself from victim-perpetrator roles; resisting peer pressure; avoiding negative

people, guns, and parties with fights; leaving high-risk situations); (b) *control of anger and aggression* (e.g., avoiding arguing and swearing at teachers; controlling angry feelings and passive-aggressive behavior; and becoming more compliant and cooperative); and (c) *positive coping skills* (e.g., various forms of self-regulation, such as calming oneself without the help of others). (3) In the Relationship domain, we sought evidence for (a) a feeling of *connection* with others (e.g., awareness of others' feelings; impact of trauma on others; feelings of universality, empathy, compassion, or concern for others); (b) *trusting* (feeling safe; opening up to others); (c) *relationship repair* and improvement (e.g., repairing, negotiating, confronting and working through conflicts with peers and parents); (d) *seeking help* (e.g., talking to others and using support); and (e) *giving help* (e.g., providing support to others).

Four judges independently assessed and coded presence or absence of evidence for benefit in each subdomain for each participant's interview on the basis of interviewers' notes. The raters then conferred and achieved consensus on tabulating a given subdomain as present or absent whenever there was disagreement. A facilitator from each of these groups was present for the discussion to provide additional clinical information when needed to achieve consensus. Hence, the results are the tabulation of the consensus coding for subdomains and for each of the three overall domains.

In study 3, the senior author also interviewed each of the seven facilitators individually to determine the extent to which they used the information they learned in the psychoeducational group in other professional encounters with students. Facilitators also were asked to rate the extent of change in their feelings of helplessness and helpfulness as a consequence of leading the groups. That is, after they had conducted the groups, they retrospectively rated their initial (pre-group) feelings of helplessness and helpfulness in contrast with their current feelings. In addition, they were asked about their best and worst experiences in leading the groups.

Results

To determine the nature of the benefit participants derived from the group, we calculated the percentage of participants for whom there was evidence of benefit in each of the overall domains and the subdomains, with the following results: (1) In the Awareness and Will domain, 100% showed benefit in at least one subdomain, and 92.5% showed benefit in each of the subdomains, self-awareness and awareness of will. (2) In the Coping domain, 95% showed benefit, with the percentages benefiting in the three subdomains being 85% in trauma avoidance, 82.5% in control of anger and aggression, and 50% in developing positive coping skills. (3) In the Relationships domain, 90% showed benefit, with the percentages in the five subdomains being 65% in connection, 25% in trusting, 35% in relationship repair, 52.5% in seeking help, and 40% in giving help.

We also examined individual differences among participants in the extent of benefit as measured by the number of overall domains within which each participant gave evidence of benefiting. Eighty-five percent of participants showed at least some benefit in all three domains (i.e., showing benefit in at least one subdomain of each of the three domains); 15% showed benefit in two domains; and no participants showed benefit in fewer than two domains. More precisely, tallying within subdomains, there were no participants who showed benefit in fewer than 2 subdomains; 5% showed benefit in 2 subdomains; 2.5% in 3 subdomains; 10% in 4 subdomains; 17.5% in 5 subdomains; 22.5% in 6 subdomains; 17.5% in 7 subdomains; 12.5% in 8 subdomains; 7.5% in 9 subdomains; and 5% in all 10 subdomains. Hence the majority of participants showed benefits in 5 to 7 subdomains.

Additionally, as in the previous studies, participants showed substantial gains in knowledge about trauma. The average pretest score Trauma Knowledge and Insight questionnaire was 27% correct, whereas the average posttest score was 91%. Because participants' satisfaction ratings were consistently high in the previous two studies, we did not routinely include this measure in study 3. Satisfaction measures administered to two of these groups, however, showed comparably high levels of participants' finding the groups to be valuable.

The group participants themselves shared with us some of their perspectives on the group and its impact on their overall life. One young man stated that the group made him realize that, if he reacted to situations in life with the same kind of anger he had been accustomed to reacting with, "it was just like adding wood to the fire." He said he realized

that, if he argued with his family member, that was exactly what happened—"the situation just blew up." He said, "If I do something different, the situation calms down," adding, "I didn't know that I could actually have power in this way." Another participant who identified himself as a gang member stated, "Even if I hate someone, I now know that they might be hurting also." He commented that this was actually making him think about his actions very differently. One participant who had fully grasped the concepts of the trauma roles noted that he had been a "victim" all his life. He related a story of a disagreement at his school. He was about to jump in when he stopped and thought, "Do I want to be a victim today?" He reflected and decided that he did not want to be a victim that day, and therefore he did not get involved. He told us that he had never realized that he was playing out a victim role. He also said he never realized that this role had any connection to past traumatic experiences.

One girl said she was able to stop herself and not say immediately what came to mind, "which in the past had brought me a lot of trouble." Another young participant commented that she was at a sporting event and overheard someone saying something about her. She realized that the person was probably trying to provoke her. She decided to ignore the comments. She stated, "I really had to use my will to not jump in and try and pulverize her. I was mad. And then I thought, 'Hey, she is in the perpetrator role. She is trying to provoke me. I am not going to let her.' It took a lot of use of my will because I really wanted to hit her. I didn't." Another participant who was about to fight someone was offered a suggestion by one of his friends (another group member): "Why don't you try that compassion thing [the Compassion Exercise] instead of fighting?" The young man who was about to fight said, "Ah, man, that won't work." His friend encouraged him to "try it anyway." The young man tried and remembered a line or two, which was sufficient to actually stop him from fighting. He said, "I guess that guy has problems, too."

Qualitative information from the facilitator interviews suggests that the impact of facilitators' training and experience in the psychoeducational intervention extended far beyond the conduct of the groups. Every facilitator indicated that he or she used the information outside the group (ranging from one or two times a week to daily), and the facilitators gave numerous examples. Moreover, they used what they had learned not only in their interactions with other students but also for personal growth. One facilitator commented, for example, "I use the intervention with myself. It helps me sit with students who are in the victim role. I have a lot of trouble working with these types of kids, and I find I can sit and help them move through things." Another facilitator noted, "I use the compassion exercise daily in my personal life. It helps me a lot."

Facilitators were asked to rate the extent to which their participation in the group decreased their sense of helplessness on a 10-point scale (with 0 being the highest level and 10 being the lowest level). The responses ranged from 0 to 5 prior to the group experience and 5 to 8 after the group experience. Conversely, ratings of helpfulness on a 10-point scale (with 0 being minimum and 10 being maximum) ranged from 2 to 5 prior to the group experience and 7 to 10 after the experience. One facilitator noted that her sense of helpfulness in working with traumatized students had increased 10-fold. Six of the seven facilitators stated a willingness to continue as facilitators in subsequent groups. The remaining facilitator declined due to a major change in work responsibilities but expressed an intention to support and lobby for the group to continue in the school.

One facilitator stated that the best experience came from "knowing the kind of histories these kids have and having seen these types of children in other capacities, a growing sense that this group actually made a difference in these kids' lives." The facilitator went on to say, "I feel so much better about myself and my work." Another facilitator stated the most positive benefit as "actually having a knowledge base of something that I can do that is helpful." Another commented, "Having specific things to do, exercises that I might have at first minimized, I came to see how much benefit there was, and I started using the exercises in other situations in my life." Another stated, "The group helps the kids maintain a level playing field in life and helps the kids move out of the one-down position in life." Another facilitator commented that the best experience came from "seeing the ideas solidify for the participants and actually seeing and hearing them talk about incidents of 'thinking before acting.'" The facilitator noted, "This group is the most rewarding thing I do."

One of the facilitators stated that her worst experience came from realizing the benefit of the group and "not being able to give time to it due to the demands of my work schedule." Another facilitator stated that the most difficult thing initially was "managing my own trauma response in that, prior to the group, I hadn't thought of myself as someone with this dynamic." Another noted, "Managing certain students in the group would at times cause a lot of anxiety."

Appraisal of Effectiveness

We have been refining the protocol in conjunction with explicating a rationale for its effectiveness (Glodich, Allen, & Arnold, 2001). That is, we endeavor to help participants avert trauma-related reenactment and risk-taking behavior in three ways: first, by increasing their *awareness* that their risk-taking behavior is a reenactment of trauma; second, by fostering their *motivation* to change their self-destructive behavior; and, third, by helping them learn and practice active *coping* skills.

The single theme that runs throughout the groups is the desirability of placing reflective thought between impulse and action. As noted earlier, some participants give voice to this theme in explicating the simple maxim "Think before you act." As we, and others, have argued elsewhere, however, for persons with a history of trauma—especially trauma in early attachment relationships—developing the capacity to think about feelings and their origins is a major challenge (Allen, 2001, in press; Fonagy, Gergely, Jurist, & Target, 2002). We construe this core capacity as mentalizing, that is, understanding oneself and others in terms of intentional mental states, such as needs, desires, emotions, and beliefs. Most of us are fortunate in taking this mentalizing capacity for granted—it is part of our folk psychology (Bruner, 1990). But mentalizing has its origins in secure attachment relationships, and it is undermined by trauma in general and attachment trauma in particular (Allen, 2001, 2003).

Hence, we designed and implemented the groups to foster whatever mentalizing capacities the participants had developed. The group leaders endeavor to foster a safe, calm atmosphere that supports an attitude of curiosity and interest in the workings of the mind. First and foremost, current behavior is seen as meaningful in relation to one's prior experience. To reiterate, the educational protocol and group process are intended to increase self-awareness as well as awareness of the feelings of others. Such awareness cannot simply be taught, as one would teach mathematics. Rather, providing words and concepts that relate to trauma serves as a springboard for engaging in discourse that enhances awareness. The educational material serves as a prompt: we encourage the group members to relate to the terms and concepts by putting their own experiences into words. And we encourage them to listen respectfully to each other so as to relate to each other's experiences. Engaging them in role-played interactions—and in reflection about these interactions—provides an opportunity for them to enhance their self-awareness and their awareness of the experience of others. This awareness serves two broad aims. First, participants learn that they can use their mental capacities—for example, attention and will—in the service of self-regulation. Second, the protocol directly and repeatedly enhances awareness of others in conjunction with fostering a compassionate attitude. We also encourage participants to extend this compassionate attitude toward themselves. We intend that these shifts in awareness and attitudes will diminish the likelihood of participating in further traumatizing actions.

Notwithstanding our intensive efforts to demonstrate objectively the effectiveness of the intervention through controlled studies with objective measures, the empirical evidence for our convictions is meager. Well-designed studies with adequate power and accepted measures showed that participants understood the concepts but did not report robust changes in trauma-related problems or risk-taking behavior. Reluctantly, we concluded that standard assessments—self-report questionnaires—were inadequate for our purposes. As stated earlier, we came to question the validity of these measures on two counts. First, participants may not have completed them conscientiously; second, they may not have completed them honestly. As noted earlier, the possibility that some participants may have been more open and honest—or more aware of—their risk-taking behavior after the intervention could have worked against demonstrating changes in the expected direction.

As we conducted these controlled studies, we were increasingly aware of the discrepancy between the objective findings and our clinical impression

of the potential benefits of the group. We came to recognize that our methods were designed to reveal groupwide effects but that the beneficial impact of the intervention might be relatively individualized. That is, we concluded that there are wide individual differences in the type and extent of benefit. Hence, we shifted our strategy and decided to talk with participants individually about their perception of what, if anything, they gained from the groups. Our content analysis and coding of these brief interviews suggested a wide range of potential benefits, as well as indicating that some participants benefited in many ways, whereas others benefited minimally. These interview findings matched facilitators' clinical impressions and, to varying degrees, were informally validated by facilitators' observations of participation in the groups and their knowledge of participants' functioning in the school setting and the community more generally.

Hence, our current appraisal of the groups' effectiveness remains based on clinical experience and qualitative evidence, albeit extensive and somewhat systematized in study 3. Yet our method in study 3 is open to considerable bias. One might contend that we found just what we were looking for, in effect, by prompting students to give evidence for the conceptual framework we had been developing to articulate the effects of the group. Yet we do not find this criticism compelling. Most of these adolescents are not apt to seek approval, and it is highly unlikely that they would simply offer us what they believe we wanted. Many of these teenagers have been in gangs and difficult living situations that predispose them to be disdainful of adults. Moreover, their responses clearly indicate participants' capacity to adopt our conceptual framework and give evidence for changes within that framework, a capacity that there is no reason to believe could have developed outside the group. We believe that having a conceptual framework and the capacity to apply it to one's life inherently increases self-awareness and potentially self-control (i.e., in the service of avoiding trauma and building relationships). Clearly, participants' capacity to use the conceptual framework for adaptive purposes could be tested more quantitatively and objectively. But our qualitative findings demonstrate that participants developed a way of speaking about their experiences. Merely teaching these teenagers a conceptual framework and enabling them to describe their daily experience in terms of it can be viewed as a significant and therapeutic accomplishment. Prior to the intervention, most of the students were not even aware that they had been traumatized and hence were not on the lookout for potentially re-traumatizing situations. But once they have a con-ceptual framework, they can use cognitive strate-gies to avoid trauma, control anger and aggression, self-regulate, form trusting relationships, and give help to others.

The next step toward empirical validation would be to design more objective measures that would better fit the kinds of effects suggested by our interviews. We find it striking, however, that schools and community agencies show enthusiasm for implementing the intervention despite the min-imal quantitative evidence for effectiveness. Per-haps this enthusiasm reflects the pressing social concerns, as well as the inherent plausibility of the intervention. This tension between felt clinical need and lack of quantitatively demonstrated effective-ness is hardly new. Yet we came to believe that we were seeking evidence of effectiveness in the wrong realm. As many have argued (Allen, 2001; Bruner, 1990; Holmes, 1999), human experience is most significantly organized in terms of narrative. Holmes (1999) aptly characterizes psychotherapy as a matter of "story making" and "story breaking." Our evolving method of assessment taps into this developing narrative capacity, as we endeavor to help participants create narrative structures for their traumatic experience in the service of break-ing old patterns and creating new ones. Each story is an individual creation. Not surprisingly, we found talking to participants individually about the value of the groups to be more helpful than asking them to fill out rating scales. We might hope that this method, in itself, adds further to the narrative capacity by providing a framework for story mak-ing and story breaking.

Community Applications

Over the course of several years, what began as a clinical intervention in a hospital setting has ex-panded in the community in ever-widening direc-tions. When we first extended the clinical program into the school, we did not alter our clinical mind-set. That is, we identified community violence as a problem and focused our attention on high school

students as a vulnerable population. Through this clinical intervention, we hoped to interrupt the cy-cle of trauma and violence, and that aim has con-tinued throughout. Yet we have also broadened our purview as a result of conducting the intervention in the school setting for a number of years. That is, we now have the explicit goal of building a network of advocates for traumatized adolescents.

In the course of implementing the intervention in schools, we have undertaken the substantial task of educating a cadre of school personnel, so that they may in turn serve as facilitators in educating students. Thus we have created a parallel process in which facilitators and students learn about trauma and reenactment, as well as coping skills. The program to train facilitators is ambitious: they go through two and a half days of orientation and education in addition to the weekly on-site training in the actual groups, along with weekly post-group consultation and debriefing discussions. In addi-tion to school personnel, police officers who have an interest in working with the school system par-ticipate in some of the training, as well as in leading some of the groups. The training, along with the actual experience of leading the groups, is designed to promote awareness of violence and its effects while building advocacy for violence prevention in high schools and the community. Thus partici-pation in the program serves as a means of consciousness-raising among facilitators. To a lesser degree, given their collaboration in imple-menting the program, school administrators also become more aware of trauma-related concerns. In addition, a number of group participants volunteer to participate in subsequent groups as peer leaders, providing a model for other participants and ex-panding the network of resources to the peer level.

As facilitators learn about violence and trauma, they become better equipped to handle trauma-related problems in their work role outside of the groups. All the facilitators stated that they used the interventions they learned in the group outside the group as well—ranging from twice weekly to daily. The facilitators all reported a decrease in their sense of helplessness in working with this population, along with an increase in their ability to be helpful. Sometimes facilitators see how they have unwit-tingly perpetuated problems. For example, one fa-cilitator identified her pattern of repeatedly step-ping into the rescuing role. She had viewed the adolescents as helpless victims who were not able to advocate for themselves. As she came to understand that this perspective did not encourage the students to advocate for themselves, she shifted her strategy. She noted that this shift dramatically changed the way she viewed the students and, in turn, what they were capable of handling on their own. Moreover, as facilitators see a way out of the cycle of repetition and reenactment of traumatic scenarios, they have even more motivation to advocate for this work.

Thus, we have begun to establish a small network of advocates in the school and police department who understand the trauma-violence cycle and how to interrupt it. They are in a position to advocate for traumatized adolescents within their settings and in the community at large. And they use new skills in interacting with youth to decrease the likelihood that the cycle of violence will continue. Increased staff training concerning the impact of trauma and violence exposure can aid many additional students in the schools and community.

Future Directions

Ironically, just as we have expanded the intervention from the clinic to the community, we also see possibilities for expanding the reach of the clinical intervention beyond the hospital setting. For example, the project is being implemented in an adolescent group home facility in the local community. The adolescents who attend this group live in the group home. The adolescents attend the group if they have had exposure to violence and abuse, and if they express an interest in attending. The facilitators of the group include the director of the group home, the group home social workers, and the first author. Initial interviews with adolescent participants suggest effects comparable to those among the group members in the school setting. Consistent with a training model, we also have included the group home parents as facilitators in one of the groups. As they learn more about the impact of trauma and violence on the adolescents, the facilitators may be better able to intervene with this population, as happens with school counselors and social workers. Hence, we are exploring the possibility that the participation of the group home parents will have a positive impact on the group home itself. In addition, a local community mental health center is currently exploring the possibility of implementing similar groups with their adolescent population.

The possibility of expanding the intervention to different age-groups within the schools also merits exploring. Mabanglo (2002) is conducting a doctoral dissertation based on the adaptation of the group to the elementary school level, working with students in the fourth through sixth grades (ages 9–12) in a rural school district in northern California. More specifically, Mabanglo has developed a six-session psychoeducational approach focusing primarily on reducing feelings of self-blame but also including some attention to risk-taking behaviors (personal communication, December 28, 2003). Initial findings suggest that children in the program report an increase in knowledge about trauma. While initial findings did not find statistically significant increases in positive attitudes, the qualitative data strongly suggest a decrease in sense of isolation and an increased sense of belonging.

Plainly, the psychoeducational approach to trauma we began developing in the clinic has potentially widespread applications in the community with youngsters at risk in a wide range of settings that include mental health programs as well as schools. Yet the resources needed to implement this program are substantial. To some extent, once trained, facilitators in schools can carry out the intervention without the help of persons who developed the intervention. Yet demands on school personnel continue to escalate, and conducting these educational groups can fall by the wayside when other priorities become more pressing. Continued advocacy, along with additional efforts to document the effectiveness of the program in stemming the tide of trauma and violence, will be needed to direct the allocation of resources accordingly.

Acknowledgments

The project has relied on extensive support from the administration, counseling staff, and social work staff of the United School District No. 501 in Topeka, Kansas; the Topeka Police Department; and the Menninger Clinic research department and clinical staff. The project has been generously funded by the Juvenile Corrections Advisory Board; the Board of County Commissioners of the County of Shawnee, Kansas; and the Child and Family Center of the Menninger Clinic. In addition, the authors thank many individuals who have contributed substantially to the conceptualization, design, and clinical implementation of the project: Gerry Schamess, Harry Palmer, Beth White, Miken Chappel, Sue Miller, Avra Honey-Smith, John Pasqualetti, Rene Valdivia, Sylvia Crawford, Julie Ward, Bonnie Robles, Officer Tom Glor, Dwayne Moore, former chief of police Dean Forster, Dinah Dykes, Roseanne Habermas, Lanette Farmer, Joe Silsby, Bonnie Walker, Marge Petty, Carolyn Altman, Sara Mays, Carrie Cornsweet Barber, Regina Benalcazar-Schmidt, Kay Kent, Pat Hyland, Dev Kerin Khalsa, Shakti Khalsa, and Phil Beard.

References

Allen, J. G. (2001). *Traumatic relationships and serious mental disorders*. Chichester, UK: Wiley.

Allen, J. G. (2003). Challenges in treating posttraumatic stress disorder and attachment trauma. *Current Women's Health Reports, 3*, 213–220.

Allen, J. G. (in press). Mentalizing. *Bulletin of the Menninger Clinic.*

Allen, J. G., Kelly, K. A., & Glodich, A. (1997). A psychoeducational program for patients with trauma-related disorders. *Bulletin of the Menninger Clinic, 61*, 222–239.

Allen-Meares, P., Washington, R., & Welsch, B. (1996). *Social work services in schools*. Boston: Allyn and Bacon.

Bowen, M. (1980). Key to the use of the genogram (family diagram). In E. A. Carter & M. McGoldrick (Eds.), *The family life cycle: A framework for family therapy* (p. xxiii). New York: Gardner.

Bruner, J. (1990). *Acts of meaning*. Cambridge, MA: Harvard University Press.

Busen, N. (1991). Development of an adolescent risk-taking instrument. *Journal of Child and Adolescent Psychiatric and Mental Health Nursing, 4*, 143–149.

Busen, N. H., & Kouzekanani, K. (2000). Perspectives in adolescent risk-taking through instrument development. *Journal of Professional Nursing, 16*, 345–353.

Ceballo, R. (2000). The neighborhood club: A supportive intervention group for children exposed to urban violence. *American Journal of Orthopsychiatry, 70*, 401–407.

Davies, J. M., & Frawley, M. G. (1994). *Treating the adult survivor of childhood sexual abuse*. New York: Basic Books.

Eth, S., & Pynoos, R. (1985). *Post-traumatic stress disorder in children*. Washington, DC: American Psychiatric Press.

Fonagy, P., Gergely, G., Jurist, E. L., & Target, M. (2002). *Affect regulation, mentalization, and the development of the self*. New York: Other Press.

Gabbard, G. O., & Wilkinson, S. M. (1994). *Management of countertransference with borderline patients*. Washington, DC: American Psychiatric Press.

Garbarino, J., & Kostelny, K. (1997). What children can tell us about living in a war zone. In J. Osofsky (Ed.), *Children in a violent society* (pp. 32–41). New York: Guilford.

Giaconia, R. M., Reinherz, H. Z., Hauf, A. C., Paradis, A. D., Wasserman, M. S., & Langhammer, D. M. (2000). Co-morbidity of substance use and post-traumatic stress disorders in a community sample of adolescents. *American Journal of Orthopsychiatry, 70*, 253–262.

Glodich, A. (1999). *Psychoeducational groups for adolescents exposed to violence and abuse: Assessing the effectiveness of increasing knowledge of trauma to avert reenactment and risk-taking behaviors*. Unpublished doctoral dissertation, Smith College, Northampton, MA.

Glodich, A. (2001). Educating adolescents. In J. G. Allen (Ed.), *Traumatic relationships and serious mental disorders* (pp. 359–366). Chichester, UK: Wiley.

Glodich, A., & Allen, J. G. (2000). *Protocol for a trauma-based psychoeducational group intervention to decrease risk-taking, reenactment, and further violence exposure: Application to the public high school setting* (Technical Report No. 00-0033). Topeka, KS: Menninger Clinic, Research Department.

Glodich, A., Allen, J. G., & Arnold, C. (2001). Protocol for a trauma-based psychoeducational group intervention to decrease risk-taking, reenactment, and further violence exposure: Application to the public high school setting. *Journal of Child and Adolescent Group Therapy, 11*, 87–107.

Harter, S. (1999). *The construction of the self: A developmental perspective*. New York: Guilford.

Hastings, T., & Kelley, M. (1997). Development and validation of the Screen for Adolescent Violence Exposure (SAVE). *Journal of Abnormal Child Psychology, 25*, 511–520.

Herz, E., Goldberg, W., & Reis, J. (1984). Family life education for young adolescents: A quasi-experiment. *Journal of Youth and Adolescence, 16*, 309–327.

Holmes, J. (1999). Defensive and creative uses of narrative in psychotherapy: An attachment perspective. In G. Roberts & J. Holmes (Eds.), *Healing stories: Narrative in psychiatry and psychotherapy* (pp. 49–66). Oxford: Oxford University Press.

James, B. (1989). *Treating traumatized children*. New York: Lexington Books.

Janoff-Bulman, R. (1992). *Shattered assumptions: Towards a new psychology of trauma*. New York: Free Press.

Kivel, P., & Creighton, A. (1997). *Making the peace: A 15-session prevention curriculum for young people*. Alameda, CA: Hunter House.

Mabanglo, M. (2002). *A quasi-experimental study of a school based psychoeducational group for school-aged traumatized children and their caregivers*. Unpublished doctoral dissertation, Smith College, Northampton, MA.

Osofsky, J. (1997). Children and youth violence: An overview of the issues. In J. Osofsky (Ed.), *Children in a violent society* (pp. 3–8). New York: Guilford.

Palmer, H. (1994/1997). *Resurfacing: Techniques for exploring consciousness*. Altamonte Springs, FL: Star's Edge International.

Palmer, H. (1999). *Inside Avatar: The book achieving enlightenment*. Altamonte Springs, FL: Star's Edge International.

Pelcovitz, D., Kaplan, S. J., DeRosa, R. R., Mandel, F. S., & Salzinger, S. (2000). Psychiatric disorders in adolescents exposed to domestic violence and physical abuse. *American Journal of Orthopsychiatry, 70*, 360–369.

Perry, B. (1997). Incubated in terror: Neurodevelopmental factors in the "cycle of violence." In J. Osofsky (Ed.), *Children in a violent society* (pp. 124–149). New York: Guilford.

Post, R. M., Weiss, S. R. B., & Smith, M. A. (1995). Sensitization and kindling: Implications for the evolving neural substrates of post-traumatic stress disorder. In M. J. Friedman, D. S. Charney, & A. Y. Deutch (Eds.), *Neurobiological and clinical consequences of stress: From normal adaptation to post-traumatic stress disorder* (pp. 203–224). Philadelphia: Lippincott-Raven.

Post, R. M., Weiss, S. R. B., Smith, M., Li, H., &

McCann, U. (1997). Kindling versus quenching: Implications for the evolution and treatment of posttraumatic stress disorder. In R. Yehuda & A. C. McFarlane (Eds.), *Psychobiology of posttraumatic stress disorder* (Vol. 823, pp. 285–295). New York: New York Academy of Sciences.

Pynoos, R. S. (1993). Traumatic stress and developmental psychopathology in children and adolescents. *Review of Psychiatry, 12*, 205–237.

Pynoos, R., & Nader, K. (1992). Post-traumatic stress disorder. In L. Bralow (Ed.), *Textbook of adolescent medicine* (pp. 1003–1009). Philadelphia: Saunders.

Saakvitne, K. W., Gamble, S., Pearlman, L. A., & Lev, B. T. (2000). *Risking connection: A training curriculum for working with survivors of childhood abuse*. Lutherville, MD: Sidran.

Saltzman, W., Steinberg, A., Layne, C., Aisenberg, E., & Pynoos, R. (2001). A developmental approach to school-based treatment of adolescents exposed to trauma and traumatic loss. *Journal of Child and Adolescent Group Therapy, 11*(2/3), 43–56.

Scannapieco, M. (1994). School-linked programs for adolescents from high-risk, urban environments: A review of research and practice. *School Social Work Journal, 18*, 16–27.

Seligman, M. E. P. (1975). *Helplessness: On depression, development and death*. San Francisco: Freeman.

Twemlow, S. W., Sacco, F. C., & Williams, P. (1996). A clinical and interactionist perspective on the bully-victim-bystander relationship. *Bulletin of the Menninger Clinic, 60*, 296–313.

van der Kolk, B. (1989). The compulsion to repeat the trauma: Re-enactment, revictimization, and masochism. *Psychiatric Clinics of North America, 12*, 389–411.

Williams, S., Fanolis, V., & Schamess, G. (2001). Adapting the Pynoos school-based group therapy model for use with foster children: Theoretical and process considerations. *Journal of Child and Adolescent Group Therapy, 11*(2/3), 57–76.

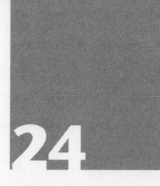

24

Jean A. Adnopoz

Working With High-Risk Children and Families in Their Own Homes

An Integrative Approach to the Treatment of Vulnerable Children

Over the past decades, increased numbers of children and adolescents have presented in schools, day care facilities, child guidance clinics, hospital emergency rooms, and courts with signs and symptoms of psychiatric distress. The service delivery systems that were designed to promote healthy development and adaptation have proved inadequate to meet the complex needs of children and families at risk. An increase in the number of children referred for placement (Knitzer & Cole, 1989), the well-publicized failures of the foster care system, and a critical shortage of child psychiatric beds have created a crisis in the mental health and child welfare systems. Traditional interventions that address specific problems in single domains of human functioning have often failed to provide an effective means of confronting the multidimensional problems that categorize vulnerable children and their families. These factors, together with the fiscal constraints imposed by managed care, have placed substantial pressure on clinicians, administrators, and policymakers to develop new models of appropriate, accessible, and fundable services capable of responding to the needs of children at high risk without removing them from the familiar world of their family and community.

The family has long been recognized as the most effective, long-term institution for raising children (Goldstein, Solnit, Goldstein, & Freud, 1996). Solnit (1976) has described the family as "the bridge from the past to the future" that provides continuity and a sense of being rooted in time, place, history, and culture. Adequately functioning families socialize children, transmit intergenerational values and beliefs, and provide a place of refuge from the challenges of the outside world. Bringing services directly into the home reinforces the importance of the family as the earliest and most significant system with which children are involved. The functional capacity of his or her family exerts a central influence on each child's ability to adapt to and cope with the vicissitudes of life. Parental capacity to think reflectively, to understand the child as a separate individual with his or her own strengths, needs, and vulnerabilities, is associated with the child's sense of competency (Tebes, Kaufman, Adnopoz, & Racusin, 1999). In cases where parental functioning is impaired and the family environment is chaotic, taking the child out of home for treatment either in traditional outpatient care or by temporarily removing him or her to a different, unfamiliar setting may fail to address the underlying systemic issues that affect the child's sense of self and ability to function autonomously.

Theoretical constructs derived from social ecology and developmental psychopathology support the view that each child's functioning is the result of the continuous interactions between his or her innate, structural capacities and the systems that constitute the social environment (Woolston, Berkowitz, Schaefer, & Adnopoz, 1998). As a result, interventions with the capacity to maintain children in the least restrictive environments, such as home and community, while addressing the interrelated needs of the child, the family, and the systems with which they interact have proliferated rapidly over the past decades.

This chapter will describe some of the characteristics of families for whom the home may be a preferred treatment site, review some of the literature on home-based preventive and intervention programs for high-risk children, and provide specific case examples drawn from both a family preservation program and a psychiatric service for children and adolescents with severe emotional disturbances that are delivered in the child and family's home.

Characteristics of Vulnerable Families

The adequately functioning family provides a safe and secure environment in which the normal developmental processes of childhood and adolescence can unfold. Within their home environment, children are likely to feel nurtured, cherished, protected, and secure. Consistent relationships with their adult caregivers enable them to explore their world and move toward eventual independence and self-sufficiency (Adnopoz, 1996).

Although the majority of children in the United States live in families able to offer children good enough care, society remains challenged by the substantial numbers of families who are unable to maintain stable, consistent, and caring relationships without assistance. Many families who require additional support or specialized services demonstrate similar characteristics that affect multiple functional domains (Geismar & Lasorte, 1964; Kaplan, 1986). These families have demonstrated inadequate coping skills in intrapersonal, interpersonal, and environmental areas and have repeated difficulty in negotiating the interrelationships between these domains. The ensuing effect can be characterized as a "web" or cluster of problems that

threaten to eventually overwhelm the family (Adnopoz & Grigsby, 2002).

Children and parents in vulnerable families may experience risks in four domains: the individual child, family, school, and broader community environment. Risk for the individual child may be associated with poor self-esteem, repeated negative parental or familial attribution, impaired impulse control, significant behavioral and health history, and unique individual personality factors or special characteristics. Risks associated with family domain factors may include interpersonal or marital conflict or violence, parental drug or alcohol addiction, abuse, isolation, and/or chronic mental or physical illness. For the child, school may pose problems of relationships with teachers and peers, poor academic performance, repeated frustration and failure, and untreated cognitive disorders. Problems in the environmental domain are likely to be influenced by the family's relationship with the wider community, neighborhoods, institutions, or systems. The complex, continuous interactions among these domains affect the family's ability to parent appropriately and determine the relative risk to the children in the family's care.

Within high-risk families, these interfamilial factors may coexist with environmental stressors such as poverty, educational failure, joblessness, homelessness, and racial or ethnic discrimination. Families coping with these stressors may be difficult to engage, distrustful of traditional clinic-based mental health services, or unable to maintain regular appointment schedules (Adnopoz & Grigsby, 2002). Many such families are more likely to become supportive of, and consistently involved in, their child's treatment and recovery when providers signal their acceptance by entering directly into their homes and local community environments, making treatment and support more easily accessible and acceptable (Adnopoz & Ezepchick, in press; Woodford, 1999). Kilpatrick (1999) argues that these families lack the leadership and control necessary to meet the basic needs of family members for nurturance, caring, safety, and protection. Few traditional institutional or examining room–based interventions have the capacity to address the constellation of internal and external factors that perpetuate the child and family's dysfunctionality and provide the level of intervention and support necessary to maintain them as a functioning unit in the community.

Family Preservation

Family-centered, home-based programs emerged as a service option for children referred to the child welfare system in the last decades of the twentieth century. The renewed interest in services to improve the capacity of parents to care for their children was attributable to the following causes: (1) The numbers of children being reported to protective service agencies across the United States as abused or neglected were growing so rapidly that their needs outstripped the capacity of the system to respond effectively. By 1995, more than 500,000 children were being placed in foster care each year (Nelson, 1996). (2) Reports of maltreatment in foster homes, combined with the knowledge that numerous children in care continued to experience additional placements and disrupted relationships, suggested that the foster care system had failed to meet the interests of the children it was designed to assist (Rosenfeld, Wasserman, & Pilowsky, 1998). An increased awareness of the psychological need of all children for a consistent relationship with a primary adult caregiver, and a focus on the multifactorial, interactive causes of child maltreatment, called some existing child welfare practices into question and led to the creation of innovative service models that would maintain family integrity while also addressing the needs of individual children.

In the past decades the United States has witnessed a rapid proliferation of services that span a wide range of purpose, goals, and clinical sophistication involving children and their parents but that share the home as the site in which they are delivered. Often based on principles first articulated by the Child and Adolescent Service System Program (CASSP) and further codified in subsequent legislation in the middle of the last decade, these services have been particularly difficult to evaluate because of the paucity of theory-driven, structured intervention models and the significant differences between models (Henaghan, Horwitz, & Leventhal, 1994). Although the site of service is clear, the services delivered there are not. Home-based service does not represent a single treatment modality; rather, it describes a systematic mechanism that is used to deliver both preventive and intervention services (Olds, Robinson, Song, Little, & Hill, 1999).

Home-visiting services had their origins in the nineteenth century when "friendly visitors" representing charitable, often religious, organizations called on families to determine their needs and offer services intended to increase their self-sufficiency. In the early years of the twentieth century, home visitation was practiced by social workers, who recognized that by entering and observing the family's environment firsthand, they were better able to assist family members to mobilize natural, community-based networks on their own behalf (Wells, 1995; Woodford, 1999). However, the home did not become a respected site of prevention and intervention services until the last decades of the twentieth century. Working with the whole family within its unique social ecology has become an essential focus of a range of programs and interventions designed to prevent negative parent and child behaviors in at-risk populations, or to ameliorate the problems of serious emotional disturbance, inadequate or abusive parenting, or delinquent behaviors that put children at risk of removal from their own homes and communities (Fristad & Marsh, 2002; Lindblad-Goldberg, Dore, & Stern, 1998).

Literature Review of Services Delivered in the Home

Sally Provence, a developmental pediatrician, initiated a theory-based, comprehensive prevention program for single, poor, inner-city mothers in New Haven, Connecticut, that included periodic home visitation. She and her colleagues found that mothers and children who received sustained services from a consistent group of providers through the child's first 30 months of life had positive long-term outcomes in several domains when compared with nonintervention controls. At the end of the intervention, children in the experimental group scored higher in language development. At 5-year follow-up, these children demonstrated higher school achievement and better school attendance and were more task oriented, while mothers had fewer additional pregnancies, were more likely to be employed, had improved their socioeconomic status, and made better use of community support resources. At 7.5 years following intervention, mothers had completed more years of education, were more likely to be self-supporting, had more satisfying personal relationships, and had waited longer to have a second child. Mothers who received the intervention were more responsive to the needs of their children and reported a more pleasing relationship with them (Provence, 1979; Provence & Naylor, 1983).

David Olds, also a pediatrician, developed a model of nurse-delivered in-home visitation for pregnant and parenting single, poor, first-time mothers with few social supports. Olds's initial study, completed more than 24 years ago, was a randomized test of a structured, curriculum-driven home visitation program designed to improve the quality of parenting, prevent abuse, and improve maternal and infant health outcomes and implemented in Elmira, New York. The study found that 2 years postintervention mothers had fewer preterm deliveries, smoked less, and had fewer kidney infections than community controls. Infants had higher birth weights and a 4.9 point increase in IQ at age 3. Experimental group mothers provided more play materials to their children and used punishment less as a means of discipline, and rates of child abuse and neglect in this group were lower than for the community control group. In addition, experimental condition mothers were better able to make use of their own partners, as well as community supports, in managing problems of everyday living. Their children were seen in the emergency room less frequently and had fewer accidents than children in the control group. These positive findings were sustained when families were reevaluated as the children turned 15 years old. Child abuse and neglect rates remained lower at 2 and 15 years. Additionally, the experimental group children were considerably less likely to have been arrested, to have used alcohol or smoked cigarettes, or to have had multiple sex partners. When the children were 15 years old, mothers in the intervention group were reported as less impaired by drug and alcohol since the birth of the index child (Olds, Henderson, et al., 1999). The initial study was replicated in Memphis, Tennessee, with a primarily urban, African American population. Some of the effects reported in the Elmira study were also found in Memphis, although the effect size was somewhat smaller. The number of health care encounters for injuries and injections were 23% lower than for the control group, and the number of hospital days required for serious injuries was significantly less. Parental reports of child behavior problems did not differ between the experimental and control groups in either study. An economic anal-

ysis conducted by the Rand Corporation found that real economic benefits were accrued by the 4th year of life for low-income children; this finding did not hold for higher socioeconomic status (SES) families and married women (Olds & Kitzman, 1993).

Heinicke and Ponce, in a review of numerous early intervention studies, found considerable evidence to support the effectiveness of home visitors in improving maternal self-concept and satisfaction and in enhancing mothers' responsiveness to the needs of their infants (cited in Cicchetti & Toth, 1998). In the UCLA Family Development Project, Heinicke and colleagues demonstrated that a randomized home visiting relationship-based intervention for third-trimester pregnant women classified as at high risk for inadequate parenting was able to increase experienced partner and family support by the infant's first birthday compared with controls (Heinicke & Ponce, 1999). In addition to home visiting, the experimental group participated in a weekly mother-infant group; the controls received regular pediatric follow-up. At 1 year of age, children in the intervention group were more securely attached and more autonomous. Heinicke has emphasized that the ability to achieve sustained effects with inadequately functioning families depends on the capacity of the intervention to address the adaptation needs of the parents.

These studies demonstrated that sustained, structured, relationship-based in-home visitation could be effective in improving maternal competence and enhancing maternal capacity to enter into positive relationships, to utilize partner and community supports, and attend to issues of self-development. In addition, preventive in-home services encouraged more effective maternal responses to limit setting, the use of appropriate controls, and the promotion of the child's autonomy, capacity for exploration and task orientation, and cognition. Process variables associated with positive outcomes have been found to include the duration of contact between the mother and home visitor, the extent of focus on parenting issues, the mother's attitude, her willingness to work with the visitor, and her view of the visitor as helpful (Korfmacher, Kitzman, & Olds, 1998).

Several models of in-home intervention services for children and families in the child welfare system have gained national attention. Home-based family preservation and support services have been available since the 1970s for families in which children are at high risk for out-of-home placement secondary to abuse or neglect. However, it has been difficult to establish evidence of their effectiveness. Homebuilders, an intensive home-based intervention developed in Tacoma, Washington, was among the first home-based treatments to use a social ecology paradigm that addressed the multisystemic interactions between the child, his or her family, and the environment. Funders such as the Edna McConnell Clark Foundation, as well as state and national policy makers, endorsed the Homebuilders model because they believed it demonstrated the ability to reduce out-of-home placement, maintain children within their families, and reduce taxpayer's costs (Adnopoz & Grigsby, 2002).

Although most studies of Homebuilder-type family preservation programs have shown that placement does not occur for the majority of children receiving services, studies to determine any further outcomes of family preservation programs have been limited by small effect sizes. The lack of randomized controlled studies and inadequate program standardization also call into question both the adequacy of the programs and the research methodologies used to evaluate them (Burns, Hoagwood, & Mrazek, 1999). Over time family-focused, in-home services have been further defined and tailored specifically to meet the needs of parents, children, and adolescents with problems such as child or parental mental illness and drug addiction, juvenile delinquency, and HIV/AIDS. A handful of randomized clinical trials have tested some of these models and found some to be effective in decreasing problem behaviors, improving family functioning, promoting the recovery of the index child, and reducing the need for more costly out-of-home placements, in either hospitals or residential programs (Henaghan et al., 1994).

Scott Henggeler and his associates at the University of South Carolina have developed a manualized, theory based, in-home multisystemic treatment (MST) that has demonstrated its effectiveness with chronic juvenile offenders, adolescent sex offenders, and substance-abusing delinquents in studies run by the program's developers. MST addresses the interpersonal and systemic factors associated with adolescent antisocial behavior (Henggeler & Borduin, 1990) and considers the child's view of his or her world, as well as the direct and persistent influence of his or her family, peer, and school environments.

The Missouri Delinquency Project examined long-term effects of MST on the prevention of criminal activity in a sample of predominantly serious juvenile offenders by comparing MST with individual therapy. This study demonstrated positive effects on perceived family relations, family interactions, parental symptomatology, interfamilial conflict, and the youth behavior problems. The intervention also produced long-term changes in the youths' criminal behaviors. Borduin suggests that improved family functioning was the primary influence on the reduction of criminal behavior in the Missouri study (Borduin, Mann, Barton, & Cone, 1995).

In an intervention for children ages 10 to 17 approved for emergency psychiatric hospitalization at the Medical University of South Carolina, Henggeler, Rowland, and Pickrel (1997) have studied whether MST could be modified effectively for use with children presenting with psychiatric emergencies. Subjects were randomly assigned either to an experimental MST condition or to treatment as usual (i.e., hospitalization and aftercare). Services were provided in the homes of family, relatives, or friends and in community shelters, respite beds, or the hospital. Caseloads were reduced from the MST standard of five families per clinician to three. Children in the experimental group had judicious but controlled access to community resources, including hospitalization and therapeutic foster care. Children in the control group received treatment as usual, often utilizing some of the same resources.

Henggeler et al. (1997) reports that MST was at least as effective, and in some cases more effective, in decreasing child symptomology and emergency psychiatric hospitalization. Rates of decreased internalizing problems were similar across the two conditions: MST was more effective in decreasing rates of externalizing symptoms. Youth in the control condition reported increased self-esteem, while families in the experimental condition showed improved cohesion and increased structure. Henggeler suggests that the treatment of youth with serious psychiatric problems and their families presents greater complexity and problem severity than he had expected based on his previous work. He proposed further study, some of which is already in progress (Henggeler et al., 1997).

The wraparound services concept, which addresses the needs of the child in the context of his or her family and broader social ecology, emerged from the Child and Adolescent Service System Program. CASSP was dedicated to the creation of interagency collaborations, community-based, advocacy-oriented systems of care, and the expansion of parental decision making and involvement to meet the multisystemic needs of children with serious emotional disturbances (Woolston et al., 1998). Theoretically rooted in environmental ecology, wraparound programs stress unconditional care and assume that changes in the environment will foster changes that persist over time for children, families, and communities. Wraparound is a strength-based intervention process that values parental empowerment, culturally competent providers, and the use of natural supports to augment professional involvement. Outcomes are measured against goals established by the family. The quality of clinical care is dependent on the resources of each local system of care. To date, there have been very few randomized trials of wraparound's effectiveness, although individual case studies have shown improvements that persist over time (Burns et al., 1999).

Although family preservation programs proliferated during the last decades of the twentieth century, there have been few attempts to examine their effectiveness. In an attempt to address this issue, the Yale Intensive Family Preservation program (IFP), a clinically informed, time-limited home-based supportive service designed by the author to maintain children at risk of placement safely within their homes and families, was selected for a methodologically rigorous evaluation (Balestracci, 2001). The primary goal of IFP was to reduce the need for placement and the concomitant disruption of the child's primary attachment when appropriate. Balestracci designed a retrospective, quasi-experimental study that included 299 intervention families and 84 wait-list controls that were identified from the 579 cases referred to IFP by the Connecticut Department of Children and Families (DCF) between 1988 and 1993. Data describing family demographics, history, maltreatment type, caregiver characteristics, service intensity, types of services provided, goals, goal attainment, and presence or absence of a therapeutic alliance were abstracted from the records of IFP for the intervention

cases, and data on history, demographics, caregiver disability, and service provision were abstracted from DCF case files for the comparison group.

Sixty-seven percent of the families in the study were found to be largely poor; only 20% included both birth parents; 40% were headed by single adults with no other adults in the home; 75% of the primary caregivers had an identified health or mental health problem; and another 40% had more than one such condition.

The most significant findings of the study were that the establishment and subsequent attainment of treatment goals were inversely related to child placement. Treatment goals were set with 96.3% of all intervention families; 22.3% fully attained them, and 63% met them partially. Six percent of families who met their treatment goals had a child placed, compared with 41.4% of families who partially met their goals and 66.7% of families who met none of their goals. A therapeutic alliance between family and at least one member of the treatment team was noted in more than 40% of the cases, although there were considerable missing data related to this variable. Importantly, the study found that when there was an existing therapeutic relationship between the treatment team and the primary caregiver, families were significantly more likely to meet their treatment goals than were those families in which no alliance was established and noted. However, Balestracci advises caution in accepting this finding, again because of missing data.

In addition, the study found that although a greater percentage of comparison families appeared to experience placement during all points of the 3-year follow-up, none of the associations was statistically significant. Strong associations were found between child placement during the 3-year follow-up and the presence in the home of children less than 5 years, a child already in placement at the time of the referral to IFP and prior DCF maltreatment, and placement history. The presence of a child under the age of 5 was a protective factor; the other factors predicted placement. Caregiver characteristics were not found to be predictive of placement, but positive associations were found between the time to the first child placement and the caregiver's secondary disabilities, such as chronic physical illness, past drug use, and child physical abuse.

Significant associations between family histories of child placement and active substance abuse by the primary caregiver, and subsequent placement in care were consistent with prior studies. In the 3-year follow-up period, children in substance-affected families were almost twice as likely to be placed outside of the home as those in non-drug-abusing families. Unlike some other studies, in this study there was no association between parental mental illness and out-of-home placement.

The strengths of the study should be noted. The sample size was larger, the follow-up period was longer, and the variety of statistical analyses broader than any other previously published family preservation evaluation. However, the small effect size points up the difficulties often found in retrospective studies of nonmanualized interventions. In fact, as this review of the literature makes clear, interventions that are theory-based, well structured according to a treatment manual, and consistently delivered in accordance with the model are those most likely to demonstrate effectiveness. Although many in-home program models have produced individual examples of clinical improvement, very few are able to qualify as evidence-based treatments. In this era of managed care and results-oriented outcomes, the challenge to clinicians and program developers is clear.

Models of Clinical Services Delivered in the Home: The Yale Family Support Service

Since 1985, the Yale Child Study Center has provided clinically informed family-focused services in the homes of children referred because of abuse, neglect, abandonment, or parental mental illness or addiction (Adnopoz & Ezepchick, in press; Gossart-Walker & Moss, 2000). The overarching goal of all Family Support Service (FSS) programs is to recognize and promote every child's need for a stable, permanent caregiving relationship by preventing unnecessary disruptions of his or her primary attachments. Interventions are designed to (1) assist parents to understand the influence their behaviors and attitudes exert upon each child's developmental, physical, and cognitive needs; and (2) address those areas that continue to place the child at risk of removal from his or her parent and family. The development of a therapeutic alliance between the clinician and the family has been found to be the essential vehicle for change in these programs (Balestracci, 2001). Through this important relationship, parents may gain the understanding

and insight necessary to bring about the behavioral and structural changes that are expected to benefit their children and themselves. Comprehensive services including evaluation, assessment, brief individual or family treatment, parent guidance, behavioral management, concrete services, transportation, advocacy, and care coordination are delivered to both children and parents. All FSS interventions are provided to families in their own homes and communities by teams composed of a master's-level social worker and a family support worker.

FSS services are governed by the following set of principles that aids in establishing practice parameters: the family system is seen as the primary unit of treatment; team members assume that change is possible within the family and pursue family strengths, not weaknesses. Although services focus on keeping families together and preventing unnecessary foster or residential placement, the programs recognize that some parents are unable to provide the level of safety and support needed by their children, often because parental and child needs are in conflict. In these cases, intervention teams work to assure permanency in another setting that has the potential to provide permanency and stability over time. All services are intensive, culturally competent, and provided on a goal-oriented, time–limited basis. Caseloads are low, averaging six to seven cases per team (Adnopoz & Grigsby, 2002).

Utilizing the home as the primary site of intervention shifts the balance of power from the service provider to the family and communicates an acceptance of the family's circumstances as long as they do not present a serious challenge to the child's well-being. The willingness of the FSS team to enter into the family's environment has other benefits as well. It allows the team to observe the family "in vivo," to assess the real world of the child and his or her caregivers, and to understand the complex, often previously unknown and unanticipated interactions that take place between the adults and their children. Within this context, the family is given support and assistance to enable them to set the agenda for intervention, identify their goals, and establish their own priorities (Adnopoz & Culler, 2000). The treatment alliance serves as a starting place for this work. It provides the base from which parents are helped to express their own wishes, fears, and disappointments and to understand how these issues have affected both their views of their children and their capacity to parent effectively. Attempts are made to identify specific tasks that can be undertaken to change family interactions based on the treatment plan and engage other members of the family network in support of the plan.

Family Preservation Services

Family preservation programs are designed for families with children who have been assessed as being at imminent risk of being placed out of the home without the provision of intensive services. Services are provided in the home by workers who have small caseloads, generally no more than six cases at one time, and are available 24 hours per day, 7 days per week, as needed by the child and family. Services are short-term, ranging from 4 to 12 weeks, depending on the program; they are designed to stabilize family functioning following a crisis and assist the family to attain a more appropriate level of functioning. A team consisting of a master's-level clinician and a family support worker provides all the services offered by the FSS Intensive Family Preservation program. Other IFP programs utilize single clinicians or paraprofessionals.

Toward an Understanding of Family Preservation

Focused on the intersection between the child's innate capacities and character structure, the quality of the parent-child relationship, and the larger ecological context of the family's community and social systems, family preservation services are characterized by both intimacy and complexity. The setting for the work is the rich, complex, and highly personal environment of the home in which the team is able to piece together a tapestry that illumines the child and family's world. IFP interventions are designed to address several problem areas simultaneously. The reverberation of changes that occur across multiple domains may serve as a catalyst or "jump start" to an improved level of family functioning. Families can then be assisted to make use of more traditional services and natural support systems to deepen and maintain the advances they have made.

Many referred families with young children exhibit significant disturbances in parent-child relationships that may inform and shape the child's self-image and lead to behavioral problems for the child. The parents of anxious or aggressive acting-out children, whose behaviors challenge and sometimes threaten to overwhelm them, often have their own problems with internal impulse controls and executive functioning. Throughout the IFP intervention, the clinical team works with parents to help them differentiate themselves and their needs from those of their children, to see the world as it is seen through the eyes of their children, and to understand the central role they as parents play in shaping that world. Parents who are able to apply positive parenting techniques and gain a basic understanding of child-specific developmental stages and phases, and the parental interaction that helps children to navigate these stages successfully, are likely to experience enhanced effectiveness, adequacy in the parental role, and closer attunement with the child. Work in this area is often focused on helping the parent to think reflexively and to understand the mind of the child as separate from that of the parent.

Parents who consistently attribute negative characteristics and behaviors to their children are assisted to recast their negative attributions into positive messages that can be expected to affect the child's self-image more constructively. Based on the team's assessment, their in-home observations, and a careful re-creation of the child and family's history, it is often critical to encourage parents to utilize direct, community-based interventions for both themselves and their children such as individual or group treatment, family or play therapy delivered in the home by the team, or referral to a more structured day treatment, recreational, mentoring, or drug and alcohol treatment program. Because all the children and families referred for family preservation services are also in the protective service system, incorporating the need for these services into the protective service plan may assure appropriate use of community services in cases where the family offers resistance to treatment. In such instances, it is the role of the IFP team to assist the family to keep appointments, transport them when necessary, and, with the parent's knowledge, reinforce the work being done by others by maintaining professional contact and clear, open channels of communication. The FSS experience suggests that direct interventions with adults and children can promote their recovery. The resulting increased behavioral control, improved capacity to understand the effect of impaired family interactions, and sense of personal competence gained by adults and children contribute to the success of the family intervention.

Family Preservation as a Means of Assessing Safety

As long as the success of family preservation is measured by its ability to prevent out-of-home placement (Nelson, 1996; Henaghan et al., 1994), its potential as a diagnostic and assessment tool may be unappreciated. Because IFP programs provide an important window into the functioning of families in which children are at risk, they can be used successfully to identify those children whose needs cannot be met by their biological parents, either because of the severity of parental problems of addiction or mental or physical illness, or because of parental difficulty in providing the intensive, specialized level of care needed by the child. In these cases, clinicians working in the home can be effective advocates for permanency, stability, and safety by documenting that the child's best interest lies in removal from the biological family and placement elsewhere.

Once it is necessary to remove a child from his or her family of origin, family preservation services should be offered to the subsequent caregiver to prevent the possibility of further placement disruption, a role played whenever necessary by the FSS program in concert with child protective services. The positive value of IFP services emerges when the service focuses on the child's best interest rather than on preservation of the family at any cost. Understanding family preservation in this context may clarify its purpose and assist its antagonists to realize its potential effectiveness.

Foster family preservation can be an effective intervention in cases where behavioral issues have developed as a result of problems of fit between a child's coping style and his or her foster parent's approach to caregiving. For example, FSS IFP teams have helped foster parents to recognize that children with a history of deprivation and neglect may feel unwanted, unworthy of adult love, and unable to trust that any adult would commit to their care. As a result, such children may challenge

their foster parents by pushing the limits and boundaries set for them and attempting to gain control over what is likely to be their worst fear, their eventual extrusion from the foster family. However, other cases have uncovered the foster parents' wish for gratification of their own psychological needs through foster parenting and the unrealistic expectations that ensue. Interventions in these cases have led to the foster parents' realization that they are not equipped to care for children with traumatic histories and psychiatric vulnerabilities. This is often followed by a request to remove these children from care. Close observation has also led to the realization that the survival strategies children have developed in neglectful or abusive homes are often discouraged or even punished in the foster home setting. For example, a 7-year-old boy who had been functioning as caretaker and cook for his younger siblings and retarded mother survived during this period by walking the streets after dark, pilfering food. Soon after his separation from his family and placement in foster care, his foster mother requested his removal after he was observed repeatedly taking food from her kitchen at night.

Close collaboration between IFP programs and the child protection programs that are likely to be the primary source of referral for IFP services is a pathway to continuous involvement with children who must move between their biological families into foster care. The IFP team is able to bear witness to the child's earlier experiences and interpret his or her behavior to the foster parent in light of the child's disrupted attachment and removal from his or her family, history, and familiar school and surroundings. Although these separations are likely to be traumatic, the continuity represented by the ongoing team's presence and their ability to provide information and support to the foster family may help in the process of the child's positive adaptation to his or her new family.

Case Illustration: The W. Family

Serena W., a 20-year-old, mildly depressed, poor, African American woman with a history of abusive relationships with men, was referred for IFP service when her 3-year-old son, Paul, suffered a broken leg after being thrown to the floor by her boyfriend in the midst of a domestic quarrel. The boyfriend was incarcerated, but concerns remained about the mother's supervision, passivity, inability to set limits, compliance with court expectations, and ability to protect Paul and his 18-month-old brother, Jeremiah.

Although Paul was frequently aggressive toward his mother and brother, there was no structure or consistency to his mother's response. She reacted to increased pressure from her child protection worker by shutting down and withdrawing further from her family. The IFP team initiated its work with Serena by engaging her as a young woman struggling to care for two children without the support and assistance of their fathers, other family members, or friends. The team viewed her as troubled, unable to make good choices for herself, and lacking confidence in her ability to manage her family. The initial twice-weekly, hour-long sessions, held in her home, were spent talking with Serena about herself, her life history, and the goals she had for herself and her family in an attempt to build a therapeutic alliance and break through her resistance to addressing the problems that surrounded her. The team was able to recognize that Serena cared for her children deeply and wanted a better life for them, but she did not know how to actualize her wish.

As the relationship deepened and she began to trust the team working with her, Serena was able to recognize that it could help her achieve her goals of a brighter future. She began by learning that her children had unmet developmental needs for an active, consistent, and involved parent. The team helped her to understand that young children are dependent on their parents to set limits and boundaries that provide a sense of order and safety in what is otherwise a frightening and chaotic world. Serena also learned that children rely on parental interaction and nurturance to gain feelings of self-worth and competence, to develop the trust and self-confidence that enables them to explore their world safely, and to promote their creativity and imagination. With the support of the team, Serena was shown specific strategies for engagement with her children. The team brought books and art materials to their play sessions, and Serena learned to enjoy participating with her children in play, reading, and art activities. The team members praised her efforts and gave her regular feedback on the good work she was doing. As she gained confidence in herself as a parent and as an individual valued by someone else, she was able to set limits and assume executive functioning. She was proud of the fact that she was able to toilet train Paul. The team worked with her to identify the community resources that could help her meet her goal of living a better, less chaotic life and went with her to introduce her to the providers. Serena enrolled Paul in a neighborhood Head Start program, joined a parenting course, and became more active on behalf of herself and her family.

In the last phase of the 14-week intervention, as she began to take pleasure in her accomplishments and gain a new sense of self-competence, Serena became available to work with the team around her history of depression, isolation, and poor choice of partners. Her willingness to confront her past at this point made it possible for her to reestablish contact with her own mother, who responded positively to her daughter's outreach to her and her more responsible behavior, and began to provide emotional support as well as child care. When the case closed, Serena's mood was significantly improved, her sense of self-efficacy was increased, her children were being provided more appropriate care, and she had joined a domestic violence support group (Adnopoz & Culler, 2000).

The success of this case reaffirms the findings of the earlier IFP study (Balestracci, 2001). The therapeutic alliance between Serena and the IFP team provided the vehicle through which Serena was able to reach her goal of creating a more structured, predictable life for herself and her two children. With the assistance of the team, she was able to more clearly understand that her children needed her, wanted her, and could not tolerate her withdrawal from them. The positive results that emerged from her active and more consistent engagement with them proved to be essential elements in helping her to gain a sense of self-competence and confidence and to address the long-standing issues that had fueled her sense of isolation and depression. The team's willingness to accept Serena as she was and to slowly engage her in a treatment relationship was a critical factor in the success of this case.

In-Home Services for Children With Psychiatric Disorders

In 1995, the Yale Child Study Center initiated a service to meet the needs of children with severe emotional disturbances who could not remain in psychiatric hospitals for more than inappropriately brief periods due to the constraints of managed care. These children, whose diagnoses include depression, anxiety, attachment, obsession-compulsive, psychotic, and stress-related disorders, among others, were at high risk of recidivism following premature discharge from treatment. Because traditional outpatient services were insufficient to meet their needs, and few other treatment options, short of institutional care, existed in the community, many of their families were unprepared to care for them. This service, which began with a wraparound plan for a single child and family, has evolved into a major, statewide replication project. The program is named the Intensive In-Home Child and Adolescent Psychiatric Service (IICAPS)

IICAPS, an intensive, in-home, goal-oriented intervention for children with severe emotional disturbance, joins the principles informing family preservation interventions with principles derived from developmental psychopathology, which view developmental progress as the result of the complex, continual interaction between the child's innate capacities and his or her environment (Cicchetti & Cohen, 1995). This view posits that changes in the child's environment can lead to positive changes in the child's developmental trajectory.

IICAPS was designed as a catalytic enhancement of outpatient services for children who are being discharged from psychiatric hospitalization or who are at high risk of hospitalization following a psychiatric crisis. The service is also appropriate for children in traditional outpatient treatment who cannot be maintained safely in their homes and community without more intensive intervention. Often utilized as a bridge between hospital and home, IICAPS interventions are guided by attachment, object relations, cognitive behavioral, family systems, and transactional theories. Services are provided by teams consisting of a master's-level clinician (social worker, nurse, or psychologist) and a bachelor's-level mental health counselor, who work under the direct, weekly supervision of a child and adolescent psychiatrist or senior clinician. Each team is responsible for delivering or linking to the services that constitute the program's core: assessment, evaluation, individual psychotherapy for children and adults, family therapy, couples counseling, parent guidance, behavioral

management, crisis intervention, and medication management. To meet the needs of each individual child and family, the intensity of IICAPS involvement can be titrated on levels ranging from 5 to 15 hours per week, depending on the particular needs of the child and family. The majority of cases require 5 to 7 hours per week; the hours represent the cumulative time spent by the team members, who see the family both individually and together depending on the work to be accomplished. To ensure caregiving continuity, teams are available 24 hours per day, 7 days per week, to intervene as family crises arise. A child psychiatrist assumes medical responsibility for the care of all patients and presides at weekly rounds. Treatment is focused on specific, defined problems that relate to the treatment goals and are viewed as amenable to measurable amelioration. The result is a program that integrates a well-defined medical model with an ecologically oriented and family-focused approach to meeting the needs of seriously emotionally disturbed children, adolescents, and their families.

The overarching goal of all IICAPS treatment is the enhancement of the "quality of fit" between the child and the systems in which he or she is embedded. Understanding that behavior and adaptation result from the complex, ongoing interactions between the child and the environment, intervention goals target four specific domains: the child and his or her inner world, the family, the child's school, and the larger systems and social environment. The parallel relationships that develop between the team members and the child and his or her parents, between the family, the child's school, and the broader systems within which they come into contact, and between the team and the team supervisor are expected to continuously reinforce progress toward the goals set by the family and lead to the desired changes in each domain.

IICAPS Treatment Phases

The initial phase of IICAPS intervention, which may take from 5 to 6 weeks, is centered on the processes of engagement and assessment. During this phase parents are expected to act as full partners with the team in identifying the "main problem," the issue that places the child at risk of psychiatric hospitalization or institutionalization, and the strengths and the barriers across all four domains that bear upon it. At this time the team also pieces together the narrative of the child and family's life, including identification of all family members and significant others and their relevance to the main problem area. In this period the family sets the goals for the intervention, develops a strategy to address problems of immediate concern, and, with the team, drafts the treatment plan.

The second phase of an IICAPS intervention is characterized by intensive work on the part of the child, the family, and the team. It is the period of greatest therapeutic action. Recognizing that goal attainment has been found to predict successful outcomes (Balestracci, 2001), this phase focuses on achieving the goals that the family has set with the assistance of the team. Possible challenges to goal setting and goal attainment are viewed as barriers to be overcome through reassessment and realignment of the treatment goals, not as rationalizations for potential treatment failure. Treatment itself is present focused, action oriented, and reality based, guided by principles that underscore the importance of continuity of caregiving, the negative consequences of relational disruptions, and multiple benefits of placement decisions that represent the least detrimental alternative (Goldstein et al., 1996). During the treatment process, the child's safety and well-being are regularly assessed in relation to the preservation of his or her primary attachments and need for continuity of family culture, history, and beliefs. In the same way, parents are helped to view the child as separate from themselves, as individuals with their own needs, capacities, wishes, and self-perceptions.

Throughout the intervention, the central focus of the therapeutic work is to bring about the smallest possible change able to exert the most lasting effect on child and family functioning, reduce the risk of future hospitalization, and optimize the child's developmental trajectory. For example, Frank, a depressed, adolescent, Caucasian male living with his grandmother, was failing in school and getting into trouble with the police. His grandmother, with whom he had been placed at the time of his mother's death 7 years previously, expressed her concerns to her protective service worker and suggested that she might have to return Frank to the care of the state. The case was referred to IICAPS for evaluation and possible stabilization. The assessment revealed that Frank's behaviors were related to his grandmother's recent hospitalization for a respiratory illness and his fears that he would be lose her to illness, and perhaps death. With this information, the IICAPS team recognized that Frank's behavior depended on the maintenance of his relationship with his grandmother. As a result, the team worked with the grandmother and protective services to help them to convey to Frank that his placement with his grandmother would continue, while also helping the grandmother to care for both Frank and herself. With this sense of stability, Frank was free to make use of other more traditional and less intensive community-based services

The third and final treatment phase is the period of ending and wrap-up. The decision of when to end the intervention is made collaboratively by the family, the child when appropriate, and the IICAPS team. Because it is likely that children and families for whom IICAPS services are appropriate will continue to need psychiatric and other supportive services postintervention, the family and team identify those resources in the community that they expect will help the family to sustain the gains they have made during the treatment. Prior to leaving the family, the team brings together the present and continuing community-based providers to ensure coordination and collaboration among those whose ongoing involvement with the child and family will be essential to the family's stability over time. For example, because it may be expected that some children will require rehospitalization at some future time, a plan to integrate such stays into a thoughtful treatment plan constitutes an appropriate task for the team during this final IICAPS treatment phase. IICAPS services are not expected to "cure" children with serious psychiatric problems. Success should be measured by goal attainment and how well the intervention has assisted the child and family to function in a sufficiently stable manner, and to be able to make appropriate use of traditional, community-based mental health and other needed resources. Although pilot, controlled studies of the intervention have begun, longitudinal data capturing long-term outcomes are not yet available.

Case Illustration: Robert and His Family

Robert, a 13-year-old Caucasian male, was referred to the Yale IICAPS program following discharge from partial hospitalization because of concerns about the ability of his family to manage his continuing depression, and the possibility of an eruption of his explosive, out-of-control behavior. Robert had been referred to the hospital initially following a verbal threat to kill his teacher. He lived in a two-bedroom apartment with his father and his mother (who were divorced from each other), his mother's boyfriend, and four brothers.

Robert's mother had been diagnosed previously as depressed, with poor ego functioning. His father, a former accountant, had been diagnosed with schizoaffective and bipolar disorders and had frequent bouts of violent and threatening behavior. His father had made six suicide attempts within the 3 years prior to the IICAPS referral. Though he was placed on psychotropic medication following these attempts, he was noncompliant with recommendations for outpatient treatment. At the time of Robert's referral to IICAPS, his father was on probation for an incident that occurred when he was actively psychotic and in which he destroyed several household items and verbally threatened his ex-wife, Robert's mother. It was evident that the circumstances of his life kept Robert's father from work, forced him to declare bankruptcy, and eventually led to the loss of his home. An intensive in-home intervention was selected for this family because of their history of noncompliance with traditional outpatient treatment and the need to address the intergenerational conflicts that seriously compromised Robert's recovery.

Although Robert lived with both parents, his primary attachment was to his father. His mother was physically residing within the household, but she had psychologically abandoned her husband and her sons many years previously. It was not surprising that Robert's mother declined to participate in any aspect of the IICAPS intervention; she did not engage in treatment planning or in the implementation of the treatment plan. As a result, the IICAPS team directed its efforts to working with Robert and his father.

During the initial treatment phase, the team assisted the family to identify the following goals related to the family's main problem, the lack of leadership and structure: (1) assist Robert, his siblings, and his father to find permanent housing away from the chaotic, sexualized environment in which they lived without privacy and support; (2) engage Robert in home-based, individual psychotherapy

with the psychologist on the team, who would focus on Robert's primary attachment to his father and help him to cope with his rage at his mother's inability to value and protect him; (3) work with the local school to enroll Robert in a program able to meet his educational and social needs; and (4) assist Robert's father to set limits and establish control over his family.

Six weeks after the intervention began, Robert's father became enraged at the lack of discipline, out-of-control behaviors, and level of dissension within his family, gathered his belongings, and sought shelter with his own parents. The IICAPS team assisted Robert's father to first find a temporary place to live and subsequently a permanent home in which he has been able to establish consistent structure and organization. Because the family had moved to another town, issues of nexus initially compromised Robert's ability to return to school and resulted in placement in a homebound program that was insufficient to meet his educational and social needs. It took the persistent efforts of the team to persuade the school administrators to enroll Robert as a classroom student. Even with their concerted efforts, it was many months before Robert was admitted as a student.

The IICAPS team worked with Robert and his family for approximately 6 months, spending 5 hours per week meeting with them in their home, working with the school system, outpatient clinicians, and others, including potential landlords, in pursuit of the goals they had set. The team helped the school understand Robert and his needs and, with the father's permission, established communication with a clinician who would become the father's prescribing physician and therapist. The treatment alliance that developed between the team, Robert, and his father allowed family members to risk failure at school and in-job training. Robert's father took cooking lessons; Robert reentered a regular classroom. Robert and his father were helped to give up their anger at Robert's mother and accept responsibility for improving the functionality of their family.

With IICAPS services, Robert and his family were able to achieve the following: (1) Robert developed a successful therapeutic alliance and was able to articulate and integrate his feelings of rage and abandonment; (2) he responded well to medication and began to feel much better; (3) he attended school regularly, and his sense of self-adequacy and autonomy improved; and (4) his father attended therapy regularly, was able to create a supportive home for his sons, and became an adequate cook. As Robert's father became more able to verbalize his affection for his sons and take pride in his ability to meet their needs, they responded more positively to him and were able to demonstrate their positive feelings for him. Robert's father's ability to control his own behavior and improve his home environment exerted a positive influence on Robert and his siblings. At the time of discharge, treatment goals had been met, and Robert and his father were stabilized and able to make good use of less intensive, community-based traditional mental health services with providers and systems that were aware of their needs.

Conclusion

The severity of symptomology presented by children and families in need of mental health treatment has threatened to overcome many traditional service providers. Many of the families who need services do not avail themselves of those that are available. Many need to be prepared for treatment before they can take advantage of its potential benefits. The services described in this chapter represent sophisticated, clinically informed treatment models that have moved from traditional examining rooms to a new venue, the child and family's home and community. By so doing, they convey a message of acceptance to the families involved in them and demonstrate a willingness to take seriously the interrelated needs of all members of the family. The IICAPS treatment model has been built upon a strongly held belief that the most promising approach to children with serious emotional disturbances lies in identifying, understanding, and addressing the complex set of internal, familial, peer, and social interactions that characterize the world of each child and family referred for care. The effectiveness of this approach remains to be tested in a methodologically rigorous manner.

The specific elements that are expected to bring about the behavioral changes leading to successful IICAPS outcomes must be examined closely. The importance of the therapeutic alliance as an instrument for change, the attainment of the goals set by the child and family, and the capacity of the parents to differentiate their children from themselves are thought to be significant contributors to successful outcomes based on clinical observation. Other hypotheses regarding the importance of duration and intensity of the intervention have also emerged from the work. Although IICAPS has been accepted as a replicable, fundable intervention by the state of Connecticut, only through randomized studies will we know the full extent of its power.

An expanding literature provides evidence of the benefits of home- and community-based interventions for high-risk, vulnerable children and speaks to the importance of providing carefully constructed and standardized programs that are monitored for treatment fidelity. The future support of effective, home-based mental health services such as IICAPS depends on the ability of program planners to develop and test interventions that meet specific, quantifiable standards while allowing for the clinical flexibility that defines the work.

References

Adnopoz, J. (1996). Complicating the theory: The application of psychoanalytic concepts and understanding to family preservation. In A. Solnit, R. Eissler, & P. Neubaur (Eds.), *The psychoanalytic study of the child* (pp. 411–421). New Haven, CT: Yale University Press.

Adnopoz, J., & Culler, E. (2000). *Multiproblem families: An update on intensive family preservation.* Unpublished paper.

Adnopoz, J., & Ezepchick, J. (2003). Family focus: A promising strategy for serving high-risk children. In National Abandoned Infants Resource Center (Ed.), *AIA best practices: Lessons learned from a decade of service to children and families affected by HIV and substance abuse.* Berkeley: University of California.

Adnopoz, J., & Grigsby, K. (2002). High-risk children, adolescents and families: Organizing principles for mental health prevention and intervention. In M. Lewis (Ed.), *Child and adolescent psychiatry: A comprehensive textbook* (3rd ed., pp. 1059–1066). Baltimore: Lippincott, Williams and Wilkins.

Balestracci, K.M.B. (2001). Intensive family preservation services: Do they live up to their name? *Dissertation Abstracts International. Section B: The Sciences & Engeneering.* Sept. 62(3-B); 1346.

Borduin, C. M., Mann, B. J., Barton, J., & Cone, L. (1995). Multisystemic treatment of serious juvenile offenders: Long-term prevention of criminality and violence. *Journal of Consulting and Clinical Psychology, 63,* 569–578.

Burns, B. J., Hoagwood, K., & Mrazek, P. (1999). Effective treatment for mental disorders in children and adolescents. *Clinical Child and Family Psychology Review, 2,* 199–254.

Cicchetti, D., & Cohen, D. J. (1995). *Developmental psychopathology; Vol. 2. Risk, disorder and adaptation.* New York: Wiley.

Cicchetti, D., & Toth, S. (Eds.). (1999). *Developmental approaches to prevention and Intervention: Rochester Symposium of Developmental Psychopathology.* Vol. 9. Rochester, NY: University of Rochester Press.

Fristad, M. A., & Marsh, D. T. (2002). *Handbook of serious emotional disturbance in children and adolescents.* New York: Wiley.

Geismar, L. L., & Lasorte, M. A. (1964). *Understanding the multi–problem family.* New York: Association Press.

Goldstein, J., Solnit, A. J., Goldstein, S., & Freud, A. (1996). *The best interests of the child.* New York: Free Press.

Gossart-Walker, S., & Moss, N. (2000). An effective strategy for intervention with children and adolescents affected by HIV and AIDS. *Child and Adolescent Psychiatric Clinics of North America, 9,* 331–345.

Heinicke, C. M., & Ponce, V. A. (1999). Relationsbased early family intervention. In D. Burak, D. Cichetti & D. Weisz (Eds.), *Developmental Psychopathology: Perspectives on Adjustment, Risk, and Disorder* (pp. 317–349). Cambridge: Cambridge University Press.

Henaghan, A., Horwitz, S., & Leventhal, J. (1994, May). *Evaluating intensive family preservation programs: A methodologic review.* Paper presented at the Ambulatory Pediatrics Association meeting, Seattle, WA.

Henggeler, S. W., & Borduin, C. M. (1990). *Family therapy and beyond: A multisystemic approach to treating the behavior problems of children and adolescents.* Pacific Grove, CA: Brooks/Cole.

Henggeler, S. W., Rowland, M., & Pickrel, S. G. (1997). Investigating family-based alternatives to institution-based mental health services for youth: Lessons learned from the pilot study of a randomized field trial. *Journal of Clinical Child Psychology, 26,* 226–233.

Kaplan, L. (1986). *Working with multi-problem families.* Lexington: Lexington Books.

Kilpatrick, A. C. (1999). Levels of family need. In A. C. Kilpatrick & T. P. Holland (Eds.), *Assessing and working with families: An integrative model by level of need* (2nd ed., pp. 3–15). Needham Heights, MA: Allyn and Bacon.

Knitzer, J., & Cole, E. S. (1989). *Family preservation services: The program challenge for child welfare and child mental health agencies.* New York: Bank Street College of Education.

Korfmacher, J., Kitzman, H., & Olds, D. (1998). Intervention processes as predictors of outcomes in a preventive home visitation program. *Journal of Community Psychology, 26,* 49–64.

Lindblad-Goldberg, M., Dore, M., & Stern, L. (1998). *Creating competence from chaos.* New York: Norton.

Nelson, H. (1996). *What is appropriate care for the children of troubled families?* New York: Millbank Memorial Fund.

Olds, D., Henderson, C., Kitzman, H., Eckenrode, J., Cole, R., & Tatelbaum, R. (1999). Prenatal and infancy home visitation by nurses: Recent findings. *The Future of Children: Home Visiting: Recent program evaluations, 9*(1), 44–65.

Olds, D., & Kitzman, H. (1993). Review of research on home visiting for pregnant women and parents of young children. *Future Child, 3,* 53–92.

Olds, D., Robinson, J., Song, N., Little, C., & Hill, P. (1999). *Reducing risks for mental disorders during the first five years of life: A review of preventative interventions.* Boulder, CO: Prevention Research Center for Family and Child Health, University of Colorado Health Sciences Center.

Provence, S. (1979, March). *Changing families and child rearing.* Paper presented at the Child Advocacy Conference of the New England Mental Health Task Force, Durham, NH.

Provence, S., & Naylor, A. (1983). *Working with disadvantaged children and their children.* New Haven, CT: Yale University Press.

Rosenfeld, A., Wasserman, S., & Pilowsky, D. (1998). Psychiatry and children in the child welfare system. *Child and Adolescent Clinics of North America, 7,* 515–536.

Solnit, A. J. (1976). Marriage: Changing structure and functions of the family. In V. C. Vaughn & T. B. Brazelton (Eds.), *The family: Can it be saved?* Chicago: YearBook Medical Publishers.

Tebes, J., Kaufman, J., Adnopoz, J., & Racusin, G. (1999). Reducing risk for children of parents with serious mental disorders through family support. *Yale Psychiatry, 8,* 115–136.

Wells, K. (1995). Family preservation services in context: Origins, practices and current issues. In I. M. Schwartz & P. Au Claire (Eds.), *Home-based services for troubled children* (pp. 1–28). Lincoln: University of Nebraska Press.

Woodford, M. (1999). Home-based family therapy: Theory and process from "friendly visitors" to multisystemic therapy. *Family Journal: Counseling and Therapy for Couples and Families, 7,* 265–269.

Woolston, J., Berkowitz, S., Schaefer, M., & Adnopoz, J. (1998). The child psychiatrist in the community. In S. Berkowitz & J. Adnopoz (Eds.), *Child and adolescent psychiatric clinics of North America* (pp. 615–633). Philadelphia: Saunders.

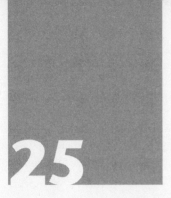

25

D. Russell Lyman and Borja Alvarez de Toledo

The Ecology of Intensive Community-Based Intervention

"He's fine at home. I don't know what you people are talking about. You just don't know how to handle him." These were words of greeting from Margarita Vega, the 26-year-old biracial Hispanic mother of 10-year-old Rashad, whose referral for intensive intervention had been precipitated by his dangling of his 2.5-year-old brother, Matthew, over the upstairs banister in the family home. Rashad, because of repeated uncontrolled, aggressive, self-destructive, and suicidal behaviors, had been psychiatrically hospitalized four times in the last year. He was enuretic and had a history of head banging, as well as a tendency to threaten to jump out of windows. He had been abusive to the family cat, which in fact had died. He had had numerous incidents of fighting with his siblings and schoolmates, when he was able to be in school. His mother, who had identified him as the problem child in a family of six children, all under the age of 11, refused to allow our intervention team member to sit during this home visit, stating, "You can come to my house to help Rashad, but don't expect me to talk to you."

Though many details of Margarita's life, her family, and her work with us have been changed to protect her privacy, Margarita is a real person who taught us a great deal about working with severely

challenged families. Her story and our attempts to partner in therapeutic work with her and her family are the cornerstone of this chapter for practitioners in intensive community-based family work. This story will help us to describe the roots, program development, and strategic clinical techniques of a service designed to maintain children who have experienced or are at risk for hospitalization or residential care. These are children who 20 or even 10 years ago would most likely be found in lengthy stays in psychiatric hospitals or languishing in long-term residential placement.

Our aim is twofold. First, as program developers we will describe the roots of our model and how it can be constructed, supported, and implemented clinically. Second, as clinicians we will seek to move beyond basic principles to describe some of the approaches we have refined over years of working with severely challenged families. These include ecological assessment, the art of intensive case management and meta-systemic family work, contingency planning for urgent intervention, and assisting families in making transitions in care. With the Vegas' help, we will also illustrate how this work can be carried out through grassroots work by a relatively small community-based agency.

The Vega Family

Rashad came to our clinic with a history of treatment failures along with family members who all had been experiencing difficulties. His mother had as a child and adolescent experienced multiple psychiatric hospitalizations but resisted family involvement, saying, "There is nothing wrong with me." Ellie, age 11, was enuretic and becoming more defiant and aggressive as she approached adolescence. Sharon, age 7, had difficulty with separation and was defiant and aggressive, as was Joshua, age 5, who also presented with separation anxiety and severe asthma. Matthew, age 2.5, presented as depressed and was aggressive toward peers in child care. He also was encopretic there and at home. John, 11 months, showed significant signs of failure to thrive.

Yet Margarita was a survivor. She showed considerable resilience, always fighting for herself and her kids to have a better life, no matter what the difficulty. Her children were engaging and personable, and they showed considerable potential for connecting with helpers. And Margarita was fully committed. In our first contact she said, "My family comes first."

Nonetheless, Margarita's style was one of mistrust and accusation. She presented to us as chronically enraged and in past treatments had received the label of borderline personality disorder, among others. She had initially been referred to our mental health clinic following one of Rashad's hospitalizations, and the school and the clinic therapist were desperate to get a team in place to help with the many needs of the family and to alleviate the responsibility and burden of being the main recipients of Margarita's rage and mistrust. Margarita reluctantly accepted our team to help with Rashad's aggression, to avoid placement (which had already been suggested by school), and to receive concrete support.

The struggle to survive was the norm in this family. Since everyone was so needy, needs were not permissible, and attention could only be attained through extreme behaviors, which included self-injurious acts and suicidal gestures. There were no rituals or routines and virtually no rules in the house. There was no such thing as a family meal. When things did not work, Margarita would yell, and different children would either act out, retreat, or quietly soil themselves again. In the midst of Margarita's resistance, it was clear that the only ticket to admission would be in providing concrete things she asked for, which included food, beds, and transportation for the children. It was also clear that none of the traditional models of clinical therapy we had been trained in would be sufficient.

Rashad's Team

Rashad and his family had been referred to the Family Advocacy, Stabilization and Support Team (FASST), a program of the Guidance Center, Inc., in Cambridge, Massachusetts. This is a highly intensive home-based team that provides family intervention services, any day of the week and at any time of day or night. Referrals target a seriously emotionally disturbed child, age 3 to 19, who is at risk of being placed out of the home. The goal of the program is to stabilize and support families so that these troubled children can remain with their families and in their home communities. Services provided to a family such as the Vegas average 12 to 15 hours a week and often include daily contact.

Rashad and his family work with a family team consisting of a clinical social worker, who serves as a therapist and clinical care coordinator, and a paraprofessional family support worker, who works with the social worker as a cotherapist and provides a range of informal supports that include respite, recreation, and transportation. The team provides services to the family wherever they are needed, including at home, in school, at residential settings, or in community settings. The program has three social workers and three outreach workers under the direction of a senior clinician who carries a beeper 24 hours a day. The program works with 14 families at a time. Full-time (full-time availability is very important) staff generally carry a maximum of six cases at any one time. The program budget is designed such that roughly 20% of program funds are reserved to purchase services such as specialized treatment, supportive recreation, or residential care.

Rashad's presentation is typical of our team's target population. These are children who are at significant risk for psychiatric hospitalization and residential placement. Many (39%) present with behavior disorders, 36% have mood disorders, and 17% show symptoms related to trauma (post–traumatic stress disorder). Psychotic disorders (5%) and other anxiety disorders (2%) are less prevalent.

Most compelling is the level of disturbance we find in the families of these children. Nearly half of them (49%) have experienced physical abuse, sexual abuse, or neglect. Only 14% live with two parents, and 26% have had previous residential treatment. Domestic violence has been reported in 59% of their families, and substance abuse in 63%.

We will find that Rashad's family is positive for nearly all these factors. Combined with our clinical intuition, this cluster of factors served as an important guide in focusing our work on the family at home and in our community. Our tracking of these and other demographics over a period of more than 6 years also illustrates the trend toward increasingly troubled children and families straining the resources of community-based services. In some cases children have entered our program with a story of 10 or more residential placements, along with the trauma of severe sexual abuse or neglect in more than one.

Our data and the experience of many community-based providers are a clear indication of a hospital and residential treatment system that has in many ways failed. Community-based systems of care are also failing families like the Vegas because there are insufficient resources to meet the needs of multiple family members, who require services that cut across multiple systems. For the Vegas a wide array of services needed to be identified, supported, and carefully coordinated in a model that was nested in the family's community, while also offering a full range of service intensity. The team we developed does this through a flexible combination of extensive advocacy and case management, stabilization through sophisticated and intensive clinical intervention, and support through a range of family-based services and supplies.

Development and Implementation of an Intensive Model

Roots of Our Community-Based Approach

Support for this model grew out of visionary thinking by our state Department of Mental Health (DMH). Analysis of the department's system indicated that it was spending significant resources ($55,000 per child per year) maintaining children and adolescents in residential treatment centers, with limited progress. Though some of the children were able to make behavioral gains while in residential treatment, our own experience indicated that some had become too comfortable with the care and attention they received, and hence were not motivated to change. Others picked up many bad habits from their peers, which made it difficult for them to shed institutional behavior when they returned to their communities. Families and their communities also often did not have the resources to provide the structure that children in placement become accustomed to. We experienced this in our own programs prior to the development of our model, when traditional outpatient therapies alone proved insufficient to hold children being discharged to us from hospitals or residential centers. A broad range of children, no matter what the degree of their own growth or lack thereof, were returned to families that were unprepared to provide the kind of holding environment afforded in residential centers, and so transitions home from placements often failed.

This also occurred because on top of logistical barriers such as the distance of the residential center from the family home, many centers tended to focus largely on their own milieu behavioral programs for the child rather than fully including the family. They did not fully support the family's development of new interactions that would actually work in the home. Insufficient attention was given to the child's pathology as at least in part a symptom of other severe challenges facing the family. Most strength building that was done targeted bolstering the child's milieu structure and treatment rather than building on family strengths. Many of us saw this in our work in the 1970s in psychiatric hospitals, where a social worker's job tended to be restricted to providing office-based family therapy and serving as a liaison between the milieu and the family, while nursing staff cared for the child, and psychiatrists attempted to cure him or her with psychoanalytic psychotherapy and medication. Two decades ago such hospitalizations could go on for a year or more without a single family session occurring in the home while the child was on leave from the hospital. Today, weeklong hospital stays do not even leave time for this, achieving only brief assessments and often heavy doses of medication, followed by discharge to an unprepared home and community.

The state mental health authority saw that this was not an effective management of resources. Multiple failures in community placement often led to entrenched pessimism and poor self-esteem in the children and their families, thus exacerbating recidivism. In our local DMH, residential services for just 10 children were costing the state more than a half a million dollars a year, with limited results. The state was also beginning to see what has now grown into a very serious social and economic issue, the "stuck kid" problem, in which children remain in restrictive placements they do not need because the supports needed to hold them in the community are lacking.

Therefore, the state made a bold and visionary move similar to new directions emerging in other areas of the country. It stopped buying ten residential beds (which today have risen to $250 to $350 a day) and redeployed those dollars to support a community-based program dedicated to supporting the children in their home communities. Following a competitive proposal process, our agency was awarded $550,000 per year to be spent on whatever staffing, services, and supplies families needed to maintain their troubled child at home. Ten families were to be served at a time, and after a highly successful first year the funds needed were reduced to $480,000 per year. No limit was placed on the duration of the intervention (given that children had been occupying beds for years in some cases), as long as the children could ultimately be maintained in the community. It was also recognized that this experiment would not always succeed, but at least in such cases the family, clinicians, and the state would know that the most intensive efforts possible had proved that the child really belonged in a residential setting.

This began as a local experiment that grew out of considerable training in systems of care work both for us as providers and for our partners in the DMH. It is a collaboration based in close dialogue that can be achieved by any agency committed to innovative practices in intensive community mental health work. Because the program is funded to serve only DMH clients, it is at a structural level elegantly simple; it serves only one master.

This stands in contrast to a growing number of statewide projects across the United States developed in the last two decades, usually through legislative action and formal interagency agreements, that pooled funds from multiple state agencies to form large systems of care for seriously emotionally disturbed children. The term "wraparound" evolved to describe this new way of surrounding a family with a community of services supported by many stakeholders. In Wraparound Milwaukee, for example, more than $30 million in annual funds, roughly $10 million each from Medicaid, child welfare, and juvenile justice programs, has been blended to serve approximately 600 children and adolescents a year (Kamradt, 2002). Evidence-based research also began to demonstrate that this systemic work could be highly cost-effective. By the year 2000, Wraparound Milwaukee involved 60 different services from 170 different providers and had reduced residential placement costs by 60% and hospitalization costs by 80% (Kamradt, 2000). At this point the program has grown to 230 different providers serving approximately 530 children on any given day (National Psychologist Staff, 2003).

Yet such projects funded by pooled funds from multiple stakeholders involve complex political processes. Oversight structures needed to be set up so that each of many stakeholders would have a voice. Many of these projects were also built on multi-million-dollar systems grants from the federal government, which specified the principles of intervention and mandated collaboration between local and state agencies and also required rigorous research components. Funded under the Comprehensive Community Mental Health Services Program for Children and Their Families through the Substance Abuse and Mental Health Service Administration, there have since 1993 been 85 systems grants serving 55,000 children and adolescents (Sondheimer, Santiago, Erickson, Herman, & Levine, 2003). These are great innovations in care that have made a difference for a number of communities, but a great many unserved communities remain.

These projects also tend to become top-heavy, since they require so many bureaucratic layers of political, financial, and operational oversight. For example, a larger pooled funding project operating in our area and others, known as Mental Health Services Program for Youth, has two levels of bureaucracy operating above the wraparound team, a large statewide steering committee that meets regularly to formulate policy, oversight, and governance, and an area advisory team composed of multiple state and third-party payers that also meets regularly to review resource allocation and quality management (Grimes & Appleton, 2003). These processes involve high-level staff and are costly.

While average length of stay in the Milwaukee project is 14 months and costs an average of $67,000 per family (Kamradt, 2000), our team's average is 8 months, with a cost of $24,038 per family. This is a significant difference, though it should be noted that neither the populations served nor the services delivered in Milwaukee and our project are fully equivalent. The Milwaukee project serves a higher proportion of adjudicated youth, and services purchased include mental health services that in our program are reimbursed by third-party health insurance.

What Margarita and her family will help to illustrate is a small, community-based, grassroots model that is implemented through a simple structure based on community relationships. It is an example of how a relatively small community-based agency can line up local funding and create an intimate team to achieve equal or better outcomes in comparison to programs such as Milwaukee Wraparound. A locally funded project can also offer distinct advantages in community rootedness, which is often a critical piece of what a family like the Vegas needs to thrive. Whether large or small, these models are built on the same principles, which have undergone a remarkable process of research, refinement, and dissemination over the last two decades.

Principles of a Wraparound System of Care

Margarita and her children presented more than the need for discrete services provided to individual family members. One of the failures of traditional methods, especially those employed in residential settings, was that children such as Rashad and his siblings were "plugged" into programs, much like pushing a round plug into a square hole. This was often in rigidified institutions that forced children to "fit" the service offered (and the funding stream supporting it) rather than adapting a range of services and supports to meet the needs of each individual child and family. As we will learn from Margarita's history, this happened to her as a child. She had been institutionalized, and there was little or no adaptation of the state hospital system routine to meet her unique and changing needs.

The wraparound concept was most powerfully articulated by mental health system researchers, who continue to have a profound influence on our system of care today (Stroul & Friedman, 1986). In their words, a system of care is "a comprehensive spectrum of mental health and other necessary services which are organized into a coordinated network to meet the multiple and changing needs of children and their families" (p. 3). This philosophy was an underpinning of a national research and training program called the Child and Adolescent Service System Program, known as CASSP (Stroul, 1996; Stroul & Friedman, 1986). CASSP articulated 10 key principles and researched what are now eight overlapping service spheres, as follows: mental health services; social services (child protection); educational services; health services; substance abuse services; vocational services; recreational services; and operational services. For systems targeting adjudicated youth, these services also include juvenile justice services (Stroul, 2002). Wraparound theory placed the family at the center of the care system, with intensive coordination of spheres of care such that they revolved cohesively around the needs of each family.

The success of the wraparound model in reducing out-of-home placement by providing high-quality and cost-effective services has been demonstrated by projects across the country, including Wraparound Milwaukee, Project Wraparound in Vermont, Kaleidoscope in Chicago, and the Alaska Youth Initiative. Numerous publications are available documenting wraparound training for work with seriously emotionally disturbed children (VanDen Berg & Grealish, 1998), as well as specific populations, such as antisocial youth (Henggeler, Schoenwald, Bordun, Rowland, & Cunningham, 1998).

This thinking followed a major paradigmatic shift in practice that had focused on family therapy as the treatment of choice. As attention turned increasingly to calls to action in children's mental health (Knitzer, 1992), the shift from traditional therapies toward what is now often referred to as "family-centered practice" began to take root in mental health, child welfare, and juvenile justice systems. This was an expansion of the family therapy movement to centering practice on all major areas of family life, not just on interactions within the family system, such that treatment took on an expanded community focus well beyond therapy sessions with the family. Concrete family support became a key element because it met enough basic needs so that the families could turn their attention from raw survival to positioning themselves for therapeutic change. As a result, professionally trained clinicians have needed to learn to welcome paraprofessional family support workers and other nontraditional community service providers as valued team members.

Recent trends include family-based services, multisystemic therapy, wraparound, family preservation, and family group conferencing (Walton, Sandau-Beckler, & Mannes, 2001). Outcomes of such services have also been studied (Epstein, Kutash, & Duchnowski, 1998), though the highly individualized nature of the wraparound model has made generalization a challenging process. National wraparound demonstration models have also tended to be possible only in large, extremely well-funded projects that leave them beyond the scope of small community-based agencies such as ours. The practical and empirical model that we have implemented offers a way that principles of care and strategic interventions can be implemented and studied, with limited resources and in grassroots settings.

What seemed one of our greatest challenges, our small size and geographic scope, has turned out to be one of our greatest strengths: Our agency is deeply rooted in Margarita's community. We know her neighborhood inside and out, and we have had carefully tended relationships with all the service providers she and her children would need. It has been an agency goal to be able to provide as many child and family mental health services as possible under one agency roof, while maintaining active linkages to other community services. Staying with these goals and strategies has served as a platform of strength on which to build wraparound principles, which target care that is community based, family focused, strengths based, individualized, culturally competent, accessible, collaborative, and accountable (Burns & Hoagwood, 2002; Stroul, 1996; Stroul & Friedman, 1986).

Community Based

A core element of the program is finding and establishing a community of supports for families so that ultimately our team will not be needed. We know that children at risk for residential placement

need more than child-specific treatments; they also need to have the factors in their home and community contexts that contributed to their difficulties addressed as well (Henggeler et al., 1998). This system must include a balance of formal and informal supports, so that structured services such as a range of outpatient mental health services can be integrated with indigenous community supports such as boys' and girls' clubs, music lessons, or even the attention of a generous neighbor. Virtually all direct work is carried out in the community (as opposed to a mental health clinic), including family homes, the child's school or residential program, youth centers, parents' places of work, recreational facilities, or wherever services are most accessible.

A critical challenge for residential centers is that often they are neither located in the child's community nor staffed to do the community work necessary to support the child's functioning in the home. Only the most progressive of centers have begun to embrace in-home family work as part of their philosophy. Margarita's family had already shown that any gains of intensive and costly interventions, such as hospitalization, could not be sustained without supports being embedded in their community. Rashad's growing pattern of revolving-door hospitalizations was a clear indicator of this.

Family Focused

Rashad, though he is the "identified patient" who was referred (and funded) for service, is not our client. His whole family is. In addition, our commitment to the whole family is unconditional, the entire intervention process is team driven, and this team is built around family partnership. For the identified patient to be maintained in the family home, relative stability of all the family members in the home must be achieved. The family must know that our work is not subject to the usual conditions of insurance or contract funding; we stay with them as long as they need us, and they will be provided with no less than all the therapeutic supports they need. They must also know that they are held by a team of multiple community providers (who are responsible to the family and each other), and that this team's main job is to partner with the family in creating and maintaining a system of care. This focus moves beyond the concept of the therapeutic alliance in traditional therapies to the development of a systemic partnership, in which the parent's voice is a critical one in working with an array of providers to plan a community of care. The family is put in charge of articulating their needs, while their strengths and problem areas are also professionally assessed. In practice it is our goal to help families to focus on hopes for the future, even in the most desperate cases, and to prioritize what they want for themselves. Margarita's goal was to keep her family intact, and this was a great asset. She also viewed Rashad's issues as being the fault of incompetent practitioners, so we made it a priority to pull the interagency service team in line and help its members get educated about how to work with the family.

Strengths Based

While reimbursement streams tend to require a diagnosis and medical model problem-oriented treatment, it is of critical importance that we identify and build on family strengths (Ronnau, 1995) and make those strengths an integral part of how we plan and deliver services with families (VanDen Berg & Grealish, 1998). Focus on strengths had been a key element of an emerging solution-focused family therapy movement, which shifted thinking from pathology and "resistance" to more positive approaches. We have found it helpful to focus on two tenets: first, that families want to change, and, second, that they have their own, if undiscovered, repertoire of solutions (De Shazer, 1985; O'Hanlon & Weiner-Davis, 1989).

Individualized

This term does not simply mean that wraparound service must attend to individual needs of each family member. Family needs occur in a complex, multidimensional and relational context that is different for every family, even if they are neighbors. This context includes not just their extended family, neighbors, and friends but also a community of resources and liabilities, as well as a community of care providers. The nuances of this system and of the family's interaction with it are the ecology in which each family must find its unique personal and community resources, in order to build something that will last beyond the course of our intervention. Hence, we have a different protocol with every family, and this approach changes as the family and our understanding of them evolve over time.

We also seek to identify in each family "differences that make a difference" based on our experience of each family's uniqueness, and work to create together a new family narrative, both for them and for those working with them. In the beginning, "individualized" with Margarita meant bringing food and beds, rather than trying to do any kind of therapy. It also meant understanding her relationship to providers in the context of her history with them, which we will discuss later.

Culturally Competent

Margarita expressed deep mistrust of the "white man's system of care." She also had contempt for African Americans who had taunted her because of her biracial heritage. We knew that her workers could be neither white nor African American, and felt fortunate to have Hispanic workers on our team. Understanding a family's cultural beliefs is a key challenge, as is finding the right match of team members with them. In addition to matching families for language and culture with their team, we compose teams that are often balanced according to gender as well as ethnicity. Thus, a family team often has a member who is a close cultural match with the family and another who brings some degree of difference, so that they can model bridge building between different points of view. Family traditions and beliefs are seen both as extremely important in understanding the family culture and as potential catalysts for positive change.

The family's cultural understanding of what "mental health" and mental health services means is especially important. One example is a Haitian girl whose mother eschewed treatment in favor of herbal cures; the team asked the mother to educate them, read up on herbal treatments, and went with the mother to purchase them. Cultural sensitivity and acumen are critical elements in ensuring that services will be accessible for the families, and in the case of this Haitian family provided the only door through which this girl, who in fact actually wanted psychotherapy, would be allowed to enter by her mother.

To understand the family's culture is also to know and feel where and how they live. The Vega family culture was one of competition for scant attention and resources. This was due both to physical limitations such as inadequate space and to a psychological mind-set that there could never be enough for everyone. Visiting the Vega home meant seeing firsthand that family members were stacked in bedrooms together and struggled constantly for attention in an apartment where at times there was also nothing to eat.

Accessible

Though at first Margarita would not let our team sit down in her home, she also made it clear that she would not meet anywhere else. This was her territory, so we met her there. The wraparound team is a mobile one that will bring services to families or families to service in whatever way is most useful. Language of the providers and culturally acceptable services are also key components of accessibility, as is the scheduling of services. Support is available at key times, such as at dinnertime or bedtime, or when it is time to get up and off to school. Financial access to services is also facilitated, so that if ancillary services increase access for families, we either purchase them or find available resources in the community. The deep community roots of an agency committed to one circumscribed area greatly enhance such access.

The program is also nested in a comprehensive agency continuum of services that can be accessed for children of all ages and at all levels of community-based treatment intensity. A child under 3 years of age who is struggling to develop can be treated in our early intervention program; another can benefit from Head Start, domestic violence services, our therapeutic family after-school program, or numerous other family-based services. All of the Vega family members received a comprehensive array of such services, and our close relationships with other community providers made it possible for us to access any services our agency could not provide.

Flexible

The need for flexibility lies at the core of creating the intervention team, funding it, delivering the services, and modifying the approach as family and contextual factors change. Staff disciplines and scheduling must be flexible, such that staff can interchange roles and responsibilities and do their work wherever and whenever needed. Hence the social worker may at times provide respite or transportation, and the paraprofessional support worker may conduct counseling sessions. Support workers share in beeper rotations and do emergency interventions just as a clinical professional would. This flexibility is made possible by the intensive consultation and supervision the team receives, such that

they brainstorm and learn together and come to trust one another's competencies. It requires a special kind of mind-set that comes with being part of a team that shares everything. Social workers in particular must have a flexible approach to their sense of their own professionalism, so that they are not threatened by the idea that a person with other life experience can be a competent therapist without having gone to graduate school.

Funding must also be flexible, such that services are not constrained by categorical funding streams that will or will not reimburse for one service or another. In a small program such as ours, this includes reserving flexible funds for the purchase of any service or item that the team and family determine is appropriate. Achieving funding flexibility also involves committing considerable case management time, as well as executive advocacy at all levels, to ensure that every appropriate funding stream is blended to support a broad menu of services.

Collaborative

In addition to collaborating with families, we clearly define our role as supporting the work of other agencies involved with a family, since they are key players in the family's adjustment after our work is done. Analysis of early programs such as the Ventura project in California underscored that collaboration in how decisions were made and coordinated was a key to success (Hernandez & Goldman, 1996). Our collaboration is metasystemic in that it recognizes that each provider and agency is nested in a context and brings a unique perspective to understanding the family and intervention goals. Each community partner brings value; however, multiple players also can have potential for doing damage if they are not actively engaged in collaboration. Considerable surrounding work is done before and after interagency planning meetings to help providers identify divergent agendas, as well as common themes and shared goals. Margarita, who had a tendency to be explosive and blaming in collaborative care planning meetings, presented special challenges in this area.

Accountable

We are accountable to families in helping them to define and address goals and evaluate progress in reaching them. We are also accountable to our funding source for all expenditures, to our local service system for our coordination, and to the professional community for the contributions we can make to improving systems of care. For this reason and because we are committed to bridging the gap between science and practice, we have collected and analyzed extensive data on family demographics, functional assessment, and service utilization. This work enables us to assess Margarita's family characteristics in relation to empirical norms, track their progress over time, and link these outcomes to the type, cost, and duration of services.

Team Structure

The team may work with a family as many as 7 days a week. One session a week is considered a minimum. Contacts with other care providers, especially in settings such as schools where children may be having behavioral issues, occur as often as multiple times a day. On average, nearly equal amounts of time are spent in family support, case management, and direct therapeutic intervention. Average treatment duration is 7 months, though there is no limit on length of stay, which has ranged from 1 to 27 months.

All team members are intimately familiar with the entire program caseload and review the cases on a regular basis in weekly team meetings of at least 1½ hours in length. They receive weekly one-on-one supervision and have access to the program director by beeper and cell phone 24 hours a day, 7 days a week. On a regular basis the team receives case consultation from senior psychologists and social workers, as well as from a psychiatrist, who conducts psychopharmacological evaluations and consultations when appropriate. The team is also backed by a small team of senior clinicians from key community mental health agencies, who meet regularly to review problematic cases and community systems issues. This grassroots connection is critical in supporting the overall provider community as a collaborative care system.

In structuring the home-based team, the aim is for them to live their professional lives together as if they were members of a healthy family, supported by the same kind of communication structures, skill building, resources, and mutual support that families need. Team cohesiveness, planning, mutual support, and supervision must be supported at a level of intensity not found in traditional outpatient mental health services (Archacki-Stone,

1995). During their work hours our team members literally live together, sharing the same office space, bathroom, and kitchenette. Each pair assigned to a family is nested in the close and cohesive system of the overall team. For peer support, they can lean across their desk to the person next to them and ask for what they need. All their intervention planning is developed by consensus. To address systems issues and special challenges in their work, the team members take half-day retreats at least twice a year.

The clinical care coordinator is a special kind of licensed social work clinician who has had intensive training in wraparound care and has ingrained flexibility. In the case of the family support worker, the term "paraprofessional" does not do justice to this person's discipline. The family support worker, because of the amount of time he or she spends with the family, brings an essential perspective to our understanding of their functioning. In the course of teamwork, the support worker becomes a talented co-therapist, as well a training expert for parents in child behavior management techniques. It is also helpful if this person is a parent, and better yet one who has been a consumer of family services.

The partnership between the support worker and the clinician is an equal one, in which often the more informal work of the support worker is the critical element in developing a working alliance with the family members. This is especially true for families needing child protection services. They tend to feel less threatened by a person who wears fewer trappings of authority.

The family service worker provides respite for parents, as well as companionship and recreational support for any of the children in the family. The family also comes to know the rest of the program team, who provide backup and crisis intervention as needed. This includes senior program managers, who step in to assist the family team in emergencies or act as clinical consultants to intervene with the family or the service system in particularly delicate situations.

Strategic Practical Approaches in Ecological Work

The integration and coordination of these services with indigenous community supports and the services of other agencies represent a change from what has been known as a "service-centered approach." In the service-centered approach, the family was expected to come to the center and fit into the services, just as we had seen in past experience in inpatient work. In the wraparound model, a "natural support ecology" is created. In this ecology the family lives at the center of interlocking spheres of support, which are nested within each other across levels of intensity and systemic complexity, described by Bronfenbrenner (1979) as micro-and macrosystems (figure 25-1). The work of the family team is "metasystemic" in which they work strategically as catalytic and cohesive agents across systems to facilitate movement and glue components together in a supporting ecology.

Work with the Vegas and families like them has led us to refine a number of strategies in wraparound work. Specific approaches include ecological assessment, the work of the "systems doctor" in case management, and strategic planning for contingencies and facilitating transitions.

Ecological Assessment

The work of ecological assessment has its roots in systems theory articulated by Piaget (1976) in cognitive theory, by von Bertalanffy (1968) in general systems theory, and by Bronfenbrenner (1979) in psychosocial theory. A key aspect of systems theory is the importance of interaction between an organism and its environment. Piaget's initial fascination with mollusks and how they adapted by bringing water with elements of nutrients and waste in and out in interaction with their environment formed a basis for his theories about the development of intelligence, in which the feedback loops of new information between the individual and his or her environment spurred cognitive restructuring. Von Bertalanffy, in his analysis of cybernetics, described the dynamic interactions of components within a feedback cycle that was necessary to the life of a system.

Bronfenbrenner applied these ideas to psychosocial theory by focusing on the ways in which a series of exchanges between an individual or his or her family and the context around them became determinants of family structure and behavior. Smaller systems, such as interactions between siblings, all take place within a macrosystem that in-

cludes social norms and culture; these interactions build on each other to form a complex history that underlies successive interactions. As portrayed in figure 25-1, each system is nested within the context of another, and the relationships within and between these systems must be assessed. Ecological approaches to working with networks of community resources is well articulated in theory underlying family-based services (Imber-Black, 1992; Kim Berg, 1994; Nelson & Allen, 1995).

In ecological assessment all aspects of the family's life are evaluated, including basic needs such as food and shelter, functioning in key areas such as at home, in school, at work, or within the rules of society, and in relationships between family members and with peers and helpers. In each area, it is especially important to assess both strengths and liabilities. For example, Rashad had significant difficulties in school, but a gym teacher there took special interest in him and had begun to help him gain confidence in mastering wall climbing. In the community context the most important influence often is the relative, friend, or neighbor who might be able to help in times of stress or crisis. These people can be immensely useful in, for example, providing a safe haven for the child when a cooling-off period is necessary. Introduction of such a person into the intervention context can also be that critical catalyst that pushes the system to operate in a more adaptive way. It was one of Margarita's strengths that she had maintained relationships with members of her extended family, about whom we would not have asked if we had not taken an ecological approach to understanding Rashad in community context.

The ongoing presence of the family team in the home is especially helpful in assessing this relationship domain. They are able to feel firsthand the quality of sibling relationships, so very troubled in Rashad's family. They are also able to assess, in the context of the home environment, the areas of strength and need for support in the caregivers. These include firsthand experience of the quality of parents' love, attachment, and commitment, as well as their real-life ability to provide structure, monitoring, and limits for their children (Ziegler & Bush, 1999).

Equally important is the transgenerational history of the family's history with care providers. The foundations for this approach had been developed

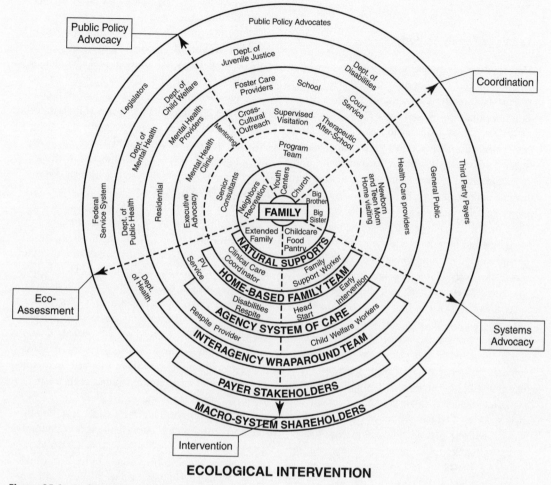

Figure 25.1. Ecological Intervention

by early family therapists such as Whitaker (1976), Bowen (1978), and Imber-Black (1992). The wraparound team puts more effort than the average outpatient clinician into getting information reaching back at least two generations, focusing particularly on relationships both with and around the extended family and with the mental health system. The team routinely does genograms with the family, which are useful visual aids both for encapsulating history and current relationships and for constructing blueprints for change (McGoldrick & Gerson, 1985).

In the case of Margarita, the transgenerational assessment process meant delving into her early history as a child of troubled parents and as a con-

sumer of mental health services. This was important enough that our team went to the trouble of going to a psychiatric hospital out of state where Margarita had spent an extended period in her childhood to obtain clinical records. Traditional training has ingrained in us that understanding a troubled person's early relationships with primary figures is key in determining the course of treatment, but the wraparound team also looks at the history and texture of a family's interactions with the caregiving system to strategically plan how to join with the family and build consensus in the interagency wraparound team. Many families come to us with a history of having been abused or at least disrespected in the system, and they themselves often have burned many bridges with care providers.

The Vega Family Ecology

Margarita is a classic example of a person whose outcome would have been vastly different if her parents had received community-based services. From her first day in New York State, Margarita's natural caretakers had been abusive and neglectful, both physically and emotionally. Her father was an alcoholic laborer who abused her mother in front of Margarita and her four siblings. Her mother, who became addicted to heroin when Margarita was in utero, fled the family when Margarita was 3, and her father died of liver disease when she was 4. Margarita had been born addicted and was a temperamental child, so no one would adopt her. She was made a ward of the state, and in her first foster placement was sexually abused at the age of 5. She spent the next 5 years acting out in as many different foster homes, and after several intermittent hospitalizations was at the age of 10 declared persistently mentally ill and placed in a state mental hospital. In the hospital, though she was able to make at least transitory relationships with milieu staff and therapists, Margarita had frequent outbursts, some of which got out of control, and she was injured several times. She was placed on heavy doses of psychotropic medications and was discharged at the age of 14 to a foster placement that failed. Because of troubles with the law, she was then put in a juvenile justice placement. Shortly after discharge at 15, she became pregnant with her first child by a Hispanic man who left immediately. Most of her relationships with men were tainted with domestic violence, in which she was often the aggressor. Rashad's younger siblings were the product of two other relationships. Margarita's history was one of a young woman who had every reason to have hatred and mistrust for the caregiving system, yet she had also never been taught how to live without it.

In the face of such histories it is easy to lose sight of family strengths. Interactions with the family chaos and Margarita's rages were overwhelming, and her team was susceptible to despair about what it could possibly work with. Through objective supervision and intensive consultation with the larger program team, the team members were able to put together a list of Margarita's strengths. This strength-based assessment served to plant seeds of self-confidence in Margarita and a sense of resilience in her team.

First, Margarita loved her children in a healthier way than one might expect from someone who had been so neglected, abused, and abandoned. Though she showed limited capacity for mirroring their achievements, disappointments, and emotions to her children, she was aware of their different needs and was absolutely committed to them. "My kids belong with me," said Margarita. "They are not going to be placed like they did with me." Margarita was also highly resourceful in the system and was able to use her rage to her children's advantage by wearing down state agencies and educational authorities to get what she thought her children needed. She was also at times aware of her limitations and learned to use the team to calm herself down when she was losing control with her children. And she had, though it was caustic and sporadic, a wonderful sense of humor. Despite her outbursts, she had a capacity for laughing at her own behaviors after the dust had settled. It was the team's job to speak to these strengths, to assist Margarita in building on them to create her own community of care, and to remind each other of them whenever the going got rough.

Ecological assessment must target every family member in the home, as well as every significant person in their family life. Rashad had been identified as the problem (in addition to his behavioral issues, he had been diagnosed with failure to thrive in infancy, and with depressive disorder and a learning disability as a child); yet it could be seen as a strength that he had been resourceful enough to call attention to the needs of his siblings through his symptomatology. In-depth assessment revealed that the oldest sister, Ellie, though competent, warm, and engaging, had lost some of her childhood because she was co-parenting with her mother She had not had her emotional needs tended to and was now beginning to show signs of anger and defiance.

Sharon, the younger sister, in addition to being defiant, was emotionally labile, and referral for clinical evaluation revealed that she had been sexually abused by a babysitter and suffered from post–traumatic stress disorder. Referral for preschool special education assessment indicated that 5 year-old Joshua had cognitive delays, and special needs assessment of Matthew pointed to the likelihood of attention deficit disorder. Developmental assessment of John indicated that he had nutritional deficiencies, as well as delays in psychomotor skills and receptive and expressive language. The father of the youngest three children, though he was in and out of the house in between incarcerations related to his chronic substance abuse, was able to be supportive (though not committed to Margarita) when he was present. Margarita had also found a biological brother, who though he had been diagnosed as schizophrenic and incarcerated for assault in the past, was sometimes able to take care of the children.

Creating a Community of Care Through Intensive Case Management

Case management includes advocacy with schools, treatment providers, and legal institutions as needed to ensure the client and family are receiving required assistance and their rights are being respected. Advocacy addresses virtually all aspects of the family's life, including financial assistance for the impoverished, health benefits, food assistance, educational planning for special needs, employment, funding for therapeutic intervention, and other needs as they are identified. Equally important is lining up informal supports, such as food banks and fuel assistance, Big Brother and Big Sister programs, martial arts or computer lessons, or local youth centers for activities after school and on weekends. In some cases the team in effect builds on the capacity of the communities to support children and families (Schorr, 1997). Our home-based team maintains an updated, written community resource manual, and actively researches new avenues for support based on each family's needs. In contrast to other family support teams that are contracted on a short-term basis by health insurers and in our area are spread across as many as 65 different cities and towns, our team's deep community roots greatly enrich the potential for finding any and every available community resource.

Case management is blended with family support in such a way that the establishment of healthy community relationships is managed. After months of trust building in the Vega family, the family support worker was allowed to take groups of the children to recreational activities such as trips to the movies, the park, and ultimately the local youth center. The paternal grandmother was paid to provide in-home respite so that mother could have time for herself or to go to meetings. The team provided transportation, taking mother and children to medical and therapy appointments, team meetings, and even grocery shopping (rather than shop sensibly at the store, Margarita had tended to spend her welfare check on fast food). Taxi vouchers were provided when needed, and Margarita was accompanied on the bus to learn new routes. Adequate health insurance was obtained for the children, and Margarita was accompanied to the local welfare office to secure financial assistance. Advocacy with the local housing authority was also carried out, so that the children, who lived three in one bedroom and four in another, could sleep in a larger apartment, two to a bedroom, matched appropriately for gender and age.

When Rashad was referred to our wraparound team, the only intervention the family was receiving was individual therapy and medication for him and sporadically for his mother. Ultimately wraparound work facilitated the following: consistent psychotherapy and medication for Margarita, Sharon, and Joshua; early intervention developmental assessment and treatment for Matthew and John, who also received nutritional consultation; therapeutic day school for Rashad, who also was placed in a therapeutic after-school program along with his sister Sharon; and therapeutic day care for Matthew through our child welfare office. Short-term residential placement was also utilized for intensive assessment of Rashad and his family context, and strategically for the family as breathers during instances of intolerable family stress. The presence of the team both at the residential center and in the home afforded multidimensional assessment of Rashad and his family, both together and apart.

Work as "Systems Doctor"

Review of the Vegas' menu of services might suggest that community wraparound is simply a process of throwing every possible resource at the family. Yet early research in national wraparound demonstration projects such as those in Ventura County and Fort Bragg suggested that "more is not always better" (Bickman, 1996). Results from the Fort Bragg project, which put out a smorgasbord of services that were sampled by professionals and families almost buffet style, demonstrated that coordination was the key to ensuring both the effectiveness and the cost-efficiency of services. This is essential because complex families require service from as many as a dozen or more agencies (Friesen & Poertner, 1995). In such cases it is easy to duplicate services in some areas and to miss gaps in others, and we have countless times worked with a family for months and then found by chance that a service such as home visits were being provided by an agency we did not know about. Surveys of parents indicate that poor communication across agencies is reported as among the top three barriers to care (the other two being distance and scheduling) experienced by parents (Friesen, Robinson, Jivanjce, Ruzich, & Pullman, 2003).

Our experience has led us to label a significant portion of the work our team does as that of "systems doctor." Basic work in this area can involve strategic realignment of existing therapeutic relationships. The team does cotherapies with other therapists working with the family, building a bridge to therapies that will last beyond the team or working to reorient stuck relationships. Community-based outpatient therapists are often overwhelmed by the needs of such families. In some cases the families are not showing up at appointments or are having difficulty engaging with a new therapist, while in others they may have reached a therapeutic impasse with the therapist. Because of the amount of contact they have with families and the amount of resources they provide for them, the team members often have an especially intensive relationship with families, which can be used constructively to support their connections with other treatment providers.

In Margarita's case, racial differences were getting in the way of family therapy. With support the team arranged the transfer of family work to a Hispanic woman of color, to address Margarita's mistrust of the "white" system. This senior social worker understood how key Margarita was in this system and wanted to do home-based family sessions, but this was extremely difficult given the chaos of six children in the home. As a solution, an outreach worker was engaged to work with the clinician in cotherapy. The outpatient clinician would work with Margarita and some combination of older kids while the outreach worker did activity therapy with the younger ones. This was the only way to get Margarita's attention and focus, and the outreach worker could serve as a pressure release mechanism when participants in sessions began to

have difficulty. On the way home, the therapy team would compare notes to understand the dynamics of the sessions.

This work can also be extremely complex, and the care manager can feel as if he or she is navigating a labyrinth with the family (Imber-Black, 1992). The work of Haley (1980) pointed to the fact that with severely troubled families, their "helping ecology" often shows confusion in roles and responsibilities. A family's service system can in fact be quite dysfunctional. In our experience, often different agencies are at odds with one another, have misperceptions of each other's point of view on a family, and may not even embrace the same basic goals. At times providers, despite good intentions, lose sight of the goals and responsibilities they agreed to and head off in a different direction. Parents are also often blamed and disempowered (Fox, 1995) by systems of care. Like the institutionalized mental patient who must buy in to the institution's perception of him or her (Goffman, 1961), they are often forced to accept the system's perception of them as bad parents, sometimes to the point of accepting relinquishment of custody of their children in order to gain needed services.

We are grateful to Margarita that she wore these issues right out front. Hospital records from almost 20 years earlier illustrated a long-term pattern of very conflicted relationships with both caretakers and service providers. She needed them and at some level recognized how important they were in her life, yet at the same time they were a reminder of her sense of abandonment, isolation, and dependence. This conflict was played out in how she related to providers. A veteran in the system, she always managed to get services but then would be aggressive and reject them because they made her feel too dependent. She would then alienate everyone and lose the services, become enraged, feel abandoned, and retreat to her sofa. In response to her withdrawal, her children would compete for attention by acting out, forcing her to start the process over to access the services she knew she needed.

An example of this systemic issue was Margarita's relationship with the local child welfare office. She wanted it out of their life, and complained about it all the time in aggressive, defiant, and inappropriate ways. Yet she also repeatedly initiated services to get specific needs met that she knew she could make that office pay for, such as day care for Matthew or after-school services for Sharon. The child welfare worker was at the end of her rope and periodically threatened to place the two youngest children in foster care and Rashad in residential placement. Our team structured the situation by developing objective benchmarks for evaluating Margarita's progress in parenting over time, expanding the focus of workers to understand episodic blowouts in the context of a larger pattern of growing competence. They also spent considerable consultation time analyzing Margarita's fluctuating ambivalence and carefully strategized an approach that was empathically respectful of both her need to reject help and her significant drive and ability for obtaining it. After firing our team once, she came back a year later, saying, "I need your team again. They are the only ones that have helped me; they understand my family."

Consistent reminders of the deeply troubled history of these dynamics, given during team supervision, were critical in supporting their survival during Margarita's counterdependent rages. One of these rages, during an hour-long ride from an especially contentious wraparound provider meeting, was so vitriolic that the social worker considered leaving her own car and fleeing. Clinicians who are subjected to a therapy client's borderline rage can find refuge in the fact that the session is only an hour long or can be ended early. This is not so during a long drive. By asking for help in repeated team consultations, the therapist was able to find the support she needed and develop strategies for dealing with future rages. These strategies were endorsed and followed through by everyone else on the team who dealt with Margarita.

At one point the team had decided to hospitalize and then place Rashad in a residential center for short-term evaluation. Because of his level of dangerousness, the team took this action without Margarita's consent. She was furious with the team. She would start meetings with raging monologues that included accusations against the "white system" and blasphemy toward different providers who had called her too much or too little. She needed to vent her rage, but it was abusive and alienating to her service providers. Yet there was meaning behind it, coming from a woman who gave a strong sense that surrendering Rashad to placement meant losing all her children, the heart of everything important in her life. With much supervision the team was able

to reframe this rage as Margarita's way of expressing her affection toward her child in placement, and so gradually was able to speak to this as a strength. The team was then able to influence the caregiver system to accept that this strength was worthy of the respect of all its members.

The systems doctor does regular checkups on the care network. It is essential that interagency wraparound team meetings occur with parents at least every 4 to 6 weeks, with telephone contact as often as daily between the clinical coordinator and specific providers. We have found this work to be most intensive in the beginning of intervention, at moments of crisis during its course, and during the termination phase when step-down supports are being arranged. We have also designed a useful one-page grid that defines each target problem, outlines related family strengths and resources, articulates a specific goal, defines the roles and activities of each professional in the family's system of care, and assesses progress on a 4-point scale on each goal. Every person present, including the parent, contributes to the grid, signs it, and receives a copy. In this way everyone is held accountable for what the team and family have agreed should be done.

Much of systems doctor's work is conducted outside of meetings. Providers who are at odds with each other may need individual or paired meetings in addition to phone calls. Too often family clinicians understand advocacy as a position of helping the family fight for its rights against the system, and hence air differences with and between other professionals and agencies in front of families. This is usually a destructive way of showing parents that we want to work with and for them. The systems doctor is one who joins with every constituent, acknowledging individual challenges and differences, offering to help, and looking for common threads in divergent points of view.

For a small community team working without the high-level blending of funding streams common in larger statewide systems of care, the systems doctor must carefully maintain ongoing relationships in different local and state agencies to ensure that payers collaborate and accept their fiscal responsibilities at the wraparound table. It is essential in this process that all stakeholders begin by establishing consensus on what the problem is (Kamradt, 2002). The case coordinator builds this consensus and offers to call a supervisor or write a letter of support for funding, or with specific players on the side develops strategies for involving other players or constructively resolving conflicts. As state agencies begin to draw their lines in the sand regarding what they will or will not pay for, the coordinator is able to remind all at the table the likely cost to them and the families if services are not rendered. Executive advocacy is called in when needed to ensure that consensus is achieved at all levels of the stakeholder system.

Another aspect of systems doctor work is assisting parents in advocating for themselves. This begins with training team staff to accept the idea that parents, not professionals, are the experts on their children and have the most potential for serving as change agents for their children (Cohen & Lavach, 1995). In Margarita's case the systems work of necessity targeted ways to support her in not speaking too abrasively. The long drives to and from meetings when Rashad was in placement, though wearing, were useful because they helped Margarita prepare for the meetings and allowed her to vent afterward.

As more providers got involved, meetings became increasingly difficult for Margarita. Her main defense was to scream insults at providers. By design, Margarita's family support worker sat next to her during these meetings, on the one hand encouraging her to speak and on the other calming her when she became enraged. We realized when Margarita refused to sit at the team table (sitting against the wall instead) that the community team, which had grown to 12 providers, had become overwhelming for her. So our team designated representatives of clusters of providers and reduced the number of participants attending those meetings. This increased the surround time needed to ensure that provider clusters were being properly represented, but it saved time and anguish in the meetings.

Strategic Planning for Contingencies

Our team develops an emergency plan for each family. In weekly staff meetings the team, on a case-by-case basis, assesses the probability of getting paged for an emergency and what it means. A "danger line" safety assessment for each family is outlined, based on history, diagnosis, and current dynamic situation, including family and community stressors, phase of treatment, and the family's style of managing crisis. One parent would page for minor conflicts and would simply need to be told, "You're in charge. Tell him to stop it and send him to his room." Other parents would page only if faced by psychotic breakdown or violence, and the team knew ahead of time that this would require an immediate visit by either the crisis clinician or the local hospital team charged with emergency admission. Layered contingency lineups are developed for each family, such that it is clear what to put in place depending on the severity of the crisis or the escalation of failure in intervention strategies attempted.

Safety assessment also includes assessment of the safety of the worker in intervening. When a worker described a refrigerator riddled with bullet holes and ducking an ashtray thrown into the wall by a mother's abusive husband, visits were suspended until he could be removed from the house. Interventions with serious crises are often by pairs of team members, who began carrying a cell phone after an angry adolescent taught us how easy it is to sever connection with backup by yanking the telephone out of the wall. Careful team consultation and training have resulted in paraprofessional family support workers who are as competent as senior clinicians in dealing with emergencies.

Margarita would initially not use the pager for crises with children, both because she was afraid that she would be labeled incompetent and have her children taken away, and because she did not want to convey a sense of crisis to authorities. This changed with time after our team got child protective services involved and coached the worker to send a clear message that calling for help when in crisis was an aspect of being a good parent. Ultimately Margarita would use the pager to calm herself down by talking to the team when she felt she could not take it any longer. Often she would page and say she was fed up and felt like hitting the kids. The team learned that at such times what she herself needed was a good parent, so the worker would remind her that if she hit the children she would be reported to the authorities, and that she had the strength to control herself.

Margarita presented her own special challenge to the team. She would page, then change her mind about wanting to talk to someone and not answer the phone. The team members would find themselves awakened in the middle of the night, knowing Margarita was having a problem but not being able to talk to her. The strategy that worked was to let her know that we would call 911 (which would result in an emergency police or hospital response to her door) if she paged and then did not answer the callback.

Transition Work

Multiproblem families such as the Vegas also need a great deal of support around transitions, because of the level of involvement with multiple systems of care. Recent research with parents indicates that among the most significant challenges to them is navigating the system of care across changes in the status of the child (Frank, Greenberg, & Lambert, 2002). As their children's needs escalate or decrease, they are forced to step up or down across systems that often do not interface well with each other.

This is especially true of transitions from out-of-home placement. Our approach is in effect to bring the family to residential treatment, and residential treatment to the family. Hence, our team joins with residential clinicians and attempts to facilitate a cotherapy partnership in ways that seek to achieve consensus on the focus of treatment (as opposed to attempting to oversee or control the treatment, which can make residential clinicians defensive). The family team helps to assess when the child is ready to go home, as well as the possible need for long-term or permanent placement. If the child is a special behavioral challenge in the residential setting, the team family support worker can join the milieu as one who knows the child, his or her context, and what strategies have tended to be successful in the past. The team targets solidifying gains on the milieu by reinforcing parenting strategies at home, supporting a bridge both to home visits on pass and to ultimate reunification with the family. In some cases it has proved helpful to bring parents or foster parents to the milieu to spend extended periods of time there, so that they can observe and integrate successful behavior management strategies.

The level of intensity of wraparound models poses a special challenge for transition work. Families benefit from resources addressing a multiplicity of needs and can become dependent on the intensive level of support the team gives. For example, team-supported trips to the grocery store so that a parent can improve skills in nutritional

planning and budgeting for food can become something a parent comes to expect. The same is true of transportation. The team makes it explicit that its work is time limited and in every case works to ensure that the necessary skills and natural family supports are firmly in place so that the team will not be needed.

Gradually, as the Vega family became embedded in a community of supports and services and grew in their confidence to manage on their own, our team began the slow process of withdrawal. Rather than consistently providing transportation, the team supported Margarita in developing the skills to find her own way. Cotherapies were decreased and eliminated as therapeutic relationships with community providers developed the strength to sustain themselves. Pager utilization was discouraged, and interventions of the clinical care coordinator were reduced to casual support by the family support worker. Family access to community supports was made routine. Achievements in family independence were celebrated. Mechanisms were set up such that community providers would communicate with each other without the coordination of our team. After 15 months of work, the Vega family was ready to carry on without intensive services.

Outcome for Margarita and Her Family

Margarita had a hard time saying good-bye. She had met her treatment goals and could not identify anything else she needed. She would often cancel family meetings, but she resisted our departure. When we offered concrete support, she proudly told us that she was able to manage. All the children had support services, which included early intervention and Head Start for the youngest children, a therapeutic after-school program for Sharon, and individual and family therapy for all of them. Rashad, our original identified patient, was in a specialized day school and was also enrolled in a therapeutic after-school program so that his free time could be properly structured. Margarita was fully engaged in the treatment the team arranged, and although she never allowed us to establish contact with her individual therapist, the therapy was clearly helping.

Margarita had enjoyed and appreciated the team's support but was not going to let the team know this directly. Rather, she showed the team members how much they meant to her by becoming upset whenever termination was mentioned. She also could not tolerate the team's attempts to recognize her family's strengths. She had not had much practice with receiving compliments. Yet when it was offered that she could call the team or the DMH if she needed more support or had an emergency, she laughed. "I am not going to call," she said,. "I told you we are fine."

After termination the team often saw Margarita in our outpatient clinic. She always smiled and before being asked would let them know that everything was fine. Almost a year later, she called requesting services for Sharon, Rashad's younger sister, by now 8 years old. Sharon was becoming more defiant and was experiencing behavioral problems in school. Her providers, concerned about her safety, were suggesting an out-of-home placement. In such cases, reopening a case is not seen as recidivism but just as natural as a follow-up visit to the doctor for a serious medical condition. This second time the team worked with Sharon for just 5 months. The team identified and arranged to fill gaps in community supports, reorganized and coordinated services already in place, and then moved on to allow Margarita to be the parent she had become.

For Margarita, special care was taken to ensure that she had integrated three areas of growth. First, through the intensity of the wraparound relationship, Margarita's team helped her to alter her perceptions of the rigidified care system that failed her as a child, so that she now perceives services as help rather than a threat. Second, the team supported her in learning to identify early signs of problems with her children, so that she can work with her systems of care to avoid crises rather than reacting to them. Finally, we have left Margarita with the conviction that she has real strengths within herself, her family, and her community and can manage on her own.

We owe a lot to Margarita and her family. They challenged us to test and refine an intensive family and systems intervention that is strategic and comprehensive at every level. They have also helped us to illustrate in this chapter what a small agency fueled by a vision and a commitment to best practices can do. The accomplishment we share with the Vegas is the knitting together of a sophisticated and deeply embedded system of care, that with the help of our wraparound team can support the most vulnerable of troubled children and families in our community.

References

Archacki-Stone, C. (1995). Family-based mental health services. In L. Combrinck-Graham (Ed.), *Children in families at risk: Maintaining the connections* (pp. 107–124). New York: Guilford.

Bickman, L. (1996). A continuum of care: More is not always better. *American Psychologist, 31,* 689–701.

Bowen, M. (1978). *Family therapy in clinical practice.* New York: Jason Aronson.

Bronfenbrenner, U. (1979). *The ecology of human development.* Cambridge, MA: Harvard University Press.

Burns, B., & Hoagwood, K. (2002). *Community treatment for youth.* New York: Oxford University Press.

Cohen, R., & Lavach, C. (1995). Strengthening partnerships between families and service providers. In P. Adams, & K. Nelson (Eds.), *Reinventing human services: Community and family -centered practice* (pp. 261–277). New York: Aldine de Gruyter.

De Shazer, S. (1985). *Keys to solutions in brief therapy.* New York: Norton.

Epstein, M., Kutash, K., & Duchnowski, A. (Eds.). (1998). *Outcomes for children and youth with emotional and behavioral disorders and their families: Programs and evaluation best practices.* Austin, TX: Pro-Ed.

Fox, M. (1995). Organizing the hierarchy around children in placement. In L. Combrinck-Graham (Ed.), *Children in families at risk: Maintaining the connections* (pp. 182–208). New York: Guilford.

Frank, A., Greenberg, J., & Lambert, L. (2002). *The experiences of Massachusetts families in obtaining mental health care for their children.* Boston: Blue Cross Blue Shield Foundation of Massachusetts.

Friesen, B., & Poertner, J. (1995). *From case management to service coordination for children with emotional, behavioral, or mental disorders: Building on family strengths.* Baltimore: Brookes.

Friesen, B., Robinson, A., Jivanjce, D., Kruzich, J., & Pullman, M. (2003, March). *Barriers and supports to family participation: What residential treatment providers need to know.* Unpublished graduate research, Portland State University, Portland, OR. Presented at the 16th Annual Research Conference, "A System of Care for Children's Mental Health: Expanding the Research Base," Tampa, FL.

Goffman, E. (1961). *Asylums: Essays on the social situation of mental patients and other inmates.* New York: Anchor Books.

Grimes, K., & Appleton, A. (2003). Building on success: MA-MHSPY replication strategies for integrated systems of care for children and families. In C. Newman, K. Liberton, K. Kutash, & R. Friedman (Eds.), *A system of care for children's mental health: Expanding the research base* (pp. 79–82). Tampa: University of South Florida.

Haley, J. (1980). *Leaving home*. New York: McGraw-Hill.

Henggeler, S., Schoenwald, S., Bordun, C., Rowland, M., & Cunningham, P. (1998). *Multisystemic treatment of antisocial behavior in children and adolescents*. New York: Guilford.

Hernandez, M., & Goldman, S. (1996). A local approach to system development: Ventura County, California. In B. Stroul (Ed.), *Children's mental health: Creating systems of care in a changing society* (pp. 177–196). Baltimore: Brookes.

Imber-Black, E. (1992). *Families and larger systems: A family therapist's guide through the labyrinth*. New York: Guilford.

Kamradt, B. (2000). Wraparound Milwaukee: Aiding youth with mental health needs. *Juvenile Justice, 7*, 14–23.

Kamradt, B. (2002). *Funding mental services for youth in the juvenile justice system: Challenges and opportunities*. Washington, DC: National Center for Mental Health and Juvenile Justice: John D. and Catherine T. Mac Arthur Foundation.

Kim Berg, I. (1994). *Family-based services: A solution focused approach*. New York: Norton.

Knitzer, J. (1992). *Unclaimed children: The failure of public responsibility to children and adolescents in need of mental health services*. Washington, DC: Children's Defense Fund.

McGoldrick, M., & Gerson, R. (1985). *Genograms in family assessment*. New York: Norton.

National Psychologist Staff. (2003). Nation's mental health system more maze than help, says commission. *National Psychologist, 12*, 17.

Nelson, K., & Allen, M. (Eds.). (1995). *Reinventing human services: Community and family-centered practice*. New York: Hawthorne.

O'Hanlon, W., & Weiner-Davis, M. (1989). *In search of solutions: A new direction in psychotherapy*. New York: Norton.

Piaget, J. (1976). *The psychology of intelligence*. Totowa, NJ: Littlefield, Adams.

Ronnau, U. (1995). Family advocacy services: A strength model of case management. In B. Friesen & J. Poertner (Eds.), *From case management to service coordination for children with emotional, behavioral or mental disorders: Building on family strengths* (pp. 287–300). Baltimore: Brookes.

Schorr, L. (1997). *Common purpose: Strengthening families and neighborhoods to rebuild America*. New York: Doubleday.

Sondheimer, D., Santiago, R., Erickson, J., Herman, M., & Levine, R. (2003, March). *Exploring new directions in the Comprehensive Community Mental Health Services Program for Children and Their Families: Implications for research*. Presented at the 16th Annual Research Conference, "A System of Care for Children's Mental Health: Expanding the Research Base," Tampa, FL.

Stroul, B. (1996). *Children's mental health: Creating systems of care in a changing society*. Baltimore: Brookes.

Stroul, B. (2002). *Systems of care: A framework for system reform in children's mental health*. Washington, DC: Georgetown University Child Development Center.

Stroul, B., & Friedman, R. (1986). *A system of care for seriously emotionally disturbed children and youth*. Washington, DC: Georgetown University Child Development Center.

Van Den Berg, J., & Grealish, M. (1998). *The wraparound process training manual*. Pittsburgh, PA: Community Partnerships Group.

Von Bertalanffy, L. (1968). *General system theory*. New York: George Braziller.

Walton, E., Sandau-Beckler, P., & Mannes, M. (Eds.). (2001). *Balancing family-centered services and child well-being*. New York: Columbia University Press.

Whitaker, C. (1976). A family is a four-dimensional relationship. In P. Guerin (Ed.), *Family therapy: Theory and practice* (pp. 182–192). New York: Gardner.

Ziegler, R., & Bush, A. (1999). *Sharing care: The integration of family approaches with child treatment*. Philadelphia: Bruner/Mazel.

26

Katherine Gordy Levine

Creating a Community of Care for Seriously Emotionally Distressed Youth

The Mott Haven Initiative, a Systems of Care Experience

I am because we are and because we are, therefore, I am.
African proverb

This chapter describes the Visiting Nurse Service of New York's Mobile Community Support Service's (MCSS) creation of a caring community for emotionally distressed youth based on recognizing that we are one; we are family. The MCSS is a component of Families Reaching in Ever New Directions, Inc. (FRIENDS, Inc.). FRIENDS is a mental health agency located in Mott Haven, a part of the South Bronx, New York. This agency was created by a federally funded grant for the express purpose of establishing a family-driven system of care. In family-driven programs, families are partners in all decisions; no treatment meetings are held without family members. Moreover, at FRIENDS, family members constitute half of the agency's board of directors.

The MCSS service seeks to form what Madsen (1999) calls "appreciative alliances" with families. At FRIENDS the MCSS staff and the rest of the caring adults, including the specialized caretakers, function as a youth's extended family. The term "family" is used as described by a group of family members from the federal government's Comprehensive Community Mental Health Center for Children and Families Program. This group, lead by Trina Osher, sought to establish the concept of family as including those who defined themselves as a

family member. According to this team, "Families can include biological or adoptive parents and their partners, siblings, extended family members (called kinship caregivers), and friends who provide a significant level of support to the child or primary caregiver" (Osher, de Fur, Nava, Spencer, & Toth-Dennis, 1999, p. 32).

The team is encouraged to think of the youngsters in the MCSS's care as "our youth," as this promotes a greater sensitivity to the concept of family and shared responsibility for meeting the needs of young people. The terms "client," "patient," "delinquent," and "case" are avoided. Families do not talk of cases, clients, patients, or delinquents but of daughters, sons, sisters, brothers, aunts, uncles, nieces, nephews, and cousins. "What would you want for your child?" is a frequently asked question during supervision. So is "What would you want to hear if you were this youth's parent?"

In the same spirit, the term "seriously emotionally distressed" replaces the more traditional term "seriously emotionally disturbed." We believe the word "distressed" offers greater recognition that the family and youth are responding to multiple stressors. This stance suggests that the situation creating such stress needs changing as much as, if not more than, the families or youth.

A related assumption driving the MCSS is that the stress our families and youth face is traumatic stress. Such stress can come from directly witnessing one act of violence or from dealing daily with abuse and other traumatizing events. We believe all those living in Mott Haven have been traumatized in one way or another. For many, the traumas have been so embedded in their lives as to seem normal. More and more theorists are viewing such stress as a major contributor to mental illness (Garbarino, 1999; Kessler, 2000; Perry, 2001; Seikkula, Alakare, & Aaltonen, 2001; Terr, 1990; van der Kolk & Fisler, 1995).

According to this theoretical perspective, the agency and community serve as the treatment medium, not just for the specific child dealing with serious emotional distress but also for the child's entire family, for all the service providers serving the child, and for the community at large. Community-based clinical care cannot stop with one-on-one care or with the relationship between client and clinician. Adequate clinical care for those living in trauma-filled communities must tend to the youth, the family, and the community. The MCSS has translated this perspective into action primarily through use of a tri-level intervention model of care.

The chapter will (1) briefly review the theoretical changes leading to the current emphasis on community-based, family-driven care; (2) describe key components of the tri-level intervention model of care; (3) illustrate use of the model and discuss outcomes, including difficulties as well as successes; and (4) review lessons learned.

Theoretical Changes

Analytic theories, social-biological theories including genetic determinism, and learning theories came of age in the same century, each hoping to scientifically explain human behavior (Bronfenbrenner, 1979; Germain, 1991; Pinker 1997; Potkay & Allen, 1986). Like siblings seeking parental love, these various mental health models have long competed with each other. Proponents of each theory have proclaimed effectiveness while loudly or subtly denigrating other theories (Duncan, Miller, & Sparks, 2000; Miller, Duncan, & Hubble, 1997).

As efforts to effectively help the seriously emotionally distressed have grown, it has become increasingly clear that like the proverbial blind men grasping separate parts of the elephant, early practice theorists were correct in their theorizing for what was in their immediate grasp, but no one had the final answer. Fortunately, some have begun to see the whole and to take a "yes/and" rather than an "either/or" approach to understanding human behavior (Duncan et al., 2000; Gergen, 1994; Kagan, 1984; Meyer, 1983; Morgan, 2000). As Kagan (1984) notes, "It is almost a general truth that the understanding of every complex phenomenon requires a simultaneous appreciation of complementary concepts" (p. xii).

As some theorists have moved toward broader approaches, so have practitioners worked to discover better ways of helping. Since the 1960s, the number of therapies has grown from 60 to more than 250. Simultaneously, as recent evidenced-based efforts have shown, no one approach has been found to be more effective than another. Some approaches might prove better in some situations, but no one approach works for all (Burns, Compton, Egger, Farmer, & Robertson, 2002; Duncan et al., 2000; Henggeler, Schoenwald, Bourdin, Rowland, & Cunningham, 1998; Lambert & Bergin, 1994; Miller et al., 1997).

Families as Partners

As mental health practitioners struggled to figure out how best to help, many began to partner with the very people they sought to help—consumers. In terms of children's mental health services, this has meant partnering with families. During the development of mental health services, parents have been blamed for creating the youth's problems or impeding his or her treatment. The child was the identified patient and symptom bearer for the family. The family's dysfunction caused the child's problems (Haley, 1997). Moreover, in spite of mounting evidence to the contrary, families continue to carry most of the blame for a youth's mental health problem (Schopler, 1971; Schriebman, 1988; Thomas & Chess, 1984),

This blaming and exclusion of caregivers from the treatment process runs counter to acceptable practices for a mildly physically ill or injured child. In such situations, caregiver knowledge, what the narrative therapists describe as "local knowledge" (Morgan, 2000), is expected to suffice (*Miller &*

Diao, 1987). A child or adolescent suffering a minor sprain might never reach the attention of specialists. Experienced parents or caregivers familiar with life's everyday injuries treat such injuries without benefit of professional advice. If the injury is such that local knowledge does not suffice, then the child is taken for medical care. This care might be provided through an office or, if the injury is more serious, say, a compound fracture of the leg requiring complicated surgery, through hospitalization where a system of specialized care can be called into action. If hospitalization is required, the goal, however, is always to return the child home as soon as possible. Unfortunately, long after it was realized physically ill children did better cared for at home when that was possible, the treatment of choice for seriously emotionally distressed youth has too often been removal from home, school, or community.

The Systems of Care Approach

Since at least the 1960s, government policymakers and others have raised concerns about the mental health treatment of children, including the tendency to pursue placement and to exclude families from planning or participating in their child's treatment (Duchinowski, Kutash, & Friedman, 2002; Knitzer, 1982; Koop, 1987; U.S. Department of Health and Human Services, 1999). As noted by the Joint Commission on Mental Health of Children (1969), the services available in the 1960s did not adequately serve youth in need. Not only were the desired results lacking, but care was fragmented as various providers, often at odds with each other, competed and failed to communicate with one another or with parents and caregivers. No continuum of care and no intermediate community-based treatments existed; youth with serious emotional distress were generally to be found in restrictive settings, while other treatment choices were limited to outpatient care. These complaints were repeated again and again (Knitzer, 1982; Koop, 1987; President's Commission on Mental Health, 1978).

Fortunately, as the inadequacy of traditional approaches to treating seriously emotionally distressed youth became more apparent, the willingness of families to be relegated to a backseat eroded. Families began to challenge the experts and to exert a greater influence on policymakers. In 1979 the National Alliance of the Mentally Ill was established, followed in 1989 by the Federation of Families for Children's Mental Health. Such politically active family-driven organizations have played an important role in shaping what has come to be known as the systems of care approach. Systems of care emphasize community-based care, comprehensive and individualized services, extensive use of supports, including the use of local and family-identified supports, full participation of families, coordination among child-serving agencies and programs, and cultural competency (Friesen & Stephens, 1998; Henggeler et al., 1998; Osher et al., 1999; Stroul & Friedman, 1994).

Discussion surrounding the need for this systems of care approach has existed since the Joint Commission on the Mental Health of Children in 1969. Movement toward meeting that need has been slow. A major step in that direction was taken when the Child and Adolescent Service System Program (CASSP) was initiated in the early 1980s. Initially, small-capacity funding grants were issued, but in 1992 Congress created the Comprehensive Community Mental Health Services and Their Families Program. This legislation funded 67 large demonstration grants through the Center for Mental Health Services. In 1994, New York State received a $17 million grant to develop a mental health–based system of care for the youth of Mott Haven, a section of the South Bronx, New York. The Mobile Community Support Service became one of the components of the Mott Haven systems of care projects. During the initial grant period, the other components included case management, family support, youth leadership, and a respite and recreation program, with local mental health clinics serving as part of the broader systems of care. A homework help program was added to the grant after 3 years of operation.

The core FRIENDS staff currently consists of an executive director, a deputy director, an access coordinator, an office manager, a financial director, an administrative assistant, a director of family support, two parent consultants, a director of homework help, three homework help tutors, three youth leaders, a receptionist, and a file clerk. Three of the staff have advanced degrees. Half of the staff, including the executive director, live in Mott Haven. As previously noted, one half of the board of directors is composed of family members. Since federal funding ended, primary financial support for FRIENDS has been provided by the New York State Office of Mental Health.

Mott Haven

Mott Haven was selected for this grant because it was a triple-jeopardy community known for its high prevalence of mental illness, substance abuse, and physical illness. Moreover, at the time of the grant, existing services were inadequate, particularly for children, and competed with one another. Finally, the fact that it was the poorest community district in the United States also played a part. Kozol (1995), in his book *Amazing Grace,* says this about Mott Haven:

> I walk for hours in the neighborhood, starting at Willis Avenue, crossing Brook, and then St. Ann's, going as far as Locust Avenue to look at the medical waste incinerator one more time, then back to Beekman Avenue. In cold of winter, as in summer's heat, a feeling of asphyxia seems to contain the neighborhood. The faces of some of the relatively young women with advanced cases of AIDS, their eyes so hollow, their jawbones so protruding, look like the faces of women in the House of the Dying run by the nuns within the poorest slum of Port-au-Prince [Haiti]. It's something that you don't forget. (p. 8)

Visiting Nurse Service of New York Programs at FRIENDS

The Visiting Nurse Service of New York (VNSNY) is funded to provide two services by FRIENDS. One contract provides a specialized respite and recreational (R&R) service for those youngsters not able to utilize traditional recreational services. The primary goal of the service is to teach the youngsters the skills needed to make use of traditional services. The R&R service also provides respite care to FRIENDS families in crisis. The R&R team consists of a respite coordinator and four respite workers who serve 50 youths a year, in addition to providing twice-monthly events for a larger number of youth and their families.

The MCSS, which is the focus of this chapter, provides consultation, clinical assessment, and crisis stabilization services for FRIENDS families and youth. The MCSS consists of a program director, a program coordinator, a half-time child psychiatrist, a community mental health nurse, two team leaders, three bachelor's-level social workers, two parent advocates, two case aides, and an administrative assistant. The MCSS team serves 150 youths and families a year and provides 500 consultations to community residents and service providers a year.

The MCSS was initially designed to provide a traditional mobile crisis and home-based crisis intervention (HBCI) service using the Homebuilder's model (Kinney, Haapala, & Booth, 1991). The Homebuilder's model provides intensive crisis services in the home over a 6- to 8-week period. Each service provider works with only two youngsters and their families at a time. Families are seen four to five times a week for an average of 4 to 5 hours per visit. Finally, service providers are on call around-the-clock. Skills teaching serves as the primary treatment modality. Since the early 1990s, VNSNY had run several successful HBCI programs and had participated in research involving those services (Evans, Boothroyd, & Armstrong, 1997, 1999).

In planning for the MCSS, family members soon made it clear they wanted something more than a traditional crisis team or Homebuilder's service. As one parent noted, "Crisis intervention is too late. If we are in a crisis, we know where to go for help. What we need is help before the crisis. We need help when things are starting to get tough or when our children begin to have trouble in school" (Levine, 1999, p. 72).

Family members also made it clear they wanted more flexibility than traditional HBCI services provided. Over the course of the first year, a number of changes were made that brought the MCSS into better alignment with family desires. The first change involved the ability to see families in an office, as well as in the home or school, as long as safety did not require home visiting. Direct services are provided in the home or the office depending on what the family wants. This offers greater flexibility and more choice to both caregivers and youth. Another change has been in the frequency of services. MCSS visits are scheduled frequently but only until safety is established. Thereafter, the family has greater input in determining the service plan, including how often visits should be made.

Another change involved the ability to stay involved with a family even if hospitalization or another placement proved necessary. Traditionally, HBCI services end if a youngster is hospitalized or placed. This leads to families and youth feeling abandoned by the team when it is most needed. The MCSS stays involved with hospitalized family and youth until the child is safely returned home and long-term services are in place, or until long-term placement becomes the discharge goal. Even if long-term placement becomes necessary, the MCSS will be available to help whenever the youth returns home.

The final way the model was changed was the addition of support staff. MCSS added parent advocates and case aides who also serve as youth advocates. The addition of support staff to the HBCI model led to an adjustment in how many cases a worker carried. Service load is now determined by the number of hours spent on case management tasks and not just by the number of families served. Line staff are expected to provide 20 to 25 hours of service per week. Those hours include trainings, case consultations, supervision, and travel time. Sometimes a worker will carry only two cases; at other times, he or she will carry three or more cases.

Services often begin with a consultation. If it appears the child needs more immediate care than can be provided by a community mental health agency or school, a clinical assessment, including a psychiatric evaluation, is completed. Based on this assessment, intensive services are provided if needed. If intensive services are not indicated, the family is referred to appropriate community providers. Since the program started, the MCSS has served more than 800 seriously emotionally stressed youth, a third of whom have been provided with assessment services, while the remaining families have been offered both assessment and crisis intervention. The MCSS has also provided more than 5,000 consultations (see figure 26-1 for details).

The Tri-Level Integrated Model of Care

The MCSS uses a tri-level integrated model of care (see figure 26-2), which seeks to integrate various theories and treatment approaches in a flexible manner that involves partnering with families, other service providers, and systems of care. Although developed prior to the criteria for interventions that "change lives" discussed by Shorr (1998) in her book *Common Purpose*, the model meets many of her criteria. She calls for family and community-based services that are flexible, responsive, comprehensive, and staffed by individuals willing to go above and beyond traditional job requirements to help the people they serve because they have faith in what they are doing.

The tri-level model, which was first used in the VNSNY HBCI programs, was developed in response to the ever-growing knowledge about how to best treat traumatized youth. Van der Kolk, Van der Hart, and Burbridge (1995) believe the treatment of post–traumatic stress disorder must include controlling the physiological stress reaction, cognitively processing and accepting the traumatizing experience, maintaining or reestablishing safe social connections, and finally building interpersonal efficacy. James (1989) echoes these beliefs when she notes, "Trauma may assault the child physically, cognitively, emotionally, and spiritually, and therefore treatment strategies must deal with each of these areas" (p. 14).

The tri-level model seeks to meet these treatment requirements by providing three levels of care—support, sharing knowledge, and specialized care. Each level consists of six tasks. The model can be used linearly, or tasks can be bypassed, to be revisited later or eliminated completely as safety and the needs and desires of the child and family dictate.

Safety First and Last

Safety is the gateway into and out of the model's levels of service. This serves the purpose of emphasizing that safety cannot be jeopardized in the interests of providing family-friendly services or avoiding hospitalization. Although it is recognized that many of the tasks from the model are involved in establishing safety, using safety as a gateway instead of incorporating it into the first level stresses that safety issues can never be bypassed or ignored.

Staff are instructed to ask directly at the beginning of each contact, "Is everyone safe?" as well as to conduct traditional safety assessments throughout each session. Staff are also trained to repeat the question "Is everyone safe?" and to ask, "Is there something more I need to know before leaving?" at the end of each contact.

OVERVIEW OF THE MOBILE COMMUNITY SUPPORT SERVICE

MISSION

The MCSS's mission is keep youngsters safely in their current school, home or the community and to do so through use of a family friendly, individualized care, strength based service delivery model.

ELIGIBILITY

- Resident of Mott Haven
- Between ages of 5 and 21
- Currently diagnosed or evidencing behaviors that would lead to an Axis I diagnosis
- Known to child welfare or juvenile justice
- IQ above 70
- At risk of removal from home, school or community

SERVICES

Consultations to families, caregivers, service providers regarding the needs of seriously distressed youth.

Assessment services to youth whose behavior is indicative of a DSM-IV diagnosis and who cannot wait for assessment because he or she is at risk of removal from home, school or community.

Assessment services can take up to 3 weeks and include a clinical assessment, a psychiatric evaluation when indicated, and linkage to follow up care.

Intensive crisis intervention services for youth who are at risk of psychiatric hospitalization. Includes a clinical assessment, psychiatric evaluation and medication when needed, skills teaching, and Child and Family Team development. Services can last up to 12 weeks and utilize a modified Homebuilder's family preservation approach.

ALL SERVICES ARE VOLUNTARY UNLESS SAFETY ISSUES EXIST.

FAMILY CHARACTERISTICS

- 33% of caregivers speak only Spanish
- 10% of caregivers have a history of psychiatric hospitalization
- 10% of caregivers have a felony conviction
- 36.5% of families have one or another member in addition to the youth referred for services who is seriously emotionally disturbed
- 43.5% of the families have experienced some form of domestic violence
- 41.4% of the families have lived with substance abuse
- 25% of the caregivers had less than a 9th grade education
- 51% of families received some form of public assistance
- 24% live on less than $5,000 a year
- Median family income is $ 9,729 per year

CHARACTERISTICS OF YOUTH

Age
- 20.8% between 5 and 7 years
- 37.0% between 8 and 11 years
- 36.7% between 12 and 16 years
- 4.7% between 17 and 21 years

Ethnic backgrounds
- 71% Latino: 52% Puerto Rican, 13% Dominican, 4% Mexican, 1% Honduran, 1% Ecuadorian
- 22% African American
- 6% Mixed
- 1% Anglo-American

Diagnosis
16.4% Adjustment Disorders
15.0% ADHD
25.7% Behavior Disorders
12.8% Mood Disorders
4.2% Psychotic Disorders
3.9% Substance Abuse Problems
10.7% Trauma Reactions
9.7% Other

Figure 26.1. Overview of MCSS

TRI-LEVEL INTEGRATED TREATMENT MODEL

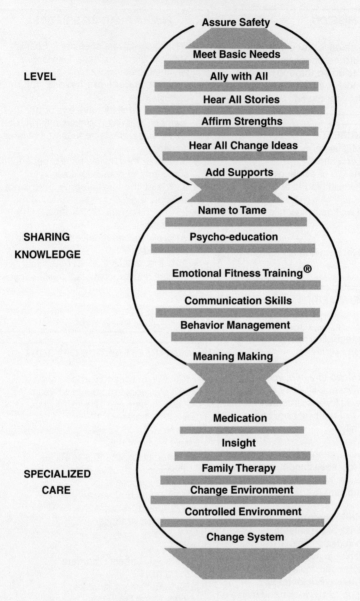

Copyright © 1989 by Katherine Gordy Levine

Figure 26.2. Tri-Level Integrated Treatment Model

Another way safety is ensured is through the use of beepers. Families are not on-call 9 to 5; a crisis can occur morning, noon, or night. All team members are expected to be available by beeper 24 hours a day, 7 days a week. Simultaneously, each family member is trained to recognize the differ-ence between a crisis for which they would page the staff and an emergency that requires them to call 911 for immediate help. An emergency is de-fined as a life-threatening situation necessitating immediate police or medical intervention: someone is locked in a room threatening suicide, someone has swallowed pills, someone has run to a rooftop, someone is physically assaulting another person or threatening others with a weapon, someone is so out of touch with reality he or she cannot be safely left alone. A crisis involves a lower level of risk. Generally, it is assumed someone in a crisis can wait 24 hours for services. A child may be talking of suicide, even have a plan, but agrees not to act on the plan and instead contact a responsible adult when suicidal thoughts intrude. A child may have done some tissue damage to another child during a fight, but the fight has been stopped and calm restored for the time being. A youth might be experiencing psychotic symptoms but not be in immediate danger. Finally, families are also assured that the MCSS staff would prefer to be beeped than to have the family worried about something.

While many of the tasks connected with the tri-level model might be accomplished as safety is being established, if safety issues exist, the model may need to be completely bypassed or jettisoned midway. For example, upon making an initial visit to a family, staff were shown a bottle of pills by a sibling and told that the client had recently taken all the pills. Ingesting pills, even being suspected of ingesting pills, demands an emergency response, and staff immediately called 911 despite the primary caregiver's protestations and the youth's denial she had taken any pills. The youth had indeed taken a liver-damaging dose of Tylenol and was hospitalized for several weeks until she was no longer considered a serious suicidal risk. Once this youth was hospitalized and safety had been assured, the tri-level model was brought fully into play. By the time the youth returned home, many tasks at the model's first two levels had been accomplished.

In another case situation, progress through the levels was proceeding step-by-step. Then the youth revealed he was being sexually abused. Although efforts were made to hear everyone's story and remain supportive of the primary caretaker, it rapidly became clear that for the youth's safety, protective services had to be brought in. The abuser, a relative of the mother, was arrested; the mother terminated services at that point. Efforts were made to reengage the mother, but this did not prove possible. Ideally, if safety issues disrupt the flow through the tri-level model, starting again at the support level allows service to continue. Unfortunately, in some situations that is not possible.

The Support Level

Once safety is established, formal use of the model begins. Most often this means starting with the Support Level. One of the goals of the tri-level model is to make certain support is seen as equal to other more traditional clinical services. Numerous studies and theorists support this idea (Beardslee, 1986; Brown, Harris, & Bifulco, 1986; Garbarino, 1995, 1998, 1999; Garmezy, 1986; James, 1989; Madsen, 1999). Garbarino emphasizes the importance of support when treating traumatized children and youth. For example, he believes one of the best hopes for troubled children lies in a connection to someone—a member of the extended family, a teacher, a child care worker, even someone the child sees only occasionally but who has absolute faith in the child's ability to succeed. Clearly, the more caring people in our youths' and our families' social circles, the more people assuming the role of extended family, the more support the family and child experience. Moreover, the more supportive people in a child's environment, the greater chances a child will experience some measure of absolute faith in his or her positive abilities. This is why the concept of agency as extended family serves as the foundation for the Support Level of Care.

There are six tasks at the Support Level. The tasks primarily involve adding supportive relationships. While essential, such relationships are not the only support offered to families. Support Level tasks include meeting concrete needs, engaging or allying with all, hearing all stories, affirming strengths, hearing all change ideas, and adding supports. The emphasis on "all" reminds staff that all family members and significant others involved in a youth's life are part of the treatment medium.

Socializing together is one way the MCSS adds support. Extended families join together for festive occasions. Extended family members eat together and play together. These everyday family experiences are not always available to families struggling with a seriously distressed youth. The VNSNY original HBCI team met in focus groups with family members regarding the needs of their seriously disturbed children and how services could be improved. Families identified a need to go out as a family. "We need to be able to relax. We don't want to always worry about what other people think of our kids" was how one family member described this need.

Through the efforts of several students and ultimately with the help of a number of other agencies, a "family fun night" was established by the VNSNY and held monthly at a local psychiatric hospital. All family members, including siblings of the youth served by the HBCI team and other participating service providers, gather for 3 hours of socializing. The night involves serving the families a light supper and then providing a choice of gym, crafts, or a family support group. The MCSS helped with the creation of a similar event at FRIENDS. This event is held at a local school and is frequently mentioned by families in consumer satisfaction surveys as a valued FRIENDS service.

Other fun events, workshops, and celebrations are also part of the FRIENDS and Mobile Community Support Service's culture of caring. Such events advance the idea that the team serves as part of an extended family and a caring community for our youth. Such events aid in promoting continuity of care. The events also ease the pain of abandonment families and youth feel when confronted with termination. Extended family members do not say good-bye, so while a family or child's involvement with the MCSS sometimes is placed on an inactive status, the relationship is never terminated. Seeing staff at various FRIENDS events maintains a connectedness valued by families, youths, and service providers.

In addition to reconnecting at various FRIENDS events, families and youth know services can begin again simply by calling for an appointment or dropping by the office. One client calls regularly from Puerto Rico to touch base with her MCSS staff-family. Recently a drop-in Staying Strong meeting, combining aspects of 12-step meetings and multifamily groups, was added to the MCSS service array (McFarlane, 2002). These meetings offer mutual problem solving in a support group consisting of other families, staff, and youth. This group offers easy access to maintaining or reestablishing contact with various MCSS service providers.

Sharing Knowledge

Support Level tasks pave the way for the model's second level—Sharing Knowledge. The Sharing Knowledge tasks include Name to Tame, psycho-education, Emotional Fitness Training,® behavior management, communication skills, and meaning making. As with Support Level tasks, the tasks at this level are interwoven.

Without the well-developed human capacity to share knowledge, civilization would not exist. Moreover, there is growing recognition that, as Lightburn and Black (2001) note,

> practitioners are engaged with clients in a learning relationship, often teaching without recognizing they are doing so, because their primary identification is that of therapists. Clinicians teach as psycho-educators, and are often mentors, guides, and coaches, whether or not they purposefully view or develop this aspect of their work. (p. 15)

The Sharing Knowledge Level purposefully develops these aspects of the helping process. The first task is Name to Tame, which involves naming not only objects but also events, feelings, and behavior. According to ancient mythology, evil spirits can be warded off by calling their names. Myths are attempts to both name and explain life events.

Without shared knowledge, accumulated knowledge would be lost. As the movie *The Miracle Worker* (Coe & Penn, 1962) so movingly described, Helen Keller eventually came to understand that the repeated sensations Annie Sullivan traced in her palm meant water. Once that connection had been made, Keller had access not only to Sullivan's knowledge but also to the accumulated wisdom of the ages. She was able to learn not just from her own experiences but from the experiences of those who came before her. She had begun to name and tame the confusion wrought by her handicaps.

Clearly, one copes better if one can name what is going on. One youth referred to the death of a younger sibling as "the day the family died." His parents had tried to protect him by not discussing the death. Both had assumed he needed no help and had tried to keep him from experiencing their pain. When he was able to name his pain so poignantly, his parents heard his anguish, and the way was paved for this youngster to mourn this loss. His and his parents' goal became "reviving the family."

In addition to providing common ground for discussing shared events, Name to Tame also involves thinking. Doing so uses the cortex—top-down processing (Ogden & Minton, 2000; Perry, 2001), which aids efforts to gain control of bodily sensations and feeling by adding reason to the decision-making process. The middle and lower brains are controlled by emotion and reflex. Without top-down processing, less control is felt, and less control is exercised. One youth struggled with owning a very considerable strength—her ability to solve problems for her friends. She also had difficulty calling on this strength for her own use. She eventually named this part of her self "Dear Abby Nicole." This Name to Tame act, a top-down processing, strengthened her ability to call on this strength for herself, putting her cortex in control.

Separating Name to Tame from more traditional, medically based psychoeducation tasks reminds all that there is specialized knowledge. Name to tame uses local knowledge. Local knowledge serves important purposes. Spiritual advisers, either from traditional churches or healers connected with Espiritismo, are important sources of local knowledge in Mott Haven. The streets are dotted with botanicas. Shrines to various Espiritismo and Santeria saints are frequently seen in homes. If a family feels a spiritual cleansing of their home is needed, the MCSS will help them provide a cleansing. Sometimes such a cleansing is carried out by a local Catholic priest, sometimes by another spiritual adviser. The thoughtful spiritual advisers know that lifting a curse or providing a spiritual cleansing is not enough to deal with psychosis or other serious emotional distress; these cases require specialized medical care. At the same time, the power of the belief in a curse may be part of the psychotic process, and then a spiritual cleansing aids the treatment. In a less dramatic and mundane example, local knowledge often suggests one can "just snap out of depression." Sometimes that works, but when it does not, specialized knowledge is needed, and then psychoeducational tasks are utilized.

The primary tools used by the MCSS in this task of sharing knowledge are "What We Think" handouts (see figure 26-3). These are one-page sheets listing, in parent- and youth-friendly language, the *DSM-IV* symptoms for the disorder the team suspects is part of the youth's distress. The handouts are first introduced to the primary caregiver during the information-gathering process as soon as staff has begun zeroing in a possible *DSM-IV* diagnosis. The caregiver is asked to see if he or she agrees with our assessment and to rate the

youth on the various symptoms. When appropriate, the same handouts are shared with the youth. Most often, the caregivers and youth agree with the MCSS's assessment. If not, other possibilities are explored. These handouts also contain the MCSS's recommendations for dealing with the distress. When the family and staff agree on a diagnosis, those recommendations are explored and ultimately incorporated into the family's action plan. Use of these handouts adds the family and youth's knowledge to the team's specialized knowledge and generally strengthens the treatment process.

A consistent recommendation on the "What We Think" handout introduces the third Sharing Knowledge task. This recommendation suggests family and youth learn another type of specialized knowledge by taking one or another Emotional Fitness Training® (EFT) course (Levine, 1997; Sunderland, 2002). EFT seeks to reduce the stigma attached to emotional distress and mental health problems. EFT programs are based on the premise that just as most people are more or less physically fit, so most are more or less emotionally fit. Physical fitness training seeks to improve physical health; EFT seeks to improve emotional health (Goleman, 1995). Each EFT program teaches and reinforces skills such as feeling awareness, feeling measurement, self-soothing, thinking before acting on negative feelings, and remembering what is important. Each skill represents a top-down approach to dealing with strong feelings.

All MCSS staff become Emotional Fitness Trainers. Three FRIENDS staff have also completed the training. Interested family and youth have recently been offered an opportunity to complete the licensing process, but none have yet completed the entire course. Part of the licensing process involves taking a Staying Strong Self-Care course. Requiring potential trainers to personally apply the concepts underscores the core EFT belief that everyone struggles with life problems and everyone needs not only support but a daily program to ensure emotional fitness (see figure 26-4).

An important aspect of each EFT program is the ability to break the curriculum down into individualized training modules based on youth and family needs and motivation. This fits in well with the systems of care principle of individualized care. The family and youth can pick and choose what aspects of EFT most appeal to their ideas of what is needed. For example, one youth was having dif-

WHAT WE THINK IS GOING ON. After speaking with you and your child, we believe he or she has a problem the doctors call **Attention-Deficit/Hyperactivity Disorder (ADHD).** This means that over the past six months, he or she has shown six of the following signs. Use this checklist to see if you agree.

Symptoms or signs	Describes my child		Severity scale 1=never 3 = weekly 5 = daily					Strengths and other comments
	Yes	No						
Fails to pay attention			1	2	3	4	5	
Can't stay at one thing			1	2	3	4	5	
Does not seem to listen			1	2	3	4	5	
Doesn't finish tasks			1	2	3	4	5	
Is disorganized, messy			1	2	3	4	5	
Loses things			1	2	3	4	5	
Is distracted easily			1	2	3	4	5	
Is forgetful			1	2	3	4	5	
Often fidgets			1	2	3	4	5	
Leaves seat or classroom			1	2	3	4	5	
Runs about a lot			1	2	3	4	5	
Feelings of restlessness			1	2	3	4	5	
Is always on the go			1	2	3	4	5	
Talks excessively			1	2	3	4	5	
Is impulsive			1	2	3	4	5	
Can't wait for turn			1	2	3	4	5	
Interrupts			1	2	3	4	5	

Youth with this problem aren't being difficult on purpose. The problem is mainly with the way their brains work. They are super charged and on high alert. Why do youth have this problem? Most often it is passed on from parents the way brown eyes or blond hair is passed on. Some think it is a response to drugs or alcohol use by the mother; some think it is because the father was a drug user or alcohol abuser. Sometimes it is a response to being traumatized. The important thing is that lots can be done to help the child with ADHD.

1. Adults need to be accepting and not blaming. Adults need to be clear about what the youth can and cannot control.

2. The youngster needs help understanding that the way his brain works makes it necessary for him to make an extra effort to pay attention. He or she needs to figure out what will help with that. Some youngsters need extra quiet when they are doing things like homework; others do better by listening to music while studying.

3. Youth need to learn to handle the bad feelings this disorder can create. Emotional Fitness Training Skills should be learned.

4. Structure is very important. Youth with this disorder need to have their lives programmed for them. Doing the same thing at the same time makes a difference.

5. Adults must learn to use TAG, STOP and CARE responses for stopping misbehaviors.

6. Adults dealing with a youth with this disorder must be emotionally strong. Practicing lots of Emotional Fitness Training® (EFT), Staying Strong and Self Soothing Skills help.

7. Medication might be necessary. Sometimes it is and when it is, it can work wonders.

This is a problem that can be solved.

Figure 26.3. Sample Treatment Sheet

Staying Strong PRACTICING A DAILY EMOTIONAL FITNESS TRAINING®
**PROGRAM KEEPS YOU EMOTIONALLY STRONG. Here is a brief description of the 12
exercises Emotional Fitness Training®suggests practicing daily.**

1. **Practice gratitude first thing every day.** Be grateful for all you have been given–Life, love, others to love, this world, and all things beautiful.

2. **Remember what is important, your mission**–Think about the kind of person you want to be: kind, caring, just. You cannot be emotionally fit if you are cruel. You cannot be emotionally fit if you are filled with anger, hate or thoughts of revenge.

3. **Be kind to another**–Being kind brings its own reward. Give a hug and get a hug. Smile and feel your spirits lift.

4. **Move your body**–15 minutes brisk exercise daily improves not only your body but your emotional fitness.

5. **Be with beauty**–Take time to look into a flower or to listen to beautiful music or to watch a bird soar.

6. **Recall someone who cared**–Too often we focus on past hurts. Remember instead another's kind act.

7. **Laugh**–Laugh with, not at. Practice laughter. Share a joke. Watch a funny movie. Have a silly face feud.

8. **Make something**–Bake some special bread, plant flowers, crochet, carve, knit, paint, make music, write.

9. **Indulge in a healthy pleasure**–A candy kiss, a bubble bath, listening to your favorite music, a cup of tea.

10. **Forgive yourself**–Accept that people, you included, are human and none of us is perfect. Stop behaviors that harm others and make amends for wrongs you have done, then let go of guilt.

11. **Forgive another**–Forgiveness is not forgetting; it is not letting another person hurt or abuse you. Forgiveness, as practiced here, refers to the forgiveness suggested by Bishop Tutu. This means stopping the circle of hurt by refusing to hurt those who have hurt you. In the long run revenge is neither healthy nor helpful.

12. **Be grateful yet again**–Every night before you fall asleep, remember and be grateful for all the good things in your life.

Practice each of these exercises daily and you will find you feel calmer, more in control, and more able to work for peace in your heart, at home, in the world.

... to appreciate beauty and find the best in others; to leave the world a bit better to know even one life has breathed easier because you have lived this–is to have succeeded.

Ralph Waldo Emerson

Visit our Web Page at www.eft.org
©Emotional Fitness Training® Inc_____♥

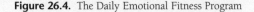

Figure 26.4. The Daily Emotional Fitness Program

ficulty controlling the impulse to run out of the school in an effort to reassure himself all was well with his mother, who suffered from asthma. He was taught a soothing and calming self-talk exercise to use whenever the urge to run back home occurred. He was also given a picture of his mother in which she wrote, "I'm taking care of me, you take care of school." This helped him remember that staying in school was his goal.

Stressed youth are usually acting-out youth.

Acting out stresses caregivers. Stress erodes the ability to manage negative feelings. If you cannot control your feelings, you have a difficult time dealing with a youth's difficult behavior. Caregivers are taught to apply EFT skills as an essential ingredient when dealing with the next Sharing Knowledge task—behavior management.

Behavior problems are the most common reasons youth are referred to the MCSS. Service providers put a great deal of emphasis on communication skills and natural consequences (Farber & Mazlish, 1980; Gordon, 1975); these contrast with the tough love approach many parents feel helps youth survive life in a high-crime area. As one mother put it, "If my child doesn't do exactly what he is told to do when he is confronted by a dealer or a cop, he's in big trouble." Tough love parents are only one part of the picture, for other parents have given up trying to control. Most frequently these are single-parent mothers from cultures in which patriarchy is strong and sons have been encouraged to dominate. Both groups need behavior management tools.

The MCSS behavior management teaching takes a "yes/and" approach. We urge parents to catch their children doing the right thing, we use behavior charts to track and reward positive change, and we urge strong responses to unacceptable behaviors. We emphasize the difference between punishment and abuse. We make it clear abuse will lead to a referral for protective services.

Youth who are ruled at home with an iron fist have a particularly difficult time behaving at school. When asked, almost every child can tell you exactly when he or she had better do what a parent wants. "She stands up." "He raises his voice." "She goes for the switch." "He gets very quiet." "His face gets red." Youth are encouraged to use that knowledge to understand that a teacher might speak more softly then Mom or Dad, but the teacher's "No" is every bit as important as a parental "No." Parents are asked to reinforce that message.

The fifth sharing knowledge task involves improving communication skills. Such efforts usually refer to teaching people to use active listening and "I messages" (Farber & Mazlish, 1980; Gordon 1975). The MCSS does a great deal of this type of teaching but also adds to this usual task improving communication by teaching the use of family meetings. In addition to serving as a tool to improve communication within the family, family meetings also help prepare youth and families for child and family team meetings. Child and family teams consisting of the family's natural supports and the service providers the family finds supportive are a major strategy of most systems of care programs. These team meetings help ensure the family's voice is heard, a strength-based approach is adhered to, and service planning is coordinated.

The goal during an intensive intervention is to hold three family meetings and three Child and Family Team Meetings. One Child and Family Team Meeting is held with the family and the referral source or child's school at the beginning of the intervention; a second meeting is held to develop the service plan after the evaluation process is completed; and a final meeting is held when the MCSS ends its intervention and the family is transitioned to another service.

Each of these tasks paves the way toward the final Sharing Knowledge task—meaning making. Emphasis on meaning making relates to the MCSS's underlying belief that the majority of our youths' difficulties are related to trauma. Trauma threatens meaning by shattering core beliefs and by destroying faith in the goodness of self and others, as well as in the possibility of living a good and meaningful life (Garbarino 1998; James, 1989; Perry, 2001; van der Kolk et al., 1995). As Garbarino (1998) notes in describing the voices that help make sense of violence:

> There is a third voice I would call soul searching. This voice begins from the realization that human beings are not best understood as animals with complicated brains but as spiritual beings who have a physical experience in the world. Once this is recognized, we can see that the world of violent trauma is not so much an injury, but a spiritual challenge that has diverted us from the path of enlightenment. (p. 28.)

Meaning making as used by the MCSS focuses on two tasks. The first is on helping families provide children with meaningful explanations for the bad things that happen, particularly the bad things people do. A strong faith is useful, and the emphasis is on life-affirming explanations that lead toward hope and connection, not despair and revenge. The second task involves restoring a sense of meaning to those who have lost theirs through trauma.

Family meetings are often used to bring up the importance of having a life-affirming explanation for why bad things happen. Most often the question comes up in relation to traumatic experiences, including the death or desertion of loved ones. Many of our youth have lost family to violence or premature death; many others have been abandoned by biological parents. One youngster fell prey to depression when his soccer ball was swept down into a storm drain. The ball symbolized the dead father he hardly knew. His one memory was of kicking a soccer ball with his father. By being helped to construct a memory book about his father, this youth was able to maintain a relationship important to his ongoing mental health (Levine, 1993). The team was able to procure a picture of the father as a boy and a number of other pictures, including one of the father holding our youth; several family memories were gathered about the father that included his hopes for his son's future. Creating the memory book not only helped the youngster maintain a meaningful relationship with his father but also involved his paternal relatives more fully in his life and helped him make sense of his loss.

The Specialized Care Level

When support does not work, sharing knowledge might succeed; but when neither support nor sharing knowledge is sufficient, more is needed. The time has come to utilize the Specialized Care Level. The tasks at this level may include development of insight; medication; family therapy; having the child live with another family member or placed in an open settings such as a therapeutic foster home or group home; placement in a controlled environment such as a psychiatric hospital, residential treatment center, or detention center; and, finally, changing systems affecting the youth and his family—what the entire systems of care movement seeks to do. Specialized Care Level interventions involve use of broader systems of care, often involve people licensed or otherwise acknowledged as being able to provide special care, or involve teams of people directed by a licensed professional.

Although the primary work at this level is not carried out by the MCSS team but through referral or collaboration, that work is augmented and integrated into each family's action plan by the back-and-forward flow through the tri-level model of care. For example, when a youth needs an emergency placement in a controlled setting, the family is offered additional support through the crisis, the youth is supported as the placement occurs, and the team remains involved and ready to accept the youth back into care when the emergency passes.

The Tri-Level Model and the Systems of Care Movement

Seeking to become part of a systems of care movement fit well with the tri-level model of care's attempt to integrate various treatment approaches and theories into a more coherent whole for practitioners and families. In addition to guiding individual efforts, the tri-level model can be used to guide all change efforts. Establishing alliances, hearing everyone's story, affirming strengths, and adding support are all steps to both system and individual change. Sharing knowledge is pivotal. Even something as simple as labeling the inability to get required services (a name to tame intervention) as a system problem is useful. Having families facing such problems write letters of complaint to appropriate change agents, including legislators, empowers families and adds support and legitimacy to all efforts to improve systems. Some families can write such letters without help, others need help writing, and some need the letters written for them. Finally, encouraging political action at all levels, from inviting legislators to speak to families to helping register families to vote, was an important part of the FRIENDS systems of care and MCSS action strategies.

The Colon Family: A Case Example

This family has two youngsters: Jason, who was 8 years old at the time of referral, and his 13-year-old half sister, Lizette. Jason was referred first. He lives with his mother Maria C., a 48-year-old white woman, in a one-bedroom apartment in one of the more dangerous and semideserted areas of Mott Haven. Joseph H., Jason's 50-year-old African American father, currently lives nearby. Both parents were thought to be former heroin addicts; this was not admitted by either. The marriage of these two was very much on again, off again, and at the time of the referral, they were separated. This separation was reported by the mother to be permanent, as she had "had enough of the father's abuse." The mother was employed by a needle exchange program and has since had several similar jobs. The father is on disability and now helps with child care.

Jason was referred to the MCSS by his school.

He suffers from a genetic disorder that makes him unusual in appearance and can cause severe hyperactivity. Jason was given to darting out of the classroom and school. More problematic, he was fascinated with electrical plugs, and the teacher had to be constantly alert to the possibility that Jason would try to put pencils and other objects into a classroom plug. He had already succeeded in shorting out the electricity at the school. According to his mother, only one or two of the plugs in the apartment worked because he had shorted them out, or she had been forced to block them. Although considered dangerous to himself and others, Jason was not deemed at immediate risk of placement in a psychiatric hospital. He was, however, considered at sufficient risk of removal from his home that an intensive intervention seemed appropriate.

Mrs. C. made it clear when first contacted that she wanted Jason placed and was only seeking services to get a psychiatric evaluation to facilitate this. She was reluctant to invite the team to her home because of her shame at the damage created by Jason. The initial work involved hearing her story, honoring her desire to receive services in the office, affirming her strengths, and hearing her ideas (see figure 26-5). Three team members were initially assigned to help: a nurse, a case aide, and the parent advocate.

Following the tri-level model, establishing safety became the first concern. The primary strategy involved a behavioral management task dubbed the STOP plan (Levine, 1997). This technique is to be used only when a child is involved in behaviors that are dangerous or hurtful to others in the parent's presence. The plan involves four steps based on the word "STOP":

S = Saying the word stop loud and with a hint of anger
T = Telling the child what to stop
O = Offering an acceptable alternative behavior
P = Physically intervening if necessary to force compliance and then praising the compliance

The mother had given up trying to control Jason's behavior, believing that efforts on her part were futile. Based on her relationship with the parent advocate, who formed a strong alliance from the first interview, Mrs. C. eventually agreed to permit team members to spend time at her apartment to demonstrate the STOP plan, a behavior management task. While the parent advocate took Jason and his mother out for breakfast, three team members gathered at the house to prepare for the demonstration. Having obtained Mrs. C.'s permission, the team moved the furniture and unblocked a number of plugs. Upon his return home, Jason spotted the changes and headed straight for a plug. The loudest staff person instantly commanded, "Jason, *stop* playing with that plug. It's dangerous. Play with the box." Jason stopped and looked up in surprise. He was instantly praised and then gently but forcibly led to "the box," a series of mechanical plugs, lights, and buzzers staff had devised hoping it would offer a safer alternative to the electric plugs. As Jason played with the box, he was praised and told this was a safe way to exercise his curiosity in mechanical things. Anytime Jason returned to a plug, the STOP plan was repeated. Mrs. C. eventually took over as the STOP commander. By the end of the day, she felt confident in her ability to keep Jason from playing with plugs. The STOP plan was augmented by teaching Mrs. C. a number of other behavioral tools, including catching and praising good behavior, use of a behavior chart, and time out for unacceptable behavior.

The success of the STOP strategy made the MCSS team and Mrs. C. partners. It was not long before Mrs. C. shared with the team her concerns regarding Lizette. Initially, she had claimed Lizette had no problems. It was not unusual for the MCSS, once an alliance has been established with the family, to discover siblings of the child initially referred to them also suffered from severe emotional distress. Once an alliance forged between Mrs. C. and the team, Mrs. C. described Lizette as being irritable and argumentative. Of more concern was that Lizette had run out of the apartment on a number of occasions, each time threatening to kill herself. On those occasions, she fled to her paternal grandmother's house and stayed there for several days.

When team members talked with Lizette, she was found to be severely depressed. She was actively contemplating suicide by taking some of her mother's pills. She felt abandoned by her birth father, Mrs. C.'s first husband. Mr. C. called sporadically but never visited. Lizette felt her mother cared only about Jason and wanted her daughter in the

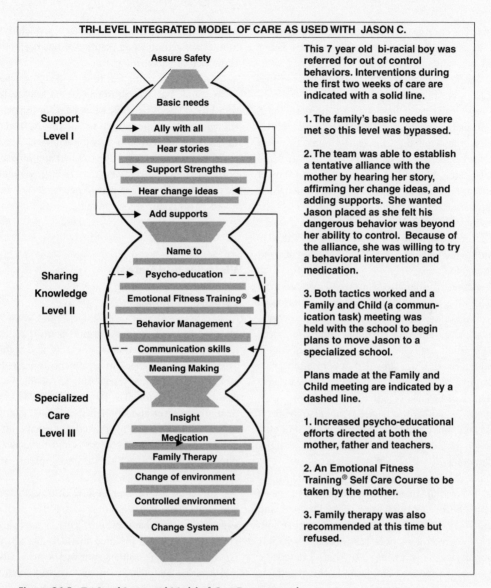

TRI-LEVEL INTEGRATED MODEL OF CARE AS USED WITH JASON C.

Assure Safety

Basic needs

Support Level I
- Ally with all
- Hear stories
- Support Strengths
- Hear change ideas
- Add supports

Name to

Sharing Knowledge Level II
- Psycho-education
- Emotional Fitness Training®
- Behavior Management
- Communication skills

Meaning Making

Specialized Care Level III
- Insight
- Medication
- Family Therapy
- Change of environment
- Controlled environment

Change System

This 7 year old bi-racial boy was referred for out of control behaviors. Interventions during the first two weeks of care are indicated with a solid line.

1. The family's basic needs were met so this level was bypassed.

2. The team was able to establish a tentative alliance with the mother by hearing her story, affirming her change ideas, and adding supports. She wanted Jason placed as she felt his dangerous behavior was beyond her ability to control. Because of the alliance, she was willing to try a behavioral intervention and medication.

3. Both tactics worked and a Family and Child (a communication task) meeting was held with the school to begin plans to move Jason to a specialized school.

Plans made at the Family and Child meeting are indicated by a dashed line.

1. Increased psycho-educational efforts directed at both the mother, father and teachers.

2. An Emotional Fitness Training® Self Care Course to be taken by the mother.

3. Family therapy was also recommended at this time but refused.

Figure 26.5. Tri-Level Integrated Model of Care Demonstrated

home only to babysit. Lizette was tearful during the initial interview but agreed to a safety contract and to see the team psychiatrist.

At the psychiatric evaluation, Lizette's three wishes included spending time with her birth father, having a room of her own, and spending time with other girls her age. Mrs. C. had told the team she thought the father was living in a flophouse in lower Manhattan and was addicted to heroin. She did not want this information shared with her daughter. In helping Lizette make a different mean-

ing of her father's absence, staff explained that it sounded as if he just did not have the strength to be the kind of father she wanted at the moment, nor was it clear why. She shared her idea he might be sick. The parent advocate agreed, saying it might be a physical illness or some kind of mental illness. Later on during an outing, the case aide was able to share that her own father had never been in her life, and she had finally decided it was her father's loss; she had to get on with her life without his support. The case aide's self-disclosure brought tears to Lizette's eyes but also marked the beginning of her ability to stop idealizing her absent father and fantasying his return.

Several possibilities for meeting her other two wishes were discussed, including buying a screen to block off part of the living room or buying a bunk bed in an effort to give her some private space. She liked the idea of the bunk bed and claimed the top bunk as her private retreat. Some shelves were placed high on the wall, and part of the bunk bed was enclosed. These efforts delighted Lizette. She was also signed up for an art class she was interested in taking; she was taught a number of self-soothing skills; she was referred to FRIENDS Youth Leadership program; finally, she was referred for ongoing therapy.

Helping this family involved tasks drawn from each of the tri-level model's levels. In addition to those described above involving allying, hearing change ideas, affirming strengths, adding supports, self-soothing, and meaning making, psychoeducation information was provided to both Jason's parents and his school. The parents also learned a number of EFT skills, Jason was placed on medication, the mother was helped to hold family meetings and family and child team meetings, and Mrs. C. and her daughter were referred for conjoint counseling.

As the MCSS intervention ended, the family was referred for ongoing case management, Jason to the FRIENDS Homework Help Program and Youth Connection Programs, and the mother continued to receive services from FRIENDS Family Support. Lizette was referred to Youth Leadership. That was 3 years ago, and Jason is doing well. He is in a good special education program, is properly medicated, and attends the Youth Connection, Homework Help, FRIENDS Connection, and various other special programs at FRIENDS. He is accepted by the other youth served in the agency. Although it is possible that because of his appearance major difficulties lie ahead as he enters adolescence, he is stable and doing well within the protective circle of his special extended family. Hopefully, his strong connections at FRIENDS will serve to buffer him from any difficulties he faces as an adolescent.

Lizette eventually moved in with her paternal grandmother but stays connected to the FRIENDS Youth Leadership program and periodically comes to the FRIENDS Family Connection. She and her mother are getting along better. She has been told about her father's many problems.

Mrs. C. is working full-time, and she and her ex-husband have established a "friendly relationship." They are both involved in Sharing Knowledge workshops and attend the FRIENDS Connection, and have also become politically active to the point where they have testified at a number of fact-finding hearings. Mrs. C. sees FRIENDS and its various MCSS staff as part of her family. As she noted, "This is our second home."

Victories and Defeats

FRIENDS Outcomes

Starting new programs is difficult. Starting a new agency, combining five new programs, and incorporating major changes in treatment approaches and governance while researching the whole process begs description. The fact that FRIENDS ultimately came to be and still remains a growing force in Mott Haven speaks to its victory over its difficulties. The fact that the MCSS is and remains an important part of the FRIENDS systems of care speaks to the MCSS's success.

Success is always a process, with times of forward movement and times of retreat. FRIENDS has experienced its share of problems. Established community agencies resented the idea that a new community mental health agency was being created and funded. Each felt the money would be better spent improving existing agencies. Because of these concerns, the Mott Haven Agenda for Children Tomorrow, an active political force for Mott Haven residents and service providers, withdrew support from the project. Other community leaders joined forces to block referrals. The local school board was particularly active in this protest movement, and school principals were told not to permit FRIENDS into the school for outreach and not to refer families to FRIENDS.

Efforts to find adequate housing for the program bogged down because of a dispute between the landlord and the funder. For the initial 5 years of service, case management and respite and recreation were located in separate buildings, while

FRIENDS and the MCSS operated out of inadequate quarters in a third-floor walk-up.

Leadership changes have been problematic. Some of those changes have involved changing leadership at the state level. As the program was starting up, a new governor was elected, and the various commissioners involved in developing the Mott Haven project moved on to new jobs. All those involved in creating the project, including the initial grant writers, research personnel, and proposed state-level overseers, also moved to new jobs. After 2.5 years, the director at FRIENDS also moved to a new job. It was nearly a year before a new director was hired. Finally, difficulties existed in terms of the various service providers. The case management program had five changes of leadership during the 7 years of the demonstration project. The Family Support and Youth Leadership programs saw three leadership changes. Of the initial service providers, only the VNSNY had stable leadership and currently is the only service to remain under contract to FRIENDS.

Despite these difficulties, FRIENDS exists, now located conveniently and in an attractive space with rooms for its programs and for community meetings and workshops. Positive relationships have been established with the school board, with 52% of the referrals coming from the local schools. The fact that 31% of referrals are made by families speaks to the success of FRIENDS within the community.

Positive relationships have been established with an important array of community service providers. The executive director of FRIENDS is a cochair of the ACT Collaborative. The director of visiting nurse service programs at FRIENDS chairs the ACT Collaborative Community Building Committee and is cochair of the Bronx Borough Based Council. The council is one of a number of similar councils established with consumers throughout New York State in an effort to further the development of systems of care approaches. Cochairs attend a citywide oversight committee that is also attended by a variety of high-level city and state officials.

MCSS Outcomes

To date the MCSS has served nearly 900 families and children. As measured by the follow-up sur-

veys, consumer satisfaction runs high: 91% of the families report being satisfied or very satisfied with the services. Improvement in symptoms related to the reason for referral was noted in 80% of the youth served. Other outcomes such as hospitalization and placement rates have also been positive, although a growing number of youngsters have been hospitalized during recent months. The increase is thought to be due to the willingness of referral sources to refer more disturbed youngsters to the MCSS. That may or may not be the case. Although many funders measure success by reduction in psychiatric hospitalization, the MCSS believes this ignores an important fact. Safety is risked if clinicians are being rated on hospitalization rates. Success should be determined by whether or not avoiding hospitalization is in the best interest of the child and whether it occurs as an unplanned or unjustified hospitalization.

Systems of Care Outcomes

Finally, the victories and defeats of the MCSS and FRIENDS cannot be completely separated from the systems of care movement. According to the 1997 System of Care Annual Report to Congress, the overall systems of care outcomes have been mixed (U.S. Department of Health and Human Services, 1997). Initial findings as measured by symptom and functional scales did not exceed care provided by more traditional services, while functional outcomes have shown notable improvements. However, as English (2002) noted:

> Findings indicated notable improvements for children after one year of service, including (1) reductions in law enforcement contacts, (2) improved grades and fewer absences from school, (3) improved behavioral functioning, and (4) more stable living arrangements achieved. Furthermore, after 1 year in services 71% of the children's caregivers were "satisfied" or "very satisfied" with their children's progress. (p. 307)

The initial outcomes of both FRIENDS and MCSS were included in these findings. MCSS consumer satisfaction ratings have consistently been in the 90% rating for "satisfied" or "very satisfied."

Lessons Learned in Building Community-Based Clinical Practice

Lesson 1: Use the Start-Up Period Wisely

New programs are graced with a start-up period. Time is needed to hire, train, and bring staff on board with the program's vision and goals; develop and establish practice procedures, paperwork, and accountability documentation; find and furnish space; and, finally, do the social marketing necessary to gain referrals. Taking advantage of this time is vital. FRIENDS did not hit the ground running. The mission was not articulated, specific goals and objectives were not clearly communicated to service providers, accountability including paperwork was not in place, and office space for the program had not been obtained.

Starting with practice procedures and accountability documentation in place would have been wiser. Then, when something was not working, collaboration and negotiation could have been brought into play to make needed changes. Such an approach would have been similar to the type of one text negotiation employed in hammering out the Camp David Accords. In that type of negotiation one party draws up the plan and then asks the other participants for revisions. The revisions are combined and used to develop a second one-text plan. The process is repeated until all agree (Fisher & Ury, 1983).

For example, one hope of the project was to pilot the use of a unified record—a record the family could have, and that would follow the child from service to service. The hopes for such a record were to prevent duplication, to eliminate the need for families to tell their stories over and over again, and to reduce paperwork for service providers. This hope was never fulfilled. A unified record might exist now if, during the start-up period, a record had been put together that met various state regulations, as well as the families' desires. Before the doors were opened to receive clients, service providers could have been told that this was the record of choice and given an opportunity to criticize and suggest change, but with the expectation that by the start-up of services this was the record that would be used by all. Service providers were asked to create such a record only after services had begun and never came to an agreement as to what should go in the record.

Lesson 2: Market and Sell Services During the Start-Up Period by Stretching Eligibility Criteria

A steady flow of consumers is essential for the success for any endeavor. In the human services field too many new programs fail to attract clients because of rigid adherence to eligibility criteria. It is particularly important during start-up to figure out how to say yes when a family or youth does not meet the eligibility criteria. For the MCSS this meant expanding the definition of risk during the start-up phase. Traditional definitions of risk generally referred to someone actively suicidal, homicidal, or dangerously psychotic. During the start-up period, this definition of risk was expanded to deal with youngsters displaying lesser symptoms of psychosis, murderous intent, or suicide. The MCSS also accepted several 4-year-olds into care during the start-up period.

A second way the MCSS stretched the eligibility requirement during the start-up phase was to agree to work with some situations in which the problem was probably not the child's serious emotional distress but a stressful family situation. To maintain research fidelity, stretching the eligibility criteria needs to be carefully monitored and seen as a start-up strategy only. The MCSS was able to stop stretching eligibility criteria after 5 months.

Lesson 3: Strategize to Include Silenced Voices

At the same time one is starting strong, it is equally important to privilege the quieter voices. This is particularly important when attempting to partner with families. Professional and expert voices are accustomed to dominating. Encouraging the setting aside of those voices so the family and youth voices could emerge challenged all. Adding to this challenge was the fact that all change ventures require certainty in order to gain acceptance. When new ways challenge old ways, most cling to the old ways. This plays into the natural tendency to polarize and assume an either/or stance that too often leads to blaming others rather then seeking solutions.

Clinical staff worried about families' refusal to follow best practice guidelines. As one staff member asked, "Should we just let a child commit suicide because the parents don't think she is depressed?"

Another staff member noted, "So we let the child fail because the mother doesn't believe in medication when we know it is what make the difference?" The answer to both questions is no. Collaboration does not mean submerging one voice at the expense of another. It means hearing all voices.

One way to strengthen the less heard voices is to hire staff, including clinicians, who have been there and done that. The MCSS sought to hire staff who were parents, lived in or near Mott Haven, grew up in Mott Haven, had a relative who lived in Mott Haven, had a relative who suffered from serious emotional distress, or had been involved in mental health treatment of one form or another. Such staff are generally more family-friendly and less likely to stigmatize serious emotional distress. Such staff also can join with families and youth with greater authenticity than someone who has not experienced such life stressors. While not essential, such experience, particularly in a climate of respect for families and the struggles facing those living with serious emotional stress, improves services. If a team member can say, "My brother has been hospitalized," "I've had therapy," or "I grew up around the corner," it usually opens a door for families and youth to feel more comfortable entering the conversation.

Top-down modeling was an essential ingredient in building staff comfort and disclosing how staff's personal experiences were in one way or another similar to those facing family and youth. When the program director causally dropped into a conversation how she had felt as a child when her family was evicted from their home, jaws dropped, but the director used this opportunity to open discussion on the importance of well-planned and thoughtful self-disclosures in building alliances.

Administration and clinical staff found it particularly difficult to let go of their knowledge in order to privilege family voices. Administration worried about diminished professionalism. Three strategies reduced these worries: (1) The VNSNY had in place a generous reimbursement schedule for ongoing training. A number of MCSS employees have been able to move forward educationally because of these benefits. (2) Because of concern about maintaining clinical professionalism, the director of Community Mental Health Services (CMHS) at the VNSNY established a CMHS University. All CMHS employees are required to complete its 4 days of training. The curriculum includes establishing safety, learning the ins and outs of the *DSM-IV,* and learning to writing clinically effective reports. (3) Finally, maintaining a supervisory ratio of one clinically sound supervisor to no more than four staff also eased administrative concerns.

A number of other strategies also proved pivotal in allowing all voices to be heard. One was absolute transparency about when clinical knowledge would be privileged and when family wishes would predominate. Families and youth were told from day one that safety was the MCSS's primary concern, and once we deemed all were safe, family and youth preferences took over. Teaching families what we considered a safety issue, as well as the use of the "What We Think" handouts, helped with this task.

Yet another strategy for including parental voices was to use round-robin instead of popcorn processing at every meeting. In popcorn processing people speak at random; this often means the strongest voice dominates. Round-robin processing requires that each participant be asked to contribute. No one is forced to speak, and passing is possible, but each person must be asked to contribute. Sometimes it might take a number of go-rounds before previously silenced voices would choose to enter the conversation, but without round-robin processing such voices might never be heard.

Lesson 4: Satisfy Your Customers

The need to include silenced voices is also involved in the issue of consumer satisfaction. Quality work based on consumer satisfaction demands being clear about expectations, measuring performance, checking outcomes, and dealing with problems. This means speaking up and encouraging others—staff and consumers—to speak up rather then assuming all is well. People who do not speak up are on what management consultant Hersey (1988) calls a bus trip to Abilene—too many people going where they don't want to go because everyone keeps quiet for fear of offending one or another person.

VNSNY emphasizes pleasing customers. Customer means not only those thought of traditionally as patients or clients but also funders, the people who supervise you, the people you supervise, referral sources, and those who work with you. As part of this focus, VNSNY staff are trained to view all service requests the way a concierge at a hotel views a request for help. The customer must leave the hotel satisfied. For families and youth this means whether they are receiving a full array of services or a quick assessment and referral to another service, all parties, at the end of an intervention, need to feel the MCSS had done all that could be done to help. When dealing with a stigmatized service such as mental health services, this is particularly important.

However, for oppressed minorities, speaking up to authority has always held dangers. Staff, as well as families and youth, when asked about satisfaction with services, preferred "going along to get along" to being direct about what was working and what was not. As one valued and trusted staff member noted during a VNSNY code of honor training that encourages reporting of wrongdoing, "I don't want to be responsible for getting someone fired. If I know someone is doing something wrong, I won't report them. Administration has to catch them, not me."

Realizing the power of such constraints doubled for families and youth was one reason the MCSS undertook to develop a consumer progress note (see figure 26-6). The note was developed by the staff and used to record all face-to-face contacts with the primary caregiver. The note measures not only goal progress but also consumer satisfaction. The original note is placed in the chart, and a copy is given to the family. A parallel effort to encourage staff openness regarding the usefulness of supervision was instituted at the same time. Both notes successfully served to encourage families and staff to become more open about complaints.

Although initially reluctant, staff and managers ultimately found the use of such a note improved their ability to provide family-sensitive services. Staff's primary unhappiness with the note was that the consumer satisfaction components tended to become rote. At the same time, there was an immediate awareness of when a family was not satisfied, as apparent in comments such as "Forced me to listen more, and I knew if a family was not satisfied" and "I got my recording done on time."

Administrative staff found the forms extremely useful in tracking staff time and accountability. Most important, families were pleased with this type of recording. Caregiver comments included the following:

"I could see how my child was doing visit by visit."
"I could prove to my other worker [a child welfare staff person] that I was working hard to help my child get better."
"I felt respected and like my ideas mattered."

Following the demonstration project, staff and administration elected to continue using the consumer progress note. In addition, other accountability efforts also kept the MCSS on target. These included focus groups, audits, and end-of-service consumer surveys.

Lesson 5: Ethical Behavior Safeguards All Family Members

Prevailing clinical wisdom often views seeing clients as family as an invitation to boundary violations. Families, youth, and nonclinical staff had fewer difficulties with the idea of becoming part of a larger extended family than did clinical staff. MCSS management believed boundaries were not the issue, but that ethical behavior was. All families face boundary issues. All families deal with what is proper behavior in close and distant relationships. Healthy families know which lines are never to be crossed.

Nevertheless, for some, the concept "We are family" felt dangerous. Two strategies helped ease such concerns. One was transparency—the willingness to take an open stance about relationship expectations and about roles. Staff were family, but they were extended family, living apart. The roles were seen as similar to those of distant family members with specialized knowledge, such as a cousin who also happens to be a plumber and can be relied on to fix a stopped drain when asked to by members of his extended family, or one who joins the family again when invited to celebrate milestones or holidays. Such relatives come when invited, are delighted to be part of the family, enjoy helping, love celebrating, expect little beyond a thank-you in return, never overstay their welcome, and live separate lives.

The second strategy was the use of thoughtful supervision regarding appropriate and ethical behavior. Because so much of the work done by all the VNSNY happens in people's homes, the agency is particularly attuned to the potential for taking advantage of service consumers' vulnerability and

```
F.R.I.E.N.D.S                                              Primary Caregiver's Progress Note

Youth's name    Jason C            Primary Caregiver's name   Marta C           ID#  F292
Date 5/22/2001       Length  1.5     Location     Home  Wrap funds: 12.50 for purchase of snacks
```

Reason for referral: **Dangerous and out of control behavior**   Occurred **10 Xs a day**   Occurs **10 Xs a day**

Check number you feel is closest to the truth: 5 is true, 3 is true some of the time, 1 is not true at all.		
(1) My child got along well at home. 1 2 3 x 4 5	(4) My child was happy. 1 2 3 x 4 5	
(2) My child did well in school. 1 2 3 4 x 5	(5) My child is doing better. 1 2 3 4 x 5	
(3) My child stayed calm. 1 2 3 4 5 x	(6) I worked on my goals. 1 2 3 4 x 5	

Current goal(s): *Stop Jason's playing with electric plugs. Such behavior occurs at least ten times a day and when Mother forcibly stops him, Jason has a temper tantrum lasting 10 minutes. Today's goal demonstrates use of the STOP plan.*

What occurred during session: *Mom, parent advocate and Jason went to McDonald's. Rest of team stayed home and moved the furniture blocking plugs. When family returned, demonstrated use of STOP PLAN and repeated it until Mom took over. Mom implemented plan 3xs and stated, "I can't believe this worked." Reminded to use it only with the behavior related to electric plugs as overuse makes it less effective.*

Talked briefly about holding a family meeting to begin preparations for a Family and Child Meeting with the school.

Next steps: *Mom will continue to use the STOP plan. Team will return on Friday and will hold a family meeting. Mother will invite father and daughter to attend this meeting. Case aide will visit Thursday to reinforce STOP Plan with Jason. Mom needs someone to help her with Jason's medical appointment. Parent advocate will accompany her. Case Manager will schedule meeting with school.*

Consumer Feedback Rating Scales:
Circle number you feel is closest to the truth: 5 is true, 3 is true some time, 1 is not true.

(1) I was listened to 1 2 3 4 5 x	(3) My strengths were recognized 1 2 3 4 5 x
(2) I could talk about my concerns 1 2 3 4 5 x	(4) I helped decide what to do 1 2 3 4 5 x

Consumer signature   Read by consumer __X_ Read to consumer____

Staff signature/Title
Date   Supervisor signature

Staff Safety /Risk of Removal Rating:
Circle number you feel is closest to the truth: 5 is high risk, 3 is some risk, 1 is no risk.
Self 1   2   3   4 x 5 Others 1   2   3 x 4 5   Home 1 2 x 3 4 5 School 1 2 3 4 x 5

Figure 26.6. The Consumer Progress Note

trust. Part of the Visiting Nurse Service code of honor training involves a clear articulation of how to handle the ins and outs of being a guest in someone else's home. For example, staff are allowed to accept small gifts as tokens of appreciation but are never to accept cash tips. Finally, the agency also offers sexual harassment training, which proved useful in discussing the importance of being attuned to inappropriately sexualized behavior between staff and clients. For example, in many cultures family members are greeted with a hug and a

kiss on the cheek. Not accepting a hug when it is offered is seen as rejecting. Offering a hug, on the other hand, is less appropriate. So is a kiss on the lips. Open discussion of such issues and permission to air concerns keep everyone safe.

Lesson 6: Attend to Staff Morale

Because of the inherent difficulties in start-up programs and in working with the seriously emotionally distressed, attending to staff morale is essential.

One of the benefits of requiring all MCSS staff to become licensed Emotional Fitness Trainers (EFT) and to take an EFT self-care course has been the side benefit of maintaining MCSS staff morale. A core aspect of the Self-Care Course is the practice of a daily Emotional Fitness Program that consists of 12 exercises (Levine, 1997). Staff are encouraged to practice each of these exercises (see figure 26-5).

One exercise focuses on what is working—Practice Gratitude. Five focus specifically on self-care—Be With Beauty, Move Your Body, Laugh, Indulge in a Healthy Pleasure, and Make Something. Finally, the remaining exercises focus on dealing with difficulty—Remembering What Is Important, Practicing Kindness, Remembering Someone Who Cared, Practicing Forgiveness of Others, and Practicing Forgiveness of Self. To encourage their use, Emotional Fitness exercises are practiced at a staff meeting, nonoffensive jokes are posted on the bulletin board, and inspirational sayings are posted around the office. In addition, staff and families are offered a variety of Emotional Fitness outings, including Move Your Body workshops featuring various physical fitness exercises and Be With Beauty Walks.

MCSS staff morale and loyalty have been consistently high. Staff see themselves as family, and turnover has been minimal, and then only when better advancement opportunities or higher salaries were offered. Staff who have left maintain contact, work per diem, and when their new jobs permit, attend staff events and celebrations, as well as various FRIENDS events.

Lesson 7: Work to Reduce the Stigma Attached to Serious Emotional Distress

According to Kessler (1994), at one time or another 50% of the population suffers from one or another mental illness—a figure many dispute and find shocking. Kessler, however, believes that if he said 99.9% of the population had been physically ill at some time in their life, no one would be shocked. Therefore, it should not be surprising that 50% of the population has been mentally ill at some time in their life. Kessler sees the reason for this as the investment of the phrase "mentally ill" with negative meaning.

The MCSS joined in a number of efforts to reduce the stigma attached to mental illness. The use of Emotional Fitness Training® programs helped with this task in a number of ways. One was the emphasis on the idea that emotional health impacts physical health, as inversely physical health impacts emotional health. Similarly, the linking of EFT to the idea of physical fitness training further normalized emotional problems. Finally, the fact that everyone involved with the child, including MCSS staff, family members, classmates, and teachers, learned the core EFT skills normalized the idea that everyone needs to strengthen the ability to manage stress and other negative feelings.

This idea was further emphasized during consultations. Many consultations consisted of self-care workshops directed toward staff of various providers within the community, as well as foster parents, child care staff, and teachers. Particularly popular were appreciation sessions involving self-soothing skills, including aromatherapy.

Another way serious emotional distress was normalized was having staff at a consultation site involved in programs offered youth. In one successful intervention in a school, two youngsters involved in bullying were matched with less troubled youngsters in a workshop called Young Ladies of Strong Feelings. The school social worker co-led the group, and two teachers participated with the youth and MCSS staff as "people with strong feelings." The 6-week workshop not only helped the bullies but, according to the involved teachers, changed the atmosphere in the school.

Lesson 8: Work to Change Conditions Creating Serious Emotional Distress

Mott Haven's high level of crime, unhealthy air, overcrowding, and lack of green space contribute to our families and youths' distress. Although many families manage to stay healthy and to raise healthy children in such communities, those continuously bombarded by one trauma after another do not fare so well. The more the stress of a community affects a family, the greater the likelihood one or another family member will suffer from symptoms of serious emotional distress. All our work is in vain if we do not also work to change the conditions that stress our families and our youth.

Both VNSNY programs at FRIENDS have been active in community efforts to reduce the level of crime and violence through the Camino de Paz/

Peace Walks Labyrinth project. A labyrinth is similar to a maze but has no blind turns or dead ends (see figure 26-7). Following a labyrinth's path takes you to the center and back (Curry, 2000).

The Camino de Paz project originated as an outgrowth of the R&R team's efforts to teach some of the children a walking meditation. A portable labyrinth was created and then taken by various VNSNY programs to a number of street fairs. The project now has a larger canvas labyrinth and three permanent outdoor labyrinths. Most have been built with community help and input by the families and youth the VNSNY have served at FRIENDS. The project also provides conflict resolution workshops run by the MCSS consultation teams. The workshops are held at the labyrinths and in local schools.

Ultimately, this project lent support to other community efforts to transform Mott Haven's image from one of violence. Community leaders sought to attract visitors from outside of Mott Haven. Because labyrinths are often a tourist attraction, the Camino de Paz project has served to attract some visitors to the area. The labyrinths also have been used by community leaders as one focus for special community events.

Lesson 9: Expensive Programs Work, but Costs Are High and Sustainability Difficult

As indicated previously, the MCSS program is successful. Families believe so, staff believe so, and referral sources believe so. Youth and family stress decrease; youths' symptoms decrease; family and youth functioning improves. However, the cost of this success is high. The annual budget for both VNSNY programs at FRIENDS is $851.157.82. Of that, $29,655.44 goes directly to families as wraparound dollars. Salaries for both programs add up to $548,811.86. The cost of the psychiatrist and nurse combined are $160,417.14. Even with what seems like a generous budget, the MCSS salaries are lower than comparable city and state salaries. Recruiting staff is difficult because of salary differentials, program location, the nature of the work, and the need to hire Spanish-speaking staff. The upside is that staff who do come aboard are committed to the work, and staff commitment is an important ingredient in the MCSS successes. Currently, all costs, except for involvement in the Camino de Paz project, which is supported by private donations, are funded through FRIENDS by the New York State Office of Mental Health (NY-

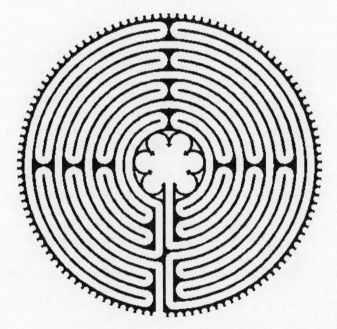

Figure 26.7. A Labyrinth

SOMH). The contract for continuing the services comes up for renewal yearly. The NYSOMH is eager to find others to share the funding. Hopefully, the successes of the program will be built on and not lost.

In achieving sustainability, one must serve the designated population and serve it well. One must also prove one serves the designated population well. As indicated by consumer satisfaction and other measures of success, the MCSS not only has served the designated population but has served it well. Unfortunately, the successes do not meet evidenced-based practice criteria that involves control groups and replication.

Meeting evidenced-based practice would require ongoing research funding, which is not currently available. Data are being collected but not systematically analyzed. In addition to attempting to include consumer voices in the treatment process, the consumer progress note was specifically designed with the hope that it would provide a user-friendly research tool for consumers and service providers. The consumer progress notes are data rich. Staff use the information to guide services, but the ability to systematically analyze the data requires more time and more research-specific knowledge than is currently available at either FRIENDS or VNSNY.

The difficulty of systematically analyzing data is not an uncommon one for most service providers. As one participant in the Chinesegut Out Retreat at the University of South Florida reported: "Service information is there. I mean, it's in the child's record. Now, how you do you extract it? What do you do with it? A lot of it depends on your staff" (Hernandez, Hodges, Nesman, & Ringeisen, 2001, p. 16.)

A lot also depends on finding sources of funding for ongoing research efforts. Once federal funds are withdrawn from a grant site, research capabilities are also withdrawn. As a result, fidelity to the original model begins to fade; equally important, the opportunity for long-term follow-up is lost. The MCSS has watched its youth mature and age. Some of our youth have been part of the FRIENDS extended family since we opened. Some of them have only moved beyond their problems as they have moved into their 20s. Some of the youth who were helped when they were 6 or 7 now need intensive help getting through adolescence. Becoming all you can become is a process that takes far longer than the few years involved in systems of grant funding for outcome research.

Finally, sustainability also depends on maintaining positive relationships with funders. The tri-level model's Support and Sharing Knowledge levels provide as useful a strategic guide when applied to funders as when applied to families and youth. The most important strategy has always been to provide gold standard services to the population the funders pay to be served. Other strategies include sharing knowledge by giving presentations at various national, state, and local sites; information sharing through monthly reports discussing both successes and concerns; and, finally, offering support to the funders in the form of serving on various committees, providing training to other programs, and recruiting family members to tell their stories to legislators. Hopefully, this will be sufficient to sustain this valuable community-based clinical service in a way that meets the needs of the Mott Haven community, its families, and its youth.

Lesson 10: Change Is Possible

Change comes slowly, and the broader the changes sought, the slower the progress. Nevertheless, the more good people of good intent work together, the more inevitable the positive progress. Caring works. When the caring extends to the community, its effectiveness multiplies.

When we step out of our offices and walk the streets leading to a family's home, we see more. When we enter a home to visit one of our families, we know more. When we are with our families for more then a 50-minute hour, we understand more. The more we understand, the more we can help others understand. Our work cannot stop with our families, for we must carry our knowledge back to the world of politicians and policymakers, hear their stories, and support their efforts. As we reach out into the community and back to the power brokers, our connection grows, and we better understand we are all of the same family. We see that our differences are small when measured against the sameness of desires, hopes, and experiences. The stronger our connections, the deeper our desire to help one another, the broader our capacity to do so.

References

Armstrong, B. (1978). The president's commission on mental health: A summary of recommendations. *Hospital and Community Psychiatry, 29*(7), 468–474.

Beardslee, W. R. (1986). The need for the study of adaptation in the children of parents with affective disorders. In M. Rutter, C. Izard, & P. Read (Eds.), *Depression in young people: Developmental and clinical perspectives* (pp. 189–204). New York: Guilford.

Bronfenbrenner, U. (1979). *The ecology of human development: Experiments by nature and design.* Cambridge, MA: Harvard University Press.

Brown, G., Harris, T., & Bifulco, A. (1986). Long-term effects of early loss of parent. In M. Rutter, C. Izard, & P. Read (Eds.), *Depression in young people: Developmental and clinical perspectives* (pp. 251–296). New York: Guildford.

Burns, B., Compton, S., Egger, H., Farmer, E., & Robertson, E. (2002). An annotated review of the evidence base for psychosocial and psychopharmacological interventions for children with selected disorders. In B. Burns & K. Hoagwood (Eds.), *Community treatment for youth* (pp. 212–276). New York: Oxford University Press.

Coe, F. (Producer), & Penn, A. (Director). (1962). *The Miracle Worker* [Motion picture]. United States: MGM/UA Studios.

Curry, H. (2000). *The way of the labyrinth.* New York: Penguin Compass.

Duchinowski, A., Kutash, K., & Friedman, R. (2002). Community-based interventions in a system of care and outcomes framework. In B. Burns & K. Hoagwood (Eds.), *Community treatment for youth* (pp. 16–38). New York: Oxford University Press.

Duncan, B., Miller, S., & Sparks, J. (2000). *The heroic client: Doing client-directed, outcome-informed therapy.* San Francisco: Jossey-Bass.

English, M. (2002). Policy implications relevant to implementing evidence-based treatment. In B. Burns & K. Hoagwood, (Eds.), *Community treatment for youth* (pp. 301–326). New York: Oxford University Press.

Evans, M., Boothroyd, R., & Armstrong, M. (1997). Outcomes of three children's psychiatric emergency programs. *Journal of Emotional and Behavioral Disorders, 5,* 93–105.

Evans. M., Boothroyd, R., & Armstrong, M. (1999). *Outcomes of an experimental study of the effectiveness of intensive in-home crisis services for children and their families: Final report.* Tampa: Center for Nursing Research, University of South Florida.

Farber, A., & Mazlish, E. (1980). *How to talk so kids will listen.* New York: Avon Books.

Fisher, R., & Ury, W. (1983). *Getting to yes: Negotiating agreement without giving.* New York: Penguin.

Friesen, B., & Stephens, B. (1998). Expanding family roles in the system of care: Research and practice. In M. H. Epstein, K. Kutush, & A. Duchnowski (Eds.), *Outcomes for children and youth with behavioral and emotional disorders: Programs and evaluation best practices* (pp. 231–259). Austin, TX: Pro-Ed.

Garbarino, J. (1995). *Raising children in a socially toxic environment.* San Francisco: Jossey-Bass.

Garbarino, J. (1998). Finding meaning in a socially toxic environment. *Reaching Today's Children, 2*(2), 27–30.

Garbarino, J. (1999). *Lost boys: Why our sons turn violent and how we can save them.* New York: Free Press.

Garmezy, N. (1986). Developmental aspects of children's responses to the stress of separation and loss. In M. Rutter, C. Izard, & P. Read (Eds.), *Depression in young people: Developmental and clinical perspectives* (pp. 297–324). New York: Guildford.

Gergen, K. (1994). *Realities and relationships: Soundings in social construction.* Cambridge, MA: Harvard University Press.

Germain, C. (1991). *Human behavior in the social environment: An ecological view.* New York: Columbia University Press.

Goleman, D. (1995). *Emotional intelligence.* New York: Bantam Books.

Gordon, T. (1975). *Parent effectiveness training.* New York: NAL Dutton.

Haley, J. (1997). *Leaving home: The therapy of disturbed young people* (2nd ed.). New York: Taylor and Francis.

Henggeler, S., Schoenwald, S., Borduin, C., Rowland, D., & Cunningham, P. (Eds.). (1998). *Multisystemic treatment of antisocial behavior in children and adolescents.* New York: Guilford.

Hernandez, M., Hodges, S., Nesman, T., & Ringeisen, H. (2001). Findings from the Chinesegut Outcomes Retreat. In M. Hernandez & S. Hodges (Eds.), *Developing outcome strategies in children's mental health* (pp. 3–20). Baltimore: Brookes.

Hersey, J. (1988). *The Abilene paradox and other meditations on management.* New York: Wiley.

James, B. (1989). *Treating traumatized children: New insights and creative interventions.* New York: Lexington Books.

Joint Commission on Mental Health of Children. (1969). *Crisis in child mental health: Challenge for the 1970s.* New York: Harper and Row.

Kagan, J. (1984). *The nature of the child*. New York: Basic Books.

Kessler, R. (1994). Lifetime and 12-month prevalence of DSM-III-R psychiatric disorders in the United States: Results from the National Co-morbidity Study. *Archives of General Psychiatry, 51*, 8–19.

Kessler, R. (2000). Posttraumatic stress disorder: The burden to the individual and to society. *Journal of Clinical Psychiatry, 61*(Suppl. 5), 4–12.

Kinney, J., Haapala, D., & Booth, C. (1991). *Keeping families together: The homebuilders model*. Hawthorne, NY: Aldine de Gruyter.

Knitzer J. (1982). *Unclaimed children: The failure of public responsibility to children and adolescents in need of mental health services*. Washington, DC: Children's Defense Fund.

Koop, C. E. (1987). *Surgeon General's report: Children with special health care needs*. Washington, DC: U.S. Department of Health and Human Services.

Kozol, J. (1995). *Amazing grace*. New York: Harper-Collins.

Lambert, M., & Bergin, A. (1994). The effectiveness of psychotherapy. In A. Bergin & S. Garfield (Eds.), *Handbook of psychotherapy and behavior change* (4th ed., pp. 141–150). New York: Wiley.

Levine, K. (1993). Memory books: Helping children cope with loss. *Caring Magazine, 12*(12), 71–73.

Levine, K. (1997). *Parents are people too: An Emotional Fitness Program for parents*. New York: Penguin.

Levine, K. (1999). F.R.I.E.N.D.S, Inc. Mobile Community Support Service: Building bridges between parents and schools (pp. 71–76). In National Resource Network for Child and Family Mental Health Services at the Washington Business Group on Health (Ed.), *Systems of care: Promising practices in children's mental health, 1998 Series* (Vol. 7). Washington, DC: Center for Effective Collaboration and Practice, American Institutes for Research.

Lightburn, A., & Black, R. (2001). The client as learner and the clinician as teacher: Working with an educational lens. *Smith College Studies in Social Work, 72*, 15–33.

Madsen, W. (1999). *Collaborative therapy with multistressed families: From old problems to new futures*. New York: Guilford.

McFarlane, W. (2002). *Multifamily groups in the treatment of severe psychiatric disorders*. New York: Guilford.

Meyer, C. H. (1983). The search for coherence. In C. H. Meyer (Ed.), *Clinical social work in the ecosystems perspective* (pp. 5–34). New York: Columbia University Press.

Miller, M., & Diao, J. (1987). Family friends: New resources for psychosocial care of chronically ill children in families. *Children's Health Care, 15*, 259–264.

Miller, S., Duncan, B., & Hubble, M. (1997). *Escape from Babel*. New York: Norton.

Morgan, A. (2000). *What is narrative therapy? An easy-to-read introduction*. Adelaide, Australia: Dulwich Center Publications.

Ogden, M., & Minton, K. (2000). Sensorimotor psychotherapy: One method for processing traumatic memory. *Traumatology, 6*(3), article 3.

Osher, T., de Fur, E., Nava, C., Spencer, S., & Toth-Dennis, D. (1999). New roles for families. In U.S. Center for Mental Health Services, Child, Adolescent, and Family Branch (pub.) *Systems of care: Promising practices in children's mental health, 1998 Series*. Rockville, MD: U.S. Department of Health and Human Services.

Perry, B. D. (2001). The neurodevelopmental impact of violence in childhood. In D. Schetky & E. Benedek (Eds.), *Textbook of child and adolescent forensic psychiatry* (pp. 221–238). Washington, DC: American Psychiatric Press.

Pinker, S. (1997). *How the mind works*. New York: Norton.

Potkay, C., & Allen, B. (1986). *Personality: Theory, research, and applications*. Monterey, CA: Brooks/Cole.

Schopler, E. (1971). Parents of psychotic children as scapegoats. *Journal of Contemporary Psychotherapy, 4*, 17–22.

Schorr, L. (1998). *Common purpose: Strengthening families and neighborhoods to rebuild America*. New York: Doubleday.

Schriebman, L. (1988). *Autism*. Newbury Park, CA: Sage.

Seikkula, J., Alakare, B., & Aaltonen, J. (2001). Open dialogue in psychosis I: An introduction and case illustration. *Journal of Constructivist Psychology, 14*, 247–265.

Stroul, B., & Friedman, R. (1994). *A system of care for children and youth with severe emotional disturbance* (rev. ed.). Washington, DC: Georgetown University Children Development Center, CASSP Technical Assistance Center.

Sunderland, J. (2002). Fit to go. *New Therapist, 17*, 28–29.

Terr, L. (1990). *Too scared to cry*. New York: Basic Books.

Thomas, A., & Chess, S. (1984). Genesis and evolution of behavioral disorders: From infancy to early adult life. *American Journal of Psychiatry, 141*, 1–9.

U.S. Department of Health and Human Services. (1997). *Annual report to Congress on the evaluation of the Comprehensive Community Mental Health*

Services for Children and Their Families Program. Atlanta, GA: Macro International.

U.S. Department of Health and Human Services. (1999). *Mental health: A report of the Surgeon General.* Rockville, MD: U.S. Department of Health and Human Services, Substance Abuse and Mental Health Services Administration, Center for Mental Health Services, National Institutes of Health, National Institute of Mental Health.

Van der Kolk, B., & Fisler, R. (1995). Dissociation and the fragmentary nature of traumatic memories: Overview and exploratory study. *Journal of Traumatic Stress, 8,* 505–525.

Van der Kolk, B., Van der Hart, O., & Burbridge, J. (1995). *Approaches to the treatment of PTSD* (Vol. 1). Washington, DC: Center for Effective Collaboration and Practice, American Institute for Research.

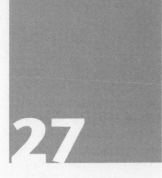

27

Steven Marans and Miriam Berkman

Police–Mental Health Collaboration on Behalf of Children Exposed to Violence
The Child Development–Community Policing Program Model

For too many children in the United States, exposure to interpersonal violence is part of the daily fabric of life. Violence affects children in their homes, their schools, and their neighborhoods. For example:

- In 1998, more than 2.7 million youths between the ages of 12 and 19 were victims of violent crime, including assault, rape, and robbery (Rennison, 1999).
- Children and adolescents are 4.5 times more likely than adults to be victims of serious crime (Centers for Disease Control, 1997).
- Each year, 1 million children are substantiated victims of abuse and neglect. At least 130,000 are sexually abused, and 2,000 die as a result of child abuse (Bash, 1997).

Many more children are witness to episodes of violence:

- It is estimated that between 3 and 17 million children per year witness a physical assault between their parents (Carlson, 2000).
- Young children are disproportionately affected by exposure to domestic violence. In a study of police records from five cities, children under the age of 5 were more likely to be pres-

ent at incidents of domestic violence and were more likely to be exposed multiple times within a 6-month period (Fantuzzo, Boruch, Beriama, & Atkins, 1997).

- A 1998 survey of 2,869 students in the 6th, 8th, and 10th grades in New Haven, Connecticut, demonstrated significant declines in children's exposure to violence compared with previous years; however, 50% of students reported seeing someone beaten or mugged, 24% reported seeing someone attacked or stabbed with a knife, 43% have seen someone seriously wounded, and 35% have seen someone shot at or shot with a gun (Schwab-Stone, Muyeed, & Voyce, 2000).

- In a survey of parents conducted in the pediatric primary care clinic at Boston City Hospital, 1 out of 10 reported their children had witnessed a shooting or a stabbing before the age of 6, half in the home and half in the community (Taylor, Zuckerman, Harik, & Groves, 1994).

It is well documented that exposure to interpersonal violence disrupts the basic preconditions for optimal child development. Children may be traumatized in the face of stabbings, beatings, and shootings because they are unable to contain the stimulation within existing psychological and neurophysiological structures. The disruption of psychological and biological systems may lead to symptoms of hyperarousal, withdrawal, and reexperiencing of traumatic events, or to circumscribed symptoms, such as disruptions in sleeping, eating, toileting, or separating (Boney-McCoy & Finkelhor, 1996; Foy & Goguen, 1998; Gorman-Smith & Tolan, 1998; Graham-Berman & Levendosky, 1998; Marans & Adelman, 1997; McCloskey & Walker, 2000; Pynoos, 1993). Children may become distracted and unable to concentrate, leading to difficulties at school. They may become irritable, aggressive, or oppositional, leading to difficulties in relationships with parents, teachers, and peers. Transient symptoms may represent the child's efforts to cope with anxiety and to reassert a sense of power and mastery in the face of feeling vulnerable and small.

When children are exposed to chronic violence, however, they may develop enduring symptoms and chronic maladaptations. Exposure to chronic violence has been associated with increased depression and anxiety, alcohol use, and lower school achievement (Garbarino, Dubrow, & Kostelny, 1992; Martinez & Richter, 1993; Pfefferbaum, 1997; Widom, 1999). Studies of children exposed to domestic violence document increased prevalence of a range of internalizing and externalizing symptoms, including post–traumatic stress disorder, depression, low self-esteem, increased aggression, and oppositional behavior (Carlson, 2000; Edelson, 1999; Jaffe, Wolfe, & Wilson, 1990; Kolbo, 1996). Tragically, another long-term adaptation to violence is the perpetration of violence. Children who witness violence are at heightened risk for later engaging in the sorts of violent behavior that once were so terrifying. For example, a longitudinal study conducted in Rochester, New York, reported that children who had been victims of child abuse were 24% more likely to report engaging in violence as adolescents than children who were not maltreated; children who were not themselves victimized but who grew up in families in which intimate partner violence was present were 21% more likely to report use of violence as adolescents than those not exposed; youth exposed to multiple forms of family violence reported twice the rate of adolescent violence as compared with those raised in nonviolent families (Thornberry, 1994).

Despite the well-known potential negative consequences of children's exposure to violence, many children and families at high risk have limited access to or inclination to use mental health services. Children's exposure to violence often occurs in a context of multiple risks. Poverty alone imposes a constellation of barriers to service, including poor health insurance coverage, lack of transportation, inflexible work schedules, and lack of child care for siblings. Other family factors, such as drug abuse, parental depression, or other psychopathology, and repeated family separations or dislocations may further undermine parents' ability to attend to their children's mental health needs in the wake of violence. Experiences of racism and discrimination may also engender distrust of official "helping" systems. In the case of domestic violence, parental fears that contact with any professional helper may lead either to increased violence and danger from the abuser or to intrusive action by child protective services (CPS) may further limit children's access to supportive mental health interventions (Peled & Edelson, 1999). In addition, when both parents and children are exposed to chronic violence, either in the community or within the family, the parent's own sense of helplessness, terror, or defensive denial may inhibit her from recognizing and addressing her children's immediate symptoms and seeking assistance (Peled & Edelson, 1999; Marans & Adelman, 1997). For a complex combination of reasons, many of the children at highest risk of serious long-term difficulties are never seen in traditional mental health clinics until months or years later, when they are referred by schools or courts due to academic failure, delinquent behavior, or entrenched psychological and behavioral symptoms.

While mental health professionals may have limited opportunities for early intervention with children and families exposed to violence and trauma, other professionals do respond immediately to scenes of violent crisis, most prominently the police. As first responders, police officers have unique opportunities to initiate processes of psychological stabilization, triage, and linkage to other community resources, including mental health services. The Child Development–Community Policing program (CDCP) is an innovative collaboration between police and child mental health professionals that aims to coordinate clinical approaches to intervention for children exposed to or involved in violence with police activities that contain the external sources of danger in the child's world. This chapter will describe the theory and practice of CDCP and the impact of this unusual interdisciplinary partnership on the delivery of policing, mental health, and other social services for children and families exposed to violence and trauma.

Development of the Police–Mental Health Collaboration

The Child Development–Community Policing program is a partnership between the Yale University Child Study Center and the New Haven Department of Police Service. Begun in 1991, the program was developed out of shared concerns of police leaders and Child Study Center faculty regarding the psychological impact on children of their frequent exposure to violence in their homes and neighborhoods (Marans, Murphy, & Berkowitz, 2002; Marans, Berkowitz, & Cohen, 1998; Marans et al., 1995; Marans & Cohen, 1993). At the time of the program's inception, New Haven, like many other American cities, was experiencing high rates of gun violence as a result of competition among rival drug gangs. In addition, nearly a third of the calls for police service involved incidents of family violence, with children present or involved in approximately half of these situations (New Haven Department of Police Service, 1995).

Police officers knew from experience that children were often present at scenes of crime and violence, and that the children they encountered at these scenes were often visibly distressed. Officers were also familiar with the experience of seeing the same children they first met as witnesses later engaged in delinquent behavior or involved in violent incidents themselves, either as victims or as aggressors. While many individual police officers cared deeply for children, most officers did not conceptualize their official law enforcement roles to include intervention on behalf of children who were not direct victims, suspects, or essential witnesses to crime. Moreover, they did not have the special training and expertise, the time, or the resources to address the psychological needs of these children.

Mental health clinicians were also increasingly concerned that they were seeing more children and

adolescents who had long histories of exposure to and victimization by violence (Marans et al., 1995; Marans & Cohen, 1993). While mental health professionals may have the skills and training to understand and respond to children's psychological distress following episodes of violence, clinicians had no contact with these children and families at the times of the events, when the violent crisis might create a window of opportunity to stabilize the child's environment and to engage the child and family in supportive and therapeutic services. CDCP brings together the immediate presence and authority of the police with the developmental and therapeutic expertise of psychodynamically oriented child mental health professionals, with the goal of creating new and potentially more effective approaches to intervention.

Foundations of the Police–Mental Health Collaboration

From the perspective of law enforcement, the CDCP model has its foundations in the community policing movement (Marans et al., 2002; Marans, 1996; Marans et al., 1995). This philosophy conceptualizes police officers as members of a community rather than as outside enforcers of law, and as creative problem solvers rather than as reactive to specific circumscribed incidents of crime (Goldstein, 1990; Kelling, 1988; Thurman, 1995). Officers are placed on long-term assignment to specific communities, where they get to know local residents, institutions, neighborhood problems, and resources. This mode of policing confronts officers more closely with the complexity of issues facing children and families and places new demands on them to expand their repertoire of responses beyond standard criminal justice interventions. For example, frustrated parents may seek out a familiar patrol officer for help in dealing with an oppositional child or an adolescent on the edge of a delinquent peer group. Similarly, battered women who see the same patrol officers responding to repeated incidents of violence against them may begin to reveal more to these officers about the developing course of violence and the ways in which they find their options for safety limited. Officers' greater awareness of the context of crime and violence often leads them to appreciate the limits of arrest and prosecution as a solution, and motivates them to collaborate with other institutions and professionals in the interest of addressing some of the social problems that underlie crime and delinquency.

From the perspective of clinical intervention, CDCP draws from several streams of theory and practice. CDCP extends the long-standing practice of child psychoanalysts and other clinicians at the Yale Child Study Center and elsewhere in applying principles of child development based in psychoanalytic observation to the work of other professionals who have an impact on children, such as child care workers, teachers, pediatricians, and child protection workers (Freud & Burlingham, 1973; Goldstein, Solnit, Goldstein, & Freud, 1996; Solnit, Nordhaus, & Lord, 1992; Lewis, 2002). These applied clinical approaches are based on the recognition that adults outside the child's family who are a regular part of the child's life, or who have critical decision-making authority regarding the child's care, can, through the nature and quality of their interactions with the child, or the decisions that they make, have enormous effects on the child's experience, which may ameliorate the negative consequences of environmental stress and deprivation, lessen the need for intensive clinical intervention, or provide sufficient external support to enable the child to make use of psychotherapy when it is needed. Mental health professionals inform the work of nonclinical professionals by appreciating the complexity of the child's experience of the world and translating that experience into language and observations that are accessible to nonclinicians (Marans, 1996). Applied clinical practice through other professionals who have ongoing contact with children can bring basic support and stabilization to many more children than will need or engage in direct clinical treatment, and may be the only way to provide intervention for some children who live in stressful or chaotic environments that cannot support psychotherapy.

The CDCP program's focus on acute response to violence is based in developing knowledge about psychological traumatization, including the biological aspects of the stress response (Marans et al., 1998). Studies of posttraumatic responses in both adults and children give reason for concern that psychological and neurobiological changes will have enduring consequences for children's development when trauma responses go unrecognized and untreated. Studies indicate long-term altera-

tions in neurotransmitter systems and neuroanatomy, which have implications for dysregulation of arousal states, cardiovascular changes, and changes in the processes of creating and retrieving memory (Bremner et al., 2003; Perry, 1996; Southwick, Bremner, Krystal, & Charney, 1994; Yehuda, Giller, Southwick, & Lowery, 1991). In general it seems that chronic exposure to violence may prime the central nervous system to be more vulnerable to a myriad of psychiatric symptoms and disorders (Bremner, Southwick, Johnson, & Yehuda, 1993; Perry, 1996). These data support the development and implementation of systems for early identification and intervention for children exposed to violence, with the goal of preventing the acute stress response from becoming permanently dysregulated. It is hoped that by intervening immediately after the violent event, the integration of the experience for the child and family may prevent the perpetuation of fear and stress that can exacerbate acute maladaptive coping responses.

The Process of Collaborative Program Development

CDCP began in a series of conversations among police supervisors and Child Study Center faculty. While the initial idea was to train police officers to recognize and refer potentially traumatized children to a specialized clinical service, it soon became clear that mental health clinicians had no basis for "training" police officers as long as they had little understanding of what police officers did or how they came in contact with children. Likewise, police officers could not be expected to facilitate children's immediate access to mental health intervention when they had little knowledge of what clinicians did or how they thought about children and families. For a viable partnership to develop, representatives of both professions needed to learn about each other's work and develop a common language for discussing their concerns. What emerged was a series of reciprocal tutorials, which involved officers in observation of case conferences and videotaped and live interviews of children, and involved clinicians in ride-along observations of police patrol and investigative interviews. The process identified members of both professions as equal partners, both teachers and learners. It also provided a forum in which participants from both institutions could gradually discuss and revise their preconceptions of the other.

CDCP Program Elements

Initial conversations and observations led to the establishment of several interrelated training and service components that promote the development of a shared frame of reference, close working relationships, and exchange of information between professionals responding collaboratively to children and families victimized by violence. Training and service components to include the following:

- Child development training for police officers: Police officers receive training in basic principles of child development and their application to child-oriented community interventions. Seminars are based on scenarios drawn from the daily work of police with children and families exposed to violence and trauma at different developmental stages. Training is co-led by a team composed of an experienced police supervisor and child mental health clinician. Increased knowledge about children's development and the potential impact of trauma allows police to take children's needs into account as they do their work.
- Police training for clinicians: Clinicians participate in a related training designed to familiarize them with community policing and law enforcement strategies. Clinicians learn about police roles in the community and protocols for police practice through seminars and regular observational "ride-alongs" with patrol officers. Greater familiarity with the potential uses and limitations of police authority expands clinicians' options in designing and implementing effective intervention strategies.
- 24-Hour consultation service: A key component of the CDCP program is a 24-hour consultation service staffed by mental health clinicians who are available to respond immediately to police requests for consultation and intervention with children and families exposed to violence. Clinicians respond to a range of police cases at any time of day or night, providing immediate intervention for children who otherwise might not be identified for mental health services, as well as con-

sultation to officers regarding their own responses to children and families.
- Weekly program conference: Clinicians, officers, and other collaborators discuss cases referred to the consultation service during a weekly program conference to develop, review, and evaluate planned responses. The program conference fosters consistent and open relationships across disciplines and provides a forum for discussing systemic and organizational issues that may interfere with effective intervention on behalf of children affected by violence.

The program is staffed by an interdisciplinary group of social workers, psychologists and psychiatrists, police patrol officers, detectives, and supervisors. Though initially developed as a partnership between police and mental health, the collaboration has since expanded to include representatives from other professions and agencies that have frequent contact with children and families acutely affected by violence. Expansion of the collaboration has been driven by experience in which existing team members found they could not adequately respond to particular types of cases without engaging additional partners. Ten years after its inception, the team includes battered women's advocates, juvenile probation officers, CPS supervisors, and representatives of the New Haven school system. The program has become a national model for police–mental health collaboration and has been replicated in 12 communities around the country, including urban, suburban, and rural sites.

CDCP Training: Establishing a Common Frame of Reference

While all the program elements are essential to the ongoing collaboration, the seminars on child development and human behavior most clearly demonstrate the shared conceptual framework that guides observations, discussions, and interventions (Marans, 1996). The central task of the seminars is to engage officers and other partners in examining how an understanding of emotional, interpersonal, cognitive, and motor development can enhance law enforcement responses to children and families. Particular attention is paid to the ways in which traumatization may be experienced and demonstrated by children at different phases of development. Exploring the range of psychological and physiological responses to overwhelming, traumatic events prepares officers to recognize those situations that may place children at the greatest risk for acute and long-term consequences.

Proceeding along a developmental sequence, the seminars highlight the ways in which phenomena originating in earlier phases of development may be observed in various forms throughout the life cycle. Seminar leaders rely on scenarios encountered in police work, films and videotapes about children, and cases from the acute consultation service to demonstrate that a greater understanding of human functioning does not mean inaction or decreased vigilance with regard to personal safety. Rather, the goal of the seminars is to help officers and others to discover new ways of observing and formulating responses to children that are informed by their development. In addition, officers have the opportunity to establish a more realistic appreciation of the impact they can have on the lives of children and families with whom they interact.

Discussions begin about early development. The supervisory officer who co-leads the seminar introduces the topic of infancy by describing the following scene:

> You have responded to a complaint of breach of peace and arrive at an apartment where music is blaring. An angry young mother greets you. The apartment is disheveled and dirty, and three children, ranging from several months to four years, are in similar disarray. Diaper changes for two of the children appear long overdue. What is your reaction?

The officers often begin the discussion by expressing their feelings of despair and anger about a scene that is all too familiar. As the instructors begin to probe the nature of these reactions, the group begins to identify concerns about the babies who are unable to fend for themselves, about the children's physical discomfort, and about the notion that the mother is overwhelmed. What emerges from the discussion is the group's awareness of an infant's physical and emotional needs and the role of the mother in mediating distress and providing crucial care and affection. The seminar leaders ask, "What happens to the infant if those basic needs are not met?" The answers suggest that the baby will be overwhelmed with pain, discomfort, and despair because it is not yet equipped to feed, clothe, or comfort itself or satisfy the demands of its feelings on its own. The leaders ask for more details, and participants respond by identifying developmental capacities and vulnerabilities—the absence of verbal language, motor maturation, and cognitive processes for problem solving, and, finally, the utter reliance of the infant on the mother for the experience of physical and emotional well-being.

Attention is then focused on the young mother. The leaders ask, "How can we understand her apparent insensitivity or incompetence?" The discussion must first address her surly response to the officers and their indignation. Seminar leaders introduce clinical phenomena that underlie parenting behavior, and participants begin to discuss symptoms that they quickly recognize but have not necessarily associated with depression and stress. This provides an opportunity to discuss the complex relationship among stress, anxiety, depression, and substance abuse.

The concept of displacement and externalization is introduced. The leaders ask, "How might this young woman feel about herself?" The answers vary. "Like a failure. . . . Maybe she just doesn't care." The leaders ask, "How might she feel when two police officers come to her door?" Officers respond, "Like we're going to tell her off, tell her what she should be doing, how she should behave." "And who are you to her at that moment? Who tells you you're not getting it right, messing up? Parents? Teachers? A critical boss?" In one session, an officer jumped in and offered, "Right, and then when she feels criticized, she takes on an obnoxious attitude and treats us like dirt." Another officer added, "As though she already knows who you are." In this session, the clinical co-leader suggested that perhaps from the moment of their arrival, the officers represented a familiar voice of authority that agreed with the woman's own sense of incompetence and self-criticism. Her surly and combative response then serves a defensive function that is triggered by the officers, but not about them personally. The discussion often ends with some greater appreciation for the complexity of the situation, but with the residual wish to do something concrete for the babies—either to implore the woman to take better care of them or to remove the children so that they can have a better home.

The film *John* (Robertson & Robertson, 1969) is shown in the following session. In the discussion that follows, seminar members describe the 17-month-old's efforts to soothe himself in the midst of a 9-day separation from his parents. They note John's attempts to reach out to the child care nurses, cuddly toys, and the observer, and his utter despair when these efforts fail. The discussion also compares John with the other children who have spent their entire lives in the residential nursery. Seminar members often observe that while seemingly unfazed by the limited attention and multiple changes of nursing staff, these children, in contrast to John, appear dominated by aggressive, driven, and need-satisfying behavior. Slowly, and often painfully, as the discussion continues, the simple solution of removal from care when parenting seems inadequate fades. The idea that removal always represents rescue is replaced by a growing appreciation for the complexity of the child-parent relationship. This includes recognition of the developmental significance of the continuity of care and the impact of disrupting it. In addition, seminar members have a fuller understanding of the balance between the child's needs and capacities and the distress that follows when needs are not met.

Similar discussions occur as the seminar continues through subsequent phases of development. Throughout, the seminar aims to increase officers' appreciation of children's experience and to apply this understanding to inform their own daily interactions with children and families. Seminar members often bring examples from their own experience and use the group as a forum for exploring ways in which attention to children's needs may inform police strategy. In these discussions, the active participation of a police supervisor sends the clear message to officers that the police leadership will support their efforts to take the perspective of children into account while maintaining a focus on safety and essential law enforcement procedures.

Collaborative Intervention on Behalf of Children Exposed to Violence

The cornerstone of the CDCP program is the 24-hour consultation service. Any officer within the police department may initiate a call when he or she becomes concerned about a child or family following a violent event and after obtaining consent

from parents or guardians. The primary goals of the acute intervention are to initiate a process of psychological stabilization and to allow the child to regain a sense of control in the wake of a potentially traumatizing experience (Marans et al., 2002). In this context, realistic concerns about safety are intimately intertwined with psychological response. Therefore, the police officer and clinician work closely together to assess and address both physical and psychological safety. Immediate safety-enhancing police interventions may include moving the child and family to another location, contacting CPS, or contacting judicial authorities to assure temporary detention of an arrested suspect. Direct communication with the child and family about issues of safety facilitates the reestablishment of psychological security.

The police officer serves as the conduit for introducing the CDCP clinician to the child and family. This allows the officer and clinician to be viewed as a team and reinforces the connection between concerns for physical and psychological safety. The clinician meets first with the parents or other adults to establish a beginning relationship and to obtain preliminary information about the child's current experience and previous functioning. To help the child gain a sense of control in the face of potentially traumatic violence, the clinician typically follows the child's lead as expressed in words, play, or drawing and helps the child express and elaborate his or her concerns. Associations to other events or internal psychological dangers are frequently more pressing than those related to the event that precipitated the referral. Phase-specific concerns about separation, bodily integrity, or competitive strivings often permeate the child's communication about their experience of violence.

The clinician's ability to listen quietly and empathetically, without telling or cueing the child about what the clinician might wish to hear, permits the child to assume control in metabolizing the event. Children are encouraged to adopt an active role in communicating their unique concerns, which may or may not resemble the factual events that they have witnessed. The clinician listens actively, asking for clarification when needed, and provides information to the child and family about a range of expectable responses and possible interventions. Clinicians arrange for follow-up contact and ongoing intervention in accordance with the needs and wishes of the family.

Officers have contacted CDCP in a wide variety of circumstances in which children and adolescents have been exposed to or involved in violence or other potentially traumatic events, either as witnesses, victims, or perpetrators. During the 3-year period from 1998 to 2001, a total of 2,443 children were seen through the consultation service (Murphy, Marans, Berkowitz, & Casey, 2002). Police referred children of all ages, with a concentration of school-age children and early adolescents. Race and ethnicity were varied; 12.8 % of those referred were Caucasian, 55.6% African American, 26.4% Hispanic, and 5.2% other, which constitutes a somewhat higher representation of minority children than the general New Haven population (approximately 40% Caucasian, 40% African American, and 20% Hispanic). A substantial majority of the children seen through the program were from poorer neighborhoods within the city. The racial and geographic distribution of CDCP calls was congruent with the general distribution of calls for police service (New Haven Department of Police Service, 2002).

The majority of CDCP calls concerned criminal incidents, including assaults, robberies, homicides, arsons, burglaries, and threats. In keeping with the overall volume of calls to the New Haven police, approximately 30% of referrals to the CDCP consultation service concerned domestic violence incidents. In addition to criminal incidents, police utilized the service for assistance in dealing with traumatic accidents, psychiatric emergencies, noncriminal juvenile conduct, and a variety of social problems In approximately 50% of the cases referred to CDCP, a clinician met with the child or family less than an hour after the incident that prompted the call. Half of the remaining families were seen within 24 hours. Most children were seen at home, though clinicians also provided acute intervention at a variety of community locations, including schools, hospitals, and neighborhood centers.

Clinical responses have taken many forms, depending on the request of the referring officer and the needs and wishes of individual families. Most cases have involved one or more mental health professionals in acute psychological intervention with a child or family following a violent event, according to the model described earlier in this chapter. In other cases (approximately 18% of referrals), response was limited to telephone consultation to the officer without direct clinical contact. Follow-up intervention tailored to individual cases has included home- or clinic-based assessment, psychoeducation for children and parents regarding expectable responses to traumatic events, regular follow-up from neighborhood officers, case management, referral, and coordination with a wide range of social services, including ongoing psychotherapy. From the beginning and throughout the CDCP intervention, the team attempts to develop an integrated understanding of the internal and environmental factors affecting a child's experience and to address the interrelated needs for physical safety, environmental stability, and psychological support in a coordinated fashion.

Case Example: Acute Collaborative Response

Police were called to a domestic disturbance. A man had stabbed a woman with a meat cleaver in the presence of their two children, ages 2 and 8. When police arrived, they found the adults still arguing and the children curled up on the couch, splattered with blood. The woman was transported to hospital by ambulance, and officers arrested the man. Police called CPS and brought the children to police headquarters. They also called the CDCP clinician on call and the children's grandmother, and requested that both respond to the police station. Officers understood that the best thing they could do to help these children regain a sense of safety and security was to arrange for them to be cared for by a trusted and familiar adult, and so they did not wait for CPS but called the grandmother immediately.

At the police station, officers brought the children food and found a comfortable, quiet place for them to wait for their grandmother, the clinician, and CPS. As they waited, the 2-year-old, Erica, complained that she "had blood on her" and became agitated that it would not come off. In consultation with the on-call clinician, officers helped Erica to wash the blood from her hands and provided her with a clean shirt. This stopped the child from being visually confronted at that moment with such a powerful reminder of the overwhelming incident and allowed her to calm down. An officer then held Erica in his lap and let her fall asleep. Meanwhile, other officers worked closely with CPS to investigate the safety and appropriateness of the children's grandmother as a temporary guardian.

Upon arrival at the police station, the 8-year-old, Sarah, cried inconsolably, but she began to regain her composure as she greedily devoured the food provided by the officers. One officer sat next to her as she ate, and she began to recount the details of the incident she had witnessed. One striking feature of Sarah's story was that she stated several times that she could have stopped them from fighting if only she had gotten the baseball bat from the closet and threatened to hit her stepfather. She also asked repeatedly what was going to happen to her mother and stepfather. She was concerned that she would never see them again.

The officer understood that Sarah's wishes to have heroically stopped the fighting were an expression of her attempt to avoid feeling so helpless and small. He therefore responded by emphasizing the action she did take and told her, "I know you wish that things were different, but you did the right thing by keeping yourself and your sister safe." In consultation with the clinician, the officer also provided honest answers to Sarah's questions about her parents. The officer obtained a medical status report from the hospital and told Sarah her mother was being treated and would most likely be returning home the next day. He also told her that her stepfather was arrested and was staying in jail for the night because what he had done was dangerous and against the law. A judge would see him in the morning and decide when he could come home. Although it was difficult for the officers to discuss such unpleasant issues with a young child, they understood that it was better to tell the truth than to leave the questions unanswered, so that the child might imagine facts even worse than reality.

Eventually, CPS approved the grandmother as temporary guardian, and she took the children home. Before she left, the clinician met with her to discuss the reactions she might expect from both children and the ways in which she could best support them. The clinician also offered follow-up meetings with the children and family. On telephone follow-up a few days later, the mother had been discharged from the hospital. She reported the children were doing fine, and there was no further clinical contact. Neighborhood officers made several unscheduled follow-up visits to the home to check on the mother's safety and the children's reactions. The mother reported being grateful for the officers' support but declined referrals for any ad-

ditional services. There have been no further calls for police services to the address.

In this case, well-trained officers, aided by the on-call clinician, were able to provide immediate support to the children and their grandmother at the moment of acute crisis. The immediate intervention focused on the children's developmental needs for stability and familiarity, as well as age-appropriate information to correct misperceptions and diminish the anxiety fueled by imagination. The team provided support and information for the children's caregivers to assist them to provide the necessary support and nurturance for the children. The follow-up contacts with police patrol emphasized ongoing concern for the safety of mother and children and availability of the police to act on their behalf, both as enforcers of the law and as brokers of service.

In other CDCP cases, police contact with children and families in an acute moment of crisis provides a link to ongoing clinical treatment for children and adults. Officers facilitate parents' engagement with clinicians by respectfully communicating their concerns for the children's vulnerability and by making services accessible. The following case presents an example of extended treatment and collaborative intervention.

Case Example: Police Referral Followed by Extensive Clinical Treatment and Collaborative Intervention

Police responded to a call from a young woman reporting a threat to her life by her estranged husband. When officers arrived, the man was gone, and Darlene, the victim, gave a disjointed and highly emotional account of the incident. Her husband, Mark, had broken into her apartment, pointed an automatic handgun at her head, threatened to kill her if she had another man in the house with his children, and then left the scene. Darlene was obviously terrified, both for her own safety and for the safety of her three young children. She was also enraged and verbally abusive to the responding officers. She had difficulty paying any attention to the children, who clung mutely to her legs as she swore and berated the officers to do something. Officers took a description and put out a broadcast for Mark. They offered to assist Darlene in arranging temporary placement in a battered women's shelter, but she declined in a fury that she should not be forced to leave her home. Officers then left the scene to respond to other calls.

Over the next several days, officers in the neighborhood received repeated complaints from Darlene that Mark was in the area, but each time they responded to the house, she was not able to report any new assault or threat, and he was nowhere to be seen. As the days wore on and Mark remained at large, Darlene became more frustrated and rageful, directing her anger increasingly toward the police who could not protect her. In turn, officers became more curt and dismissive of her complaints. From the perspective of the patrol officers, there was nothing they could do prior to the court's issuance of an arrest warrant, unless they were able to apprehend Mark in the course of new criminal activity or its immediate aftermath. They experienced Darlene's desperate demand that they do something to protect her as an attack on their competence, which they defended by distancing themselves. From Darlene's perspective, the system had failed her. She began carrying a knife to protect herself.

A detective from the Domestic Violence Unit was assigned to investigate the case. The detective, who had completed CDCP training and worked closely with the CDCP clinicians, was able to listen in more detail to Darlene's story, not only in relation to the current incident but also in relation to the whole course of her abusive relationship with her husband, including a history of serious physical abuse of her son and removal of all three children by CPS. Darlene explained to the detective that her greatest fear was not physical injury to herself but loss of her children to CPS, which had just returned them to her custody contingent on her maintaining no contact with Mark. Her aggressive and demanding stance with the police could then be understood as a plea for help in keeping her children with her. The detective, who was herself a single mother, was able to begin building a working relationship with Darlene by recognizing and supporting her commitment to keep her children safe. With this basis of understanding, the detective worked closely with Darlene to obtain necessary information to expedite Mark's arrest and assure his pretrial confinement. The detective also helped her to obtain a transfer to a different apartment complex, where Mark would not be able to find her.

In addition, the detective was attentive to Darlene's concern about the psychological needs of her oldest child, Arthur, age 5. Arthur had been physically abused by Mark (not his father), had repeatedly witnessed Mark's abuse of Darlene, and had just returned to Darlene's care following a year in foster care. He not only was acutely terrified by Mark's latest threats but also was reported to be fearful, demanding, aggressive, and disruptive at home and school. The detective contacted a CDCP clinician and arranged a home visit to introduce the clinician to the family. The detective knew that Darlene was overwhelmed and hesitant to trust people, but she also believed that Darlene really did want and need help for her son. The detective used the relationship she had developed with Darlene to facilitate a connection with the clinician.

A clinician started to work with Darlene and her family, beginning with a clinical evaluation of Arthur coupled with support for his mother to stabilize their environment. Arthur presented as a bright and engaging child who was preoccupied with thoughts of violent attacks, chaotic disruptions, and fears that he would be sent back to foster care as punishment for "being bad." He graphically demonstrated his experience through play. For example, in one early session, a play family moved into a carefully arranged new house only to have a hurricane destroy the house and hurl the people and furniture out into the wind. At school, Arthur had difficulty paying attention or complying with instructions, though he responded well to individual attention from the teacher. When not closely supervised, he would wander about his classroom, eventually settling in the doll corner to play. At home, he squabbled constantly with younger siblings and competed for his mother's attention. When his attempts to engage her were unsuccessful, he responded with angry defiance or regressed behavior. Having fought long and hard for his return from foster placement, Arthur's mother was bitterly disappointed that there were so many problems associated with having him home. In frustration, she often threatened to send him back, which only made matters worse.

For Arthur and for Darlene, the most important first goal was to achieve a sense of immediate safety and stability that could provide a foundation for psychological recovery from years of traumatic experience. During the period of initial contact, the clinician frequently acted as liaison between Darlene, police, and battered women's advocates. Active advocacy on Darlene's behalf assisted her not only in enhancing her family's safety but also in achieving a greater sense of control and competence in protecting her children. A second immediate goal was to help Darlene to separate her own sense of vulnerability from Arthur's and to develop some empathy for him, so that she could begin to rebuild a maternal relationship with him. The clinician helped Darlene to understand how important it was for Arthur that she was taking thoughtful steps to keep him safe and encouraged her to let him know that he could continue to rely on her. In working with Arthur the therapist made clear that her role was to listen, to understand his experience, to help his mother to understand, and not to assume the functions of a substitute mother.

Therapy was slow and periodically disrupted by repeated crises in the family. The therapist was able to maintain Darlene's engagement in her son's treatment, however, by continually reinforcing her desire to avoid repeated separations of the family and helping her to understand her son's aggressive and disruptive behavior as a response to his experience of helplessness and loss. In this context, it was sometimes helpful to engage Darlene in remembering her own experiences of lashing out at others when she was feeling fearful and helpless.

The relationship between Arthur's therapist and his mother also provided an opportunity to monitor the family's safety and to reconnect Darlene with police and advocates periodically, as her former husband's legal status changed. For example, Darlene became noticeably agitated and irritable as her former husband neared his release date from incarceration. She was short-tempered with her children and picked fights with her boyfriend. She was terrified that Mark would come looking for her immediately upon his release from jail, and that he would be outraged and violent when he learned that she was pregnant. She knew she should protect her son from the knowledge that Mark was getting out of jail, but she was too overwhelmed to contain her conversations with family members until Arthur was asleep. As Arthur saw his mother more and more upset, he attempted to cope with his own helpless feelings by becoming defiant and aggressive. This only fueled his mother's sense that everything around her was out of control and led her to become harsh and punitive in an effort to restore her authority. The only option Darlene could think of was to run, but she felt helpless and overwhelmed when she thought of leaving her apartment and her job and removing her son from school and therapy, which had finally helped him feel more secure.

When Arthur's therapist learned what was happening, she was able to arrange a meeting with Darlene and the battered women's advocate who had worked with Darlene prior to Mark's incarceration. The meeting focused on examining Darlene's options for safety once Mark was released. The advocate reminded Darlene that she had a right to be informed of Mark's impending release. She reviewed with Darlene the conditions of Mark's probation and their divorce, which prohibited his contact with Darlene and the children. The advocate provided police with copies of the court orders to facilitate their enforcement. Together, the clinician, advocate, and the police detective discussed with Darlene the relative risks and benefits of flight to another jurisdiction as opposed to remaining in New Haven, where police were prepared to work with her to keep her as safe as possible. The detective installed an electronic system in Darlene's apartment, which would alert police immediately if Darlene pushed a panic button. Police supervisors arranged for the patrol officers in Darlene's neighborhood to introduce themselves to her and to visit her regularly to monitor her safety. With these safeguards in place, Darlene felt she no longer had to run but could keep her job and her connections to family and other supports in New Haven. This allowed her to protect her children from one more dislocation and disruption.

None of the therapist's work with Darlene or Arthur would have been possible without the detective's introduction or the coordinated involvement of the interdisciplinary team. For families such as Darlene's, immediate concerns for physical safety are so intertwined with emotional experience that attention to the family's urgent physical needs becomes a central component of clinical care. At the same time, attention to Darlene's sense of terror and emotional vulnerability helped her to make more productive use of the legal and environmental supports that were available. For Arthur, who had experienced so many disruptions, it was imperative to achieve greater environmental stability as a foundation for his continued development. Because the police are so centrally involved in establishing physical safety and security in the wake of violence, they can play an invaluable role in supporting a more extended therapeutic process.

From the perspective of the police, this case provides an example of the frustrations commonly experienced by officers and the potential benefits of coordinated interdisciplinary response. First-responding patrol officers, who did not understand the context of the case and did not have any other professional support to help them intervene with the victim, became embroiled with her in a mutually frustrating cycle of miscommunication, disappointment, and anger. In contrast, the Domestic Violence Unit detective was able to use the CDCP consultation service along with her own knowledge of children and parenting to establish a working relationship with Darlene. This enabled the detective to facilitate successful prosecution of the criminal case, to assist the family to immediate safety, and to make connections with other service providers. Together, the coordinated group of advocates, therapist, police, and court personnel could address the complex and interrelated legal, environmental, and psychological issues presented by the family. Though the detective did not have time to maintain a consistent long-term relationship with Darlene, she did assume personal responsibility for the policing aspects of the case and remained available as needed. By broadening her role beyond traditional law enforcement boundaries to include service coordinator and sisterly authority figure, this detective was able to see her intervention as far more successful than the more limited patrol response.

Impact of CDCP on Police Practice

The CDCP program has had a profound effect on police policy and practice, as demonstrated by the following specific changes:

- Before the establishment of CDCP, police had not referred any children for clinical services.
- From 1995 to the present, clinicians have received an average of 10 referrals or requests for consultations per week (Child Development–Community Policing Program, 2002).

- All new police recruits receive a 1-day course in developmental issues for children, and all supervisory officers have received the full developmental seminar.
- There is a police officer either assigned to or responsible for every New Haven public school.
- CDCP clinicians' names and pager numbers are listed at every dispatch station in the police department's central communications unit and in every police substation.
- The CDCP clinician is listed as an essential contact in the police department's formal notification system for serious events. Since 1998, the police reporting form requires that all children present at a crime scene be listed, and there is a check-off box for contact with a CDCP clinician.

In addition, the partnership has affected the ways in which officers conceptualize their own roles in the lives of children and families. Traditionally, police officers have viewed their purpose as protecting or enhancing physical safety, and investigating and documenting criminal activity. Officers ordinarily do not see themselves or wish to be seen as therapeutic agents. However, at times of crisis and trauma, police officers' job of restoring order often constitutes the most important immediate psychological intervention. Most police officers remain unaware that they are serving this role; however, New Haven's experience demonstrates that officers can become more conscious of the stability they represent, and that officers can often tailor their responses to maximize their reorganizing effect.

Unlike other professionals, whose first contact with children and families affected by violence may not come for days or weeks after a violent incident, police officers respond to the scene immediately and are therefore present during the acute moment of crisis or soon after. As a result, police officers have unique opportunities to intervene at a time when many parents and children may be most receptive to accepting assistance because they are so acutely overwhelmed. In these moments, officers can provide a voice of reality that confirms for children and adults that something very serious and wrong did in fact take place. Officers thus assist children to be less alone with frightening and overwhelming feelings and support parents to engage with supports outside the family, which might otherwise be rejected in favor of efforts to keep thoughts of the event at bay.

Impact of CDCP on Clinical Practice

Clinical thinking and practice have also changed dramatically as a result of the CDCP partnership. For example:

• Establishment of 24-hour on-call service staffed by Child Study Center faculty and clinical trainees makes clinical consultation and emergency response available as requested by police.
• Clinicians' frequent presence at scenes of violence and trauma has increased their knowledge about the details of children's exposure to violence and its aftermath.
• Children acutely and chronically exposed to violence have received clinical intervention beginning moments after the potentially traumatic event. This has provided clinicians with the opportunity to learn more about the natural course of children's reactions as they unfold.
• Senior faculty psychiatrists, psychologists, and social workers have received training as CDCP fellows; all CSC clinical trainees (including medical students) are oriented to police and judicial policy and protocols as part of their training.
• Clinical rotation in the CDCP consultation service is available as a training elective.

Perhaps most important, as the partnership between mental health professionals and police has provided opportunities for clinicians to observe police officers interacting with children and families, it has increased their appreciation of the potential therapeutic uses of police authority. Though it is common clinical practice to collaborate closely with professionals from other social service institutions, few mental health professionals consider the police as potential participants in interdisciplinary case plans. Experience with CDCP has demonstrated, however, that in situations where a child's environment is dangerous and unstable, police can not only assist in addressing the realistic sources of danger but also act as consistent representatives of benign authority, which help to contain the child's anxiety and provide external behavioral limits when the child lacks sufficient internal impulse controls.

Based on this perspective, clinicians involved in CDCP have increasingly coordinated their work with the efforts of police, as well as other figures of authority such as probation and child protection, which affect the essential environmental foundations for clinical intervention. Coordination with police and other legal authorities has resulted in earlier clinical access for acutely traumatized children and has permitted some families to sustain clinical treatment, which would have been unlikely absent the involvement of law enforcement or governmental authority. In addition, by developing relationships with other professionals, clinicians have been able to affect the experience of many children and families that could not support regular involvement in psychotherapy but do have ongoing contact with professionals in other domains. Rather than seeing these external governmental forces as completely outside the clinical sphere, CDCP has expanded the notion of what constitutes "clinical intervention" to include developmentally informed activities of the police and others.

Note

1. Portions of this chapter have appeared previously in other publications: S. Marans, Psychoanalysis on the beat: Children, police and urban trauma, *Psychoanalytic Study of the Child, 51* (1996): 522–541; and S. Marans, R. A. Murphy, & S. J. Berkowitz, Police-mental health responses to children exposed to violence: The Child Development–Community Policing program, in M. Lewis (Ed.), *Comprehensive Textbook of Child and Adolescent Psychiatry* (Baltimore: Williams and Wilkins, 2002).

References

Bash, C. (1997). *New directions from the field: Victims' rights and services for the twenty-first century.* Washington, DC: U.S. Department of Justice Office for Victims of Crime.

Boney-McCoy, S., & Finkelhor, D. (1996). Is youth victimization related to trauma symptoms and depression after controlling for prior symptoms and family relationships? A longitudinal prospective study. *Journal of Consulting Clinical Psychology, 64,* 1406–1416.

Bremner, J. D., Southwick, S. M., Johnson, D. R., & Yehuda, R. (1993). Childhood abuse in combat-related post traumatic stress disorder. *American Journal of Psychiatry, 150*, 235–239.

Bremner, J. D., Vythilingam, M., Vermetten, E., Southwick, S. M., McGlashan, T., Nazeer, A., Khan, S., Vaccarino, L. V., Soufer, R., Garg, P. K., Ng, C. K., Staib, L. H., Duncan, J. S., & Charney D. S. (2003). MRI and PET study of deficits in hippocampal structure and function in women with childhood sexual abuse and posttraumatic stress disorder. *American Journal of Psychiatry, 160*, 924–932.

Carlson, B. E. (2000). Children exposed to intimate partner violence: Research findings and implications for intervention. *Trauma, Violence and Abuse, 1*, 321–342.

Centers for Disease Control and Prevention. (1997). *National summary of injury and mortality data, 1985-95*. Atlanta, GA: National Center for Injury Prevention and Control.

Child Development-Community Policing Program. (2002). *Case Activity and Patient Electronic Recording System (CAPERS)*. New Haven, CT: Yale University School of Medicine.

Edelson, J. (1999). Children's witnessing of adult domestic violence. *Journal of Interpersonal Violence, 14*, 839–870.

Fantuzzo, J., Boruch, R., Beriama, A., & Atkins, M. (1997). Domestic violence and children: Prevalence and risk in five major U.S. cities. *Journal of the American Academy of Child and Adolescent Psychiatry, 36*, 116–122.

Foy, D. W., & Goguen, C. A. (1998). Community violence related PTSD in children and adolescents. *PTSD Research Quarterly, 9*, 1–6.

Freud, A., & Burlingham, D. (1973). Infants without families. In *The Writings of Anna Freud* (Vol. 3, pp. 3–664). New York: International Press.

Garbarino, J., Dubrow, N., & Kostelny, K. (1992). *Children in danger: Coping with the consequences of community violence*. San Francisco: Jossey-Bass.

Goldstein, H. (1990). *Problem-oriented policing*. Philadelphia: Temple University Press.

Goldstein, J., Solnit, A. Goldstein, S., & Freud, A. (1996). *In the best interest of the child: The least detrimental alternative*. New York: Free Press.

Gorman-Smith, D., & Tolan, P. (1998). The role of exposure to community violence and developmental problems among inner-city youth. *Developmental Psychopathology, 10*, 101–116. Graham-Berman, S. A., & Levendosky, A. A. (1998). Traumatic stress symptoms in children of battered women. *Journal of Interpersonal Violence, 13*, 111–128.

Jaffe, P. G., Wolfe, D. A., & Wilson, S. K. (1990). *Children of battered women*. Newbury Park, CA: Sage.

Kelling, G. L. (1988). The quiet revolution in American policing. *Perspectives on Policing*, no. 1. Washington, DC: U.S. Department of Justice Office of Justice Programs National Institute of Justice.

Kolbo, J. R. (1996). Risk and resilience among children exposed to family violence. *Violence and Victims, 11*, 113–128.

Lewis, M., & Leebens, P. K. (2002). Consultation process in child and adolescent psychiatric consultation-liaison in pediatrics. In M. Lewis (Ed.), *Comprehensive textbook of child and adolescent psychiatry* (pp. 935–940). Baltimore: Williams and Wilkins.

Marans, S. (1996). Psychoanalysis on the beat: Children, police and urban trauma. *Psychoanalytic Study of the Child, 51*, 522–541.

Marans, S., & Adelman, A. (1997). Experiencing violence in a developmental context. In J. Osofsky (Ed.), *Children in a violent society* (pp. 202–222). New York: Guilford.

Marans, S., Adnopoz, J., Berkman, M., Esserman, D., MacDonald, D., Nagler, S., Randall, R., Shaefer, M., & Wearing, M. (1995). *The police-mental health partnership: A community-based response to urban violence*. New Haven, CT: Yale University Press.

Marans, S., Berkowitz, S. J., & Cohen, D. J. (1998). Police and mental health professionals: Collaborative responses to the impact of violence on children and families. *Child and Adolescent Psychiatric Clinics of North America, 7*, 635–651.

Marans, S., & Cohen, D. J. (1993). Children and inner-city violence: Strategies for intervention. In L. A. Leavitt & N. A. Fox (Eds.), *The psychological effects of war and violence on children* (pp. 281–301). Hillsdale, NJ: Erlbaum.

Marans, S., Murphy, R. A., & Berkowitz, S. J. (2002). Police–mental health responses to children exposed to violence: The Child Development-Community Policing program. In M. Lewis (Ed.), *Comprehensive textbook of child and adolescent psychiatry*. Baltimore: Williams and Wilkins.

Martinez, P., & Richter, J. (1993). The NIMH community violence project: II. Children's distress symptoms associated with violence exposure. *Psychiatry, 56*, 22–35.

McCloskey, L. A., & Walker, M. (2000). Posttraumatic stress in children exposed to family violence and single event trauma. *Journal of the American Academy of Child and Adolescent Psychiatry, 39*, 108–115.

Murphy, R. A., Marans, S., Berkowitz, S., & Casey, R. L. (2002, November). Mental health and police responses to children exposed to violence. In R. A.

Murphy (Chair), *Evaluation and treatment of childhood violent and medical trauma.* Symposium presented at International Society for Traumatic Stress Studies, Baltimore.

New Haven Department of Police Service. (1995). Computer Aided Dispatch Records.

New Haven Department of Police Service. (2002). Computer Aided Dispatch Records.

Peled, E., & Edelson, J. (1999). Barriers to children's domestic violence counseling. *Families in Society, 80,* 578–586.

Perry, B. D. (1996). Neurobiological sequelae of childhood trauma: PTSD in children. In M. Murburg (Ed.), *Catecholamine function in posttraumatic stress disorder: Emerging concepts* (pp. 223–225). Washington, DC: American Psychiatric Press.

Pfefferbaum, B. (1997). Posttraumatic stress disorder in children: A review of the past 10 years. *Journal of the American Academy of Child and Adolescent Psychiatry, 36,* 1503–1511.

Pynoos, R. S. (1993). Traumatic stress and developmental psychopathology in children and adolescents. In M. Oldham & A. Tasman (Eds.), *Review of Psychiatry, 12,* 205–238.

Rennison, C. M. (1999). *Criminal victimization 1998: Changes 1997–98 with trends 1993–98.* Washington, DC: U.S. Department of Justice Bureau of Justice Statistics.

Robertson, J., & Robertson, J. (1969). *John, seventeen months, in residential nursery for nine days.* Distributed by New York University Film Library.

Schwab-Stone, M., Muyeed, A., & Voyce, C. (2000). Report on the Social and Health Assessment (SAHA): Trends 1992–1998. New Haven, CT: New Haven Public Schools.

Solnit, A. J., Nordhaus, B. F., & Lord, R. (1992). *When home is no haven.* New Haven, CT: Yale University Press.

Southwick, S. M., Bremner, D., Krystal, J. H., & Charney, D. S. (1994). Psychobiologic research in posttraumatic stress disorder. *Psychiatric Clinics of North America, 17,* 251–264.

Taylor, L., Zuckerman, B., Harik, V., & Groves, B. M. (1994). Witnessing violence by young children and their mothers. *Developmental and Behavioral Pediatrics, 15,* 120–123.

Thornberry, T. (1994). *Violent families and youth violence.* Washington, DC: U.S. Department of Justice, Office of Justice Programs, Office of Juvenile Justice and Delinquency Prevention.

Thurman, Q. C. (1995). Community policing: The police as a community resource. In P. Adams & K. Nelson (Eds.), *Reinventing human services: Community and family centered practice* (pp. 175–187). New York: Aldine de Gruyter.

Widom, C. S. (1999). Posttraumatic stress disorder in abused and neglected children grown up. *American Journal of Psychiatry, 156,* 1123–1129.

Yehuda, R., Giller, E. L., Southwick, S. M., & Lowery, M. T. (1991). Hypothalamic-pituitary-adrenal dysregulation in PTSD. *Biological Psychiatry, 30,* 1031–1048.

28   Roni Berger

It Takes a Community
to Help an Adolescent
Community-Based Clinical Services
for Immigrant Adolescents

Fourteen-year-old Yelena is an eighth-grade student who participates in a weekly acculturation
group conducted during lunchtime at her heavily
immigrant-populated junior high school in New
York. She came to the United States 3 years ago
with her parents and her maternal grandparents,
who took advantage of the opportunity opened for
Jews to leave the former Soviet Union to pursue a
better future for their daughter and gain freedom
from anti-Semitism. Her father, a physicist by training, held a high government position in his homeland. In New York, after a long period of unemployment and temporary jobs, he was hired for a
technical position, which offers him a social status
and salary considerably below what is typical for
someone with his education. Her mother, who was
a music teacher, now works as a cashier in a local
supermarket. The five family members live in a
crowded two-bedroom apartment. In the group,
Yelena reports conflictual relationships with her
parents, who do not allow her to date, demand that
she stay home at all times except school hours, forbid her to invite friends over, and criticize her appearance. She feels angry, guilty, misunderstood,
and depressed.

Yelena is not alone. The already large population of immigrant adolescents is growing. The concept "immigrant adolescents" has been used to describe three different subgroups: (1) those who
immigrated as children and grew up in the receiving country (also called the 1.5 generation); (2)
those born in the absorbing culture to immigrant
parents; and (3) those who immigrated during their
adolescent years. The latter group has traditionally
been identified as high risk and is, therefore, the
focus of this chapter.

My familiarity with this population group results mainly from 5 years of service as a trainer and
supervisor of youth workers serving the community of immigrants from the former Soviet Union
in Brighton Beach in Brooklyn, New York. My role
there was to provide weekly supervisory sessions
for workers. The goal of this supervision was to
enhance workers' professional knowledge and
skills, specifically in relation to serving adolescent
immigrants. Strategies included educating workers
about principles and techniques of assessment and
interventions, application of relevant practice models, and helping them process their own biases and
projections to the clients and develop appropriate
ways for coping with these reactions. Evaluating
workers' performance and providing support involved intimate knowledge of their work with adolescents. Supervision was conducted individually

or in small groups with two to three participants. In addition, I facilitated a weekly group supervision, which offered workers an opportunity to share information, ideas, and concerns and develop skills of collaboration and teamwork. This experience taught me about these youngsters' needs, struggles, strengths, and resilience in coping simultaneously with the challenges of two transitional processes—the developmental passage from childhood to adulthood, and the relocation from culture of origin to a new culture—while demonstrating what we as practitioners can do to help them in their struggle.

One of the first and most important things I learned was that regardless of the severity of their distress, adolescents like Yelena and their parents are not likely to seek help. This underutilization of mental health services is well documented in the professional literature (Bemak, Chung, & Bornemann, 1996; Gottesfeld, 1995; Hoberman, 1992; Logan & King, 2001; Nguven, 1984; Pumariega, Glover, Holzer, & Nguyen, 1998; Tabora & Flakerud, 1997; Woodward, Dwinell, & Aorns, 1992). However, I would like to argue that immigrants' need for mental health services can most effectively be met by community-based services that respect and integrate aspects of their culture of origin.

The chapter includes three sections. First, unique characteristics of adolescent immigrants and their special needs are reviewed and illustrated. The second section reviews hallmarks of community-based practice, discusses and illustrates principles generated from successful community-based mental health services for adolescent immigrants, and argues why such services are better equipped than traditional services to meet their needs. The focus is on *what* proved helpful and *how* it can be done. Finally, the third section presents one example of a community-based mental health service. While this chapter is based on my experience with one specific group of adolescent immigrants, I believe that many of the ideas, principles, and strategies presented here are applicable and relevant, with adaptations, to other adolescent immigrant populations.

Immigrant Adolescents: Characteristics and Issues

Recent waves of immigrants, mostly from Central and South America, Asia, and the former Soviet Union, are presenting new challenges for service providers and policymakers in the United States, Canada, and Australia, where these immigrants are settling (Schuck, 1999; Shen-Ryan, 1992). It is estimated that about 7% to 10% of the immigrants are adolescents, ages 12 to 18 (Castles & Miller, 1998; Hernandez & Charney, 1998).

While each adolescent immigrant has unique characteristics and personal, family, and ethnic-cultural background, they also share some general features and issues. Adolescent immigrants experience immigration-related losses and numerous changes in all aspects of their life, leading to social, economic, and cultural insecurity. At the same time, they are struggling with age-related physical, cognitive, emotional, and social changes and new roles, responsibilities, and expectations (Berger, 1996, 2005; Baptiste, 1990; Furnham & Bochner, 1986; Mirsky & Prawer, 1992; Stewart, 1986; Waters, 1996). All adolescents face the developmental task of exploring and making major decisions for their future. Immigrant adolescents frequently need to make such decisions under more stressful conditions, and often with less help. Many of them also experience marginalization and discrimination because of minority status. Even more challenging is the psychological burden of preimmigration traumas of war, natural disaster, torture, oppression, and persecution.

The combination of these various stressors contributes to the unique vulnerabilities in adolescent immigrants, which can result in a range of mental health problems such as anxiety, confusion, disorientation, identity crisis, helplessness, decreased self-esteem, a sense of existential vacuum, insecurity, inadequacy and alienation, personal annihilation, emptiness and meaninglessness, frustration, anger, loneliness, and depression (Baider, Ever-Hadani & Kaplan-DeNour, 1996; Berger, 1996, 1997; Drachman & Shen-Ryan, 1991; Garza-Guerrero, 1974; Glassman & Skolnik, 1984; Goodenow & Espin, 1993; Harper & Lantz, 1996; Hernandez & Charney, 1998; Hulewat, 1996; Lee, 1988; Liebkind, 1992; Stewart, 1986). Clinical expressions of these problems may be evident in children as young as 13 who demonstrate reckless behavior such as extensive drinking, sexual acting out, self-mutilation, and suicidality.

Immigrant adolescents have limited resources to help them cope. They have been cut off from friends and other familiar peer groups they might normally turn to for support. Like many adolescents, these youngsters tend to have negative stereotypes of mental health services and are fearful that they will be stigmatized and considered "crazy." Furthermore, strong beliefs in the original culture of many adolescent immigrants include disapproval of self-disclosure and sharing of feelings and intimate information with extrafamilial sources.

Their parents and other older relatives are often not available to provide the necessary help because of their own struggles with immigration-related challenges and their lack of familiarity with the new culture. For example, the concept of adolescents' struggle for autonomy and normative rebellion against authority, with which American parents are very familiar, is an alien notion in many of the immigrant cultures. Therefore, behaviors that may be tolerated by Western parents are perceived differently and judged much more harshly by immigrant parents. Their reaction to their child's behavior may further escalate conflicts in the family.

Adolescents are known to acculturate to their new environment faster than their parents. This creates an intergenerational gap that broadens (Gold, 1989; Landau-Stanton, 1985) and often results in role reversal, with adolescents becoming translators and interpreters of the new environment for their parents. This role reversal may interfere with adolescents' seeking help from their parents to cope with the same environment that they are helping their parents understand and manage. In addition, tense relationships are not uncommon because adolescents are often angry with their parents for imposing immigration without giving the young people an opportunity to participate in the decision process. They are often torn between a sense of obligation and responsibility for the parents, on the one hand, and resentment and striving for autonomy, on the other hand. Parents feel that they sacrificed their careers to ensure their children better social prospects and to save them from anti-Semitism and discrimination, and that they therefore have the right to continue to make decisions about their social relationships. This complex and painful dynamic often remains unresolved until a later phase when the children move out and become young adults.

In spite of the identification of immigrant adolescents as high risk, recent studies show that "the mental health and adjustment of children and youth in immigrant families appears to be similar to, if not better than, that of U.S.-born children and youth in U.S.-born families in most respects" (Hernandez & Charney, 1998, pp. 83–84). This indicates that in addition to considerable risk factors, many adolescent immigrants also possess a resiliency that helps them cope with the multitude of changes, stressors, and hardships of the immigration experience and to actually prosper. One role of the community-based practitioner is to identify and cultivate these strengths.

It is helpful to remember that immigrant adolescents choose different paths to cope with their challenges. Gibson (2002) demonstrated this in interviews with five Bosnian adolescent refugees who presented "a wide range of responses to questions about how individuals identify themselves culturally or nationally" (p. 41). Berger (1997) observed patterns of coping with identity among immigrant adolescents. Some reject their culture of origin, "erase" it, and fully embrace the new culture. They maximize their adoption of the new culture's norms, dress style, behavior code, and music. English is preferred to their original language. They hang out with American-born friends, change their names, and try to eliminate their accent to "pass" for nonimmigrants. Others "cling" to their culture of origin and reject the new culture. They often live in ethnic enclaves, socialize mostly with other immigrants from the same country, and minimize their interaction with noncompatriot youth. Yet another group alternates between the two cultures, trying to combine parts of the past and present and create a "new me." These adolescents speak both languages, have friends from both cultures, and consume a mix of food and other material goods.

Semyon's story is not uncommon. He was raised by his maternal grandmother while his divorced mother worked to support the family. He has not seen his father since he was a toddler. Divorced families in the former Soviet Union were not uncommon. When Semyon was 12, an uncle sponsored the migration of the family to the United States. The mother now works two low-paying jobs to put food on the table. The grandmother does not speak English. Teachers here have much less authority over youth than in Semyon's homeland. All these changes have resulted in Seymon's becoming "a street kid." He is often truant from school, has been involved in petty crime, and experiments with drugs. He frequents the local community center, where, together with several other rough young-sters, he terrorizes other kids. He spends endless hours at the pool table, brutally chasing away any-body else, using bad language, and refusing to be-have in a more collaborative way, despite pleas and threats by staff.

When a social worker based in a community mental health service first approached him, Sem-yon responded with a dismissive, disrespectful, and provocative style. But the worker, himself an im-migrant from the former Soviet Union, did not give up. He spent hours at the pool table, declined to respond to provocation from Semyon and his "gang," and did not try to push any behavior changes. Gradually Semyon and his friends toler-ated him as a part of the landscape. One evening the social worker noticed that Semyon was missing, and that his young friends were nervous and rest-less. He managed to find out that Semyon had been arrested by the police and volunteered to negotiate the situation. In the process of helping Semyon during his arrest, it became clear that his macho facade was a disguise for a frightened, disoriented, and scared kid who felt lost and helpless in this foreign environment. This became a pivotal point in their relationship. Following the resolution of the arrest incident, Semyon slowly started to be more responsive to the worker's efforts to engage him. When the social worker came to the com-munity center where Semyon and his friends were hanging out, Semyon was now willing to talk to him, first about his day and practical issues (e.g., problems encountered at school), and then gradu-ally about his family, his concerns regarding his future, and his relationships with girls. Initially all these conversations took place in a casual manner by the pool table. One evening Semyon agreed to the worker's suggestion to sit at a quiet corner in the center, which then became their routine. Some-times they would go out to talk while strolling the neighborhood or in a local coffee shop. The worker made a deliberate effort to keep the meetings in-formal for fear that structuring them more "profes-sionally" would scare the youngster away. Gradu-ally the worker became Semyon's new hero, to whom he remarked, "You are like a big brother that helps me with my troubles." The following months became a long and bumpy road. This road was not free of "relapses," times when Semyon refused to see the worker, used inappropriate language, or ac-cused him of "doing this because this is your job

for which they pay you; you do not really care for me." However, the social worker never gave up. During the following year, he helped Semyon enroll in a local alternative school, find a part-time job, and start to turn his life around. Throughout the process the social worker encouraged him and ex-pressed trust in the youngster's ability to achieve his goals.

In this example, the key to the social worker's ability to help Semyon was the combination of per-sistence, availability in a nontraditional way, and familiarity with the community. These are some of the factors that have proved helpful in working with immigrant adolescents. Trial and error in real-life situations rather than a traditional approach to office-based work help practitioners involved in servicing this population to gradually develop guidelines for what works, and learn how to adjust general principles of intervention to fit the unique needs of these youngsters. Empirical evidence sug-gests that when such a nontraditional model is adopted, minority clients tend to stay in treatment (Gottesfeld, 1995). The following section presents and illustrates what we learned.

Community-Based Mental Health Service: A Viable Approach

Our experiences from serving adolescent immi-grants suggest that community-based mental health services offer an effective alternative to traditional mental health services. An important characteristic of community-based services is that they are pro-vided *within the context of the client's natural envi-ronment* rather than in the context of a specialized professional structured organization such as a hos-pital or a mental health clinic. These natural envi-ronments may include schools, community centers, clubs, parks, and other "hangout" locations.

Adolescent immigrants are living between dif-ferent worlds, confused about their "previous me" and "current me," and are often lost, existing on the margins of these worlds because they do not fully belong to any. However, helping them within their own ethnic community has been demonstrated to be the key that enables them to thrive in the context of their other communities.

The advantages of community-based mental health services for adolescent immigrants are two-fold. First, developing community-based services involves working with the ethnic community's strengths to enhance its potential as a source of support for its troubled youngsters. Second, community-based services are less encumbered by many of the cultural and institutional barriers created by traditional services in serving this population group. Some of the advantages of community-based services include culturally acceptable problem definition, normative venues for help seeking behavior, nonstigmatized context, accessibility, feasibility, affordability, culturally competent service providers, nonthreatening services, culturally appropriate models, and linguistic relevance.

Culturally Acceptable Problem Definition

The definition of mental health–related needs has been discussed by Cox and Ephross (1998) as culture specific. Immigrants do not always share the Western view of what constitutes a mental health problem. This requires practitioners to be receptive and nonjudgmental rather than critical when immigrants have their own view of the situation. Some behaviors that would be a reason for seeking or referring to professional help in our culture are accepted as normal in other cultures. For example, physical disciplinary methods common in the Russian culture are defined as punishable child abuse in the United States. These differences can create discrepancies in identifying situations that require professional intervention.

Even when immigrants agree with the social worker that there is a problem, their perception of the nature of the problem is often different. Practitioners need to demonstrate sensitivity to this by using terms that are acceptable to the target population, such as "acculturation stress" rather than "mental health issues," "coping with transition" rather than "emotional problems." Such neutral and stigma-free language is more feasible in the context of the community than in the context of medical or other problem-focused specialized settings. The ethnic community provides the practitioner with vocabulary one can use to frame and address a problem ("we call this so and so," "in our culture this is viewed as such and such"), whereas medical settings are dominated by pathology-saturated jargon and are often informed by models that embrace a deficit rather than a strength perspective (e.g., *DSM-IV* language). The latter tends to alienate immigrants.

What does this mean for the practitioner? How can the principle of culturally acceptable problem definition be translated into practice? First, the worker needs to recognize that the clients may have a different perspective on their situation and that this perspective is valid and important. Having given up the belief that their own view on the situation is the "correct" and "true" perspective, practitioners should seek to gain understanding from clients, their families, and people in the community regarding such issues and their meaning in the context of the clients' culture. This can be done by interviewing the adolescents themselves, people in their environment, and key people in the community and by seeking translation of media (newspapers, radio, and TV shows) regarding relevant issues (e.g., the advice column is a treasure of knowledge regarding the culturally appropriate approach to personal and interpersonal issues).

Normative Venues for Help-Seeking Behavior

Even when immigrants perceive a situation as problematic, they may address it in ways that differ from the norms in the culture of resettlement, since help-seeking behavior is also a cultural product. Immigrants are often reluctant to seek help or even cooperate when a school or medical staff refers them for help because the stigma attached to personal-emotional problems and mental health issues casts a shadow of shame over the whole family in ways not fully appreciated by those outside their culture. The effects can be long-standing and may compromise the status, welfare, and even prospects for marriage for all family members within the community. Thus even serious mental health problems are often kept as private family secrets (Berger, 1996; Harper & Lantz, 1996; Sandhu, 1997; Slonim-Nevo, Sharaga, & Mirsky, 1999).

The case of Irina illustrates this. Irina is a talented and ambitious student, a gifted violinist, and by Western criteria, a very disturbed girl. She has a history of self-mutilation and suicide attempts. When she shared her suicidal thoughts with the social worker, including a specific plan for killing herself, the concerned worker initiated a hospitalization in an adolescent ward of a psychiatric hospital. The family refused to approve the hospital admission, criticizing the social worker as an ignorant person who was overstepping her boundaries. They demanded that no further efforts be made to engage Irina to prevent self-harm.

In contrast to this direct mental health intervention, community-based services allow immigrants to be more receptive to help within the parameter of their culture. Working with resources of the community, such as religious leaders and other key authority figures, enables practitioners to reach out to immigrant adolescents and their families in a way that does not put the family in a precarious social position, to receive help without losing face. In Irina's case, the social worker developed a relationship with Irina's music teacher. Together they organized a series of lectures about psychological aspects of relocation for young musicians. This served as a springboard for reaching out to students who experienced difficulties, among them Irina.

Nonstigmatized Context

To enhance the prospects of mental health services being used by immigrant adolescents, it is useful to locate them in their natural environment. A neutral, nonstigmatized, friendly, and nonthreatening setting is of paramount importance for providing effective services to them. Immigrants tend to be suspicious about public mental health services, perceiving them as part of an established authority capable of taking away freedoms. Because of political and authoritarian abuses, asking for help with emotional and psychological problems in their country of origin could result in a person's losing a job or a much-needed driver's license (Berger, 1996; Cox & Ephross, 1998; Handelman, 1983). Therefore, "safe" environments such as community centers, schools, vocational training centers, and social clubs offer opportunities for reaching out and providing clinical services in a useful and client-friendly manner.

The language used to conceptualize services is of utmost importance. Such services need to bear nonthreatening, stigma-free descriptions such as "discussion group" or "acculturation services" rather than any language that implies pathology, mental illness, or emotional problems. Hardly any immigrant is likely to set foot in an "outpatient service" because "patient" implies that one is sick and that something is wrong with that person. A title that builds on the community affiliation, such as a

"center for Russian youth," has a positive identification and would more likely engage young people who could benefit from services. In this type of setting, the encounter between the adolescent and the social worker occurs within the context of the community rather than a sterile and impersonal professional environment; the worker can use the social fabric of the community, as well as real-life opportunities, to help meet the needs of the adolescent.

Another useful way to create a less formal environment that helps "defrost" suspicious attitudes and enhance trusting relationships is by going with clients to the theater, to museums, and on other field trips. Ana, a social worker with Russian adolescents, found that visits with her clients to the Jewish Museum in New York stimulate vivid discussion in relation to clients' identities, their confusion about who they are and who they wish to be. Spending an hour on the trip in a social situation allows her to assess clients' interpersonal issues and enables her to offer information about social norms in their new culture.

Working within the community can achieve two goals: helping immigrants learn about American norms, and helping their American-born counterparts learn about the immigrants' cultures and the experiences that influence their behavior. By raising mutual understanding, community-based services can help to combat negative attitudes such as "immigrants invest all their time studying, thus taking away places in selective schools and scholarship money from American-born youngsters," "immigrants refrain from socializing with others and prefer to create their closed groups," and, following 9/11, "immigrants of Middle Eastern origin, especially Muslims, are not to be trusted."

One example of such an activity that countered immigrants' stereotypes was the development of a relationship between a mostly immigrant high school in Brooklyn (in which the largest group of immigrants included Jews from the former Soviet Union) and an upper-middle-class Orthodox Jewish high school in Manhattan. The social worker in Brooklyn contacted the principal of the Manhattan school and negotiated a visit of a group of his students to celebrate together the Jewish holiday of Hanukkah. The hosts, in a somewhat patronizing manner, prepared a ceremony and traditional refreshments but were surprised by a rich musical performance by their guests. The atmosphere quickly warmed, producing an unanticipated request by the host students for a visit to Brooklyn. Such encounters are beneficial in reducing distances and serves as a springboard for ongoing collaboration between students in developing joint projects for national science competitions, artistic performances, and so forth.

Accessibility, Feasibility, and Affordability

Experience with the Russian Adolescent Project showed that use of mental health services by immigrant adolescents is determined to a large degree by the location, scheduling, and price of services. Community-based services address these logistics with their flexibility and user-friendliness to engage youth in nontraditional ways.

Location

Location of services needs to be carefully planed. Immigrant adolescents are more likely to use services within their local ethnic community rather than ones in difficult-to-reach locations. Fugita (1990), who studied use of mental health services by diverse ethnic groups, found that having locations that are not accessible by public transportation reduces utilization, while having locations in the ethnic or racial community decreases the chances of clients' dropout. The importance of accessibility was demonstrated by a campaign for early detection of breast cancer in an ethnic enclave. A free examination by top experts using state-of-the-art instruments in a prestigious university hospital was offered. However, this required an hour-long subway ride into Manhattan. Many women expressed interest, but only a few actually showed up to be tested. A social work student who was placed in the setting for her fieldwork practicum suggested that women were reluctant, anxious, and uncomfortable in negotiating the ride to the city and the maze of the hospital. A local examination site set for 2 days in the neighborhood health club brought more than 80 women to the test. Although this is an example of a physical health issue, the same applies to mental health—local and accessible services within the community are more likely to meet the needs of the youth.

Locating a service in the traditional community, however, may make potential clients concerned about their privacy, especially in small, close ethnic communities. Barriers to using these services include a fear of being seen entering the building or meeting somebody they know in the waiting room, both of which could lead to being negatively labeled, ridiculed, and rejected by other community members. Developing services that are based in culturally acceptable settings in the community offers a solution that addresses both accessibility and stigmatizing issues. The staff are perceived as part of the normative acculturation services rather than as mental health professionals. They are viewed as the people who help with "legitimate" difficulties such as employment, training, and negotiating the system. Thus, they are easily accessible while minimizing the negative stigma.

Scheduling

Many adolescent immigrants need to hold part-time and/or random jobs to help their families make ends meet. Coping with both school- and job-related demands, adolescent immigrants have a hectic life that requires services with flexible scheduling, including evening and weekend options. Such flexibility is easier to achieve in innovative, responsive services in the community rather than in traditional prescheduled services that typically require observing regular appointments.

Walk-in and by-demand services have been most successful. They offer an opportunity for adolescents to come and participate whenever they feel the need and have the time, without being forced to commit to a fixed timetable. In addition to compatibility with their schedule, such services also validate the independence and self-determination of youth ("I decide when to come rather than having to commit to a certain time at the professional's availability").

For example, lunch hour support groups (called discussion groups to avoid the connotation of immigrants as in need of support, i.e., incapable of making it independently) in local middle and high schools successfully mushroomed. This model is described in detail in the Russian Adolescent Project case example later in this chapter.

Art, who has attended such groups and claims to have benefited from them, explains: "Just knowing that there is someone available for me every Wednesday at noon is helpful. It is comforting and supporting to be sure that if I need her [the social worker], she is there and I can come and talk about what bothers me and get advice. Just this knowledge helps even when I do not show up."

Affordability

Even modest fees and sliding scales are often beyond the ability of immigrants to pay. An amount of $100 a month can be unaffordable to someone who struggles just to pay the rent and buy food. Marina, a recent immigrant from Russia, recounted how her request to try on used jeans at a garage sale was met with an unbelieving sneer. "They could not understand that for me spending $3 on trousers that won't fit was a big deal." Of particular importance is adequate support for services that are funded in ways that protect the freedom to provide creative services (e.g., fee-for-service).

Culturally Competent Service Providers

Community-based services are more readily culturally sensitive services when provided by staff members who are bicultural. Such workers, themselves often immigrants of the clients' culture of origin, are aware of cultural taboos and acceptable patterns of interaction. They can provide a powerful role model and a supportive adult figure to inspire youth, support figures that have may been lost during immigration (Glassman & Skolnik, 1984), and also serve as a bridge from the adolescent's culture of origin to the new culture.

Immigrants lack familiarity with most Western mental health concepts, disapprove of sharing private and family information with strangers, and expect personal matters to be kept within the family. Therefore, they often prefer informal help from relatives, religious leaders, and compatriots (Fuller Hahn, 1992). Workers who are familiar with these cultural norms can frame their services in ways that are acceptable. For example, an extremely orthodox Jewish family from an Eastern republic refused to allow a social worker to build a therapeutic relationship with their very troubled daughter, claiming that all is in the hands of God. The worker managed to gain access to the girl when she suggested that God has different ways of helping, and maybe sending a social worker is the way he has chosen in this particular case.

Furthermore, providing service providers who are members of the same community as their clients stimulates a process of capacity building and en-

hances the sense of efficacy. However, while coethnic service providers are knowledgeable about the culture of the clients, some clients might view being served by people of their own culture as inferior, and prefer service providers from the new culture. In addition, similarity in immigration experience and ethnic-cultural background of client and worker may create unresolved issues of countertransference.

Since providing services by bicultural clinicians is not always feasible, it is imperative that clinicians who are not bicultural be trained to work with the immigrant population. For both groups of clinicians, supervision is helpful, although the supervisory role is different for each.

In supervision of bicultural clinicians, major tasks are education about social and professional norms of the absorbing culture and the role of social workers, and helping the adjustment of their knowledge and skills to the new culture. A parallel process is created, in which the supervisor fulfills for the worker many of the functions that the worker fulfills for clients. These functions include education, guidance, modeling, support, and counseling.

In training clinicians who are not bicultural, the focus of supervision is on adjusting their knowledge and skills to specific client populations. This involves self-reflection and awareness of their own values, assumptions, and biases. It also requires developing understanding of the immigration experience and its effects and acquiring knowledge about and respect for the specific culture of their clients. Service providers often react with anger, intolerance, and reluctance to be responsive to immigrants' needs and requests. Fadiman (1997) documented in detail the clash between medical staff in a California hospital and a refugee Hmong family from Laos, whose young daughter was diagnosed with severe epilepsy. From her doctors' perspective, the origin of her condition is biological, and they prescribe multiple drugs to help control her seizures. The parents, who believe the disease is caused by spiritual forces, gradually develop doubts about the benefits of the medications and eventually refuse to administer them. The girl is declared brain dead, but the family continues to care for her, harboring hopes that her soul will be reunited with her. Although this may be an extreme case, many of the misunderstandings described in the book accurately reflect the cultural issues that might impede immigrants from receiving appropriate treatments.

Recent years have witnessed increased recognition of the importance of cultural competence and a growing body of knowledge about building capacity for assessment and intervention strategies with diverse groups (Lum, 1999; National Association of Social Workers, 1996). Main principles of cultural competence include combining knowledge about clients' cultural heritage and values with understanding between groups and individual differences, imperative for success with an immigrant population. Clinical knowledge and skills relevant for culturally competent practice can be developed by client-worker collaboration. The supervisor plays a central role in helping clinicians explore and figure out how such collaboration can be developed in a way that is acceptable to clients' culture.

Nature of Services

"Talk therapy" is viewed as futile in many cultures (Nguven, 1984). Somatization of stress is not uncommon in various cultures, and accordingly, "just talking" is not considered helpful; people expect tangible, concrete services (Chandras, 1997; Fugita, 1990; Rodriguez & O'Donell, 1995). Providing specific advice and explanations on practical issues, and through them indirectly addressing underlying problems, often fits better with the expectations in different cultures.

The following example illustrates this point. When I was first hired to train and supervise staff in two programs in South Brooklyn, I facilitated a discussion with them to clarify their expectations from their supervision group. The American workers unanimously wished to have an opportunity to reflect on clinical issues and dilemmas they experienced in their daily practice and receive collegial feedback; the Russian workers preferred that I present a structured didactic lecture because "for us just exchanging ideas is not real learning; you are the expert so we would like you to tell us what we should do in given situations."

Adolescents in general, and immigrants in particular, are often reluctant to seek or accept traditional processing of feelings in a therapeutic context where the therapist is in an authority position. Innovative approaches to engage the youth are nec-

essary. To help them deal with feelings such as mourning, loss, anger with parents, and so on, indirect and action-focused approaches proved to be beneficial. For example, a group of adolescents who opposed efforts of the social worker to process their emotions were instead able to discuss their impressions and thoughts about the effects of being uprooted in connection to an exhibition that they saw in the Jewish Museum in New York. Later in this chapter I describe in detail the use of community theater as a way for adolescent immigrants to address and cope with their feelings.

Community-based programs can offer integrative models of care that combine services for skills development, help in acculturation, and counseling. Mastery of social knowledge and skills helps clients gain a sense of control over their life, raises their self-confidence, improves their acclimatization to the new culture, and empowers them (Berger, 1996; Furnham & Bochner, 1986; Glassman & Skolnik, 1984). These capacity-building programs and the content focus create a "basket of care" that helps with developmental issues and has therapeutic effects without being defined as therapy.

Culturally Appropriate Models

Brief, strengths-based, psychoeducational, action-oriented, solution-focused and cognitive-behavior models that focus on helping immigrants regain autonomy and address practical issues proved to be more useful than traditional therapeutic approaches in working with adolescent immigrants (Berger, 1996; Slonim-Nevo et al., 1999). For example, teaching techniques for prioritizing issues and stress management is effective because it is much more compatible with the strong emphasis that Chinese, Japanese, Korean, and other cultures put on cognition than the traditional models that emphasize the processing of emotional experiences.

Most traditional mental health services are based on problem-oriented models, which conceptualize immigration exclusively as a trauma and focus on its posttraumatic devastating effects. While immigration is indeed a highly stressful experience with possible detrimental effects on individuals and families, pathology has been overemphasized and salutary effects minimized (Witmer & Culver, 2001). In the last decade, the potential for both negative and positive effects of trauma has been documented (O'Leary, Alday, & Ickovics, 1998). Empirical research has shown that traumatic events create not only the danger of emotional distress and functional decline but also the opportunity for personal growth (Tedeschi & Calhoun, 1995; Weiss, 2002). Survivors of natural disasters, war experiences, violent victimization, and life-threatening illnesses such as breast cancer reported personal benefits as a result of their struggle to cope with the trauma (Calhoun & Tedeschi, 1999; Cordova, Cunningham, Carlson, & Andrykowski, 2001; Weiss, 2002). Immigration, like other traumas, includes resilience and a potential for posttraumatic growth (Berger, 2005; Berger & Weiss, 2002; Calhoun & Tedeschi, 1999; Gibson, 2002).

Although some writers acknowledge the existence of resilience among adolescent immigrants (Harker, 2001; Hernandez & Charney, 1998), empirical research on the topic is very scarce. One exception is the comprehensive study of Muslim Bosnian adolescent refugees by Weine and associates (1995), who reported "adaptive flexibility" and "notable resilience." In another study, Chavkin and Gonzalez (2000) identified among Mexican immigrant youth who lag behind other immigrant groups in educational completion and achievement, personal family and community protective factors that enhance academic resilience. However, in spite of these few voices that have started to explore resilience in recent years, most of the literature about immigrant adolescents still focuses on problems and deficits.

Portraying the immigration experience as exclusively problematic without recognition of immigrants' resilience, and failure to balance risks of posttraumatic stress with the benefits of posttraumatic growth may inflict unnecessary stigmatization on immigrants. Mental health assumptions and interventions that have been developed within the context of mainstream Western culture without appropriate modifications may cause more harm than help. The *DSM-IV* suggests a diagnosis of adjustment disorder "when an identifiable stressor leads to impaired relationships in the patient's work or social life" (Morrison, 1995, p. 454). This seems to include most, if not all, immigrants. Using standards of Western middle-class white culture as a yardstick against which behaviors are measured, and failure to recognize certain behaviors as normal reactions to an abnormal situation may lead to bi-

ased diagnosis. Applying a psychiatric diagnosis pathologizes appropriate reactions to the stress of immigration, thus potentially presenting an added burden, rather than support, to the immigrant's mental health. The pathologizing effects of assigning psychiatric labels to refugee-related loss and distress were recognized by Bracken and Petty (1998), who remind practitioners "not to inadvertently impose Western discourse on trauma centralized around the concept of post–traumatic stress disorder (PTSD), on other cultures' experiences" (quoted in Gibson, 2002, p. 33). In a recent conference on trauma, participants noted less use of the diagnosis of PTSD in Europe than in the United States and expressed concern in regard to what they perceived as "unhelpful over diagnosis" (Joyce & Berger, 2003). Because of this, immigrants are often misdiagnosed and offered interventions that are not helpful.

Community-based programs foster the positive powers of immigrants by focusing on adjustment, education, skill development, enhancing language proficiency, job seeking and vocational training, and drug abuse and sexually transmitted disease prevention programs—all of which offer a validating framework for provision of services in a way that is relevant to clients. Stress research indicates that action helps to cope with trauma, regain control over one's own life, and reinforce a sense of self-worth.

While traditional mental health services are structured hierarchically, with the service provider as the expert and the immigrant as the recipient, community-based services that are collaborative enable the adolescents to do for themselves and give back to their community rather than being passive recipients of services. Activities such as learning the language and vocational training can help youth recognize that at least part of their problems is caused by objective circumstances rather than their own failure. Participation in collaboratively designed programs enables them to regain mastery, thus restoring their sense of self-esteem (Berger, 1996; Leader, 1991).

For example, in one enclave of immigrants from the former Soviet Union, a worker helped a group of high school students establish an affordable summer day care service for young children of working mothers in their community. An adolescent complained in a group about conflicts with her parents, who work long hours and demand that she babysit her younger sister during the summer because they could not afford a camp. This led to a discussion of participants' summer plans, in which many group members expressed anger and frustration over their failure to get a summer job. This discussion paved the road for expressions of resentment toward their parents' decision to immigrate, dissatisfaction with life in the new environment, and despair. The social worker facilitated a discussion of alternative approaches to address their concerns. Gradually a plan evolved for group members to organize a babysitting service in which group members could share the responsibilities, make money, maintain some free time, and address the needs of working parents in their neighborhood. The group activity focused for several months on looking for an appropriate location and developing a schedule for activities with the preschoolers and a schedule of "shifts" for group members. Six adolescents successfully collaborated in running the service for a whole month, after which they expressed feeling encouraged by their success and by the community's appreciation. This active engagement in community problem solving increased skills and competencies in restless young people, giving them purpose as well as fulfilling responsibilities to their families.

Linguistically Relevant Services

Language has been identified as a barrier to use of mental health services. Providing services in the immigrants' language is much more feasible and common in community-based services because of a greater availability of bilingual personnel. Lack of fluency with the English language is a major stressor for immigrants in general (Zapf, 1991). It becomes even more of an issue in therapy, which addresses sensitive topics. Having to address such issues in a language in which one lacks fluency intensifies the difficulties and limits the ability of immigrants to express delicate nuances of their feelings.

Offering the service in the immigrants' "mother language" facilitates self-expression and communication, enhances efficiency and comfort, and validates and reflects respect for the cultural roots of the clients, which in itself has a therapeutic effect. Marina, a recent immigrant explains, "I can discuss the history of the United States and the Civil War in English, but it is much more natural and easy to explain my tensions with my parents in Russian. I would not even know how to say in English some of the things we yell at each other."

A Case Example: The Russian Adolescent Project

The Russian Adolescent Project (RAP) is an example of a community-based mental health service for adolescent immigrants. It provides group, family, and individual acculturation, preventive, and therapeutic services to youth who emigrated from the former Soviet Union and their families.

Mission

The mission of RAP is to develop and deliver mental health services that are tailored to address the unique needs of immigrant adolescents from the former Soviet Union in a manner that is acceptable to the youngsters and their families and compatible with their culture.

History

Since the early 1980s, political upheaval has swept away the Communist government in the former Soviet Union. One result of these changes was a wave of families, mostly Jewish, who moved to the United States. These immigrants had grown up in a totalitarian, repressive Communist, antireligious regime that practiced total control over the life of the individual from cradle to grave. Mental health services were abused and used punitively for purposes of political control. Key to survival was maintaining mistrust of strangers beyond the immediate family (even family members sometimes squealed on each other) and a close circle of friends. This was especially the case regarding suspicion of professionals affiliated with the establishment (Ivry, 1992). Consequently, in the immigrants' culture of origin, therapy, especially traditional talk therapy, has been seen as useless and "just talking," not valued as a strategy for solving problems. In contrast, education was a central value; schools and teachers have been powerful and influential in the lives of students and their families.

These adolescents and their families faced multiple adjustment challenges when they arrived in the United States. Schools in the southern parts of Brooklyn, particularly Coney Island and Brighton Beach, reported encountering a growing number of immigrants from the former Soviet Union who were presenting with mental health problems. These problems, which were created or exacerbated by the hardships of immigration and the clash between the newcomers' culture of origin and the more liberal culture of resettlement were compounded by normal developmental issues.

It also became clear that traditional mental health services were not equipped to address the newcomers' unique needs, as there was an absence of services to facilitate acculturation. The Jewish Board Family and Children Services (JBFCS), one of the nation's largest nonprofit mental health and social service agencies with a strong clinically oriented culture, quickly identified and responded to these gaps in services. The director of their Madeleine Borg outpatient mental health clinic, who was especially sensitive to the challenges involved in engaging youth, initiated the establishment of an adolescent unit to provide clinical services for immigrant adolescents in response to this new wave of immigration from the former Soviet Union.

The unit was initially launched as a branch of the mental health clinic in Coney Island. Two workers, both immigrants themselves from the former Soviet Union, were hired to reach out to the Russian-speaking community. One was pursuing his college education but lacked training in the helping professions. He was assigned the reaching-out activities; the other had professional experience as a psychologist in her country of origin and was responsible for clinical aspects of service provision.

A lucky combination of circumstances—the willingness of schools to open their doors for acculturation services and availability of funding—set the stage for developing this modest start into a full program titled the Russian Adolescent Project as an integral part of the new clinic. This clinic became licensed for providing mental health services. The idea was that school-based workers would have a double role of providing adjustment-facilitating services and mental health screening. While they helped émigrés with acculturation, they were to use a clinical lens to identify youth and families at risk and refer them to clinical services. Thus, these workers became a bridge between the troubled youth and the clinical settings.

Gradually a functional division of time evolved, in which the same workers performed reaching-out and clinical roles. This model has been the modus operandi of the project for the last decade and will be described later in the section on structure. RAP has been developed with no protocols or guidelines for practice. Practice principles emerged and were shaped by trial and error as a collaborative effort of the leadership of the program, the professional supervisor, the workers, and key people in the community. A director and a group of clinicians who have been involved with the project for many years secured consistency in application and transmission of these principles to new personnel.

Goal and Objectives

The overriding goal of the project is to identify immigrant youth in distress and help them cope with their situation so that they can continue to pursue their education, and to enhance their emotional, psychological, and social well-being and functioning. To achieve this goal, the program has defined several objectives:

1. To provide acceptable, affordable, and non-stigmatizing services of information and support to adolescent immigrants to help them cope effectively with their unique stresses;
2. To provide assistance to parents and educators to enable them to help the adolescents; and
3. To identify adolescents who struggle with more severe mental health problems and provide appropriate culturally sensitive and culturally relevant services.

Conceptually the program is informed by immigration theory, a rehabilitative-supportive approach and a strength perspective (Portes & Rumbaut, 1996; Saleebey, 1997). This means that when a worker in the program encounters an adolescent, the focus is on "How is this youngster resilient?" rather than "What is wrong with this young person, and how can it be fixed?" Such a frame of reference often differs from what clinicians have learned in their professional training and requires of practitioners and supervisors a deliberate and challenging effort to refocus.

Context

Services have been offered within the context of public schools, parochial Jewish schools (the "Russian yeshivas"), and community centers under non-stigmatized, positively oriented labels (e.g. "discussion groups," "acculturation services") because

Russian immigrants tend to be suspicious of mental health professionals, value educational task-oriented activities, and do not readily accept the possible benefits of traditional talk interventions.

Structure

A structure designed to support the objectives was developed. The same social workers facilitated the acculturation groups and worked in the mental health clinic. Thus, if an adolescent is identified in the context of the group as requiring more intense, specialized, or individualized help, the same worker with whom the adolescent has developed a relationship and a certain degree of trust in the context of the group will provide the mental health services in the clinic. This decreases reluctance to seek help. Sacha, age 14, participated in a lunch hour group in his middle school. Sacha attended sporadically. When he was present, he told dirty jokes, interfered when others spoke, and challenged Vladimir, the social worker, himself an immigrant from the former Soviet Union. Attempts to involve Sacha in any productive interaction within the group proved futile. The staff of the school reported that his behavior in class was equally destructive, but his single mother had rejected any previous suggestions for referral to mental health services. She declined to cooperate with efforts to address her son's issues, stating, "You are the teacher; you should find ways to deal with him." With the supervisor's support and encouragement, the worker continued to welcome Sacha in the group, made efforts to involve him in group discussion, and ignored his acting out.

The worker made deliberate efforts to engage Sacha by expressing confidence in him and awarding a "special" status. For example, he would request Sacha to help with organizational aspects of the group (e.g., get crayons from the secretary). On one occasion Vladimir handed Sacha his car keys and a note permitting the youngster to access the car and fetch a box that contained materials for group activities. Sacha was appalled, "You are giving me your car keys? What if I take it?" Vladimir shrugged and expressed his belief that Sacha would bring the box in a responsible manner.

Gradually, in response to Vladimir's expression of trust, Sacha began to reciprocate with a certain degree of trust in Vladimir. When at the end of the year Vladimir expressed his wish to continue to meet with Sacha during the summer, the boy and his mother agreed. At this point, Vladimir's suggestion was not perceived as a referral to a mental health service; rather, it was viewed as going to meet Vladimir in his other office. This was an action that the family felt comfortable with.

Service Providers

The workers in the project are immigrants from the former Soviet Union, with training and professional experience in education, psychology, and psychiatry, who are going back to school to pursue a degree in social work. Both the youngsters and their families feel more comfortable sharing their concerns with workers who speak their native language and who understand many of their experiences and underlying and unspoken themes. However, because clients and workers belong to the same community, informal encounters in the supermarket, at the theater, and at social occasions are unavoidable. Therefore, a certain degree of concern regarding confidentiality persists and needs to be repeatedly addressed. The contract includes clear statements followed by frequent reminders that the worker will "ignore" clients on nonprofessional occasions and will not initiate a communication, leaving the client free to decide whether to acknowledge the worker.

Types and Models of Services

The project provides preventive, diagnostic, therapeutic, and psychoeducational services. Clients are recruited by reaching out through direct advertisement in places where youngsters hang out, such as clubs and community centers, and by referral from guidance counselors and teachers of English as a second language (ESL). Services include groups, individual and family counseling, and community activities.

Groups

An important modality of service provision is group work. This choice has been informed by several considerations. First, group work has been documented to be very useful with adolescents because of their age-related tendency to associate in groups and preference to turn for support to peers rather than to adults (Henry, 1992; Leader, 1991). Lopez (1991) illustrated how social group process acts for adolescent immigrants as a protective factor, which promotes a capacity for competence and mastery over their new environment. The group helps participants gain a more realistic perception of their difficulties, as they are able to recognize that many of their experiences are shared with others and are related to objective circumstances rather than to their personal failure. The group also provides participants a safe place for mutually learning norms of the new culture and nonthreatening ways to gain experience with new ways of interaction that build competence in negotiating it successfully. Group work is also considered to be an effective modality in serving immigrants because it provides them with a support system that substitutes for social networks lost to immigration and with positive role models that can instill hope and empower (Glassman & Skolnik, 1984). Homogeneous groups have been documented as most helpful in rebuilding young people's sense of identity (Berger, 1996; Halberstadt & Mandel, 1988; Mirsky & Prawer, 1992).

The program offers groups for both adolescents and their parents. A number of efforts have been made to facilitate groups for educators. Adolescent groups are typically open, with no preregistration or prescreening required. The only condition for school-based groups is that the student has a free period or a lunch period when the group meeting is scheduled. Each session is an independent unit, so that new or infrequent participants do not feel excluded. However, experience has indicated that most participants tend to attend consistently for the duration of a full semester. Participants are welcome to express themselves in Russian, English, or a combination of the languages.

Groups focus mostly on normative acculturation- and relocation-related issues involving identity, parent-adolescent relationships, and crossgender relationships. In accordance with their cultural tradition, the focus is usually on "practical" issues of learning to adjust to American norms that will result in improving their academic performance. These issues serve as a springboard for discussing related emotional and psychological issues that may hinder adjustment.

Parent groups are dedicated mostly to psychoeducation and mutual support. Parents resent Western liberal parenting styles and consider them inappropriate because their parenting style in the former Soviet Union had been quite authoritarian. The groups provide an opportunity to learn about American normative adolescent development. They discuss adapting parenting practices to the new en-

vironment. Processing these cultural differences with others who share the same experience provides parents with an opportunity to be exposed to diverse ideas about resolving these differences and get support. As a result, they are able to decide which are nonnegotiable expectations and come to terms with some inevitable compromises.

Individual and Family Counseling

In cases of more severe problems such as chemical dependency, mood disorders, psychotic disorders, eating disorders, and so forth, individual and/or family counseling services are offered. Although traditional psychodynamically oriented therapy is also used in some cases, clinicians tend to favor cognitive-behavior and solution-focused approaches that are more compatible with the Russian emphasis on practical solutions. A deliberate effort is made to use all models in a culturally sensitive way (e.g., respect for the discourse of suspiciousness that is characteristic to this population).

Community Activities

Health fairs, holiday parties, and a community theater are part of the services offered in the context of RAP. These activities help further introduced immigrants to the norms of their receiving culture and enhanced their connection to their new social environment. This increases their feeling of integration and helps restore their sense of competence and self-worth. Of particular interest, the community theater grew out of an activity group in a local community center frequented by many immigrant adolescents. During a group meeting in which relationships with parents were discussed, the worker used role-playing as a means to help participants express their feelings and gain understanding of their parents' position.

Group members gradually became very excited and involved in the role play. The social worker, who had a background in theater studies, introduced them to basic principles of Stanislavsky's method for getting ready to play a role. With enthusiasm and excitement, the group decided to expand their creation into a play. Rumor about the activity soon spread, and more youngsters joined. The Russian tradition of theater and its usefulness as a vehicle for masked social criticism contributed to the enthusiasm toward the project. With the direction of the social worker, a large group of adolescents worked for 8 months to develop an elaborate script with a plot that focused on relationships and intergenerational conflicts in an immigrant family from the former Soviet Union. They rehearsed, composed and practiced music, and prepared costumes. The play, presented to an audience of parents, members of the community center, and the Russian community as a whole, was received very positively. The participants gained much-desired recognition and self-esteem, in addition to developing collaborative relationships.

Parents were especially proud of their children. The content of the play was discussed in several parent groups. Presentation of the issues and feelings indirectly in the context of a play rather than in angry encounters with their children allowed parents the necessary distance to understand the youngsters' experiences. A number of families reported that the play helped parents and adolescents communicate with a higher degree of mutual understanding.

The community theater is one example of fostering posttraumatic growth by community-based services. The momentum that developed and stimulated a process of meaning making and harvesting positive changes from painful experiences of loss and living in conflicting worlds. This process involved working out issues of continuity and constancy, new role models, and issues of identity. In the theater the youth created a safe haven, which allowed them to be critical and set the stage for a dialogue that felt safe for them and was also acceptable to their families.

Outcomes

Although RAP operated for more than a decade, a systematic evaluation of its outcomes was not conducted. However, anecdotal data suggested that the project benefited participating adolescents and their families. Principals, guidance counselors, ESL teachers, and additional school personnel who work with this particular group of adolescent immigrants consistently reported improvements in individual cases. Workers in the program cited numerous success stories. Youngsters kept attending programs and reported their satisfaction with it. When budgetary constraints threatened to discontinue the project, there was strong vocal resistance in the community.

It is conceivable that as the wave of immigrants from the former Soviet Union decreases, many of the clients will adjust while others move to receive services within general non-immigrant-specific settings, and this special project for immigrants from the former Soviet Union will fade.

Conclusion

Traditional mental health services have often failed to help immigrant adolescents because of cultural, institutional, and personal barriers. Community-based services offer an alternative approach that can meet the needs of this population group. This chapter has reviewed characteristics of this high-risk target population and discussed how community-based services can be integrated into the community for its youth. The Russian Adolescent Project in Brighton Beach, Brooklyn, illustrates how a community-based mental health service offers a viable alternative to traditional mental health services by providing group, family, and individual acculturation, prevention, and therapeutic services to immigrant and refugee youth and their families within a culture-sensitive setting.

Essentials of this emergent practice of community-based clinical services for immigrant adolescents are multidimensional. The backbone of such services is the emphasis on capacity building, the strength perspective, and collaborative work with the community. Culturally and linguistically relevant approaches to assessment and intervention models, creative techniques for outreach, and use of the natural, stigma-free settings for service delivery by culturally competent service providers are of utmost importance. Accessibility, affordability, flexibility, feasibility, and use of creative arts are crucial in developing successful services.

While clinical impressions point to the success of this program, a systematic evaluation of the intervention process and clients outcomes is yet to be conducted. Such an evaluation can help identify and develop evidence-based knowledge about the best practices and interventions for working with immigrant adolescents. It will also help us to understand which of the principles of community-based service used in this program can be applied to other immigrant groups, and what modifications are necessary. Differentiating aspects of the programs that are unique to particular groups of immigrant adolescents from those that apply to other populations of youth will help us to develop guidelines for helpful community-based services.

References

Baider, L., Ever-Hadani, P., & Kaplan-DeNour, A. (1996). Crossing new bridges: The process of adaptation and psychological distress of Russian immigrants in Israel. *Psychiatry: Interpersonal and Biological Processes, 59*, 175–183.

Baptiste, D. (1990). The treatment of adolescents and their families in cultural transition: Issues and recommendations. *Contemporary Family Therapy, 12*, 3–22.

Bemak, F., Chung, R. C-Y., & Bornemann, T. H. (1996). Counseling and psychotherapy with refugees. In P. B. Pedersen, J. G. Draguns, W. J. Lonner, & J. E. Trimble (Eds.), *Counseling across cultures* (pp. 243–265). Thousand Oaks, CA: Sage.

Berger, R. (1996). Group work with immigrant adolescents. *Journal of Child and Adolescent Group Therapy, 6*, 169–179.

Berger, R. (1997). Adolescent immigrants in search of identity: Clingers, eradicators, vacillators and integrators. *Child and Adolescent Social Work Journal, 14*, 263–275.

Berger, R. (2005). *Immigrant women tell their stories.* New York: Haworth.

Berger, R., & Weiss, T. (2002). Immigration and posttraumatic growth: A missing link. *Journal of Immigrant and Refugee Services, 1*(2), 21–39.

Bracken, P., & Petty, C. (1998). *Rethinking the trauma of war.* New York: Free Association Books.

Calhoun, L. G., & Tedeschi, R. G. (1999). *Facilitating posttraumatic growth: A clinician's guide.* Mahwah, NJ: Erlbaum.

Castles, S., & Miller, M. J. (1998). *The age of migration: International population in movements in the modern world.* New York: Guilford.

Chandras, K. V. (1997). Training multiculturally competent counselors to work with Asian Indian Americans. *Counselor Education and Supervision, 37*, 50–59.

Chavkin, N. F., & Gonzalez, J. (2000). *Mexican immigrant youth and resiliency: Research and promising programs.* Washington, DC: Office of Educational Research and Improvement.

Cordova, M. J., Cunningham, L. C., Carlson, C. R., & Andrykowski, M. (2001). Posttraumatic growth following breast cancer: A controlled comparison study. *Health Psychology, 20*, 176–185.

Cox, B., & Ephross, P. H. (1998). *Ethnicity and social work practice.* New York: Oxford University Press.

Drachman, D., & Shen-Ryan, A. (1991). Immigrants and refugees. In A. Gitterman (Ed.), *Social work practice with vulnerable populations* (pp. 618–646). New York: Columbia University Press.

Fadiman, A. (1997). *The spirit catches you and you fall down.* New York: Noonday Press.

Fugita, S. S. (1990). Asian/Pacific American mental health: Some needed research in epidemiology and service utilization. In F. C. Serafica (Ed.), *Mental health of ethnic minorities* (pp. 64–83). New York: Praeger.

Fuller Hahn, D. (1992). Soviet Jewish refugee women: Searching for security. In E. Cole, O. M. Espin, & E. D. Rothblum (Eds.), *Refugee women and their mental health: Shattered societies, shattered lives* (pp. 79–87). New York: Haworth.

Furnham, A., & Bochner, S. (1986). *Culture shock: Psychological reactions to unfamiliar environments.* New York: Methuen.

Garza-Guerrero, A. C. (1974). Culture shock: Its mourning and the vicissitudes of identity. *Journal of the American Psychoanalytic Association, 22*, 408–429.

Gibson, E. C. (2002). The impact of political violence: Adaptation and identity development in Bosnian adolescent refugees. *Smith Studies of Social Work, 73*, 29–50.

Glassman, U., & Skolnik, L. (1984). The role of social group work in refugee resettlement. *Social Work with Groups, 7*, 45–62.

Gold, S. J. (1989). Differential adjustment among a new immigrant family members. *Journal of Contemporary Ethnography, 17*, 408–434.

Goodenow, C., & Espin, O. M. (1993). Identity choices in immigrant adolescent females. *Adolescence, 28*(109), 173–184.

Gottesfeld, H. (1995). Community context and the underutilization of mental health services by minority patients. *Psychological Reports, 76*, 207–210.

Halberstadt, A., & Mandel, L. (1988). Group psychotherapy with Russian immigrants. In D. Halperin (Ed.), *Group psychotherapy: New paradigms and perspectives* (pp. 311–325). Chicago: Yearbook Medical Publishers.

Handelman, M. (1983). The new arrivals. *New York Association for New Americans Practice Digest, 5*(4), 3–22.

Harker, K. (2001). Immigrant generation, assimilation, and adolescent psychological well-being. *Social Forces, 79*, 969–1004.

Harper, K. V., & Lantz, J. (1996). *Cross-cultural practice: Social work with diverse populations.* Chicago: Lyceum.

Henry, S. (1992). *Group skills in social work.* Pacific Grove, CA: Brooks/Cole.

Hernandez, D. J., & Charney, E. (Eds.). (1998). *From generation to generation: The health and well-being of children in immigrant families*. Washington, DC: Committee on the Health and Adjustment of Immigrant Children and Families, National Research Council and Institute of Medicine.

Hoberman, H. M. (1992). Ethnic minority status and adolescent mental health services utilization. *Journal of Mental Health Administration, 19*, 246–267.

Hulewat, P. (1996). Resettlement: A cultural and psychological crisis. *Social Work, 41*, 129–135.

Ivry, J. (1992). Paraprofessionals in refugee resettlement. In A. Shen-Ryan (Ed.), *Social work with immigrants and refugees* (pp. 99–117). New York: Haworth.

Joyce, P., & Berger, R. (2003, May). *What language does PTSD speak? Clinical social work, cultural competence and diagnosis*. Paper presented at VIII European Conference on Traumatic Stress, Berlin.

Landau-Stanton, J. (1985). Adolescents, families and cultural transition: A treatment model. In A. Mirkin & S. Koman (Eds.), *Handbook of adolescents and family therapy* (pp. 363–381). New York: Gardner.

Leader, E. (1991). Why adolescent group therapy? *Journal of Child and Adolescent Group Psychotherapy, 1*, 81–93.

Lee, E. (1988). Cultural factors in working with Southeast Asian refugee adolescents. *Journal of Adolescence, 11*, 167–179.

Liebkind, K. (1992). Ethnic identity: Challenging the boundaries of social psychology. In G. M. Breakwell (Ed.), *Social psychology of identity and the self concept* (pp. 147–185). London: Surrey University Press.

Logan, D. E., & King, C. A. (2001). Parental facilitation of adolescent mental health services utilization: A conceptual and empirical review. *Clinical Psychology: Science and Practice, 8*, 319–333.

Lopez, J. (1991). Group work as a protective factor for immigrant youth. *Social Work with Groups, 14*, 29–42.

Lum, D. (1999). *Culturally competent practice: A framework for growth and action*. Pacific Grove, CA: Brooks/Cole.

Mirsky, Y., & Prawer, L. (1992). *Immigrating as an adolescent, being an adolescent as an immigrant*. Jerusalem, Israel: Elka and Van Leer Institute (Hebrew).

Morrison, J. (1995). *DSM-IV made easy*. New York: Guilford.

National Association of Social Workers. (1996). *The National Association of Social Workers code of ethics*. Washington, DC: Author.

Nguven, S. D. (1984). Mental health services for refugees and immigrants. *Psychiatric Journal of the University of Ottawa, 9*, 85–91.

O'Leary, V. E., Alday, C. S., & Ickovics, J. R. (1998). Models of life change and posttraumatic growth. In R. G. Tedeschi, C. L. Park, & L. G. Calhoun (Eds.), *Posttraumatic growth: Positive changes in the aftermath of crisis* (pp. 127–151). Mahwah, NJ: Erlbaum.

Portes, A., & Rumbaut, R. C. (1996). *Immigrant America*. Berkeley: University of California Press.

Pumariega, A. J., Glover, S., Holzer, C. E., & Nguyen, H. (1998). Utilization of mental health services in a tri-ethnic sample of adolescents. *Community Mental Health Journal 34*, 145–156.

Rodriguez, O., & O'Donell, M. (1995). *Help seeking and use of mental health services by Hispanic elderly*. Westport, CT: Greenwood.

Saleebey, D. (Ed.). (1997). *The strength perspective in social work practice*. White Plains, NY: Longman.

Sandhu, D. S. (1997). Psychocultural profiles of Asian and Pacific Islander Americans: Implications for counseling and psychotherapy. *Journal of Multicultural Counseling and Development, 25*, 7–22.

Schuck, H. P. (1999). *Citizens, strangers and in-betweens: Essays on immigration and citizenship*. Boulder, CO: Westview.

Shen-Ryan, A. (Ed.). (1992). *Social work with immigrants and refugees*. New York: Haworth.

Slonim-Nevo, V., Sharaga, Y., & Mirsky, J. (1999). A culturally sensitive approach to therapy with immigrant families: The case of Jewish emigrants from the former Soviet Union. *Family Process, 38*, 445–461.

Stewart, E. C. P. (1986). The survival stage of intercultural communication. Tokyo: *International Christian University Bulletin, 1*, 109–121.

Tabora, B. L., & Flakerud, J. H. (1997). Mental health beliefs, practices, and knowledge of Chinese American immigrant women. *Issues in Mental Health Nursing, 18*, 173–189.

Tedeschi, R. G., & Calhoun, L. G. (1995). *Trauma and transformation: Growing in the aftermath of suffering*. Thousand Oaks, CA: Sage.

Waters, C. M. (1996). The intersection of gender, race and ethnicity in identity development of Caribbean American teens. In B. J. Ross Leadbeater & N. Way (Eds.), *Urban girls: Resisting stereotypes, creating identities* (pp. 65–81). New York: New York University Press.

Weine, S., Becker, D., McGlashan, T. H., Vojvodka, D., Hartman, S., & Robbins, J. P. (1995). Adolescent survivors of "ethnic cleansing": Observations on the first year in America. *Journal of the American Academy of Child and Adolescent Psychiatry, 34*, 1153–1159.

Weiss, T. (2002). Posttraumatic growth in women with breast cancer and their husbands: An inter-subjective validation study. *Journal of Psychosocial Oncology, 20,* 65–80.

Witmer, T. A., & Culver, S. M. (2001). Trauma and resilience among Bosnian refugee families: A critical review of the literature. *Journal of Social Work Research, 2,* 173–187.

Woodward, A. M., Dwinell, A. D., & Aorns, B. S.

(1992). Barriers to mental health care for Hispanic Americans: A literature review and discussion. *Journal of Mental Health Administration, 19,* 224–236.

Zapf, K. M. (1991). Cross-cultural transitions and wellness: Dealing with culture shock. *International Journal for the Advancement of Counselling, 14,* 105–119.

Paula Armbruster, Laura Ewing,

Virginia DeVarennes, Abigail Prestin,

Lisa Lochner, Ursula Chock,

and Saglar Bougdaeva

The Neighborhood Place
An Alternative Mental Health Program

This chapter describes the Neighborhood Place, an innovative prevention program with two primary goals: to engage children from marginalized, disenfranchised families in constructive activities outside of the school day, and to give them a voice for the expression of their thoughts and emotions. By engaging these children in positive activities, routines, and structures in a stigma-free environment, problems, should they emerge, could be addressed on-site without the customary referral to a "clinic." Additionally, children would learn pro-social skills and have an opportunity to channel their talents and energies in ways that are socially acceptable and appropriate. Implicit in the development of the Neighborhood Place was the belief that a community-based program, in which the portal to services was not mental health but a more culturally accessible intervention interwoven with a psychiatric component, would be effective for these families. Mental health professionals administered this program so that although the entry point is an after-school as well as summer arts and athletics program, psychiatric intervention is embedded in its implementation. This chapter comprises four components: background, literature review, program description, and summary. Specifics of the program

are addressed so that it can be adapted or replicated in various environments.

Background

The Neighborhood Place was developed as a result of a study that examined treatment outcome before and after the introduction of managed care in an urban, university-based children's psychiatric outpatient clinic. It was found that managed care had little clinical impact on clients, as indicated by standardized measures of general functioning (Armbruster, Sukhodolsky, & Michelson, in press). The decrease in the average number of overall sessions from 15 to 10 was not the result of managed care, as 20 sessions are approved initially by the behavioral health managed care organizations in our state, but may be attributed to the fluctuations of attrition patterns within the clinic, which has varied over the years (Armbruster & Fallon, 1994; Armbruster & Schwab-Stone, 1994). Furthermore, 10 sessions met the criteria for an appropriate dosage of intervention, which is considered to be a minimum of 9 sessions (Andrade, Lambert, & Bickman, 2000; Angold, Costello, Burns, Erkanli, & Farmer,

2000). Regarding the clinical measures, however, the mean Global Assessment Functioning (GAF) score (American Psychiatric Association, 1994), which measures the highest level of functioning, was 48 upon admission to the clinic and 52 at discharge, representing minimal improvement. The results of the Children's Global Assessment Scale (C-GAS; Shaffer et al., 1983), which measures the lowest level of functioning, were a mean score of 48 at entry and 50 at termination, again, a negligible change. Diagnoses remained unchanged from entry to discharge.

In response to these findings, the authors raised the following questions: First, was the objective of the clinical interventions to simply maintain these children and prevent further regression? Second, were the standardized measures used in the study inadequate to measure outcome? Third, did the findings reflect the need for earlier identification and prevention or for alternative interventions? In answer to our first question, if, indeed, our task was to prevent these youth from developing more severe problems, the results indicated that this goal was achieved; the children did not regress further, according to the measures. The second query led us to a review of standardized measures used to evaluate outcome, and new questionnaires have been selected. Another outcome study will be implemented to determine if there is any difference in results. In response to the final question, an alternative intervention called the Neighborhood Place was developed. This program focused on prevention and provided mental health services to children and families through a culturally accessible gateway. Such an intervention would identify children with mental health problems before they developed acute symptoms and needed to seek treatment. Additionally, since the majority of the children who compose the population are severely disadvantaged, we questioned whether once-a-week psychotherapy in an unfamiliar setting was the optimal intervention, particularly since these children return home, often to violent and chaotic neighborhoods. Hence, a site in the neighborhoods that are home to these children was considered as an alternative location.

Before proceeding further, it is useful to describe the clinic population and the environment in which these children live. The clinic and the children and families it serves are located in one of the most economically and socially polarized cities in the nation. Close to 30% of the city's population lives in public housing (Housing Authority of the City of New Haven, 2003), in contrast to the six institutions of higher learning that reside within its borders. The publicly funded clinic serves the city's disadvantaged population: 65% to 70% are on Medicaid (Title IXX), 83% are single-parent families, and 61% are minority (41% African American and 20% Hispanic). The combined attrition rate of the clinic is 45%, measured by different clinic phases (e.g., dropout after completing telephone intake prior to in-person contact, dropout after one session, dropout during evaluation, dropout after completion of evaluation, dropout during treatment; Armbruster & Fallon, 1994; Armbruster & Schwab-Stone, 1994). The clinic is representative of the children attending the city's public schools in that the majority of the students are poor and minority, and, unfortunately, with a few exceptions, parent involvement is one of the main challenges faced by the schools. For example, in an elementary school with a population of 400 to 500 students, fewer than 10 parents consistently attend parent-teacher organization (PTO) meetings.

This disconnection from mainstream organizations, such as educational and mental health services, is reflected in the health care arena as well. For example, the Connecticut Medicaid Managed Care Council found that 15% to 20% of this economically depressed population utilized hospital emergency departments for health problems, consistently did not show up for appointments, or were absent when managed care outreach workers arrived at their homes for appointments (Connecticut Medicaid Managed Care Oversight Quality Assurance Subcommittee, 2002). These observations prompted additional questions regarding the provision of service interventions: Is there a cohort of families, the "truly disadvantaged," who believe they have been dismissed by the "system"? Do these same individuals, in turn, dismiss the system because they feel that "there is nothing in it" for them (Wilson, 1998, p. 276)?

To create effective interventions, the mental health delivery system may benefit from examining these issues from sociological or anthropological in addition to, or rather than, psychiatric or medical perspectives. This recommendation was also made by the Surgeon General's Conference on Children's Mental Health, which suggested the shift from a medical framework to an ecological framework

(U.S. Public Health Service, 2000). The Child and Adolescent Service System Program, or as it is now known, the system of care, has supported this recommendation as well (Stroul, 1993). A medical perspective isolates symptoms such as aggressive, antisocial behavior and depression, often without considering the context of those symptoms. The disciplines of sociology and anthropology consider the cultural context of behavior and examine values, norms, and expectations. Such frameworks are not new to mental health professionals: social work utilized these theories with its espousal of the "person-in-the-environment," or ecological, viewpoint (Germain & Gitterman, 1995, p. 816). The environmental perspective has also been adopted by other mental health disciplines (psychology, psychiatry, psychiatric nursing) to understand challenges facing impoverished populations so that effective interventions may be created. Marginalized groups, no matter how handicapped they may be, are often reluctant to seek help from "mainstream" institutions. Such institutions are often perceived as stigmatizing, unwelcoming, and judgmental. Leaf and colleagues found that those with acute mental health needs were the most reluctant to seek services and were part of a severely disadvantaged population (Leaf, Bruce, Tischler, & Holzer, 1987). Hence, how services are framed is key to successful implementation.

Literature Review

According to Wilson's (1998) findings on the effects of neighborhood disadvantage on adolescent development, high population turnover, poverty, drug use, delinquent youth, and single-parent families frequently characterize disadvantaged neighborhoods. This environment creates conditions that limit residents' ability to create or adhere to conventional or "mainstream" norms. Instead, numerous risk factors and high mobility of residents often lead to a condition where strong peer groups rule the neighborhood. The emergent peer systems operate outside of the mainstream and thereby create both a physical and an ideological distance between members of these communities and mainstream institutions. Therefore, weekly psychotherapy may not be as effective for either the child or the family existing within these peer groups. If teen pregnancies, high school dropouts, criminal behav-

ior, and drug use are part of the culture of some communities, suggestions and admonitions by educators or health and mental health professionals may not resonate beyond school or clinic walls.

Garbarino (1998, 2001) suggests that social forces interact with or involve a degree of violence and poison the environment, decreasing the well-being of the community's residents. Children in these communities, overwhelmed by risk factors, are often unable to create meaning in their own lives. Instead, left with a sense of hopelessness, they may look to deviant or antisocial peer groups to provide meaning. Whereas many youth look to involvement in a "mainstream" gang, such as a sports team or a school band, as a means to explore identity and gain peer group acceptance, children without these community resources may find that affiliation with a deviant "street gang" provides them with "power, status, peer group acceptance [or] a surrogate family where close attachments with parents do not exist" (Gordon, 1999). Services need to replicate the street "gangs," which offer structure, identity, and support, in a pro-social way; otherwise, little connection will be made between provider and recipient.

Given the circumstances of these communities, the implementation of an alternative intervention may prevent problems from occurring or identify them early and increase the effectiveness of later treatment. Therefore, to help disadvantaged children succeed in "toxic environments," interventions situated directly in their neighborhoods can provide a number of advantages by supplying alternative social experiences, responsible adults, and resources (Garbarino, 1998; Rutter, 1999). Community-based interventions have cycled through periods in which they have lacked support; within the past 15 years, however, they have regained popularity. This growth has emerged within the context of federal, state, and local grant money aimed at promoting collaborative community-based care and the systems of care model within communities (Burns, Hoagwood, & Mrazek, 1999; Stroul, 1993).

Despite a great deal of variability depending on the ecology of particular communities, the common element of the system of care is to join service providers with families within the context of their communities. For example, some of the more established programs include multisystemic therapy (Henggeler, Schoenwald, & Borduin, 1998), comprehensive school programs or "full service schools" (Dryfoos, 1998; Franklin & Streeter, 1995), and intensive "wraparound" services, which is a "system of coordinated care" that brings families together with multiple mental health service provider agencies that offer a wide range of approaches to care (Lightburn, Olson, Sessions, & Pulleyblank-Coffey, 2002). However, a limitation of many such programs is that the service providers leave the communities after service is delivered or the grant funding has ended (Burns et al., 1999).

Among the model programs of community-based service providers that have been sustained are Community Assessment Centers and Communities in Schools (CIS). The Community Assessment Centers were established by the Office of Juvenile Justice and Delinquency Prevention (OJJDP) and offer a single point of entry into the juvenile justice system, immediate and comprehensive assessments, integrated case management, and comprehensive management information systems at a single site within the community (Oldenettel & Wordes, 2000). As a result, juveniles involved with the justice system receive integrated services and the presence of service providers within their communities. Likewise, CIS repositions existing community resources at local school sites (Communities in Schools, 2002). With services located at schools, residents are able to have both integrated and locally available services within their communities. These programs, which have succeeded in engaging the support of their communities, have been able to sustain themselves over time because they have been effective in meeting the needs of their target populations.

Although there are a number of community-based interventions, there is still a need to design and implement more programs that provide children in disadvantaged communities with committed adults, alternative social experiences, and safe spaces in which they can develop. Currently, research on the efficacy or effectiveness of these services is sparse (Burns et al., 1999). Furthermore, these programs are often fragmented and time-limited. Community-based care is needed to improve outcomes for children from disadvantaged communities; yet, to reach this goal, mental health providers must commit not only to designing quality programs but also to assessing the effectiveness of their designs.

After-school programs make sense intuitively

and carry with them potential benefits such as additional time for academic instruction, cultural enrichment, and increased adult supervision. Fashola (1998) highlights three primary reasons for after-school care: (1) additional supervision during a time when children might engage in antisocial or destructive behaviors; (2) provision of enriching experiences; and (3) improvements in socialization and academic achievement. Posner and Vandell (1994) looked at the academic and emotional adjustment of low-income children attending formal after-school programs. They found that children's participation in such programs, which provided academic and enrichment activities that increased their pro-social engagement with peers and adults, was positively correlated with academic grades, peer relations, and emotional adjustment.

Another outcome study of low-income youth attending after-school programs specifically focused on the effects of an after-school educational enhancement program on a group of adolescents living in a public housing project (Schinke, Cole, & Poulin, 2000). The authors report that program participants demonstrated higher scores on reading, spelling, history, science, and social studies, higher overall grade averages, and improved school attendance than a control group living in the same public housing project.

Fashola (1998), who reviewed 34 after-school programs reports a variety of positive outcomes, ranging from improved academic performance to increased feelings of safety and positive peer relationships. A number of studies point to a correlation between after-school program involvement and a decreased incidence of drinking, smoking, drugs, sex, and violence and improved social and behavioral adjustment, better peer relations, and more effective conflict resolution (Miller, 2001). It is noteworthy, however, that many of these studies contained limitations such as lack of a control group or selection bias.

However, after-school programs offer no panacea for at-risk youth: the literature reports negative findings as well. Pierce, Hamm, and Vandell (1999) studied the emotional climate of after-school programs. They report that negative peer interactions in after-school programs were correlated with increased internalizing and externalizing behaviors and poor social skills for boys, and increased externalizing behaviors for girls. Furthermore, boys who experienced negative staff regard and who were presented with a higher number of choices for activities exhibited increased internalizing and externalizing behaviors and decreased reading and math grades. These results focus on correlations; consequently, causation cannot be implied. However, the studies suggest that students are more likely to succeed in programs where staff exhibit positive regard, where there is a high degree of program structure, and where activity choices are limited.

Vandell and Corasaniti (1998) also report that children who attended community center-based after-school programs were stigmatized in school and were not presented with age-appropriate activities. Rosenthal and Vandell (1996) found a negative correlation between overall center climate and total enrollment. According to Fashola (1998), the negative correlations associated with different aspects of after-school programs demonstrate how simply offering after-school programs may not be enough: These programs must be of high quality and must contain certain elements deemed to be essential to effective programs, such as access to academic instruction, including qualified instructors, recreational, and cultural components; effective program development and management; well-trained staff with lower rates of turnover; a solid, clear program structure; positive discipline; frequent evaluation and assessment; an advisory board; and inclusion of families and children in the planning process.

Finally, Dynarski (2003) notes that first-year findings for the examination of the 21st Century Community Learning Centers Program (21st Century), a nationwide school-based after-school program, were mixed. For the black and Hispanic middle school participants, there was an increase in grades and scores, as well as a decreased level of absenteeism and tardiness. Homework turned in by participants was more likely to be satisfactory to teachers. Participants in general spent more time under adult supervision, and their parents were more likely to volunteer or engage in their child's academic life. However, for the program as a whole, the study reported that overall attendance was low and inconsistent; grades and test scores of attendees were not higher than those of nonattendees; participants were no more likely to complete homework or school assignments than nonparticipants; attendees did not report a greater feeling of safety as a result of their involvement with 21st Century, nor

did exposure to working in groups help them feel more competent in their social skills in terms of planning, implementing, and meeting goals within a team setting.

The discrepancy among the previously mentioned studies highlights the complexity of research evaluating after-school programs. Assessment of after-school programs presents a number of difficulties, including the type of student served, a wide variation in program quality, and divergent program goals. For example, programs frequently attempt to achieve a number of contrasting goals, ranging from access to cultural or recreational activities, improved grades, and better peer relations. Posner and Vandell (1994) highlight the contrasting program goals and outcomes for low-income versus middle-class children. They argue that after-school programs may help low-income children but may provide little benefit to middle-class children based on differential access to other sources of enrichment activities. They posit that middle-class children can often afford enrichment activities such as music and art lessons, whereas low-income children often do not have this opportunity. For those children who have access to and can afford lessons, center-based after-school care may not be beneficial. According to Posner and Vandell's findings, a critical task in after-school care for low-income children is to offset negative effects of poverty. Consequently, the program goal for low-income children may be to increase attendance in order to decrease unsupervised time spent in dangerous neighborhoods, whereas for middle- and upper-income children, goals may vary from enrichment to enhanced social status.

Despite the limitations and mixed results of current research, the few studies available do highlight a number of potential positive outcomes, specifically for low-income children who attend after-school activities. However, the current body of literature points to the need for methodologically sound studies that not only further assess the effectiveness of current programs but also explore differential pathways to achieving these outcomes. Knowledge of what works could help to increase funding, improve programs, and create quality programs. The research on the potential negative outcomes for children in after-school care suggests that without quality programs, after-school time may simply continue to represent a time when children are at risk.

Building on this knowledge base, we identified the seven following ingredients essential to the Neighborhood Place:

1. Accessibility: Culturally neutral medium accessible to all racial, ethnic, and socioeconomic groups;
2. Inclusiveness: Open and free of charge to children and families from the community, irrespective of background;
3. Activity: After-school hours infused with the highest quality of enriching activities (arts, athletics) that engage diverse groups of participants;
4. Structure: High adult-to-child ratio to provide structure and supervision;
5. Parent involvement: Strong element of parent participation, support, and engagement;
6. Location: Sites in familiar community locations, such as schools, neighborhood centers; and
7. Mental health: Clinicians fully integrated into the program as secondary service providers

The Neighborhood Place

The Neighborhood Place, emerging from our experience and our findings regarding treatment outcome, as well as the results of other studies, was particularly inspired by the work of Garbarino and Rutter. Their research has concluded that a committed adult and an alternative social experience are the critical ingredients for children to lead productive lives and to emerge from the "toxic environments" in which they live (Garbarino, 1998; Rutter, 1999). The program was also driven by the belief that any mental health intervention must be culturally acceptable to the community it serves.

These principles were the basis for the Neighborhood Place, an after-school program and summer program that was launched on July 1, 2000, open to the community and free of charge. The primary function of the Neighborhood Place is to engage children and families in positive "mainstream" activities that potentially hold relevance for them. The program is built to foster the growth of relationships between staff and participants, as well as to increase interest and participation in prosocial activities. Such activities need to serve as a cultural bridge, so that children and families per-

ceive the activities as welcoming, and on culturally neutral ground where their values and norms do not clash with those of the service providers. Engaging children and families through such a conduit has the potential to form new, positive connections with individuals and organizations that represent "the system." In this way, the Neighborhood Place seeks to offer an "alternative social experience" in which at-risk children can begin to develop the skills to become constructive adults. According to Garbarino (1998), it is important that youth learn to form positive relationships with adults, because children in toxic environments often are not given a sense of security from the adults in their communities. Adults, overwhelmed by stressors such as poverty and violence, are often unable to shield their children from the same stressors. Children may then internalize the message that adults are unreliable and powerless (Garbarino, 2001).

Rutter (1999) believes that alternative activities should be provided to children who may be seeking affiliation with a peer group. These activities carry significantly less risk than those of the deviant peer groups but can still be as attractive to the program's participants as the activities promoted by the deviant groups. In other words, youth need an alternative to the "gangs," but one that provides them with the positive ingredients that the gangs offer, such as support, identity, and belonging. Many of these children perceive adults as uncaring and disinterested in their lives and believe mainstream organizations such as schools, mental health, and health to be irrelevant. Therefore, with a high adult-to-child ratio, a "committed adult" is more likely to emerge in the child's life (Garbarino, 1998; Rutter, 1999).

Finally, the Neighborhood Place exposes children to activities that are outside of their daily routines in order to broaden their perspectives and help them become familiar with heretofore alien individuals, organizations, and experiences. By providing activities that are generally offered only to "mainstream," or more economically secure, children, we hope to bridge the gulf between marginality and mainstream. In this way, the resentment and dismissal of services offered by the "establishment" may be diminished.

The second task is to give children an outlet for their emotions and thoughts, so that they have a "voice" that is heard and valued. Offering a pro-social vehicle for expression could be a deterrent for negative behavior. The arts appeared to be the most appropriate vehicle to achieve these two goals, as they are culturally neutral in that African American, Hispanic, Asian, and European artwork is universally admired. Also, the arts provide a full range of media for creative and constructive self-expression. A Stanford University anthropologist has found in her evaluation of programs for at-risk, disadvantaged youth that the arts are the most effective intervention for this group. Improvements in behavior, self-esteem, and academic performance are among her findings (Brice-Heath, Soep, & Roach, 1998).

To address the many social and emotional needs of these youth, mental health permeates the entire program and is used both to identify severely emotionally and behaviorally disturbed children and to provide intervention as needed. The Neighborhood Place is propelled by the belief that within the context of these children's environments, a core of committed staff members, partnered with mental health professionals, working together to provide positive alternative experiences, can help redirect the energies of these youth so that they can lead productive lives.

The summer 2002 program was 8 weeks long and ran from 9:00 A.M. to 5:00 P.M., Monday through Friday, at a public school and a community center, both of which were located in the most crime-ridden, disadvantaged, "toxic" neighborhoods. The population of the community center was primarily Hispanic, and the public school population was predominantly African American. Although this schedule met the needs of parents of latchkey children, it was difficult to secure artists and staff for these time frames, and younger children found the long day problematic. Ongoing schedule flexibility such as rest periods, half-day options, and flexible dismissals will help to maintain younger children during a lengthy curriculum.

On the premise that children will act out less if they experience more success, the curriculum grouped children based on their ages and developmental capabilities. For example, early latency age children ages 6 to 8 were given a curriculum that encouraged fine motor skills such as drawing a portrait of themselves, family, friends, or their homes but that limited the expectations requiring expertise in these skills such as the integration of foregrounds and backgrounds. As opportunities for success were presented, a noticeable decrease in self-deprecating statements and more positive behaviors occurred.

The cost of operating this program was high, and administrators face the pressure of "an ever-present demand [to] . . . find new ways of attracting funds to meet the needs of the client population" (Lightburn et al., 2002, p. 290). In the case of this program, state departments and foundations to which the founders applied showed no interest in contributing to its funding. The program obtained funding though the political negotiations of its cofounder, a state senator. This illustrates the importance of developing and engaging legislative allies with access to state budgets. Funding also determined the duration of the program and number of participants: The longer the program ran and the higher the quality, the more expenses it incurred. Funding was public, which is often unsustainable or subject to fiscal cuts. Other resources must be explored so that the program is less vulnerable to state fiscal crises and able to maintain high standards for quality services. Staff with grant-writing skills or those who are willing and able to lobby legislatures and private foundations would be an asset to future programs.

Due to the current economic climate, the program's budget was cut completely in late 2002. Fortunately, many of the program's affiliates offered their services free of charge, allowing the program to continue *without funding*. Therefore, the Neighborhood Place and the local arts organizations with which it partners stand together through this fiscal crisis in a united effort to offer these children resources generally available only to children of privilege. Since there is an effort for museums and other art institutions to move from an elitist/exclusive to an inclusive/outreach position, these organizations welcomed an agency that offers them the opportunity to have a presence in the community. This situation also demonstrates the critical importance of networking and building partnerships. As a result of the positive acclaim that the program received, and the networks developed, we have reason to believe funding will be reinstated.

Program Evaluation

The program evaluation comprises two components. The first is a set of questionnaires regarding different aspects of the program, which were administered to children, parents, and staff involved with the summer 2002 program of the Neighborhood Place. The questionnaires, which were developed by the program administrators and linked to the goals of the program (e.g., pro-social behavior), functioned as a rating of the program by both participants and all components of the staff (art and athletic instructors, junior counselors, mental health clinicians). The response to the program was very positive by both parents and children; overall, staff response was positive as well, with helpful, concrete suggestions for improvements.

The second component of the program evaluation consisted of standardized measures. The goal of administering standardized measures was threefold: to enhance the child profile beyond demographics; to assess the level of disturbance of the children; and to compare the children with those at the clinic. Since the mission of the program was prevention, it was important to know if the participants were at risk and comparable to the clinic clients psychologically. Two of the measures selected are given routinely at the outpatient clinic: the Child Behavioral Checklist (CBCL; Achenbach & Edelbrock, 1983) and the Global Assessment of Functioning. Additionally, the Piers-Harris Self-Concept Scale (PHSCS; Piers-Harris, 1986) was given to children on the first day of the program. The CBCL was completed by the parents at the onset of the program. The mental health staff assessed each child on the GAF, arriving at a consensus score for the child. By using two measures given at the clinic, we believed we would be able to compare clinic and Neighborhood Place children on levels of impairment.

The mean CBCL score for the Neighborhood Place was 50, whereas, in the clinic, the mean CBCL score was 64. Thus, the children from the summer program were identified as being within the normal range of functioning by their parents, while those from the clinic were not. Clinicians rated more than half of the children who attended the Neighborhood Place with a mean GAF score of 58; approximately 60% these children were rated as severe to moderate in functioning. This indicated that the Neighborhood Place population was as poorly functioning as the clinic children, who had a mean GAF score of 53.

A sample of 25 cases was assessed by using the three standardized measures: GAF, CBCL, and PHSCS. The mean scores for the CBCL and PHSCS based on both the parents' and children's perceptions were in the normal range and were significantly different than the clinicians' mean score, which indicated that the children were below the range of normal functioning.

The self-esteem measure showed no change, but it was given at a 7-week interval, which is inadequate time to register impact; however, it was part of the effort to describe the program participants. We plan to administer it after a year to children who continue with the program. The evaluation is being redesigned for next summer.

An evaluation that measures the impact of community programming on children is difficult to implement. Families resist completing standardized measures and disclosing information about their children to people they do not know. Our data indicate that there is a discrepancy between how the parents view their children and the perspectives of the clinicians regarding these children.

Whereas the perception of the parents of the children at the clinic indicated that they were concerned about their children's behavior, neither parents nor children involved with the Neighborhood Place viewed the children's behavior as impaired; if they did observe problems, they did not wish to disclose them to individuals they did not know. Whatever the reason, this may explain why, in part, the majority of the children had no clinical contact. According to the clinicians, however, these children had serious behavioral and emotional difficulties that were going untreated. An example of these differing perceptions may be noted in case example 2.

If violence, drugs, and poverty are everyday occurrences in their community, it is not surprising that a parent may not believe his or her child's acting-out behavior to be unusual or inappropriate, as a clinician would. This discrepancy illustrates the chasm that often exists between the service provider and service utilizer, one that must be addressed to obtain reliable measures of outcome.

Because this is a community-based program that is presented as arts and athletics, families bring their children to the Neighborhood Place without concern about stigma. However, since mental health is integrated into the program, children and families receive services, either directly or indirectly. Hence, the Neighborhood Place is a true prevention program because it serves youth whose need for mental health intervention might otherwise be unidentified until it may be too late.

Program Components

Arts

The arts are seen as the medium that has the potential to overcome cultural barriers. Thus, they are the gateway through which these children may be engaged and may access mental health services in a nontraditional setting, as well as be exposed to creative and constructive activities. Additionally, the arts provide a means of expression through which they can voice their emotions and concerns.

The program partnered with all the arts organizations in the city and its surrounding area. Local artists gave the children instruction in activities such as drama, music, creative writing, drawing, painting, photography, and ceramics. Children interacted with artists whose racial and cultural backgrounds were similar to their own. Many children identified talents and interests that they may not have discovered were it not for the activities that the program offered. Additionally, the role of the art instructors included mentoring, chaperoning on trips, and serving as a link between children, parents, and staff. Often, the benefits extended to their families, who took pride in their children's work or performance. With the passage of time, the children began to demonstrate more confidence and competence in their activities and social interactions.

Case Example 1

One of the Neighborhood Place's participants was a 9-year-old Hispanic girl whose father had a terminal illness. She was worried and anxious about her father's health, did not engage in extracurricular activities, and consistently expressed a desire to stay at home to assist her mother with her father's care.

As she was exposed to art through the activities of the Neighborhood Place, particularly drawing and painting, the girl experienced multiple developmental gains. The clinicians and mentors encouraged her peer interactions and enhanced her

social competence by decreasing isolation, increasing her communication skills, and expanding the focus of her empathy and caring to others outside of her father and his illness. While she had been defended against the challenges of traditional therapy in verbalizing her emotions, art classes challenged her in a less intimidating manner to look beyond her usual methods of self-expression and problem solving to alternative means, which enhanced her resiliency.

In addition to the arts, the inclusion of parents in program activities helped to promote bonding between the girl and her mother. The gardening project enhanced their communication and problem-solving skills through planning and work division. Gardening also gave both a venue outside of a therapy office to internalize and practice the behavioral skill of "being in the moment," rather than worrying about an illness they could not control. This child was offered an alternative at which she could succeed. Through the arts, she gained an outlet for her anxiety by sublimating it through constructive media such as art and gardening.

Specific expectations, organization, structure, adequate training, and role definition were critical to the success of the arts program. Artists who expressed a clear understanding of their role in the program fulfilled their proposed curricula and experienced little frustration with children's behavior. Regarding the management of acting-out behavior, artists reported many benefits from the involvement of clinical social workers in the classrooms, and many of them asked to be paired with a clinical social worker in class to assist with problematic children.

Athletics

The sports staff succeeded in engaging children throughout the summer. Most of the children were initially reluctant to participate in the sports activities, which were unfamiliar to them. By the end of the summer, they were enthusiastically participating in all the athletics and learning new sports.

However, the competitive nature of sports prompted increased acting-out behavior among the children, which the instructors were unprepared to handle. In the future, sports instructors will be trained in behavioral management techniques and instructed to keep these techniques consistent throughout the duration of the program; athletic instructors may each be paired with a clinician.

Case Example 2

A 9-year-old Hispanic boy, who resided with his brother, two sisters, and both parents, participated in the summer program. He was extremely aggressive and frequently ran away. He had difficulty using verbal means to express himself, and while he may not have been impaired, his cognitive performance was difficult to evaluate due to his inability to remain in class. Although he had been seen by the school-based health clinic clinical social worker for 2 years, his mother, who seemed overwhelmed at home, continued to be contacted frequently regarding his behavior problems at school. These behavior problems continued while the boy participated in the Neighborhood Place. In spite of his father's refusal to participate, a clinical social worker and the sports coordinator worked with his mother to create a behavioral plan, which allowed him to do only one of three warm-up athletic activities rather than all three warm-ups required for sports participation.

He responded well to this flexible plan, yet his level of aggressively expressed anxiety proved to be more difficult to maintain during the arts activities, which did not meet his needs for gross motor stimulation. In addition, his home life remained overwhelming for his entire family, including his usually absent father. Following his decompensation, his two sisters also began having behavior problems, and his mother decided to remove all her children from the program. She felt as overwhelmed during the summer as she did during the school year in dealing with behavior problems.

This example illustrates the difficulty of engagement and the need for increased mental health support. Perhaps adding a home visitation component to assess the best way for the family to meet success may have been more effective. In addition, increased assistance of clinical social workers may have helped the boy's two sisters to better cope with expectations of their family and the program. Finally, this child's involvement should have been limited to only his success (athletics), and he should have been allowed to attend half days. In fact, as administration learned of the challenges facing families, an increasing number of children were given a half-day option.

As this example illustrates, the parent was more disturbed by the perceived criticism of her child's behavior than by the behavior itself. Yet this highlights the importance of the environmental contexts of these children. They all lived in violent, impoverished, crime-ridden neighborhoods where they often faced abuse, lack of supervision and structure, and low expectations at home. Since this was the familiar "culture" of the family, often what might be considered antisocial or undersocialized in other contexts, such as school, was not a cause for concern.

Trips

Each Friday, the children visited an arts or outdoor site. Children were divided into groups of four, with two adults per group; generally, a parent was paired with an instructor. These trips were opportunities for children to explore the city beyond their communities, and many later returned with their families to parks or museums that they had been introduced to by the program. Visits to local parks provoked a new appreciation of and interest in nature in many of the children, who are often confined to concrete and asphalt outdoors. Everyone involved with the program—children, parents, and staff—reported positively on the trips.

Case Example 3

An 11-year-old Hispanic girl living with her mother, two brothers, and her mother's boyfriend participated in the summer program. The child's mother had a history of substance abuse and inappropriate boundaries with her children, and her family has been involved with the state's child protection services, the clinic, and other agencies. The child had difficulty with anger management and physical aggression. Her mother attended parent workshops, in addition to working with the clinical social workers and the coordinator to create a behavior plan, providing the child with alternatives to physical aggression.

The child loved horseback riding but could not go on trips if she acted out three times in one week. She managed her behavior for 2 weeks after the behavior plan was created, but on the third week, she had more than three incidents of acting-out behavior. She was not allowed to go horseback riding that week and was extremely upset. Afterward, she discussed alternative ways to handle her aggression with the clinical social worker and decided to leave the classroom if she felt angry. A few days later, the clinical social worker saw her sitting outside of the classroom, looking stern, and asked what she was doing. She replied, "I was getting angry and about to hit someone, but I want to go horseback riding so I left the classroom." The child never missed another horseback-riding lesson.

This case exemplifies the positive impact that exposure to new interests and challenges can have on a child. Her new love of horses motivated her to change her behavior, and a flexible behavioral plan allowed her to do so. Again, this example transcends the boundaries of traditional intervention.

Adolescents

Local adolescents were engaged in the summer 2002 program as junior counselors in an effort to provide them with a positive work experience, for the benefit of the children who live in a peer culture with a paucity of well-functioning adults in their lives. These youth struck a balance between peer and role model and formed unique relationships with the children and the adult staff. They also provided valuable feedback about the Neighborhood Place during weekly meetings and received positive ratings on the questionnaires.

Case Example 4

One of the summer program's participants was a 13-year-old Puerto Rican boy whose father and brothers were incarcerated. None of his family members participated in the program. In spite of this, he attended the program every day and expressed the desire to be different from the rest of his family. He was very creative and enjoyed the one-on-one attention that he received from the program and the opportunity for an alternative focus for his energies and self-expression. The program built on and expanded his strengths. He received accolades and support for his commitment and achievement in both arts and sports. Hence, his sense of self shifted to a positive, competent one.

Through the individual attention from the staff, he was able to bond and learn coping and problem-solving skills and translate them to new experiences, which broadened his view of the world. For example, through self-talk and verbal communication of his feelings he was able to tolerate new activities such as sailing and horseback riding, which he previously would have dismissed as "un-

cool" due to his anxiety with experiences outside of his norm. As he became more comfortable with the exposure to new and different activities, his awareness of the alternatives to the inner city increased without intimidation. By utilizing experiential activities as well as traditional mentoring, he was able to internalize options to the world he currently lives in and improve resiliency. His enthusiasm for the program motivated other children to participate, and next summer he will be recruited and trained to be a junior counselor.

Mentoring

The mentoring component was built into the arts and athletic components to provide a one-on-one relationship between each child and an artist or athletic instructor and to link the young participant, his or her parents(s)/guardian(s), and program staff. This aspect of the program was one of its biggest successes, with children and parents all reporting on its benefits. Children had a resource they could go to with problems, parents had a consistent contact person within the program, and lines of communication were opened between children, staff, and parents.

Case Example 5

One African American female joined the summer program in the third week of July. As a 14-year-old, she was the oldest participant, which made her uncomfortable. Given the importance of peers in teen culture, this girl felt that she would be better able to form a relationship with someone closer to her age. She requested to be paired with a junior counselor. It was unusual for a junior counselor to serve as a mentor, a role that was reserved for the adult clinicians and instructors. However, given the participant's age and request, the exception was made. Allowing the teen this choice gave her positive control over one aspect of her life. She also received positive feedback and a sense of self-determination for her judgment in her selection; indeed, her choice was a tribute to her innate psychological health, as she selected a mentor who had significant strengths.

The junior counselor was also from the same background as the teen and was a high achiever. In the junior counselor, the teen found someone with whom she could identify, respect, and trust. For instance, the teen was able to seek out her junior counselor for help coping with the death of a close friend. With the help of the junior counselor's nurturance of the teen's ego, the program was changed to accommodate her need to be treated less as a young child and more as an increasingly mature adolescent. By having an opportunity to take on more sophisticated roles in the program, she was able to increase her comfort within the program and gain a positive sense of self.

Mental Health

Five clinical social workers constituted the mental health staff for the summer 2002 program. With only one exception, the mental health staff consisted of individuals from the same ethnic groups as the population the program served. They assisted artists with acting-out children, co-taught arts and athletics activities, and worked with children who were referred by the artists, athletes, and parents. They were also integrated into groups with high-risk children to intervene when a child acted out, where they could either initiate a group intervention or remove the child from the group to deal with him or her one-on-one.

Arts and athletics instructors with less experience dealing with acting-out children frequently requested the aid of the clinical social workers. To counteract this trend, clinical social workers discussed individual cases in the context of child management and group dynamics with staff members. The clinical social workers were well received by the children, parents, and staff.

Case Example 6

One child was a patient at the clinic before she participated in Neighborhood Place summer 2002 program. Clinic treatments for her included individual therapy, pharmacological intervention, and in-home services. The clinical social worker who had been working with this child spoke to her mother about the Neighborhood Place and the benefits it could offer her and her daughter; hence, participation at the Neighborhood Place was added to her other treatments. Since the clinician at the Neighborhood Place knew the other service providers, no communication barrier existed.

Although her mother was interested in the program, she was unable to commit to her own participation. In spite of this obstacle, the administrators allowed the child to remain in the program. A clinical social worker was assigned as a point person for the girl's individualized program plan and managed the different interventions used to help her stay an active participant. For instance, to address her running away, the social worker walked her to activities, utilizing the walk, unlike traditional psychotherapy, to talk about what was going well that day and problem solving on what could be done to make it better. Because her acting-out behavior seemed to result from poor self-esteem in addition to psychiatric issues, a reward system was created to acknowledge good choices in behavior without focusing on the poor behavior.

Work with her mother continued; however, contact was initially kept to brief discussions on her daughter's progress at the Neighborhood Place in order to respect the mother's defenses. All progress was reported in a nonjudgmental, nonconfrontational, matter-of-fact manner, with a few ongoing suggestions to help educate the mother on alternative parenting methods, child development, and establishing a trusting relationship with her child.

Focusing on strengths and using a nonjudgmental stance with both the child and mother enabled them to experience success where they previously had none. The child remained in the program successfully. The child's mother was pleased with her daughter's accomplishments and with the program itself. The intervention was successful because it utilized a gradual approach that helped the mother become a more effective parent.

Adequate mental health staffing is key to the overall quality of the program. Clinical staff must be competent in their knowledge of child development, child psychiatry, crisis management, and the engagement of parents. Awareness of these concepts allows staff to tailor the curriculum and create behavior plans to meet the needs of the families and children who are experiencing difficulty participating in the program. These concepts are also actualized in the daily program to address psychiatric emergencies that arise and work with parents who may be inconsistent in their involvement with their child's programming. In addition, this knowledge helps clinical staff to educate not only program participants but also artistic and athletic staff.

Parents

More than 70% of the parents who completed the questionnaire expressed positive feelings about staff effectiveness, communication, and the involvement of clinical social workers. The majority of parents believed the program was a safe, healthy environment for their children and would have them return. Similarly, more than 78% of the children would attend the program again. Parent involvement in the program was a priority. Parents were asked to chaperone on trips and to assist instructors for art or athletic activities, and they were required to attend orientation sessions and weekly parent support meetings. The topics of the meetings were generated by the parents and included but were not limited to discipline, academics, peer pressure, and loss. On average, more than one third of the parents attended the 7 weeks of parent meetings. These parents were active and interested in the concerns of the staff members and the successes of their children and the program. They actively discussed their children and difficulties that they had both inside and outside the home. Many parents provided valuable suggestions for the program and indicated interest in volunteering during future programs.

Staff noted that while all parents and guardians attended the mandatory initial orientation, 65% of the parents did not attend other mandatory programs such as workshops. In the future, administrators will supply parents with multiple and varied options for participation. One option will be to participate in meetings, groups, or parent workshops, which meet to support parents, help them cope with daily and unexpected stressors, and increase parenting skills. Another option will be to volunteer as a helper in one of the many activities in the program. In this role, parents would assist instructors and, by being exposed to behavior management alternatives through the examples set by the clinical staff, would have the opportunity to model more effective child-adult interaction. Parents will also be encouraged to form a relationship with the clinical staff that would create a less intimidating environment in which they would be more at ease seeking help for their children and themselves. Early engagement with parents at the start of the program will give staff the opportunity to explain to the parents the expectation that parents will be an integral part of the program and that their role will include participation in the various activities, as well as problem solving with staff members when issues arise for their child or other children.

Although few in number, some parents did not provide assistance to staff members in dealing with their acting-out children. They were not involved for a variety of reasons, including conflicting work schedules, apathy, lack of outreach, lack of consistent follow-up communication, and frustration regarding reoccurring behavioral concerns. These reasons point to the need for an increased commitment to outreach communication efforts of the staff.

Case Example 7

One of the program's participants was a 9-year-old African American boy who lived with his mother and older brother. His father had been in and out of prison for 5 years due to drug charges. The child had been seeing a school social worker for 3 years, with treatment focusing on aggression and his insecure attachment with his father. In spite of the school social worker's attempts, he was unable to internalize the behavior regulation skills he learned in therapy and continued to be aggressive and disruptive in school. He was referred to the Neighborhood Place by his social worker, who worked in conjunction with staff to create a structured environment to practice communication and emotion regulation skills. The supervision the program provided was also a safe alternative to the intermittent supervision his mother tried to secure while she was at work.

Multiple efforts were made to help this boy translate his skills from therapy session to real-world interactions, including his mother's attendance at parent workshops and extensive behavior plans that rewarded him at home, as well as at the program. The behavior plan consisted of a points and rewards system in which he would receive points for following the rules in each activity and would be rewarded accordingly. He was also able to earn rewards at home, which consisted of valuable one-on-one time with his mother. In spite of these attempts, he continued to act out by leaving the classroom, disobeying staff, and getting into fights. In addition, it was unclear if his mother was able to follow through with rewards at home for good behavior. As the behavior problems continued, both he and his mother became discouraged with the behavior plan.

Since his negative behavior continued, it became evident that he was unable to tolerate a full 8-hour day at the program. As a result, he was allowed to attend half days, and the activities he attended were those that were strengths rather than

Table 29-1. Child Demograpics of the Neighborhood Place (N =63)

	n	%			n	%
Gender				Ethnicity		
Male	41	65		African American	21	33
Female	22	35		Latino	34	54
				Caucasian	5	8
Age				Other/Mixed	3	5
6- to 14-years-old	63	100				
				Child Education		
Family Status				K to eight	63	100
Mother & Father	20	32				
Single Female	23	37		Parent Education/Employment		
Single Male	0	0		High School	29	46
Mother & Stepfather	12	19		Some High School	30	48
Father & Stepmother	1	2		Some College	28	44
Other Relatives	3	5		No College	24	38
Foster Home	1	2		Employed	37	59
Caretaker	1	2		Unemployed	20	32
Other	1	2				

challenges. As the focus shifted from his behavior problems, he became less anxious and consequently less agitated and able to engage in the program. By the end of the summer, he was one of the Neighborhood Place's star musicians. This is one example of the need for flexibility in both parent and child engagement, as well as communication and follow-through by staff and outside clinicians.

While the paucity of parent responses to questionnaires indicates the difficulties inherent in obtaining information in naturalistic settings, the parents who responded did so favorably. Parents stated that the Neighborhood Place provided those who worked with a safe place for their children to be during the workday. Those who did not work also felt comfortable leaving their children at the program so that they could use the day to run errands, go to class, or look for employment. Several parents reported that their children returned from the program tired from a full day of activities and therefore spent less time out late playing in the street. Parents attributed a decrease in their children's attention to television and video games to their new interests in the activities that they learned while at the Neighborhood Place, and many also reported that children showed interest in reading and going to the library.

Finally, the children who participated in the

Neighborhood Place came from a range of family situations, with slightly more than one third from two-parent households, and almost 40% from single-parent homes. In addition, 48% of the parents had not completed high school, 38% had high school education only; 32% were unemployed, and 10% declined to provide information. These statistics indicate that the majority of families served by the Neighborhood Place were disadvantaged (see table 29-1). The level of distrust and fear is high among such families, and, as reported by Ireys, Devet, and Sakwa (2002), they may view acts of altruism with suspicion, which would lead them to question both the motives of the care providers and the message implicit in the extension of the assistance. Providers need to assure their target population that their motives are positive and that they are offering services to help families combat stressors, not because they believe the families to be "incompetent" (Ireys et al., 2002).

Training

A 2-week training period for all staff members was held prior to the start of the summer 2002 program and continued throughout the summer. Staff met regularly to discuss ongoing issues of programming, behavior management, and interpersonal issues. These meetings took place in two venues: one with clinical staff and the other with the entire staff, including administrative, arts and athletics staff, and junior counselors. The clinical staff meeting addressed the behavioral health component of the program, whereas the larger staff meeting served to ensure consistency of programming across all components of the curriculum. Training was also accomplished informally in multiple areas of the program via modeling, shadowing, consultation, and supervision. In addition, the consistency of those working with the groups of children gave arts, athletics, and clinical staff members a chance to form working relationships, exchange ideas, and implement new procedures during the course of the program.

In future programs, the 2-week preliminary training will be extended. Also, to prepare the youth who will participate as junior counselors in the summer 2003 program, we have partnered with Strive, a national boot-camp-style program that challenges youth by taking them out of their known environments and teaching them skills of problem solving, self-esteem, teamwork, and empathy. These skills are then refined in trainings that will be given prior to and during the program, where clinical staff will teach junior counselors active listening skills and behavior management.

Conclusion

The Neighborhood Place is an alternative intervention and prevention program for meeting the mental health needs of disadvantaged children whose needs might not be met in more traditional settings. Limitations within the traditional model, as identified by Lightburn and colleagues, include "fragmentation of services, disconnection between policy and practice, parent alienation, culturally irrelevant services, high staff turnover, poorly trained staff and poor integration of cost-effective, evidence-based treatment" (Lightburn et al., 2002, p. 282).

In an effort to meet this challenge, the Neighborhood Place enlisted highly trained professionals in their respective fields to offer pro-social activities and to provide an alternative mental health intervention to at-risk children and families living in "toxic" environments. In an effort to provide the social and emotional supports offered by the gangs, the Neighborhood Place offered an alternative to the streets by engaging these children in productive "mainstream" activities relevant to their backgrounds and establishing trust between these individuals and the "mainstream."

The program adopted a strength-based approach, which diverges from the medical model of diagnosis and treatment of pathology and instead focuses on engaging clients and helping them develop skills (Lightburn et al., 2002). We believe that these goals were met, as measured by responses to the questionnaires administered to the parents, children, and staff. We also believe that we provided services to a percentage of those youth who constitute the two thirds of the U.S. children who have unmet mental health needs (U.S. Public Health Service, 2000). Nevertheless, we did not anticipate the degree to which these children were both antisocial and undersocialized. This provided a major challenge, even though seasoned clinicians experienced in working with difficult children administered and were an integral part of the program.

Additionally, the administrators of the program realized that the art and athletic instructors, as well as other staff, must possess certain attributes to successfully fulfill their roles in the program. Characteristics of community-based mental health practitioners have been described elsewhere (Armbruster, Andrews, Couenhoven, & Blau, 1999), but the essential ingredients of flexibility, motivation, and commitment to this population should be applied to all staff members. Furthermore, staff should match the ethnic composition of children and families participating in the program as much as possible. As mentioned earlier, experience is not enough. Dedication to working with marginalized children and families is key. We have learned that experienced clinicians without the other necessary attributes will not succeed, whereas younger and less experienced individuals with such attributes will enhance the program.

Replicating such a program may be difficult in rural areas, owing to distance and more limited resources. However, in urban areas, with the range of resources generally available (mental health, arts, athletics), the possibility of implementing a similar program would appear realistic. Nevertheless, two issues must be considered with particular caution when planning a program like the Neighborhood Place: the number of children served at a site and the mode of interacting with such vulnerable children. Based on our experience, we recommend that no more than 25 children be served at a particular site. To provide a program for 100 participants, the children should be divided among four sites rather than meeting all at one location. Administration and management of the program will be much more successful and the impact on the children more positive if the groups are small. Concerning the daily interaction with these children by administration, clinicians, as well as other staff, generally the assumption is to support pro-social behavior by making consistent, positive statements to the children. However, we learned that compliments were so alien to these children that when they were praised, they became very anxious and would act out. As a result, we suggest relinquishing previous assumptions regarding clinical interventions and proceeding slowly in order to understand what will be the most effective means to support pro-social behavior. We found that if given the opportunity, the program participants often will educate the staff regarding the optimal mode of interaction.

A paradigm shift from "business as usual" to a commitment to providing mental health service that is culturally acceptable and accessible to the population in need is required. Again, the context is the art class or the athletic arena, not a child psychiatric clinic. Before mental health services, which are often viewed as "mainstream" by disadvantaged children and families, can be effectively offered, it is necessary to frame the services so that trust and engagement are established. No matter how well-intentioned the practitioners may be, mental health service cannot be offered in a cultural vacuum; it must be part of the fabric of the individuals' lives. Given the enthusiastic response by children and their parents to the Neighborhood Place, especially its socialization, education, and mentoring aspects, our original premise was confirmed: Children and families were hungry for the opportunities the program provided and were open to mental health interventions when offered within this context.

References

Achenbach, T. M., & Edelbrock, C. (1983). *Manual for the child behavior checklist and revised child behavior profile.* Burlington: Department of Psychiatry, University of Vermont.

American Psychiatric Association. (1994). *Diagnostic and Statistical Manual of Mental Disorders* (4th ed., rev.). Washington, DC: Author.

Andrade, A. R., Lambert, E. W., & Bickman, L. (2000). Dose effect in child psychotherapy: Outcomes associated with negligible treatment. *Journal of the American Academy of Child and Adolescent Psychiatry, 39,* 161–168.

Angold, A. E., Costello, J., Burns, B. J., Erkanli, A., & Farmer, E. M. Z. (2000). Effectiveness of nonresidential specialty mental health services for children and adolescents in the "real world." *Journal of the American Academy of Child and Adolescent Psychiatry, 39,* 154–160.

Armbruster, P., Andrews, E., Couenhoven, J., & Blau, G. (1999). Collision or collaboration? School-based mental health services meet managed care. *Clinical Psychology Review, 19,* 221–237.

Armbruster, P., & Fallon, T. (1994). Clinical, sociodemographic, and systems risk factors for attrition in a children's mental health clinic. *American Journal of Orthopsychiatry, 64,* 577–585.

Armbruster, P., & Schwab-Stone, M. (1994). Sociodemographic characteristics of dropouts from a child guidance clinic. *Hospital and Community Psychiatry, 45,* 804–808.

Armbruster, P., Sukhodolsky, D., & Michelson, R. (in press). *The impact of managed care on children's outpatient treatment: A comparison study of treatment outcome pre and post managed care.*

Brice-Heath, S., Soep, E., & Roach, A. (1998). Living the arts through language and learning: A report on community-based youth organizations. *Americans for the Arts Monographs* 2(7), 1–20.

Burns, B. J., Hoagwood, K., & Mrazek, P. J. (1999). Effective treatment for mental disorders in children and adolescents. *Clinical Child and Family Psychology Review, 2,* 199–254.

Communities in Schools. (2002). *Mission Statement.* Alexandria, VA: Communities in Schools National.

Connecticut Medicaid Managed Care Oversight Quality Assurance Subcommittee. (2002, November). Hartford, CT: Connecticut State Legislature.

Dryfoos, J. G. (1998). *Full-service schools: A revolution in health and social services for children, youth and families.* San Francisco: Jossey-Bass.

Dynarski, M. (2003). *When schools stay open late: The National Evaluation of the 21st-Century Community Learning Centers Program.* Washington, DC: U.S. Department of Education.

Fashola, O. (1998). *Review of extended-day and after-school programs and their effectiveness.* Report 24. Baltimore: Johns Hopkins University, Center for Research on the Education of Students Placed at Risk (CRESPAR).

Franklin, C., & Streeter, C. L. (1995). School reform: Linking public schools with human services. *Social Work, 40*, 773–782.

Garbarino, J. (1998). Children in a violent world. *Family and Conciliation Courts Review, 36*, 360–367.

Garbarino, J. (2001). An ecological perspective on the effects of violence on children. *Journal of Community Psychology, 20*, 361–378.

Germain, C. B., & Gitterman, A. (1995). Ecological perspective. In *Encyclopedia of Social Work* (Vol. 1, pp. 816–824). Washington, DC: National Association of Social Workers.

Gordon, R. (1999). National Forum on Youth Gangs. British Columbia, Canada: Simon Fraser University.

Henggeler, S. W., Schoenwald, S. K., & Borduin, C. M. (1998). *Multisystemic treatment of antisocial behavior in children and adolescents.* New York: Guilford.

Housing Authority of the City of New Haven. (2003, January). New Haven, CT: New Haven City Government.

Ireys, H., Devet, K., & Sakwa, D. (2002). Family support and education. In B. J. Burns & K. Hoagwood. (Eds.), *Community treatment for youth* (pp. 155–175). New York: Oxford University Press.

Leaf, P., Bruce, M., Tischler, G., & Holzer, C. (1987). The relationship between demographic factors and attitudes toward mental health services. *Journal of Community Psychology, 15*, 275–284.

Lightburn, A., Olson, M., Sessions, P., & Pulleyblank-Coffey, E. (2002). Practice innovations in mental health services to children and families: New directions for Massachusetts. *Smith College Studies in Social Work, 72*, 279–301.

Miller, B. M. (2001). Beyond class time: The promise of after-school programs. *Educational Leadership, 58*(7), 6–12.

Oldenettel, D., & Wordes, M. (2000). *The community assessment center concept.* Bulletin. Washington, DC: U.S. Department of Justice, Office of Justice Programs, Office of Juvenile Justice and Delinquency Prevention.

Pierce, K. M., Hamm, J. V., & Vandell, D. L. (1999). Experiences in after-school programs and children's adjustment in first-grade classrooms. *Child Development, 70*, 756–767.

Piers-Harris, E. V. (1986). *The Piers-Harris Children's Self-Concept Scale, Revised Manual.* Los Angeles: Western Psychological Services.

Posner, J. K., & Vandell, D. L. (1994). Low-income children's after-school care: Are there beneficial effects of after-school programs? *Child Development, 65*, 440–456.

Rosenthal, R., & Vandell, D. (1996). Quality of care at school-aged childcare programs: Regulatable features, observed experiences, child perspectives, and parent perspectives. *Child Development, 67*, 2434–2445.

Rutter, M. (1999). Resilience concepts and findings: Implications for family therapy. *Journal of Family Therapy, 21*, 119–144.

Schinke, S. P., Cole, K. C., & Poulin, S. R. (2000). Enhancing the educational achievement of at-risk youth. *Prevention Science, 1*, 51–60.

Shaffer, D., Gould, M. S., Brasco, J., Ambrosini, P., Fisher, P., Bird, H., & Aluwahlia, S. (1983). A Children's Global Assessment Scale (C-GAS). *Archives of General Psychiatry, 40*, 1228–1231.

Stroul, B. A. (1993). *Systems of care for children and adolescents with severe emotional disturbances: What are the results?* Washington, DC: CASSP Technical Assistance Center, Georgetown University Child Development Center.

U.S. Public Health Service. (2000). *Report of the Surgeon General's conference on children's mental health: Developing a national action agenda.* Washington, DC: Author.

Vandell, D. L., & Corasaniti, M. A. (1998). The relation between third graders' after-school care and social, academic, and emotional functioning. *Child Development, 59*, 868–875.

Wilson, W. J. (1998). Inner-city dislocations. *Society, 35*, 270–277.

30

Larry Davidson, Janis Tondora, Martha Staeheli,

Maria O'Connell, Jennifer Frey, and

Matthew J. Chinman

Recovery Guides

An Emerging Model of Community-Based Care for Adults With Psychiatric Disabilities

"We're not cases, and you're not managers."
(Everett & Nelson, 1992, p. 49)

In the decade since the appearance of Everett and Nelson's article with the above phrase as its title, the field of community mental health has become increasingly dissatisfied with traditional models of case management. This same period has seen significant advances in the development of new, safer, and more effective medications, psychiatric rehabilitation strategies, disorder-specific cognitive behavioral psychotherapies, and peer-run and other innovative services. In addition, the mental health consumer/survivor/ex-patient movement has made considerable inroads into mainstream mental health practice, moving the field from a despairing view of mental illness as a progressive, degenerative disease toward a more hopeful, recovery-oriented paradigm. Despite these significant advances, it remains the case, however, that the predominant service offered to most adults with serious psychiatric disabilities is clinical case management (Sledge, Astrachan, Thompson, Rakfeldt, & Leaf, 1995). Arguably, there have been several advances in clinical case management practice during this period as well, from the intensive, team-based, and in vivo approach of assertive community treatment to the introduction of strengths-based and rehabilitative forms of case management that attempt to shift the goals of care from stabilization and maintenance to

enhanced functioning and community integration. As Everett and Nelson's title suggests, however, these approaches continue to conceptualize the person with the disability as a "case" and the health care provider as a "manager."

In this chapter, we argue that continued use of inherited models of case management limits the progress that otherwise could be made in actualizing this shift from a deficit- and institution-based framework to a recovery and community integration paradigm. We argue that this paradigm calls for new models of community-based practice that move beyond the management of cases and beyond merely semantic changes that introduce new terms for old practices (e.g., Jacobson & Greenley, 2001). We suggest that one such model that appears to be emerging in the field is that of tour guide, community guide, or, as in the title for this chapter, "recovery guide." Prior to introducing this model, we first (1) review existing models of case management that have underlain the last 40 years of community-based practice. We then (2) outline the principles of care that ground a recovery-oriented alternative; (3) describe the key components of the recovery guide model; and (4) consider some of the broader implications of this model for community-based practice.

Inherited Models of Case Management

Case management arose out of the community support program movement as an attempt to address several of the failures of deinstitutionalization (Anthony, Cohen, Farkas, & Cohen, 1988; Parrish, 1989). In addition to being inadequately funded, the community-based systems of care that were developed to enable people with serious mental illnesses to leave state hospitals were so fragmented and uncoordinated that they have been described as "non-systems" of care (Hoge, Davidson, Griffith, & Jacobs, 1998). Because it was practically impossible for people seeking care to navigate these complex and unintegrated health and social service systems on their own, the role of case manager was created and initially tasked with identifying, accessing, and coordinating various services to meet the multiple needs of individuals with serious mental illnesses living in the community (Hoge, Davidson, Griffith, Sledge, & Howenstine, 1994; Sledge et al., 1995). The primary responsibility of case managers working under these conditions was to assess client needs, attempt to link clients to appropriate services (termed "brokering"), and monitor their service use and outcomes.

When it became apparent that lone case managers could not ensure access to or coordination among services over which they had no administrative or fiscal authority, team-based approaches to case management were developed in which mental health professionals both provided and "brokered" care (Hoge et al., 1994). The most well-articulated and rigorously evaluated team-based approach to intensive case management was developed in the 1970s by Stein and Test (1980), who initially named their approach the Program for Assertive Community Treatment (PACT). PACT or ACT, as it has since come to be more commonly known, and various other derivative versions of intensive case management are characterized by the provision of comprehensive care in natural community settings enabled by lower client-to-staff ratios, caseloads that are shared among teams of professionals, 24-hour emergency coverage, and time-unlimited services (Bond, 1991; Mueser, Bond, Drake, & Resnick, 1998). As we describe later, this shift to the provision of direct care by an outreach-based team of professionals gave the first impetus to the recovery guide model of practice.

Concurrent with these developments, concerns that traditional community mental health services emphasized the impairments and areas of difficulty of people with psychiatric disabilities over their strengths and areas of competence gave rise to both strengths-based and rehabilitative approaches to case management (Mueser et al., 1998). These approaches incorporate many of the principles of psychiatric rehabilitation (Anthony, 1993), emphasizing the importance of skill building as an avenue to promoting community tenure. These approaches also allow for more input and direction by the person with the disability as opposed to being driven by mental health professionals as experts with an accumulated body of knowledge. Finally, this approach stresses that the community, where most of the contact between case manager and client takes place, offers resources for, as well as presents obstacles to, the person's continued growth and development.

While these various approaches provide clarity in terms of the case manager's responsibilities in relation to the client, they provide little direction for how the case manager is to fulfill all these responsibilities. In other words, they instruct the case manager in *what* to do but not necessarily in *how* to do it. For guidance in this regard, individual case managers are often left to their own devices, falling back either on what limited training they have received or on their own personal, largely intuitive, style of relating to others. As a result, we have found it useful in our experiences of training and supervising case managers to identify and make explicit the often implicit models that people have for how they are to do their jobs. While simplistic and reductive, these models have proved to be effective teaching tools in clarifying the various roles community providers can play in the lives of people with psychiatric disabilities. We present the most common of these models in table 30-1 and, for each model, offer a metaphor for the role of the mental health professional and describe the interventions most associated with that role.

The limitations of these various models will become apparent when viewed through the lens of the recovery movement and its community integration paradigm. To elaborate on this perspective, we offer a list of the top 10 principles of community-based care that can inform a new model of community-based practice. With this model, we present an alternative role for mental health professionals working with adults with severe psychiatric

Table 30.1. Existing Models for Clinical Case Management

Primary Role of Provider	Principal Theorist(s)	Representative Concepts and Interventions
Detective	Sigmund Freud	• Repressed memories and impulses are the primary source of psychological distress and illness, and the uncovering of these memories and impulses is essential to progress and recovery. • The central task of treatment is a focused exploration of past events and early life history and relationships.
Cultural Anthropologist	Carl Jung	• The collective unconscious, an inherited set of images and ideas common to all humans, serves as an emotional template, shaping the course of both the individual's intrapsychic and interpersonal life. • Wellness is promoted through an appreciation of trans-generational and cross-cultural common human experiences and an understanding of the current social milieu in which the client lives.
Cheerleader	Carl Rogers	• The key ingredient of treatment is the relationship between the therapist and the client where the therapist offers the client "unconditional positive regard" • Unconditional positive regard allows clients to feel accepted for who they are without any labels or conditions, and this acceptance promotes trust in the therapist and creates an environment that enables clients to take risks and to grow (Kensit, 2000).
Coach	B. F. Skinner	• Behavior is largely motivated by external rewards and punishments and not by free will. • The behavioral therapist targets current problem behaviors, adopts a directive stance, establishes explicit treatment goals, and determines the reinforcement schedules that are most likely to affect desired change (DeBell & Harless, 1992).
Teacher	Aaron Beck	• Affective distress and dysfunctional behavior are due to excessive or distorted ways of thinking about and interpreting one's experiences (Weinrach, 1988). • It is the task of the therapy to identify and restructure these distortions in thinking, often through a series of cognitive exercises and homework assignments in which clients learn to think in a healthier, more rational way.
Police Officer/ Social Control Agent	E. Fuller Torrey	• Centralized systems of care in which mental health providers have greater authority to control the lives and treatment of individuals with mental illness are necessary to protect both the individual with the illness and the general public.
(Paid) Friend	Peer Support Movement	• Placement of people in recovery in leadership positions in peer support groups, advocacy and education initiatives, and consumer-operated programs and businesses provides positive role-models and instills hope in individuals that recovery is possible for all people.

disabilities and offer a detailed metaphoric exploration of the role of the recovery guide in facilitating their recovery and community integration.

Top 10 Principles of Recovery-Oriented Community-Based Care

In contrast to the continued debate and lack of clarity over what the concept of "recovery" means in relation to severe psychiatric disability, a considerable amount of consensus has emerged on the core principles of recovery-oriented care (Anthony, 2000; Davidson, Stayner, et al., 2001; Jacobson & Greenley, 2001; Ridgway, 2001). Based on our re-

view of this literature (Davidson, O'Connell, Tondora, Staeheli, & Evans, 2003; O'Connell, Tondora, Evans, Croog, & Davidson, 2003), we have distilled the following top 10 principles by which any new, alternative model of clinical practice should be assessed. Although the principles overlap, each one addresses a unique and important dimension of recovery-oriented care.

Principle 1: Care Is Recovery Oriented

Although this principle may seem a bit self-serving (or tautologous), it nonetheless should be stated first and foremost that mental health care needs to be grounded in an appreciation of the possibility and nature of recovery in severe mental illness. As described in the recent *Mental Health: A Report of the Surgeon General*: "All services for those with a mental disorder should be consumer-oriented and focused on promoting recovery" (U.S. Department of Health and Human Services, 1999, p. 455). This dictum stands in stark contrast to the last 150 years of mental health care, an era based on a maintenance and stabilization framework, at best, or on a model of progressive deterioration, at worst. The notion that many people can recover from a serious mental illness is relatively new, and the implications of this recognition have yet to be translated fully into practice (Harding, Zubin, & Strauss, 1987).

As one implication of this shift, people need to be offered hope and/or faith that recovery is "possible for me." Having a sense of hope and believing in the possibility of a renewed sense of self and purpose are essential to recovery. This sense of hope may be derived from religious faith or from others who believe in the potential of a person, even when he or she cannot believe in him- or herself (Davidson, Stayner, et al., 2001; Deegan, 1996b; Fisher, 1994; Jacobson & Curtis, 2000; Jacobson & Greenley, 2001; Mead & Copeland, 2000; Smith, 2000). The therapeutic role of hope as an essential element in promoting recovery has been described as follows: "Hope sustains, even during periods of relapse. It creates its own possibilities. Hope is a frame of mind that colors every perception. By expanding the realm of the possible, hope lays the groundwork for healing to begin" (Jacobson & Greenley, 2001, p. 483).

In addition to hope, recovery from mental illness, broadly defined, involves a process of overcoming some of the consequences of illness; gaining an enhanced sense of identity, empowerment, and meaning and purpose in life; and developing valued social roles, citizenship, and community connections despite a person's symptom profile or continued disability (Cooke, 1997; Davidson, Stayner, et al., 2001; Deegan, 1996b). In recent years, there has been a growing emphasis on developing mental health care that supports, rather than hinders, people's opportunities to participate in such processes of healing. As a departure from earlier, less hopeful, practices that promoted low expectations for people diagnosed with severe mental illness, implementing a recovery vision requires a change in the manner in which care is conceptualized and delivered based on belief in the potential of people with psychiatric disabilities to improve over time. Recovery-oriented care would thus include practices that (1) help people gain autonomy, power, and connections with others; (2) aid in skill development, as well as symptom management and treatment; (3) focus on abilities and strengths, rather than deficits; and (4) are guided by the person in recovery. As mental health professionals, we should be asking our clients questions about their hopes, dreams, interests, talents, and skills, and perhaps the most important question—"How can I best be of help?"—in addition to assessing their problems and difficulties (Carling, 1995). As suggested by Carling (1995), when working with clients, mental health professionals can evaluate the extent to which they are providing recovery-oriented services by asking themselves, "Does this person have more or less power as a result of this interaction?" (p. 60). We recommend expanding this question to "Does this person *gain* power, purpose (valued roles), competence (skills), and/or connections (to people) as a result of this interaction?" Equally important is the converse: "Does this interaction *interfere* with the acquisition of power, purpose, competence, or connections to others?"

Principle 2: Care Is Strengths Based

A further implication of such a shift is recognition that traditional mental health services have been organized around a narrow medical model that perceives mental illness as a disease that must be "treated" and "cured" (Corrigan & Penn, 1998). By focusing on the assessment and treatment of the deficits, aberrations, and symptoms—the things that are "wrong" with people—providers have had a tendency to overlook all that remains "right" with people, that is, their remaining and coexisting areas of health, assets, strengths, and competencies (Davidson & Strauss, 1995). Because there does not yet exist a "cure" for mental illness, emphasizing the negative has led to a tremendous sense of hopelessness and despair among both clients and the mental health professionals serving them. A recovery orientation encourages us instead to view the glass as half full. Based on Rappaport's principles of empowerment (1981), this perspective allows us to see that, no matter how disabled, "All people have existing strengths and capabilities as well as the capacity to become more competent" (Grills, Bass, Brown, & Akers, 1996, p. 129). As a result of this recognition, we come to appreciate that "the failure of a person to display competence is not due to deficits within the person but rather to the failure of the social systems to provide or create opportunities for competencies to be displayed or acquired" (Grills et al., 1996, p. 130). By focusing on strengths rather than deficits, people can begin to identify and develop greater competencies, assets, and resources on which to expand their opportunities (Rapp, 1993; Rapp & Wintersteen, 1989), promoting the development of an upward positive spiral of competence, leading to increased health and increased competence (Davidson, 2003).

The process of rediscovering one's remaining areas of health and one's talents, gifts, and possibilities may begin when the individual can acknowledge and accept the limitations imposed by his or her illness (Hatfield, 1994; Munetz & Frese, 2001; Smith, 2000; Sullivan, 1994; Young & Ensing, 1999). This acknowledgment and acceptance does not mean accepting one's identity as a "mentally ill person," however. Accepting one's illness has to do with redefining how a person thinks about and understands life's challenges (Ridgway, 2001). Patricia Deegan (1988), for example, describes a "paradox of recovery, i.e., that in accepting what we cannot do or be, we begin to discover who we can be and what we can do." Gaining a sense of perspective on one's strengths and weaknesses is critical in the process of recovery because it allows the person to identify, pursue, and achieve life goals despite the lingering presence of disability (Deegan, 1988, 1993; Hatfield, 1994; Munetz & Frese, 2001; Ridgway, 2001; Sayce & Perkins, 2000; Smith, 2000; Sullivan, 1994; Young & Ensing, 1999). Within this view, limitations become the "ground from which spring our own unique possibilities" (Sayce & Perkins, 2000, p. 74). As a person recovers from illness, the illness then becomes less of a defining characteristic of self and more simply one part of a multidimensional self that also contains strengths, skills, and competencies. Care, then, to be recovery-oriented, must elicit, flesh out, and cultivate these positive elements at least as much as, if not more than, assess and attempt to ameliorate, decrease, or remediate difficulties.

Principle 3: Care Is Community Focused

Following on the heels of the early days of deinstitutionalization, the National Institute of Mental Health recognized that the multiple needs of people with serious mental illnesses living in the community were not being addressed by existing care. It thus designed and disseminated a model of community treatment that focused on housing, income maintenance, medical care, and rehabilitation in addition to traditional mental health services (Turner & TenHoor, 1978). Turner and Schifren (1979) described the resulting community support system initiative of the 1970s as promoting the development of a "network of caring and responsible people committed to assisting a vulnerable population meet their needs and develop their potentials without being unnecessarily isolated or excluded from the community" (p. 2). Somewhere along the way, however, care that was designed to be community focused became confused with care that was simply community based, with the *focus* of care being replaced by the *locus* of care (Stein, 1989).

In addition to being provided outside of hospital settings, community-focused care is that which (1) is primarily provided in a person's natural community; (2) facilitates the development of relationships with people in one's community; (3) helps people develop citizenship and roles that are of value to one's community; and (4) works with members of the general community to combat stigma and increase access to resources. Rather than simply trying to fix the individual, and as suggested in Rappaport's (1981) reframing of failure described earlier, community-focused care views the incongruence between the person and his or her environment as the target for intervention. This is done by helping the individual assimilate into his or her environment (through symptom management, skill acquisition, etc.) and by helping the community and the environment to better accommodate people with disabilities (through education, stigma reduction, the creation of niches, etc.). The goal is to develop "multiple pathways" into and between members of communities (Dailey et al., 2000).

Principle 4: Care Is Person Centered

American society places tremendous value on the freedom to exercise choice in everyday life. Constrained only by access to resources, it is assumed that all adults have the right and responsibility to make their own decisions about where they live, what they do, and how they want to be treated, as long as these decisions do not infringe on another person's rights. During the century of institutional care, these rights and responsibilities were denied to inmates of the asylum, because they were viewed as incapable of taking care of themselves. Unfortunately, this view did not disappear altogether with the downsizing of state mental hospitals but instead has been carried, to various degrees, into community treatment settings, re-creating an institution without walls in the community (Davidson, 1997; Estroff, 1995). Continuing to be viewed as largely incapacitated by their psychiatric disorder, people with severe mental illnesses have yet to be accorded the same rights to autonomy and self-determination, or the same responsibilities for self-care, as the general public. As a result, traditional mental health models still typically view clients as passive recipients of the care and ameliorative efforts of others (i.e., cases to be managed) rather than as active participants in, and agents of, their own recovery (Davidson, 1997; Deegan, 1996b).

A person-centered model of care is one that is guided by the person with the disability; reflects his or her own wants, needs, and preferences; involves primary relationships as sources of support; focuses on capacities and strengths; and accepts risks, failures, uncertainties, and setbacks as natural and expected parts of learning and self-determination (Gerteis, Edgman-Levitan, Daley, & Delbanco, 1993; O'Brien & Lovett, 1992). In such a model, providers learn to "do nothing without the client's approval, involving clients in decisions regarding every step of the process." In addition, according to this model, "opportunities to move each client closer to being the director of the case management scenario [are to] be found, created, and exploited" (Rapp, 1998, p. 374). For this model to be effective, of course, people with disabilities need to continue to feel like members of society despite their disability status, as opposed to being subsumed by their illness or diagnostic label. If the illness is allowed to rob the individual of his or her personhood and all the socially valued roles that accompany it, the patient role is often one of the few that remain (Estroff, 1989). This process neither promotes insight nor breaks through the individual's presumed denial but rather promotes the illness to a master status. But, as Deegan (1996a) observes, when the person's "identity [becomes] synonymous with a disease, then there is no one left inside to take on the enormous work of recovery" (p. 12).

Even though it often leads to the rejection of conventional mental health services precisely because of the damage they can do to a person's self-esteem and identity, people need to resist such attempts to raise the illness to master status by redefining one's self as a person of whom mental illness is simply one part. As we described in our earlier research: "The process of rediscovering and reconstructing an enduring sense of self as an active and responsible agent provides an important and, perhaps, crucial source of improvement" (Davidson & Strauss, 1992, p. 140).

Principle 5: Care Allows for Reciprocity in Relationships

The recovery process entails regaining both a sense of agency in one's life and a sense of belonging and self-worth within a community of one's peers (Davidson, Stayner, et al., 2001). Personal agency involves not only feeling effective and able to help oneself but also being able to positively impact the lives of others. We have long known that it can be therapeutic to give of oneself to others (Biegel & Tracy, 1994; Riessman, 1990). However, many clients have become so accustomed to receiving care and having decisions made for them that they may feel they have little of value to share. Furthermore, people with psychiatric disabilities may be accustomed to having their offers of reciprocity rejected because the traditional therapeutic boundaries and professional roles held by many mental health providers forbid this sort of two-way street. The largely asymmetrical and unidirectional relationships that exist between professionals and clients create a situation in which "staff hold the power to allocate or give based on their judgment" (Curtis & Hodge, 1994, p. 25) and may contribute to a passivity that carries over into other, more naturally occurring, relationships (Davidson, Stayner, & Haglund, 1998).

Providers can help clients gain a sense of agency and self-worth by treating them as "fully competent equals," by accepting appropriate gestures of reciprocity, and by encouraging participation in self-help (Mead & Copeland, 2000). In addition, it may be for this reason that the development of valued social roles and involvement in meaningful activities have been identified as cornerstones of the recovery process, as they provide people with a sense of self-worth and purpose in life (Anthony, 1993; Davidson, Stayner, et al., 2001; Ridgway, 2001; Young & Ensing, 1999). It is extremely difficult to have a sense of belonging to one's community without a sense of what one has to contribute to that community and what roles one can play in it. As summarized concisely by Jacobson and Greenley (2001): "To connect is to find roles to play in the world" (p. 483)—preferably roles that benefit others as well as oneself. This principle was articulated eloquently by a participant in an earlier study who said the following during the course of a qualitative interview:

> I could choose to be a nobody, a nothing, and just [say] "the hell with it, the hell with everything, I'm not going to deal with anything."
> And there are times when I feel like that. And yet, I'm part of the world, I'm a human being. And human beings usually kind of do things together to help each other out, that type of thing. And I want to be part of that. . . . If you're not part of the world, it's pretty miserable, pretty lonely. So I think degree of involvement is important . . . involvement in some kind of activity. Hopefully an activity which benefits somebody. I have something to offer . . . that's all I'm talking about. And I think [this project] made it a little bit easier for me to think in those terms, to not be afraid to give things to people, and not be afraid to take things from people in return. (quoted in Davidson, Haglund, et al., 2001, p. 288)

Principle 6: Care Is Culturally Responsive

As documented in the recent supplement to *Mental Health: A Report of the Surgeon General* entitled *Executive Summary. Mental Health: Culture, Race, and Ethnicity* (U.S. Department of Health and Human Services, 2001), people from ethnic and racial minority groups are both overrepresented and yet underserved among recipients of public sector mental health care. While the prevalence of psychiatric disorders may be comparable across cultural and racial groups, access to care, service use, and health outcomes are not. Significant disparities exist in each of these domains, evident in the fact that people of color are able to find few, if any, effective services that are tailored and responsive to their unique social and cultural background. These service utilization patterns also may be linked to data that suggest that some forms of traditional treatment may be less effective or even detrimental when used with ethnic minority populations. For instance, Spanish-speaking families have been found to experience an increase in symptoms when treated with highly structured family therapy and to experience a reduction in symptoms with the use of less structured case management services (Telles et al., 1995). As this example suggests, one of the reasons for the disaffiliation of people of color from mental health care is the lack of sensitivity of traditional services to their cultural and racial identity. In addition to a mistrust of the mental health system (Becerra, Karno, & Escobar, 1982; Grier & Cobbs, 1968; Gutierrez, Ortega, & Suarez, 1990; Neighbors, Elliott, & Gant, 1990), there also are characteristics of traditional services that run counter to the values of these communities. For both African and Hispanic Americans, for example, these characteristics include a reliance on institutions as opposed to personal relationships and extended peer and family networks and a focus on the individual as opposed to the group (Butler, 1992; Grier & Cobbs, 1968; Gutierrez et al., 1990; Neighbors et al., 1990).

The lack of congruence between cultural values and traditional mental health services, in combination with disparities in service access, utilization, satisfaction, and outcomes, prompted the Surgeon General to call for expanded research to clarify when and how traditional treatments ought to be adapted, or new ones developed, to meet the needs and preferences of people of color. Leaders in the field of mental health have begun to respond to this challenge by developing culturally responsive services to address some of the needs of multicultural populations (U.S. Department of Health and Human Services, Office of Minority Health, 2001). When developed programmatically, these services can be oriented to the local community and attempt to optimize use of local resources.

It is difficult, however, even for culturally responsive programs to be tailored to the unique cultural identities of specific individuals. We know from research on ethnic identity development, for example, that not all individuals from a particular ethnic background, even if it is from the same specific subgroup (e.g., Afro-Caribbean or Chilean), will identify to the same degree and in the same ways with their cultural heritage and its traditional values (Casas & Pytluk, 1995; Pope-Davis, Liu, Ledesma-Jones, & Nevitt, 2000; Vandiver, 2001).

Based on a number of factors, such as length of time in the United States and family context, tremendous variability can be found within even the smallest enclaves of ethnic minority communities, leading to the truism that no two Native Americans or Hispanic Americans will be exactly alike with respect to their ethnic identity. As a result, recovery-oriented care not only needs to be attentive to cultural differences across race, ethnicity, and other distinctions of difference (e.g., sexual orientation) but also must incorporate this sensitivity at the level of the individual client. Only an individual-level process can ensure that providers avoid stereotyping people based on broad or inaccurate generalizations (e.g., what all lesbians want or need) and enable them instead to tailor services to the specific needs, values, and preferences of each client, taking into account each individual's ethnic, racial, and cultural identification and affiliations. Although this is a relatively underdeveloped area that we feel warrants significant attention in the future, we also view the recovery guide model as providing a particularly efficient yet comprehensive framework for addressing issues of culture, race, ethnicity, and other distinctions of difference, as we describe later.

Principle 7: Care Is Grounded in the Person's Life Context

Care that is grounded in a person's "life context" acknowledges, builds on, and appreciates each person's unique history, experiences, situations, developmental trajectory, and aspirations (Davidson & Strauss, 1995). In addition to culture, race, and ethnicity, there are less visible but equally important influences on each individual's development, including both the traditional concerns of mental health professionals (e.g., family composition and background, history of hospitalizations), as well as less common factors such as personal interests, hobbies, and role models that help to define who we are as individuals. Because many people with psychiatric disabilities have found their illness to subsume who they were as people prior to becoming ill, providers often fall into viewing people as if they were born with a mental illness and did not have a life beforehand (Davidson & Strauss, 1995). Also, many people with psychiatric disabilities become accustomed to living on the margins of society and become resigned to a life of invisibility. To address both of these consequences, providers

must understand the impact that marginalization has had on the person and on his or her expectations of life; they must encourage the person to reconnect to who he or she used to be as one possible bridge to reaching life goals despite the limitations imposed by his or her disability. Appreciation of an individual's life context, too, represents an underdeveloped but important dimension of recovery-oriented care; it will be described further through the lens of the recovery guide.

Principle 8: Care Is Relationally Mediated

Recovery is not a solitary process or a journey that one traverses alone; it is a fundamentally social process (Jacobson & Greenley, 2001). Supportive relationships, whether they are with family, friends, professionals, community members, or peers, allow individuals to become interdependent in a community that can both share in their disappointments and pain and revel in their joy and successes (Baxter & Diehl, 1998; Fisher, 1994; Jacobson & Greenley, 2001; Mead & Copeland, 2000; Ridgway, 2001; Smith, 2000; Sullivan, 1994; Young & Ensing, 1999). In addition, people in recovery often describe the importance of having someone believe in them when they could no longer believe in themselves, and they often attribute their recovery, more than anything else, to someone "really believing in me" or "seeing something inside me that I couldn't see" (Davidson, Stayner, et al., 2001; Ragins, 1994). Regardless of the number of tools or interventions a service provider uses, it thus cannot be emphasized enough that at the heart of any effective intervention is the relationship between the provider and client (Anthony, 1993). Like other caring people in the person's life, mental health providers must believe in the individual even when he or she cannot believe in him- or herself and serve as a gentle reminder of his or her potential. To promote recovery, providers must be able to envision a future for the client beyond the role of "mental patient" based on the client's own desires and values and must share this vision with the client through the communication of positive expectations, optimism, and hope.

Consistent with this principle, the establishment of trusting, supportive relationships through persistence and consistency is considered by some to be the most fundamental requirement of recovery-oriented care. In the presence of such relationships, the illness no longer remains the primary focus of the person's life, and the person is then able to move on to other interests and activities (Anthony, 1993). With this kind of encouraging support, people will be more likely to expand their horizons and take risks that they have not taken before. To maximize the benefits of this process, providers must be more than just "case coordinators." They must also be willing to fill gaps in needed service areas and "to assist clients in developing their own individual visions and journeys of recovery through the process of defining meaning and purpose in their lives" p. 402). Unfortunately, but consistent with the assumptions of the models described earlier in this chapter, a major factor missing in the conceptualization of case management is often this emphasis on or permission for the development of a genuine relationship between the case manager and the client—a relationship that then mediates the process of growth and recovery. It is for this reason, among several others, that we suggest the need for alternative models of practice.

Principle 9: Care Optimizes Natural Supports

Traditional mental health systems have been described as tending to "surround people with serious mental health problems with a sea of professionally delivered services . . . which stigmatize them and set them apart from the community" (Nelson, Ochocka, Griffin, & Lord, 1998, p. 881). A recovery-oriented model of care helps minimize the role that professionals play in clients' lives over time and maximize the role of natural supports such as friends, family, neighbors, and other community members. Rather than substituting for such networks, mental health providers can help people "mobilize" their own support networks through the development of new ties and the maintenance and strengthening of existing ties (Biegel & Tracy, 1994). One strategy for expanding relationship networks is to tap into and "place a premium on the use of existing available community resources like families, volunteer opportunities, neighbors, junior colleges, sports leagues, YMCAs, faith communities, and arts centers" (Rapp, 1998, p. 371). For mental health providers to facilitate these connections, they must have an intimate knowledge of the communities in which their clients live, the community's available resources, and the people who are important to them, whether a parent, friend, landlord, or grocer. Service providers also must be knowledgeable about informal support systems in communities, such as support groups, singles clubs, and other special interest groups, and be willing to learn more about other possibilities that exist to help people connect.

This kind of knowledge is difficult if not impossible to generate from the armchair in the office. Similarly, the process of connecting people can be, and often needs to be, done through more than a referral or brokering process. Helping people optimize natural supports requires developing connections yourself, being familiar with resources and friendly spots in the community, and routinely being involved in the community. Where pathways to community life seem largely absent for the individual, it is the job of the provider to develop active, intentional relationships with a range of community members and organizations so that the individual with the disability will have access to a range of normalized activities and socially valued roles through which he or she can leave behind the identity of "mental patient" and internalize the more healthy identities offered by his or her community of membership (Gilmartin, 1997; Rappaport, 1995). Providers can then go with a client to a support group or social club or introduce a person to someone they know who is already a member (Carling, 1995). Such is the value of having providers who are well integrated into their own communities—the task becomes easier as a provider's own network expands.

Principle 10: It (Really) Is Your Job

This principle may seem irreverent, but it is borne out of many years of experience and frustration in trying to conceptualize the role of the mental health provider as recovery oriented rather than deficit oriented, and as community based rather than office based. Even after reading the first nine principles above, many mental health professionals—despite their assurances that they have in fact adopted a recovery orientation—will continue to view all these principles as somehow applying to someone else. It is good for clients to have hope for their futures, to explore community resources and activities, and to assume valued social roles through which they can contribute to the community—so this reasoning goes—but all that is someone else's concern, not mine. As a professional—the reasoning continues—my job is to conduct a thorough assessment, offer an accurate diagnosis, and provide effective treatments for my clients' disorders. It is not to ensure that they are having fun or being involved in meaningful activities, any more or any less than it is to ensure that they are living in safe and affordable housing, meeting their basic needs for food and clothing, or finding and maintaining gainful employment.

As suggested in the last principle, however, one of the more difficult, and perhaps less obvious, implications of adopting such a community focus is that mental health providers need to shift the locus of their efforts to offering practical assistance in the community contexts in which their clients live, work, and play. To effectively address "individuals' basic human needs for decent housing, food, work, and 'connection' with the community," providers must be willing to go where the action is, that is, they must get out of their offices and out into the community (Curtis & Hodge, 1994, p. 15). They must be prepared to go out to meet people on their own turf and on their own terms, and to "offer assistance which they might consider immediately relevant to their lives" (Rosen, Diamond, Miller, & Stein, 1993, p. 134). As described by Rosen, their job

is to draw all the fragments of services and resources which we find in the community into a system and safety net around the service user, and even to recreate asylum, in the best sense, in the community; that is, a haven of safety and a harbor from which to set out again. (1994, p. 48)

This safety net includes the need for supportive family and social relationships, meeting basic survival needs like food, clothing, and safe housing, and securing employment and other socially valued roles, as well as accessing appropriate and needed psychiatric and physical health care.

Unfortunately, many mental health professionals, operating within the more traditional treatment paradigms reviewed earlier (see table 30-1), prefer to work as office-based psychotherapists and to distance themselves from individuals with serious mental illness and from the problems they confront in their day-to-day lives (Rosen, 1994). When the therapist has the luxury of working with a dedi-cated case manager who is assigned to address the day-to-day issues, this also may function as a tool for distancing the therapist from the lived experience of the client and thus may remove him or her from the real world in which the clients' problems arise, resulting in the clinician having "a clear picture of neither the problems nor the solutions" (Deitchman, 1980, p. 788). One of many examples of this process is provided by vocational rehabilitation. Through the kind of distancing entailed in making referrals to vocational rehabilitation specialists, mental health providers have demonstrated an unfortunate tendency of divorcing the meaning of work for people with severe psychiatric disorders from the various meanings that work has for the rest of us. In earlier work (Strauss & Davidson, 1997), we noted that this tendency has had a dehumanizing impact not only on clients but also on the providers who serve them:

Work has been viewed primarily as adjunctive or as a support to treatment, with the expectation that recovery or cure will have to take place before work can return to playing a central role in the person's life. This view neglects the fact that the disabled person continues to live his/her life despite . . . the disorder, and that major dimensions of life such as work and social relationships may retain the meaning they had for the person prior to the onset of his/her illness. . . . As soon as we turn our back on the body of first-person knowledge, the guide derived from our own lives, we start talking about "schizophrenics" or "manic-depressives" or "borderlines". . . . Work loses its fundamental meaning and importance in human existence and comes to be seen as an adjunct or support to a person's "real" treatment. [In contrast,] work should be viewed as the bridge across which a person can travel in leaving severe mental disorder and becoming an increasingly competent, intact, human being. (pp. 107–108)

To avoid this distancing and dehumanizing tendency, we recommended that providers draw upon their own experiences when considering the critical nature of the worker role—or of any other socially valued role, for that matter—for all individuals, continuing to view the client squarely within the context of his or her daily life (Strauss & Davidson, 1997).

In addition to contributing to the dehumanizing of their clients, providers' insistence on office-based practice misses much of the significance of the shift to the recovery orientation for which we are arguing. It has not worked over the previous 25 years for many clients for their providers to postpone attending to their acquisition of meaningful and gratifying personal lives until after their illnesses have been treated (Scott & Dixon, 1995). Severe psychiatric disorders are often long-term, disabling conditions for which cures do not yet exist. People with these disorders cannot sit back and simply wait for their medications, or skills training groups, or other treatments to work before they start to attempt to get their lives back. Of course, people with psychiatric disabilities have known this all along, and many have gone about reclaiming their lives outside of, and at times despite, their mental health care. For care to make positive contributions to this process, all the strategies, goals, and interventions that providers have at their disposal must be reframed as tools to be used in the person's own recovery.

In this vein, it is not simply the psychiatrist's job, for example, to diagnose and prescribe appropriate medications for a client's condition with the assumption that the client will take the medication and improve. From the perspective of a recovery orientation, it also becomes the psychiatrist's job to understand how the medication will affect other important dimensions of the person's life (e.g., a job or relationship) and to talk with the client about how medications can be used effectively as a tool in his or her own recovery. One client who is taking a risk to start a new job may need to increase his medication to offset his increased anxiety, while another client starting a new job may need to decrease her medication to overcome its sedating effect in the morning so that she can get out of bed on time. Similarly, a client taking risks in developing a new relationship may be concerned about a medication's effect on his or her sexual functioning. Because it cannot be anyone other than the psychiatrist whose job it is to explore and understand these issues to prescribe medications effectively (Noordsy et al., 2000), it also cannot be anyone other than the guide's job to explore and understand the many other facets of the client's life in the community. Within a recovery orientation, there is no other job.

The Emerging Model of Recovery Guide

Since the introduction of Stein and Test's Program for Assertive Community Treatment in the 1970s, intensive, team-based models of community-based practice have emerged as the service of choice for people seriously disabled by psychiatric disorders, particularly for those who have been "difficult-to-engage" in, or have been unresponsive to, conventional care (e.g., those who are homeless or who have co-occurring substance use disorders; Bond, 1991). One of the major advances entailed in the ACT approach—and the one that makes ACT a particularly good point of departure for the development of recovery-oriented care—was the provision of skills training and other direct mental health services "in vivo," meaning in the natural community settings where they are actually needed as opposed to in a clinician or case manager's office. Rather than being a finished product, we suggest, this shift from office to community-based practice initiated with ACT represents a work very much in progress, with several steps still needing to be taken in fulfilling the more substantive promises of this new paradigm.

Adherents and practitioners of the ACT approach began to articulate some of these implications by contrasting the traditional role of case managers, which they likened to "travel agents," to their new role as outreach-based providers, which at first was conceptualized as that of "traveling companions." As described by Deitchman (1980):

> The client in the community needs a traveling companion, not a travel agent. The travel agent's only function is to make the client's reservation. The client has to get ready, get to the airport, and traverse foreign terrain by himself. The traveling companion, on the other hand, celebrates the fact that his friend was able to get seats on the plane, talks about his fear of flying, and then goes on the trip with him, sharing the joys and sorrows that occur during the venture. (p. 789)

As contained in this metaphor of the traveling companion, ACT staff cannot be content with sitting behind their desks and making appointments for their clients (i.e., the brokering model), as their clients may then frequently fail to show up for such appointments. Similarly, staff cannot be content with making suggestions regarding steps their clients may need to take in their lives (e.g., seeking employment), as clients may then either disregard or be unable to follow such suggestions on their own. Rather than waiting for their clients to show up at their office, the staff must meet the clients where they are in the community and facilitate their participation in such activities, to the point of actually accompanying them if necessary.

Although the traveling companion metaphor represents a significant first step toward a new model for community-based practice, it does introduce at least a couple of problems. First, as we found previously with the model of consumer or peer advocates, the traveling companion image suggests that the staff and client share a relationship of two friends traveling together. This image fails to capture the fact that staff are assigned to assess and address the client's needs and are paid for their service, suggesting a false reciprocity between the two parties. As argued by Rosen (1994) and Rosen et al. (1993)—experienced ACT proponents all— ACT staff should no more be confused with friends or peers due to their community location than should traditional office-based case managers. For this reason, they suggest the image of a tour guide as opposed to that of a traveling companion, the tour guide metaphor preserving the staff member's status as a care provider and the resulting, largely asymmetrical nature of the relationship. This notion of tour guide closely resembles the notion of "community guide" proposed by John McKnight in his work with adults with developmental disabilities. A community guide, according to McKnight (1992), is an individual who "assume[s] a special responsibility for guiding excluded people out of service and into the realm of the community" (p. 59). In addition to providing a service for which he or she is reimbursed (unlike friendship), it is important for community guides to learn, according to McKnight, "that in order for the fullness of community hospitality to be expressed and the excluded person to be wholly incorporated as a citizen they must leave the scene" (1992, p. 59). In other words, rather than becoming an enduring figure in the person's life, community guides play a transitional role in facilitating the person's engagement in social relationships with peers in the community. Guides are neither peers nor friends but

tools for the person to use in reconnecting to the things that matter to him or her.

The notion of tour or community guide in this way represents a step beyond that of traveling companion. Even this revision falls short of capturing the full flavor of community-based practice, however, in at least one important respect. Simply stated, most people with severe psychiatric disabilities do not readily or willingly seek out the assistance of a guide. The journey of mental illness is not a trip that anyone wants to take, and thus is one for which people are unlikely to contact mental health providers for assistance, at least in the early phases of the illness. These phases are more commonly characterized by confusion, cognitive interference, withdrawal, and shock. Due to the stigma that continues to accrue to mental illness in popular culture, the lack of education or information provided to the lay public regarding psychiatric disorders, and the denial and disbelief that accompany the onset of many serious illnesses, people often struggle with serious mental illness for many years before coming to understand that what they are struggling with *is* a psychiatric disorder. Another prolonged period may then pass before they can muster the courage and trust to accept their need for treatment and support. As a result, community-based practitioners cannot assume that clients will come to them of their own volition out of a genuine desire to receive guidance from a mental health expert—or, for that matter, a community guide— just as they cannot assume that clients will appreciate their efforts to offer assistance when clients do not yet accept or recognize that they need it. Should a person willingly seek out the assistance of a tour guide to navigate the complex health and social systems required to access needed services, or seek out a community guide to help him or her reclaim his or her life in the broader community, then the provider's job is made considerably easier. Early in the course of illness, however, this is more the exception than the rule.

The rule suggests instead that the first job of the provider, even prior to becoming a community guide, is to *engage* a reluctant and disbelieving, but nonetheless suffering, person in care. For this reason, we prefer the term "recovery guide" for the primary role of the mental health provider in working with people with serious mental illness, defining this role as an expansion upon the tour or community guide through explicit recognition and incorporation of the need for engagement as the first step in developing the trusting relationship that then can be put to use in guiding the person along the path of recovery. We thus begin our exposition of the roles and responsibilities of the recovery guide here, with the first lesson to be learned in working with people with serious mental illness, which we define as the following:

Lesson 1

Most people will not know that they have a psychiatric disorder at first, and therefore will not seek help on their own. The initial focus of care thus should be on the person's own understanding of his or her predicament (i.e., not necessarily the events or difficulties that brought him or her to your attention), and on the ways in which the provider can be helpful in addressing this predicament, regardless of how the person understands it at the time.

The recovery guide needs to take the prospective client's own perception of his or her difficulties as the point of departure for any efforts to be effective in developing a trusting relationship that then can serve as the cornerstone for other helping efforts. In the common parlance of community-based practitioners, this is captured by the phrase "meeting the client where he or she is at." This lesson was learned initially in conducting outreach to persons who were homeless, when outreach staff began to realize that people were more responsive to offers of coffee and a sandwich, concrete assistance with securing housing, or meeting other basic needs than to offers of psychiatric treatment or medication. Extrapolating from this rather extreme situation to more common ones, providers need to attend to what the prospective client is concerned about most, regardless of its relationship to his or her mental illness. In this respect, providers also cannot assume that everyone with a mental illness experiences the illness in the same way, or has had similar experiences of seeking or receiving help in the past. In fact, people have many different ways of accounting for the disruptions, interruptions, and difficulties brought about by the illness, ranging from the perception that he or she is being conspired against by others, to his or her unique relationship to God, to the effects of previous accidents or substance use, to punishments for earlier sins.

Rather than viewing these perceptions or beliefs as further evidence of the client's illness, we suggest that it is more useful to view them as representing the client's best efforts to make sense of her or his own experiences—without the benefit of our knowledge and expertise (Davidson, 2003). In addition, the client's attitudes toward you and the kind of assistance you have to offer will be shaped by his or her previous experiences with psychiatric treatment and the mental health system as a whole, particularly if he or she has had experiences of involuntary commitment or forced medication. Despite your most benevolent intentions, suspiciousness toward mental health services and a legitimately earned skepticism regarding providers' motives may make the engagement process complicated and protracted.

In prior research involving interviews with clients of an assertive community treatment team (Chinman, Allende, Bailey, Maust, & Davidson, 1999), we learned that clients may resist the engagement efforts and guidance of ACT staff if they perceive that they are being asked to do things by strangers who have not yet taken the time to get to know them as a person. This research suggested that while there is value in offering problem-specific psychoeducation and other clinical interventions, there is equal, if not more, value in getting to know the individual first independent of his or her illness; for example, the person may be an accomplished pianist, a lover of pepperoni pizza, or a nervous mother worried about losing custody of her children. Engaging the person around one of his or her interests or concerns may prove to be key to establishing yourself in the client's eyes as an individual who is genuinely interested in, and concerned about, his or her well-being.

In addition to meeting the client where he or she is and expressing a genuine interest in him or her as a person, efforts with prospective clients who have come to mistrust the mental health system and others in general need to be repetitive and persistent over time. Efforts to be persistent in engaging the client should not, however, supersede the overarching goal of establishing and maintaining a trusting relationship with the client. The recovery guide must be careful to allow the individual the right to decline his or her overtures, advice, and other interventions, and to enter into the relationship at a comfortable pace. In the study mentioned earlier, one ACT staff member coined this the "velvet bulldozer" approach (Chinman et al., 1999) to capture the gentle but persistent way in which he had had to pursue one of his particularly reluctant clients.

The phenomenon represented by the velvet bulldozer has been described from both the client's and the provider's perspective. From the client's perspective, this is described as people "sticking by me" or "believing in me even when I no longer believed in myself" (Davidson, 2003). When asked by the research interviewer what she thought had been most helpful about the ACT team to which she had been assigned following years of rejecting treatment, for example, the client who was being pursued by the velvet bulldozer explained: "They kept showing up . . . they didn't drop me or let me get off the medications . . . they didn't give up, they just stuck with me." It was only after several months of repeated efforts to engage this client that she first began to have some trust in the staff's concern and intentions toward her. And it was not until she began to feel understood by the staff after several more months that she began to listen to what they were saying and consider their recommendations, loosening her hold on the isolation and daily substance use to which she had become accustomed. Eventually, she was able to reveal that she had been a practicing architect before the onset of her affective disorder, showing the staff some of her sketches as she began to take on a more active role in her own recovery.

The kind of patience and persistence required by this type of work is obviously not for everyone. As described by Estroff, this type of approach "appeals to people who do not know the meaning of the word 'no.' They don't like the status quo; they will try anything to help their clients and they are not loyal to institutions or to centers, only to the people they are working with" (Estroff, cited in Rosen, 1994, p. 61). In more positive terms, the process of gentle but persistent pursuit was captured eloquently by Antoine de Saint-Exupéry in his children's tale *The Little Prince* (1943). In this story, a young prince travels the galaxy, learning important lessons from the various people, animals, and plants he meets on his way. When he reaches the earth, he learns what it means "to tame" a fox in the following passage:

"Good morning," said the fox.

"Good morning," the little prince responded politely. "Who are you?" he asked, and then added, "You are very pretty to look at."

"I am a fox," the fox said.

"Come and play with me," proposed the little prince. "I am so unhappy."

"I cannot play with you," the fox said. "I am not tamed."

"Ah! Please excuse me," said the little prince. But after some thought, he added: "What does that mean—'to tame'?" . . .

"It is an act too often neglected," said the fox. "It means to establish ties."

" 'To establish ties'?"

"Just that," said the fox. "To me, you are still nothing more than a little boy who is just like a hundred thousand other little boys. And I have no need of you. And you, on your part, have no need of me. To you, I am nothing more than a fox like a hundred thousand other foxes. But if you tame me, then we shall need each other. To me, you will be unique in all the world. To you, I shall be unique in all the world. . . . My life is very monotonous," he said. "I hunt chickens; men hunt me. All the chickens are just alike, and all the men are just alike. And, in consequence, I am a little bored. But if you tame me, it will be as if the sun came to shine on my life. I shall know the sound of a step that will be different from all the others. Other steps send me hurrying back underneath the ground. Yours will call me, like music, out of my burrow. And then look: you see the grain-fields down yonder? I do not eat bread. Wheat is of no use to me. The wheat fields have nothing to say to me. And that is sad. But you have hair that is the color of gold. Think how wonderful that will be when you have tamed me! The grain, which is also golden, will bring me back the thought of you. And I shall love to listen to the wind in the wheat . . ."

"What must I do, to tame you?" asked the little prince.

"You must be very patient," replied the fox. "First you will sit down at a little distance from me—like that—in the grass. I shall look at you out of the corner of my eye, and you will say nothing. Words are the source of misunderstandings. But you will sit a little closer to me, every day . . ."

The next day the little prince came back.

"It would have been better to come back at the same hour," said the fox. "If, for example, you come at four o'clock in the afternoon, then at three o'clock I shall begin to be happy. I shall feel happier and happier as the hour advances. At four o'clock, I shall already be worrying and jumping about. I shall show you how happy I am! But if you come at just any time, I shall never know at what hour my heart is to be ready to greet you . . . One must observe the proper rites . . ." (pp. 45–46)

In the case of community-based practice, the "proper rites" include such things as calling clients ahead of time so as not to show up unannounced, setting up regular times for contact, not giving up or becoming defensive in response to repeated rejection, and being available to assist the client with things he or she is interested in doing or needs when he or she is ready to do so.

Lesson 2

Regardless of whether or not he or she sought your help, recognize that the client had already embarked on his or her own journey before meeting you.

Once an initial sense of trust and engagement with the recovery guide is in place, staff may move to those components of their role that are more consistent with the guide metaphor. It is important to remember, however, that the client was already on his or her own journey before the onset of the illness, and before he or she came into contact with the recovery guide. As much as having a serious psychiatric disorder may have interrupted or interfered with the client's aspirations and plans, the journey that follows still has to be connected in meaningful ways to what came before. In other words, clients' lives did not begin with the onset of their disorders, just as their lives are not encompassed totally by psychiatric treatment and rehabilitation. While seemingly obvious perhaps, these points were driven home to us by some of the questions we fielded when we first started to use the tour guide metaphor in our teaching. Following an exposition of the various roles and resources of the tour guide, for example, one experienced clinician objected by saying: "That all sounds fine and good, but what if the client won't get on the damn bus?" It is not the recovery guide's job to get the client to

agree to "get on the bus." Not only might clients prefer to take a taxi, ride a bicycle, or walk, but more important, clients are already on journeys of their own when we meet them. It is we who need to join their journey, get on *their* bus, so to speak, rather than try to persuade them to get on ours.

Once we recognize that the client was already on a journey prior to the onset of his or her illness, and therefore prior to meeting us, the focus then shifts to the ways in which this journey was impacted by his or her illness. How has his or her psychiatric disorder changed the person's aspirations, hopes, and dreams? If the person appears to be sticking resolutely to the hopes and dreams he or she had prior to onset of the disorder, and despite or in denial of the disorder and its disabling effects, then what steps need to be taken for him or her to get back on track or to take the next step or two along this track? Rather than the reduction of symptoms or the remediation of deficits—goals that we assume the client will share with *us*—it is the client's own goals for his or her life beyond or despite his or her disability that need to drive the treatment planning and rehabilitation efforts.

Once these goals have been identified and articulated, recovery guides have a number of tools at their disposal to facilitate the client's progress toward achieving them. The recovery guide's professional and clinical training and knowledge provide some of these tools, helping the client work toward recovery by providing education about serious mental illness, the recovery process, coping strategies, and the person's options, and by translating mental health procedures, services, and language into understandable and usable information. The guide's expertise should not be taken as a substitute for knowing the needs, interests, and strengths of the client, however. The guide's expertise also cannot be imparted to the client in a straightforward manner, as if giving a person cognitive strategies or telling a person what to do ever leads to significant personal change. Instead, the content and course of the journey must be directed by the client's own experiences, preferences, and concerns, rather than those of the guide. The client, in consultation with the guide, can choose where to go, when, and in what manner, and whether to stroll leisurely through scenic routes or to charge ahead on a more direct but rocky path. This is partly because the client will have a better sense of his or her own stamina and energy level, his or her ability to tolerate frustration and setbacks, and the pace of change at which he or she feels most comfortable. It also is due to the fact that it is the client's life that ultimately has to change to support recovery, and thus it is the client who must do much of the hard work of recovery him- or herself. In addition to providing tools for the trek, the guide can share with the client ways of making the journey safe, sustainable, and satisfying.

Lesson 3

Rather than dwelling on the client's distant past or worrying about the client's long-term future, recovery guides focus on the next several steps of the journey and on the sites that lie ahead.

Psychodynamic approaches to psychotherapy and clinical case management have long been criticized for focusing on clients' distant pasts rather than on their present circumstances and needs. One example of this practice was given by a participant in the ACT study described earlier, who reported that she stopped seeing an office-based psychotherapist for her affective disorder and alcohol dependence when this person wanted to focus only on her childhood memories and their presumptive effects when she felt that she had pressing concerns in her day-to-day life. "She kept telling me that I hadn't gotten over my father's death," she complained. "Like whoever does?" When this clinician sent her a letter informing her that she was going to be discharged from treatment for missing too many appointments, the woman described wanting to frame the letter as her "graduation diploma," feeling that this was the only way she would be able to leave the mental health system behind.

In the opposite direction, clinical psychiatry has made profound and far-reaching mistakes in telling clients and their families that illnesses like schizophrenia or manic-depressive psychosis were death sentences from which they would never recover (North, 1987). Although perhaps no longer suggesting that families grieve for the loss of their adult child recently diagnosed with serious mental illness as if he or she had died, it is still routine for providers to inform clients that they will have to take their psychiatric medications "for the rest of your life, just like you would have to take insulin for diabetes." Not only do we lack credible evidence on which to base such statements (i.e., many people stop taking their medications later in the course

of their recovery without undue effects), but long-term pronouncements of any sort are typically not very helpful to anyone, including people receiving mental health services. As we now know that there is a vast heterogeneity in outcome for serious mental illnesses and that diagnosis can no longer predict prognosis (Carpenter & Kirkpatrick, 1988; Davidson & McGlashan, 1997; Harding et al., 1987; McGlashan, 1988), providers should refrain from pretending that they have a crystal ball through which they can predict their clients' long-term future.

It is in this respect, among others, that the recovery guide model can be particularly helpful in directing the provider's attention toward the "sites" most likely to be of interest to their clients. Tour guides neither dwell on their clients' histories prior to their current excursion nor worry about what their clients will be doing when they return home following the trip. In addition, while they may provide some overall information about the entire trip at its inception, such as listing the historical sites they will be visiting, good guides focus primarily on the next one or two sites coming up immediately so as to hold their clients' interest while not inundating them with too much information. If the bus is on the way to the Eiffel Tower, for example, the guide does not drone on about Notre Dame Cathedral or bestow praises on the Arc de Triomphe. Certainly the guide does not try to prepare his or her clients for the next leg of their trip by recounting the history of the Roman Coliseum when the tourists are still in Paris.

In this respect, the recovery guide's primary focus is on helping to prepare the client for the *next one or two steps* of the recovery process by anticipating what lies ahead in the near future, by focusing on the characteristics and challenges of the present situation, and by identifying and helping the client avoid or move around potential obstacles in the road. This idea of looking forward in the client's recovery is dramatically different from the focus of several of the previous models, as suggested previously, and is crucial to adopting a recovery orientation. Although the recovery guide deemphasizes early personal history (because it may not be relevant) and long-term outcomes (because we cannot predict them), either of these perspectives may be invoked should they prove useful in the current situation. As we will describe in more detail later, clients who become stuck in patterns of relating or failing at certain tasks may need assistance in understanding and liberating themselves from the legacy of their past. Demoralized and hopeless clients who view mental illness as a death sentence may need to be given information about the heterogeneity of long-term outcome and their chances for improvement. In general, however, recovery guides have their hands full focusing on supporting the client's efforts in the present. This forward-looking orientation requires the recovery guide to provide a context for the new experiences and learning of the client, but with a clear awareness that the journey is guided by the preferences, goals, and interests of the client rather than by some imaginary ideal of normalcy held by the provider to which the client is supposed to aspire (Davidson & Strauss, 1995).

Lesson 4

Your credibility and effectiveness as a recovery guide are enhanced to the degree that you are familiar with, and can anticipate, interesting sites, common destinations, and important landmarks along the way.

This lesson derives directly from lesson 3. As a result of the recovery guide's focus on the next one or two steps in the journey, it is helpful for guides to develop a familiarity with the territory of recovery and to be able to anticipate interesting sites, common destinations, and important landmarks that clients are likely to encounter along their way. This is not to contradict the highly personal nature of each individual's journey. Despite the unique characteristics of each individual's struggle, there remain areas of commonality and overlap, issues and concerns that may be shared among a number of people who face some of the same challenges in coping with and compensating for their disorder. Examples of such shared concerns include relevant health services (e.g., medication options, medical treatment for other illnesses) and social services (e.g., accessing entitlements or support for parenting issues), learning skills for independent living (including finding safe and affordable housing and managing the responsibilities of being a tenant), and dealing with developmental issues of separation and individuation that have been delayed or prolonged by the onset of the illness. Self-help and peer support groups might be included as a way for clients to share common experiences and gain

the support of others who are working on the same issues. Other landmarks may include finding opportunities to socialize outside of mental health centers or clubhouses. Involvement in meaningful activities, like work or education, or doing something creative and beyond the scope of traditional treatment, can help clients move beyond the relationship with the recovery guide into the broader community—the destination of choice for most people. These common destinations are outlined in figure 30-1, along with the range of resources and tools the recovery guide has at his or her disposal in facilitating the client's exploration of these and other sites of interest.

The resources and tools that the recovery guide has at his or her disposal include professional training and experience; these are not to be discounted, no matter how conventional they may be. The guide has many other resources and tools at his or her disposal, however, that have not been emphasized as much in the models described earlier. These include a hopefulness toward clients and their potential for improvement that has been lacking in earlier eras; the client's own aspirations, interests, assets, and goals, which drive the recovery and service planning activities; the observations, input, and resources of family members and other important people in the client's life and community; and the recovery guide's own personal experiences, particularly as a member of the same community to which his or her clients belong. This last point is worth noting, as it is one of the resources that is related directly to the notion of the guide as opposed to that of detective, teacher, coach, and so forth. In psychoanalytic training for example, much was made of the trainee's need to be in psychoanalysis him- or herself to become familiar with his or her own blind spots and become immersed in the analytic process. McKnight (1992) makes a parallel point about the need for the community guide to have an active investment in, and extensive familiarity with, his or her local community to make use of these resources in his or her work with clients. "Most effective guides," writes McKnight, "are well connected in the interrelationships of community life. They have invested much of life's energy and vitality in associational activity. Based upon these connections, they are able to make a variety of contacts quickly because 'they know people who know other people' " (pp. 59–60).

In addition to the client's assets, interests, and

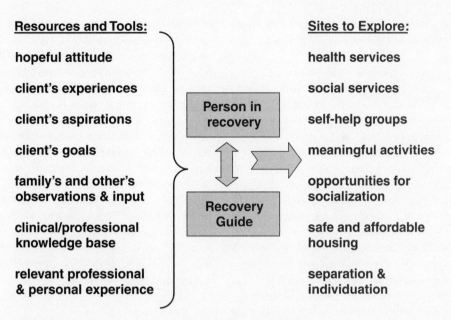

Resources and Tools:

hopeful attitude

client's experiences

client's aspirations

client's goals

family's and other's observations & input

clinical/professional knowledge base

relevant professional & personal experience

Person in recovery

Recovery Guide

Sites to Explore:

health services

social services

self-help groups

meaningful activities

opportunities for socialization

safe and affordable housing

separation & individuation

Figure 30.1. Common Components of the Recovery Guide Model

goals, the resources and input of his or her natural supports, and the guide's own professional knowledge and personal experience, it is useful for the guide to be familiar with, and be able to anticipate, the concerns and questions that commonly arise for people in different phases of recovery. Early in the course of illness and treatment, for example, people often wonder about the following issues:

- What is happening to me?
- How can I get rid of whatever this is that is happening to me? How can I make it stop?
- What can I tell my parents and other people who care about me?
- How can I catch up to my peers?
- How can I have a normal life?
- How can I keep this from happening again?

Guides can anticipate such questions as part of the preparation for the upcoming trek; knowing that these issues may be on a client's mind, and having accumulated valuable experiences with other clients who have struggled with these same concerns, will enhance significantly the credibility and trustworthiness of the guide in the client's eyes. Similarly, it is common later in the course of the recovery process for issues such as the following to emerge as the person tries to make sense of his or her past and to create a new future based on what is possible now given his or her disability.

- What happened to me?
- Why did it happen? Why did it happen to *me*?
- What is possible for me now?
- How can I get there from here?

Clearly these are difficult, and at times impossible, questions to answer. These are the kinds of questions, however, that lie at the heart of the journey of recovery—whether or not the guide chooses to attend to them. To be able to share these concerns with the guide and accept the guide's involvement in his or her struggles, the client must be able to trust that the guide has his or her best interests in mind and will not willingly or knowingly lead him or her to a dangerous place. The guide can earn this trust by not giving false information about the language or customs of the country they are visiting together, by respecting the client and his or her central role in the recovery process, and by not ridiculing, disparaging, criticizing, or judging the client. This trust also includes faith in the guide's professionalism and competence, which the client develops over time as he or she becomes confident that the recovery guide will act in an ethical and knowledgeable way, has the power and knowledge to open doors and make things work, and is aware of and open to a range of options from which the client can make meaningful choices. Without both forms of trust, the client is unlikely to invite the guide to join him or her on the next leg of the journey.

Once the journey is under way, the recovery guide must be able to assess and follow the interests and preferences of the client. Just as it would be inappropriate for a tour guide to take you to France if you want to go to India, so too would it be counterproductive and inappropriate for the recovery guide to try to get a client a job at Wendy's when he or she expresses an interest to work at Macy's. Once client preference has been made clear, the recovery guide must be willing to engage and join with the client in pursuit of the client's own goals. This may mean coordinating medical care among a number of providers, investigating employment opportunities, helping the client to enroll in classes or become involved in community activities, helping to navigate the Medicaid system, or working with family members to create a compassionate and supportive recovery environment. Through these and other joint explorations, this process is oriented toward assisting the client in creating a life outside of or beyond his or her disability.

Throughout this entire process, the issue of client choice and self-determination is key. Offering clients meaningful choices, and respecting and honoring those choices, can pose real dilemmas for recovery guides, however. For example, what if the person refuses to choose to go along with his or her physician's recommended treatment regimen? What if he or she continues to refuse all services, or insists on choosing to disregard the guide's efforts, showing what the guide considers "poor judgment"? The first step that the guide will need to consider in such circumstances is to reconsider what is being offered to, or recommended for, the client from the client's own perspective. What is being offered to the client? What is entailed in following the recommended regimen? Does it move the client in the direction of his or her own goals and interests? Does the client perceive it to be useful or helpful in achieving what he or she wants to achieve? Is it consistent with the client's own beliefs, goals, hopes, and strengths? In short, is it a tour or leg of the journey worth taking (from the client's perspective)?

If the guide remains convinced of the value of the options not taken, then he or she may need to consider the possibility that the client is already embarked on a different leg of the journey that may not be obvious to us. In other words, he or she may be too busy pursuing other options to take the detour we are recommending. Again, the guide needs to consider whether what he or she is offering will impede or facilitate the journey that the client has already begun. In the end, it is ultimately the client's life and the client's journey, so the client must decide which paths to follow and which to ignore, pass by, or try to keep in mind for a later, more fortuitous, time. In circumstances that do not pose serious and imminent risks to the client (e.g., active suicidal ideation with intent) or to others (e.g., assaultive behavior), all of us, as Patricia Deegan has reminded us, need the opportunity and freedom to learn from our own mistakes. Guides must accordingly afford their clients, in Deegan's (1996b) words, "the dignity of risk" and "the right to failure" (p. 97).

Lesson 5

Guides prepare for the journey by acquiring tools that will be effective in addressing or bypassing symptoms and other sequelae of the illness that act as barriers to the client's recovery.

A final, major area of focus for the guide involves assessing the potential obstacles that might lie in the client's path and working collaboratively with the client to find ways to address, overcome, or bypass these barriers as they arise. Many conventional clinical and psychotherapeutic skills can be incorporated into this component of the recovery guide's backpack, as long as the guide has the requisite training and supervisory resources available to deliver these interventions competently. We have found that moving what traditionally have been office-based practices into community settings requires more rather than less clinical skill, sophistication, and supervision than office-based practice. The challenges of deploying more flexible boundaries and enabling the development of a less unidirectional relationship while continuing to act in the client's best interest alone raise many thorny ethical and practical issues that have yet to be fully and adequately addressed. Without these skills and the ability to use them effectively in reducing, overcoming, or bypassing barriers to the client's recovery, however, the recovery guide will have a significantly diminished backpack, and thus a significantly depleted capacity for being truly helpful in facilitating the client's journey.

Rather than simply transferring these skills from the office to the recovery guide's backpack, preparing clinical skills for use "on the street" requires a shift in perspective. This shift entails focusing less on symptom reduction per se and more on assessing, anticipating, and addressing barriers that get in the way of what the client wants to, or is trying to, do. Obviously, this requires having a sense of what the client is trying to accomplish, as well as how specific symptoms, cognitive deficits, stigma, or other barriers get in the way of the pursuit of these goals. While it is true that conventional clinical practice has emphasized the promotion of health and competence as well as symptom and deficit reduction, it also is true that most models of serious mental illness assume that a person's symptoms and other areas of dysfunction need to be reduced or contained *before* he or she can resume normative activities such as attending school, obtaining and maintaining competitive employment, living independently, and so forth. We now know, however, that many people can live independently, attend school, work, and have gratifying personal relationships even while continuing to experience symptoms and other sequelae of their illness (Davidson, Stayner, et al., 2001). Our previous research also has suggested that to the degree that these issues are addressed, clients will be better prepared and more motivated to take an active role in their own treatment and rehabilitation (Davidson, Stayner, Lambert, Smith, & Sledge, 1997). On both humanitarian and clinical grounds, then, recovery guides understand that people need not wait until their illness has been effectively treated and reduced in order to pursue their personal goals and aspirations and to derive meaning from, and take pleasure in, life.

Consistent with this lesson is the definition of recovery emerging in the consumer/survivor and psychiatric rehabilitation literatures, which suggests that the reduction or amelioration of symptoms and deficits is not as crucial to being "in recovery" as the attitude the person takes toward his or her condition and the person's ability to lead a meaningful life despite continuing disability (Davidson et al., 2003). The recovery guide accepts this framework and then goes about the work of reframing a variety of established interventions as tools to be used in promoting the person's reclamation of a dignified and gratifying life in the community. Within a recovery perspective, for example, medications are taken not simply to treat an illness, as antibiotics are taken to treat an infection (Davidson & Strauss, 1995), but are taken in order for the person to be able to work, to attend and concentrate in the classroom, or to keep his or her own apartment. Similarly, cognitive-behavioral interventions for delusions (Kingdon & Turkington, 1994; Fowler, Garety & Kuipers, 1998) are offered to clients not only to decrease the suffering they experience due to their paranoid and persecutory ideas but also so that they may develop and maintain satisfying relationships with their peers—including peers who do not have a mental illness—rather than continuing to be shunned and rejected by others based on their alienating behavior. An increase in symptoms can often be taken as an indication of a significant event or challenge occurring in the person's life and may need to be attended to as a factor influencing the pace of the journey or the need for the person to stop at certain landmarks for rest and replenishment. Symptoms alone, however, should not be the cause of a cancellation of the journey altogether, or lead to indefinite delays in resuming the trek. On the contrary, people have been incredibly creative in finding their own ways to manage the symptoms and other sequelae of their illnesses, and guides need to learn from and be familiar with such coping strategies so that they may offer them to their clients along the way.

In addition to addressing the direct effects of the illness as obstacles in the person's path, an important component of recovery involves recovering from the collateral damage left in the wake of mental illness. Often this can mean recovering from the effects of life in the mental health system and having been socialized into the role of mental patient. This may also include dealing with the indirect effects of mental illness, like poverty, stigma, and fear. In practical terms, having a life costs money, and poverty is a major barrier to effective integration into the community. Addressing the issues of fear and stigma requires a constant awareness of their existence and of the many ways in which they marginalize and limit the opportunities of people who have a mental illness. The role of the recovery guide involves thinking and exploring with the client ways to open doors and enhance access to community involvements while remaining attentive to the ways in which stigma and fear arise and need to be addressed in the process of community (re)integration. To the degree that this at times requires broader community education, advocacy becomes an accepted part of the recovery guide's scope of responsibility.

Identifying and helping the client to overcome the various barriers to recovery that he or she encounters thus becomes an integral component of the work of the recovery guide. To do this work effectively, the guide needs to be familiar with the territory and anticipate the obstacles that people are likely to encounter, from both inside and outside of the illness. Just as a mountain guide would need to know how trails are laid out and where snow is most likely to fall in an avalanche, our recovery guide needs to be familiar with a variety of sources of information that speak to the common challenges and areas of increased vulnerability experienced by people with serious mental illnesses. In addition to the professional and clinical knowledge base they accrue in their training, this requires becoming familiar with, and seeking ways to apply, available literature on adolescent and adult development, family systems, and first-person accounts of illness and recovery. Common issues of loss and grief, separation and individuation, and the need for valued social roles add to this body of knowledge. Finally, recovery guides, as mentioned earlier, need to be intimately aware of the important community resources that will benefit or interest their clients, including informal support systems in the community that exist outside of the formal mental health system. The standard of care to which recovery guides aspire includes knowing the territory of recovery, the various paths up and down the mountain and those specific to each client, and ways to translate this knowledge effectively into practical strategies that restore hope and functioning.

Discussion

In this chapter, we have presented the recovery guide as a useful framework through which mental health professionals can understand their role as facilitators of recovery and community integration for people with serious mental illness. We have focused primarily on the ways in which the role of the recovery guide differs from traditional provider roles, and on how this role impacts the nature of the helping relationship. It also is important, however, to look beyond the immediate provider-client relationship and consider how systemic factors can either support or impede the journey of the client and his or her recovery guide.

Training and clinical supervision are areas in which mental health systems can make significant impact upon the professional development of service providers. The recovery guide model incorporates case management in the context of a clinical relationship with relaxed boundaries that must shift to accommodate each individual and his or her unique recovery journey. The guide might be called upon to help a client find furniture for a new apartment, offer testimony before the legislature, purchase a dress for Sunday services, or take a bus to visit an elderly parent. Each new situation can present a range of ambiguous and complex boundary dilemmas. In fact, such dilemmas are so inherent to community-based clinical practice that Curtis and Hodge (1993) have suggested that providers who are not facing boundary issues in their daily work are probably not doing their jobs.

At the same time, the mental health field lacks clear guidelines for what is professional and/or appropriate behavior for community-based practitioners (Carey, 1998), and "relaxing the boundaries" goes against the very grain of what most professionals are taught in training programs and clinical supervision. The adoption of the recovery guide model thus necessitates new standards not only for mental health providers but also for the institutions and supervisors that prepare them for clinical practice. Training programs must counter the pessimistic messages that are often sent to students regarding the chronic course of mental illness by presenting narratives of, and forums with, people in recovery, as well as clinical research studies which have documented that partial to full recovery is possible for at least one quarter, and up to two thirds, of people with schizophrenia and other severe psychiatric disorders. Similarly, the notion of "recovery," and the provider's role in promoting it, must be expanded beyond clinical stability and maintenance to incorporate the pursuit of a meaningful life and a positive sense of belonging in the community.

Clinical supervisors and managers in mental health systems can reinforce this perspective and support recovery guides by helping them to transfer their skills and knowledge from the classroom to the community. Often this involves drawing upon their own experiences as community-based practitioners or sharing the stories of people in recovery who speak and write about the types of relationships and services that are helpful and not helpful. For example, mental health professionals are frequently taught to maintain professional distance from their clients as a means of retaining objectivity in the helping relationship. Yet, while there are certainly negative consequences of overinvolvement for both the staff and clients, people report that "greater damage may be done by rigid enforcement of the traditional connotation of professional distance" than by boundary violations (Curtis & Hodge, 1994, p. 24). Supervisors must therefore allow recovery guides to reflect upon the "getting to know" aspect of their work, as it is this aspect— the trusting relationship between guide and client— that often makes providers uncomfortable because they might simply not know how to go about it (Chinman et al., 1999).

Individual and group supervision, in which recovery guides share their experiences with one another and have an opportunity to give and receive feedback, is a critical venue through which guides can process the range of complex issues that accompany community-based practice. Supervision may include such issues as (1) how to conduct meetings and interactions in a wide range of settings (e.g., coffee shops, soup kitchens) in such a way that both the guide and the client feel, and are, reasonably safe; (2) when and how to introduce the client to a social circle that you may already be connected to as a member of the same community (e.g., a religious parish); (3) how to decide when it is appropriate to use your personal resources to assist a client (e.g., using your own vehicle to drive the person to her daughter's kindergarten graduation when the agency van is not available); or (4) which type of personal information (e.g., the guide's own disability status) can be shared in the name of establishing and maintaining a genuine and empathic helping relationship. Supervision must address all these bends in the road of the recovery journey as well as the guide's *own personal* anxieties about the demands of the trek—especially in light of the fact that traditional training programs do not often adequately prepare providers for this type of work.

Finally, while clinical supervision can be a critical piece in assisting the guide to become comfortable in his or her role as an individual provider,

it cannot, in and of itself, address larger, systemic obstacles that might impede recovery. These obstacles include such things as (1) eligibility or entry criteria that the person must meet to be admitted to certain services (e.g., "work readiness" as a criteria for vocational rehabilitation); (2) funding structures that recognize a limited range of clinical interactions as reimbursable services; (3) inadequate community resources (e.g., a lack of affordable housing); (4) excessively high caseload sizes that prevent the development of responsive helping relationships; or (5) entrenched policies and procedures that prohibit such relationships even where caseload sizes would allow them (e.g., a rigid agency policy against accepting gifts from clients). When such obstacles are encountered on an individual's pathway to recovery, it is the job of the guide to work in collaboration with the client to identify the roadblock and to find routes under, around, over, or through it. This might mean encouraging the client to challenge the "rules" by becoming active in the agency's or the system's various decision-making bodies (e.g., a policy and procedures committee or a consumer affairs council) or becoming active yourself. Where such efforts fail, the recovery guide and the client might even find themselves tempted at times to break the rules to get around the roadblocks described here (Borg & Topor, 2002). Better yet, in proposing the recovery guide as an emerging model of community-based care, we would like to close with the question, "Isn't it time for new rules altogether?"

References

Anthony, W. A. (1993). Recovery from mental illness: The guiding vision of the mental health service system in the 1990s. *Psychosocial Rehabilitation Journal, 16*(4), 11–23.

Anthony, W. A. (2000). A recovery-oriented service system: Setting some system level standards. *Psychiatric Rehabilitation Journal, 24*, 159–168.

Anthony, W. A., Cohen, M., Farkas, M., & Cohen, B. F. (1988). The chronically mentally ill case management: More than a response to a dysfunctional system. *Community Mental Health Journal, 24*, 219–228.

Baxter, E. A., & Diehl, S. (1998). Emotional stages: Consumers and family members recovering from the trauma of mental illness. *Psychiatric Rehabilitation Journal, 21*, 349–355.

Becerra, R., Karno, M., & Escobar, J. (Ed.). (1982). *Mental Health and Hispanic Americans: Clinical Perspectives*. New York: Grune and Stratton.

Biegel, D. E., & Tracy, E. M. (1994). Strengthening social networks. *Health and Social Work, 19*, 206–217.

Bond, G. R. (1991). Variations in an assertive outreach model. In N. L. Cohen (Ed.), *Psychiatric outreach to the mentally ill: New directions for mental health services* (No. 52, pp. 65–80). San Francisco: Jossey-Bass.

Borg, M., & Topor, A. (2002). Recovery from "chronicity": Some life experiences. *WAPR Bulletin, October*. Retrieved January, 15, 2002, from http://www.wapr.net/vol14n03.htm

Butler, J. P. (1992). Of kindred minds: The ties that bind. In M. A. Orlandi (Ed.), *Cultural competence for evaluators* (pp. 23–54). Rockville, MD: Office of Substance Abuse Prevention.

Carey, K. (1998). Treatment boundaries in the case management relationship: A behavioral perspective. *Community Mental Health Journal, 34*, 313–317.

Carling, P. J. (1995). *Return to community: Building support systems for people with psychiatric disabilities*. New York: Guilford.

Carpenter, W. T., & Kirkpatrick, B. (1988). The heterogeneity of the long-term course of schizophrenia. *Schizophrenia Bulletin, 14*, 645–652.

Casas, J. M., & Pytluk, S. D. (1995). Hispanic identity development: Implications for research and practice. In J. G. Ponterotto, J. M. Casas, L. A. Suzuki. & C. M. Alexander (Eds.), *Handbook of multicultural counseling* (pp. 155–180). Thousand Oaks, CA: Sage.

Chinman, M. Allende, M., Bailey, P., Maust, J., & Davidson, L. (1999). Therapeutic agents of assertive community treatment. *Psychiatric Quarterly, 70*, 137–162.

Cooke, A. M. (1997). The long journey back. *Psychiatric Rehabilitation Skills, 2*(1), 33–36.

Corrigan, P. W., & Penn, D. L. (1998). Disease and discrimination: Two paradigms that describe severe mental illness. *Journal of Mental Health, 6*, 355–366.

Curtis, L., & Hodge, M. (1993). *Boundaries and ethics in community support services*. Unpublished training materials. Burlington, VT: Trinity College, Center for Community Change Through Housing and Support.

Curtis, L., & Hodge, M. (1994). Old standards, new dilemmas: Ethics and boundaries in community support services. *Psychosocial Rehabilitation Journal, 18*(2), 13–33.

Dailey, W. F., Chinman, M. J., Davidson, L., Garner, L., Vavrousek-Jakuba, E., Essock, S., Marcus, K., & Tebes, J. K. (2000). How are we doing? A statewide survey of community adjustment among people with serious mental illness receiving intensive outpatient services. *Community Mental Health Journal, 36*, 363–382.

Davidson, L. (1997). Vulnérabilité et destin dans la schizophrénie: Prêter l'oreille á la voix de la personne. (Vulnerability and destiny in schizophrenia: Hearkening to the voice of the person). *L'Evolution Psychiatrique, 62*, 263–284.

Davidson, L. (2003). *Living outside mental illness: Qualitative studies of recovery in schizophrenia*. New York: New York University Press.

Davidson, L., Haglund, K. E., Stayner, D. A., Rakfeldt, J., Chinman, M. J., & Tebes, J. (2001). "It was just realizing . . . that life isn't one big horror": A qualitative study of supported socialization. *Psychiatric Rehabilitation Journal, 24*, 275–292.

Davidson, L., & McGlashan, T. (1997). The varied outcomes of schizophrenia. *Canadian Journal of Psychiatry, 42*, 34–43.

Davidson, L., O'Connell, M. J., Tondora, J., Staeheli, M., & Evans, A. C. (2003). *Recovery from serious mental illness: Paradigm shift of (another) psychiatric shibboleth?* Unpublished manuscript.

Davidson, L., Stayner, D. A., & Haglund, K. E. (1998). Phenomenological perspectives on the social functioning of people with schizophrenia. In K. T. Mueser & N. Tarrier (Eds.), *Handbook of social functioning in schizophrenia* (pp. 97–120). Needham Heights, MA: Allyn and Bacon.

Davidson, L., Stayner, D. A., Lambert, S., Smith, P., & Sledge, W. H. (1997). Phenomenological and participatory research on schizophrenia: Recovering the person in theory and practice. *Journal of Social Issues, 53*, 767–784.

Davidson, L., Stayner, D. A., Nickou, C., Styron, T. H., Rowe, M., & Chinman, M. L. (2001). "Simply to be let in": Inclusion as a basis for recovery. *Psychiatric Rehabilitation Journal, 24*, 375–388.

Davidson, L., & Strauss, J. S. (1992). Sense of self in recovery from severe mental illness. *British Journal of Medical Psychology, 65*, 131–145.

Davidson, L., & Strauss, J. S. (1995). Beyond the biopsychosocial model: Integrating disorder, health, and recovery. *Psychiatry: Interpersonal and Biological Processes, 58*, 44–55.

De Bell, C., & Harless, D. (1992). B. F. Skinner: Myth and misperception. *Teaching of Psychology, 19*, 68–73.

Deegan, P. E. (1988). Recovery: The lived experience of rehabilitation. *Psychosocial Rehabilitation Journal, 11*(4), 11–19.

Deegan, P. E. (1993). Recovering our sense of value after being labeled. *Journal of Psychosocial Nursing, 31*(4), 7–11.

Deegan, P. E. (1996a, September). *Recovery and the conspiracy of hope*. Paper presented at the Sixth Annual Mental Health Services Conference of Australia and New Zealand, Brisbane, Australia. Retrieved March 1, 2002, from Intentional Care web site: http://www.intentionalcare.org/articles/articles_hope.pdf

Deegan, P. E. (1996b). Recovery as a journey of the heart. *Psychiatric Rehabilitation Journal, 19*, 91–97.

Deitchman, W. S. (1980). How many case managers does it take to screw in a light bulb? *Hospital and Community Psychiatry, 31*, 788–789.

Estroff, S. E. (1989). Self, identity, and subjective experiences of schizophrenia: In search of the subject. *Schizophrenia Bulletin, 15*, 189–196.

Estroff, S. E. (1995). Whose story is it anyway? Authority, voice, and responsibility in narratives of chronic illness. In S. Toombs, S. Kay, & D. Barnard et al.(Eds.), *Chronic illness: From experience to policy* (pp. 77–102). Bloomington: Indiana University Press.

Everett, B., & Nelson, A. (1992). We're not cases, and you're not managers. *Psychosocial Rehabilitation Journal, 15*(4), 49–60.

Fisher, D. (1994). Health care reform based on an empowerment model of recovery by people with psychiatric disabilities. *Hospital and Community Psychiatry, 45*, 913–915.

Fowler, D., Garety, P., & Kuipers, E. (1998). Understanding the inexplicable: An individually formulated cognitive approach to delusional beliefs. In C. Perris & P. McGorry (Eds.), *Cognitive psychotherapy of psychotic and personality disorders: Handbook of theory and practice* (pp. 129–146). New York: Wiley.

Gerteis, M., Edgman-Levitan, L., Daley, J., & Delbanco, T. L. (1993). Medicine and health from the patient's perspective. In M. Gerteis, S. Edgman-Levitan, J. Daley, & T. L. Delbanco (Eds.), *Through the patient's eyes* (pp. 1–15). San Francisco: Jossey-Bass.

Gilmartin, R. M. (1997). Personal narrative and the social reconstruction of the lives of former psychiatric patients. *Journal of Sociology and Social Welfare, 24*, 77–102.

Grier, W., & Cobbs, P. (1968). *Black rage*. New York: Basic Books.

Grills, C. N., Bass, K., Brown, D. L., & Akers, A. (1996). Empowerment evaluation: Building upon a tradition of activism in the African-American community. In D. M. Fetterman, S. J. Kaftarian, & A. Wandersman (Eds.), *Empowerment evaluation: Knowledge and tools for self-assessment and accountability* (pp. 123–140). Thousand Oaks, CA: Sage.

Gutierrez, L., Ortega, R. M., & Suarez, Z. E. (1990). Self-help and the Latino Community. In T. J. Powell (Ed.), *Working with self-help* (pp. 218–236). Silver Springs, MD: National Association of Social Workers.

Harding, C. M., Zubin, J., & Strauss, J. S. (1987). Chronicity in schizophrenia: Fact, partial fact, or artifact? *Hospital and Community Psychiatry, 38*, 477–486.

Hatfield, A. B. (1994). Recovery from mental illness. *Journal of the California Alliance for the Mentally Ill, 5*(3), 6–7.

Hoge, M., Davidson, L., Griffith, E., & Jacobs, S. (1998). The crisis of managed care in the public sector. *International Journal of Mental Health, 27*, 52–71.

Hoge, M. A., Davidson, L., Griffith, E.E.H., Sledge, W. H., & Howenstine, R. A. (1994). Defining managed care in public-sector psychiatry. *Hospital and Community Psychiatry, 45*, 1085–1089.

Jacobson, N., & Curtis, L. (2000). Recovery as policy in mental health services: Strategies emerging from the states. *Psychiatric Rehabilitation Journal, 23*, 333–341.

Jacobson, N., & Greenley, D. (2001). What is recovery? A conceptual model and explication. *Psychiatric Services, 52*, 482–485.

Kensit, D. (2000). Rogerian theory: A critique of the effectiveness of pure client-centered therapy. *Counseling Psychology Quarterly, 13*, 345–352.

Kingdon, D. G., & Turkington, D. (1994). *Cognitive-behavioral therapy of schizophrenia*. Notinghamshire, UK: Bassetlaw Hospital.

Lunt, A. (2000). Recovery: Moving from concept toward a theory. *Psychiatric Rehabilitation Journal, 23*, 401–405.

McGlashan, T. H. (1988). A selective review of recent North American long-term follow-up studies of schizophrenia. *Schizophrenia Bulletin, 14*, 515–542.

McKnight, J. L. (1992). Redefining community. *Social Policy, Fall-Winter*, 56–62.

Mead, S., & Copeland, M. E. (2000). What recovery means to us: Consumers' perspectives. *Community Mental Health Journal, 36*, 315–328.

Mueser, K. T., Bond, G. R., Drake, R. E., & Resnick, S. G. (1998). Models of community care for severe mental illness: A review of research on case management. *Schizophrenia Bulletin, 24*, 37–74.

Munetz, M. R., & Frese, F. J. (2001). Getting ready for recovery: Reconciling mandatory treatment with the recovery vision. *Psychiatric Rehabilitation Journal, 25*, 35–42.

Neighbors, H., Elliott, K., & Gant, L. (1990). Self-help and black Americans: A strategy for empowerment. In T. J. Powell (Ed.), *Working with self-help* (pp. 189–217). Silver Springs, MD: National Association of Social Workers.

Nelson, G., Ochocka, J., Griffin, K., & Lord, J. (1998).

"Nothing about me, without me": Participatory action research with self-help/mutual aid organizations for psychiatric consumers/survivors. *American Journal of Community Psychology, 26,* 881–912.

Noordsy, D. L., Torrey, W. C., Mead, S., Brunette, M., Potenza, D., & Copeland, M. E. (2000). Recovery-oriented psychopharmacology: Redefining the goals of antipsychotic treatment. *Journal of Clinical Psychiatry, 61*(Suppl. 3), 22–29.

North, C. (1987). *Welcome, silence.* New York: Simon and Schuster.

O'Brien, J., & Lovett, H. (1992). Finding a way toward everyday lives: The contribution of person-centered planning. Harrisburg, PA: Pennsylvania Office of Mental Retardation.

O'Connell, M., Tondora, J., Evans, A., Croog, G., & Davidson L. (2003). *From rhetoric to routine: Assessing recovery-oriented practices in a state mental health system.* Unpublished manuscript.

Parrish, J. (1989). The long journey home: Accomplishing the mission of the community support movement. *Psychosocial Rehabilitation Journal, 12,* 107–124.

Pope-Davis, D., Liu, W., Ledesma-Jones, S., & Nevitt, J. (2000). African American acculturation and black racial identity: A preliminary investigation. *Journal of Multicultural Counseling and Development, 28,* 98–113.

Ragins, A. (1994). Recovery: Changing from a medical model to a psychosocial rehabilitation model. *The Journal, 5*(3), 8–10.

Rapp, C. A. (1993). Theory, principles, and methods of the strengths model of case management. In M. Harris & H. C. Bergman, (Eds.), *Case management for mentally ill patients: Theory and practice* (pp. 143–164): Langhorne, PA: Harwood Academic Publishers/Gordon & Breach Science Publishers.

Rapp, C. A. (1998). The active ingredients of effective case management: A research synthesis. *Community Mental Health Journal, 34,* 363–380.

Rapp, C. A., & Wintersteen, R. (1989). The strengths model of case management: Results from twelve demonstrations. *Psychosocial Rehabilitation Journal, 13,* 23–32.

Rappaport, J. (1981). In praise of paradox: A social policy of empowerment over prevention. *American Journal of Community Psychology, 9,* 1–25.

Rappaport, J. (1995). Empowerment meets narrative: Listening to stories and creating settings. *American Journal of Community Psychology, 23,* 795–807.

Ridgway, P. A. (2001). Re-storying psychiatric disability: Learning from first person narrative accounts of recovery. *Psychiatric Rehabilitation Journal, 24,* 335–343.

Riessman, F. (1990). Restructuring help: A human services paradigm for the 1990s. *American Journal of Community Psychology, 18,* 221–230.

Rosen, A. (1994, April). Case management: The cornerstone of comprehensive local mental health services. *Australian Hospital Association, Management Issues Paper, No. 4,* 47–63.

Rosen, A., Diamond, R., Miller, V., & Stein, L. (1993, October). *Becoming real: How to go from model programme to enduring service.* Paper presented at the Hospital and Community Psychiatry Institute, Baltimore.

Saint-Exupéry, A. (1943). *The little prince* (K. Woods, Trans.). New York: Reynal and Hitchcock.

Sayce, L., & Perkins, R. (2000). Recovery: Beyond mere survival. *Psychiatric Bulletin, 24,* 74.

Scott, J., & Dixon, L. (1995). Psychological interventions for schizophrenia. *Schizophrenia Bulletin, 21,* 621–630.

Sledge, W. H., Astrachan, B., Thompson, K., Rakfeldt, J., & Leaf, P. (1995). Case management in psychiatry: An analysis of tasks. *American Journal of Psychiatry, 152,* 1259–1265.

Smith, M. K. (2000). Recovery from a severe psychiatric disability: Findings of a qualitative study. *Psychiatric Rehabilitation Journal, 24,* 149–159.

Stein, L. I. (1989). The community as the primary locus of care for persons with serious long-term mental illness. In C. Bonjean, M. T. Coleman, et al. (Eds.), *Community care of the chronically mentally ill: Proceedings of the sixth Robert Lee Sutherland Seminar in Mental Health* (pp. 11–29). Austin: Hogg Foundation for Mental Health, University of Texas.

Stein, L., & Test, M. A. (1980). Alternative to mental hospital treatment 1. Conceptual model: Treatment program, and clinical evaluation. *Archives of General Psychiatry, 37,* 392–397.

Strauss, J. S., & Davidson, L. (1997). Mental disorder, work and choice. In R. Bonnie & J. Monahan (Eds.), *Mental disorder, work disability, and the law* (pp. 105–130). Chicago: University of Chicago Press.

Sullivan, W. P. (1994). A long and winding road: The process of recovery from severe mental illness. *Innovations and Research, 3,* 19–27.

Telles, C., Karno, M., Mintrz, J., Paz., G., Arias, M., Tucker, D., & Lopez, S. (1995). Immigrant families coping with schizophrenia: Behavioral family intervention v. case management with a low-income Spanish-speaking population. *British Journal of Psychiatry, 167,* 473–479.

Turner, J. C., & TenHoor, W. J. (1978). The NIMH community support program: Pilot approach to a needed social reform. *Schizophrenia Bulletin, 4,* 319–349.

Turner, J. E., & Schifren, I. (1979). Community support systems: How comprehensive? *New Directions for Mental Health Services, 2,* 1–23.

U.S. Department of Health and Human Services. (1999). *Mental health: A report of the Surgeon General.* Rockville, MD: Center for Mental Health Services.

U.S. Department of Health and Human Services. (2001). *Executive summary. Mental health: Culture, race, and ethnicity. A supplement to Mental health: A report of the Surgeon General.* Rockville, MD: Center for Mental Health Services.

U.S. Department of Health and Human Services, Office of Minority Health. (2001). *A practical guide for implementing the recommended national standards for culturally and linguistically appropriate services in healthcare.* Retrieved March 20, 2002, from *http://www.omhrc.gov/clas/guide3a.asp*

Vandiver, B. (2001). Psychological nigresence revisited: Introduction and overview. *Journal of Multicultural Counseling and Development, 29,* 165–174.

Weinrach, S. (1988). Cognitive therapist: A dialogue with Aaron Beck. *Journal of Counseling and Development, 67,* 159–164.

Young, S. L., & Ensing, D. S. (1999). Exploring recovery from the perspective of people with psychiatric disabilities. *Psychiatric Rehabilitation Journal, 22,* 219–231.

31

Jaakko Seikkula

Open Dialogue Integrates Individual and Systemic Approaches in Serious Psychiatric Crises

This chapter presents the work of the Open Dialogue (OD) approach to mental health intervention in psychiatric crises developed by a team of clinicians and researchers in Finland. In Open Dialogue the first treatment meeting occurs within 24 hours after contact and includes as many significant people as possible from the patient's social network. The aim is to generate dialogue and put words to the experiences embodied in the patient's psychotic symptoms. Psychosis is a way of responding to stressful life situations, and in therapy, generating dialogue becomes the primary aim. All issues are analyzed and addressed with everyone present. Treatment is adapted to the specific and varying needs of patients and takes place at home, if possible. Psychological continuity and trust are emphasized by constructing integrated teams that include both inpatient and outpatient staff, all of whom focus on generating dialogue with the family and patients instead of trying to rapidly remove psychotic symptoms. Treatment is based on generating dialogue; a case is analyzed to illustrate this principle.

The Open Dialogue approach was initiated in Finnish western Lapland, in a small province with 72,000 inhabitants. In the local psychiatric hospital, where the author worked as a psychologist from

1981 through 1998, family- and network-oriented treatment was the goal. In 1984 the traditional manner of admitting patients was challenged. The team started to organize open meetings—referred to as treatment meetings—for analyzing the problem and preparing the treatment plan after a patient was admitted to the ward. Instead of having a staff meeting after separate individual interviews by the doctor, the nurse, the social worker, and the psychologist, the team decided to have the patient present in the meeting from the outset, together with all the professionals involved in his or her treatment. Staff members stopped having their own separate gatherings to plan treatment. At the same time, instead of inviting families into family therapy after the team had defined the problem, the team started to invite families to participate immediately after a family member was hospitalized. Gradually, it became evident that this change in working style caused a remarkable shift in the position of both the family and the patient. Families were no longer objects for staff-planned treatment; instead, they became active participants in joint processes. In many impasse situations, the team noticed that the only way forward was to change the team's own activity in the actual situation (Seikkula et al., 1995). The team began to rethink the structural paradigm on the principle that it is the team's task to intervene, which in turn effects change in the family (see Boscolo & Bertrando, 1993; Selvini-Palazzoli, Boscolo, Cecchin, & Prata, 1978). In working this way, the team was able to integrate the experience of treating psychotic patients individually with the systemic approach. In this chapter the shift from a traditional systemic family therapy approach to the idea of Open Dialogue is described. The chapter will focus on aspects of the dialogue itself and will describe a way of organizing psychiatric treatment in a Nordic social and welfare system.

Opening doors for families to participate in analyzing the problem, preparing a treatment plan, and participating in treatment meetings throughout the entire treatment sequence were the first steps in seeing all problems as problems in the patient's actual social situation. In such situations, many other aspects and other parties in the patient's social network proved to be important. In family therapy based on the structural paradigm, the nuclear family is the basic unit for treatment, since symptoms are seen as functions of the family system, be it the nuclear family or the extended family (Kemenoff, Jachimczyk, & Fussner, 1999). In the new approach, it became natural to engage all the important participants in the patient's social network as a way of increasing coping resources and opening up new constructive perspectives. Treatment was no longer aimed at finding the reason for psychosis in the family system or in the past history of the individual. After recognizing the importance of language and dialogue as specific forms of being, interventions in family meetings were changed to focus on the actual dialogue instead of on changing the family system.

In building up a family- and network-centered psychiatric system, the next step was to realize the importance of holding the first treatment meetings as soon as possible after the crisis has occurred. This led to a rapid decrease in the need to hospitalize patients (Keränen, 1992; Seikkula, 1991, 1994). Implementing this policy made it necessary to organize a mobile crisis intervention team in each psychiatric outpatient clinic in the province. Currently, all staff members in psychiatric units can be called upon to participate in mobile teams according to patients' particular needs. Regardless of the specific diagnosis, if there is a crisis situation, the same procedure is followed in all cases. If there

is a question of possible hospital treatment, the crisis clinic in the hospital will arrange the first meeting, either before the decision to admit voluntarily or, for involuntary patients, during the first day after admission. At this meeting a tailor-made team, consisting of both outpatient and inpatient staff, is constituted. The team usually consists of two or three staff members (e.g., a psychiatrist from the crisis clinic, a psychologist from the mental health outpatient clinic for the area where the patient is living, and a nurse from the ward). The team takes charge of the entire treatment sequence, regardless of whether the patient is at home or in the hospital, and irrespective of how long the treatment period is expected to last.

Current research shows that the OD approach, with its emphasis on facilitating dialogue within the treatment system, can be effective. Since the establishment of this new approach, the incidence of new cases of schizophrenia in this small and homogeneous region has declined (Aaltonen et al., 1997). Further, the appearance of new chronic schizophrenia patients at the psychiatric hospital has ceased (Tuori, 1994). In an ongoing study of first-episode psychotic patients, the need for hospitalization decreased, and it proved possible in many cases to replace neuroleptic medication with anxiolytics at the outset. Consequently, only 27% received neuroleptic medication during the 2-year follow-up period (Seikkula, Alakare, & Aaltonen, 2000, 2001b). This did not lead to poorer outcomes, given that 83% of the patients had returned to their jobs or studies or were looking for jobs 2 years later, and 77% did not have residual psychotic symptoms. A possible reason for these relatively good prognoses was the fact that the duration of untreated psychosis declined to 3.6 months in western Lapland, where the network-centered system enabled easy access to psychiatric care and an immediate start of treatment (Seikkula et al., 2001b).

Psychosis in Treatment Meeting

In the initial treatment meeting all the important members of the patient's social network, together with the patient, gather to discuss all issues associated with the reported presenting problem. All management plans and decisions are made with everyone present. The dialogic task is to construct a new language to describe the difficult experiences of the patient and those nearest him or her—experiences that do not yet have words. In analyzing this approach, Gergen and McNamee (2000) noted that it could be seen as transformative dialogue rather than disordering discourse. Although OD is not a diagnosis-specific approach for psychotic problems, treatment of psychotic crises best illustrates the central elements of the approach. In organizing open meetings, our professional understanding of the nature of psychosis began to change. Psychosis can be seen as one way to deal with terrifying experiences that cannot be expressed other than through the language of hallucinations and delusions. For example, most of the female psychotic patients who present themselves for treatment have experienced physical or sexual abuse either as children or as adults (Goodman, Rosenberg, Mueser, & Drake, 1997). In clinical situations, these traumatic experiences are often present in the hallucinations or delusions about which patients speak (Karon, 1999).

Case Study: Breaking Windows

A female patient had been hospitalized for more than 2 weeks, and a treatment meeting was organized to prepare for her discharge. In this meeting, her husband, her son, the doctor, the ward team, and a two-person team from the psychiatric outpatient clinic participated. The patient was asked to describe what happened when she was admitted to the hospital. She answered by describing how one afternoon she was at home with her son, who had suddenly asked if there was someone in the garden. She was frightened, believing someone was there, although she could not see anyone. She was convinced it was the man with whom she had lived for a 2-year period, 16 years previously. The following day, when her husband returned home from work and drove into the yard, she started to fear that he was under the influence of drugs and was going to kill her. She locked all the doors so her husband could not come in. Her husband grew irritated and started to yell on the front steps. She became terrified and, in the end, broke two large living room windows by throwing chairs through them. After this attack she was hospitalized.

The team expressed interest in her former husband and asked her to tell them about their relationship. She said that it was difficult for her to speak of it, having never done so before. The man, she said, was a narcotics addict and always, when he was under the influence, assaulted her and beat her heavily. She used to stay home long enough for her bruises to disappear so no one would know she was a victim of her husband's violence. After 2 years she managed to divorce him. They had not met since. She told the team that one night 5 years ago, while she was alone at home, the telephone rang, and she answered to find that her ex-husband was calling to ask how her life was. She became terrified while on the phone, trembling, and ran out of words. After the conversation, she remained terrified for a long time and had her first psychotic breakdown 2 months later.

Since this was now the first time she had been able to verbally express these terrifying memories, the team began to ask about concrete descriptions of how the attacks had happened, whether her husband had hit her with his fist or with an open hand. The intent was to encourage her to develop and use plenty of words to construct a story of the traumatic memory. In a stress situation, difficult and terrifying experiences in one's life may be actualized and can be relived (Penn, 1998; van der Kolk & Fisher, 1995). When encouraged to do so, people can begin to search for a way to express re-actualized experiences in the form of metaphors. In the case described, where the patient had a delusion that her husband was under the influence of drugs and was coming to kill her, the fear was not realistic at the moment but had actually happened in a previous relationship.

Dialogue Becomes the Aim of Therapy

The forum for Open Dialogue is the treatment meeting. The participants include all the authorities from different agencies who are involved in treating the specific problem, and as many people as possible who are important in the patient's social network, for example, family members, relatives, fellow employees, neighbors. This means also that different therapists are present in the same meeting. The patient's individual psychotherapist, for instance, is often invited to the meeting, to increase the likelihood that a real integration of approaches can be agreed upon. According to Alanen (1997), OD meetings have three functions: (1) to gather information about the problem, (2) to construct a treatment plan and make all needed decisions based on the diagnosis developed during the OD conversation, and (3) to generate a psychotherapeutic dialogue. Overall, the intent is to strengthen the patient's adult coping capacities and to normalize the situation rather than focus on regressive behavior (Alanen, Lehtinen, Räkköläinen, & Aaltonen, 1991).

The starting point for treatment is the family's language: How has each individual, in his or her own language, observed and named the patient's problem? The treatment team adapts its own language to each case according to need. Problems are seen as social constructs, reformulated in every conversation (Bakhtin, 1984; Gergen, 1994, 1999; Shotter, 1993a, 1993b, 1998). Each person present speaks in his or her own voice, and, as Anderson (1997) has noted, listening becomes more important than the manner of interviewing. The therapeutic conversation resembles that described by Anderson and Goolishian (1988; Anderson, 1997), Penn (1998; Penn & Frankfurt, 1994), and Andersen (1995; see also Friedman, 1995).

The meeting takes place in an open forum, too. All participants sit in the same room, in a circle. The team members who have taken the initiative for calling the meeting take charge of conducting the dialogue. On some occasions there is no prior planning regarding who will take charge of the questioning; on other occasions, the entire team decides in advance who will conduct the interview. The first questions are as open-ended as possible, to guarantee that family members and the rest of the social network can begin to speak about the issues that are most relevant at the moment. The team does not plan the themes of the meeting in advance. From the very beginning the task of the interviewers is to adapt their answers to whatever the clients say. Most often, the team's answer takes the form of a further question, which means that subsequent questions from team members are based on, and have to take into account, what the client and family members have said.

Everyone present has the right to comment whenever he or she is willing to do so. Comments should not interrupt an ongoing dialogue, and the speaker should adapt his or her words to the ongoing theme of discussion. For the professionals present this means they can comment either by inquiring further about the theme under discussion or by commenting reflectively to the other professionals about what they have started to think in response to what is said. Most often, in those comments, new words are introduced to describe the client's most difficult experiences. Frequently, the professional staff has obligations they must handle. It is advisable to focus on these issues toward the end of the meeting, after family members have spoken about what are the most compelling issues for them. After deciding that the important issues for the meeting have been addressed, the team member in charge suggests that the meeting may be adjourned. It is important, however, to close the meeting by referring to the client's own words, by asking, for instance, "I wonder if we could begin to close the meeting. Before doing so, however, is there anything else we should discuss before we end?" At the end of the meeting it is beneficial to briefly summarize its themes, especially whether or not decisions have been made, and if so, what they were. The length of meetings can vary, but usually 1.5 hours is adequate. Of course, if a large number of network members are present, more time should be taken, perhaps with a coffee break.

Psychotic problems provide an example of the most difficult crisis handled in treatment meetings. The OD process attempts to make sense of the client's experience and find ways of coping with experiences that are so stressful the client has not been able to construct a rational spoken narrative about them. In subsequent stressful situations, these experiences may be actualized and a way found to utter them metaphorically (Karon, 1999; Penn, 1998; van der Kolk & Fisher, 1995). This is the prenarrative quality of psychotic experience (Holma & Aaltonen, 1997; Ricoeur, 1992). Encouraging and facilitating Open Dialogue, without any preplanned themes or forms, seems to enable clients to construct a new language through which they can express difficult events in their lives. The events may be of any kind and may have happened at any time. Many different types of content can open up paths for new narratives.

Whatever their background, it is important to take hallucinations seriously and not challenge the patient's reality during the crisis situation, especially in the initial phase of treatment. Instead, the therapists can ask, "I do not understand how you can control other people's thoughts. I have not found that I can do that. Could you tell me more about it?" The other network members in the meetings can then be asked, "What do you think of this?

How do you understand what the client is saying?" The purpose is to allow different voices to be heard concerning the themes under discussion, including psychotic experiences. If the team manages to generate a deliberative atmosphere allowing different, even contradictory, voices to be heard, it is possible to construct narratives of restitution or reparation (Stern, Doolan, Stables, Szmukler, & Eisler, 1999). As Trimble (2000) puts it, when comparing the dialogical approach to the ideas of network therapy, "Restoration of trust in soothing interpersonal emotional regulation makes it possible to allow others to affect us in dialogical relationships" (p. 15). This may be one aspect of the process in which a patient and his or her social network can begin to acquire new words to describe and think about their problems.

Patients often start to tell psychotic (delusional, hallucinatory) stories at some specific point during the meeting when very sensitive and essential themes related to the onset or etiology of the psychosis are revealed. Team members can act on this observation. When something related to the client's not-yet-spoken experiences is touched upon, they can carefully scrutinize this segment of the dialogue. A team member may ask, for instance, "What did I say wrong, when you started to speak about that?" or "Wait a moment, what were we discussing when 'M' started to speak about how the voices have control over him?" Psychotic speech thus becomes one voice among the other voices present in the OD conversation. The "reasons" for psychotic behavior can be discerned at those crucial moments.

In general, the team's role during the meeting is (1) to allow the patient's social network to take the lead, and (2) to respond to each utterance in a dialogical way that promotes new understanding between the different participants (Bakhtin, 1984; Voloshinov, 1996). Dialogue becomes both the aim and the specific way of being in language in the therapy. Instead of primarily focusing on and aiming at changing the patient (e.g., rapidly removing the psychotic symptoms), or changing the family's interactional style, the main therapeutic effort takes place in the space between the team members and (1) the family or (2) those members of the client's social network who are present. Building up a dialogical rather than a monological dialogue means thinking carefully about how to respond to the patient's and the family's utterances. It means being

present in the actual conversation. In contrast, systemic family therapy can be seen as consisting of rather a lot of monological utterances in which team members use tactics, such as circular questioning, to initiate change in the family system. Systemic family therapy does not require answers for everything clients or family members say because the primary treatment goals (modifying family structures) are not necessarily based on themes actively under discussion.

Creating New Language for the "Not Yet Spoken"

In Open Dialogue, the "tactic" is to build up dialogical discourse. In dialogue, new understanding starts to emerge as a social, shared phenomenon. The individuals present at meetings speak about their most difficult experiences. In terms of psychotic speech, people speak about things that do not yet have any other words than those of hallucinations or delusions. Once the client's psychotic reality is shared, new resources become available. What first takes place in dialogue in the social domain may thereafter be converted into an inner dialogue. Vygotsky (1970) speaks of the zone of proximal development in the child. This means the space between adult and child, wherein the adult's more developed functioning provides scaffolding for the child to reach beyond the current limits of his or her abilities. This idea can be used to describe the psychotherapeutic situation as well (Leiman & Stiles, 2001). In a social situation, with members of the patient's most relevant social network present, the patient can "be in the dialogue" without using psychotic symptomatology. This may be one explanation of why psychotic patients frequently participate in OD during the first meetings without expressing psychotic content (Alanen, 1997). We hypothesize that such conversations are possible because team members, not having been involved in the strong emotions aroused by the crisis, can tolerate the patient's uncertainty, listen carefully to the words uttered, and, through their questions, respond in ways that facilitate the dialogue (Seikkula, 2002).

One way the team members can respond is to initiate reflective conversation (Andersen, 1995) among themselves. Without forming any specific reflective team, they move flexibly from constructing questions and comments, to having reflective discussions with each other. Sometimes this presupposes that the team will ask for permission: "I wonder if you could wait a moment so we can discuss what we have started to think about. I would prefer it if you could sit quietly and either listen, if you want, or not if you don't want. Afterwards we will ask for your comments about what we have said." Usually the family and the rest of the social network listen very carefully to what the team members say about their problems. Reflective discussions have a specific task because treatment plans are developed during the conversations. All is "transparent." Decisions about hospitalization, the rationale for medication, and planning for individual psychotherapy are examples of issues that may be addressed during reflective discussions. Overall, the purpose is to open up a range of alternatives from which choices and decisions are made. For instance, in deciding to initiate compulsory treatment, it seems important to openly state and discuss different opinions, even disagreements, among team members in regard to making that decision.

OD in Comparison to Systemic and Psychoeducational Approaches

Some ideas pertaining to systemic family therapy (Selvini-Palazzoli et al., 1978) are used in OD, but there are differences, too. Open Dialogue does not focus on the family system or even on communication patterns within the family system (Boscolo & Bertrando, 1993). The aim of OD is not "to give an impulse to change the fixed logic of the system by introducing a new logic" (Boscolo & Bertrando, 1993, p. 217) but to create a joint space for a new language, in which things can start to have different meanings (Anderson & Goolishian 1988; Anderson, 1997). In comparison to narrative therapies, both OD and narrative therapies share the social constructionist view of reality (Gergen, 1994; Shotter, 1993a, 1993b). They differ, however, in how they see the author of the narrative. Whereas the narrative therapist aims at reauthoring the problem-saturated story, in dialogic approaches the aim is to move from monologues, which are stuck, to more deliberative dialogues (Smith, 1997). Whereas, in narrative therapy, each narrative has an author, in dialogical therapies a new narrative is

cocreated in the shared domain of the participants. Gergen and McNamee (2000) have termed OD "a transformative dialogue."

Open Dialogue and psychoeducational programs (Anderson, Hogarty, & Reiss, 1980; Falloon, 1996; Falloon, Boyd, & McGill, 1984; Goldstein, 1996; McGorry, Edwards, Mihalopoulos, Harrigan, & Jackson, 1996) share the view that the family is an active agent in cocreating new narratives. The family is seen neither as the cause of the psychosis nor as an object of treatment but as "competent or potentially competent partners in the recovery process" (Gleeson, Jackson, Stavely, & Burnett, 1999, p. 390). The differences between structural and narrative approaches lie in the theoretical assumptions about the etiology of psychosis. In addition to these differences, OD emphasizes meeting during the height of the crisis, and the process involves jointly developing treatment plans.

Case Illustration

The following case is presented by way of illustrating the treatment process in OD. Treatment usually starts with the team being given a small amount of information about the case. In the present case, Seppo's father called the local mental health outpatient clinic on a Monday morning to ask for help for his son, who had started to speak of an extreme terror that a gang was going to force its way into his apartment. The nurse who answered the phone thought Seppo might be having psychotic problems and suggested a meeting straightaway, on the afternoon of the same day. Because Seppo's father did not want to have a home visit, the first meeting was organized at the local psychiatric outpatient clinic. The nurse contacted the psychiatrist of the clinic and the crisis clinic of the psychiatric hospital. Thus, a three-person team participated in the treatment. Surprisingly, Seppo's parents did not turn up at the first meeting. The following sequence consists of the very first comments made at the meeting; "S" stands for Seppo; "N1" and "N2" for the nurses.

N1: Where should we start?

S: The whole . . . I can't really remember anything.

N2: Has it been that you don't really remember anything for a long time?

S: Well . . . I don't know if it has been that way since midsummer. I do remember if I've been in contact with someone and all the things that have happened. But then I find I've left my own place and don't know if I was even there. Suddenly, I come into being and find myself wherever it is and so . . .

N2: Whom are you living with?

S: I'd been living by myself, but now I've gone to my parents.

N1: Whose idea was it that you came here?

S: Well . . . my mother's.

N2: And what was your mother worried about?

S: I don't know if I've spoken about it with her. I really can't remember anything. I have a feeling that I may even have hit someone, but I just can't remember.

N2: Has anyone said this to you?

S: No . . . I am paranoid and so I think something has happened.

N2: What about Father; is he worried about any particular matter?

S: I don't know, but yesterday evening when we were watching TV he went to bed and in the morning he had gone to work.

N2: And what was it like then?

S: I was afraid, I was quarrelling with that guy. They have a key to my place and they . . . they were asshole fucking in July and did all these kinds of things.

N2: In July?

The discussion began with Seppo's comment, and the team members continued it by adapting their questions to what was said previously. The team strove to capture Seppo's experience in his own terms. Seppo's story became more and more violent; simultaneously, the structure of his sentences dissolved, a sign of his overwhelming fear and confusion. In the beginning the team asked very concrete questions about his life, and the story was coherent and comprehensible. Initially, dialogue was possible, but that radically changed after he remembered his father being absent that morning. The story became more and more threatening and psychotic, and the team's confusion grew in the course of the discussion. One way out might have been for the team to use internal reflective discussion, but the team did not attempt to intervene in that way.

At the end of the first meeting it was agreed that the next meeting would take place the following day at Seppo's parents' home. In that meeting his parents and sister were present. The discussion was continued fluently as if it were a continuation of the first interview. Family members spoke in a nonpersonal way, which was quite difficult to follow. They sounded as if they were presenting a report without any personal emotions, although they reported their idea that Seppo had probably been assaulted. The team did not view these as symptoms but remained curious about the assaults.

The treatment process continued with very closely spaced meetings. Initially, Seppo calmed down to the extent that he stopped speaking about his fears, but at the same time he also stopped going out, gradually keeping apart from his friends. Family problems rapidly began to emerge. The father had left the family, as they stated, "for Seppo's sake." Gradually the family began to talk obliquely about the father's drinking problem, which did not, however, come into the open so discussion about it would be possible. After 6 months of treatment the process was bogged down so that referring Seppo to the hospital was seen as the only alternative. After a 1-week period in hospital, a treatment meeting was organized with the family, the treatment team, and the ward team present. At the end of the meeting the team initiated a discussion about the difficult situation regarding both the family and the treatment.

N2: What do you, Lisa [the mother], think about this?

M(other): Well . . . (Seppo stands up).

F(ather): You're the one who has quite a lot to say in this matter, who is living here . . . (gives a deep sigh).

M: It's like everyday life, I think he will manage by himself there [at home], but he hasn't made any progress (laughing).

Psych1: Matti [the father] has quite clearly presented his own thoughts, but Seppo's mother's opinion is still rather unclear (turns to the ward psychologist; Seppo sits down).

N1: Her opinion is that no progress has been made.

Psych2: Lisa has said Seppo could come home, but no progress has been made.

M: Will there ever be any progress where nothing else can happen?

S: If now I am in a state that no more progress can happen.

M: Yeah . . .

Psych2: Paavo [the team's psychologist], do you think that Matti clearly expressed his point of view?

Psych1: Well, Matti clearly said that the situation can't continue where Seppo only stays in bed, since this makes Lisa angry.

Psych2: But, on the other hand, Matti is asking why don't we take Seppo home. He says it both ways, yes and no and, I think, Seppo's mother also says yes and no.

Psych1: But, I think, Matti is looking for some solution that could happen if Seppo goes back home. Matti would like to guarantee Seppo's mother some rest. Seppo could be in his own place, as well.

N2: It might be good for Lisa's rest, but would it be good for Seppo?

After a long meeting it was agreed to meet again the next day. The discussion was now dialogical, with joint understanding being constructed together. When someone said something, he or she formulated the utterance so a response to it was necessary. Without this, the dialogue could not proceed. However, the interaction within the family was so difficult that even within this dialogue permanent solutions to the problem could not be found. It was not possible to bring the conflicts into the open through discussion. The only alternative had been for the father to leave home.

Seppo went home but very soon returned to the hospital because his fears had become even more intense. For instance, he described how NATO's agents were haunting him and how two nuclear warheads were aimed at the hospital from northern Norway, and most of the people outside the hospital had been killed. The discussions on the ward did not calm him but, instead, stimulated him even more, so that one day he assaulted a doctor. He said that this doctor was a Russian agent who wanted to kill him. Actually, this doctor had participated in the first treatment meeting but not subsequently.

During the 2.4-month period that Seppo stayed in the hospital he began to calm down a little, but he still spoke a lot about his fears. Neuroleptic medication was started, but this did not have any rapid effect on his fears. He continued talking about powerful external threats. The family discussions were continued, and as his father began to talk about his drinking problem, he became very de-

pressed and began to talk about suicide. He was hospitalized for a couple of nights. After this episode the family's situation began to improve so that the parents decided to buy a larger residence in order to move back together and to have Seppo with them. After this, Seppo was discharged from the hospital, and during this phase the first noticeable improvement toward a more secure reality occurred. He rapidly began to calm down and to visit his friends.

Two years after the outset of treatment, Seppo was living at home with his family without expressing any obvious psychotic ideas. Family meetings continued on a monthly basis. He participated in individual psychotherapy for a year but then wanted to discontinue. The 5-year follow-up interview indicated that Seppo had not had any psychotic symptoms for the previous 3 years, and that his treatment had continued in the form of psychological and vocational rehabilitation. He had taken a couple of vocational rehabilitation courses organized by the state employment agency. The treatment meetings were organized to support Seppo and his family in building their new life.

Several of the main treatment principles of OD can be illustrated by this example. Treatment was started immediately, with the first meeting called within 6 hours after the initial contact made by the mother. The nurse who was contacted took responsibility for organizing the first meeting, and those who participated were the main team members for the entire course of the treatment. This was one factor in providing psychological continuity. A second factor was that the team working with the family in its home participated actively in ward meetings, as well. One problem in maintaining responsibility and psychological continuity in this case was that the doctor who participated in the very first meeting was not present at subsequent meetings. This was not discussed in meetings and may have raised questions in Seppo's mind, since he attacked that doctor.

The treatment plans were adapted to the specific and varying needs of the family. In the crisis phase, daily meetings were organized at their home; hospitalization was decided upon when needed; neuroleptic medication was prescribed after Seppo's initial temporary progress gave way to relapse; individual psychotherapy was recommended and provided; and during the final phase of treatment, rehabilitation services were offered.

Throughout treatment, the team tolerated uncertainty. This was seen in the content of the dialogue, where efforts were made to understand the problems of the whole family in the context of their lives as they were living them, instead of in "disordering discourse." It was also seen in the team's response to the difficult situation during the first 6 months of treatment, when Seppo's condition improved, but the conflict between mother and father became increasingly evident.

The main problems during treatment were, perhaps, in not fully including the social network perspective. With hindsight it can be argued that there should have been meetings with the network, especially those with whom Seppo had encountered violent problems. During the treatment process it became evident that he did, in fact, have serious problems with the gang he belonged to, which led to a court summons to answer charges in connection with drug abuse and theft. The problems experienced in generating dialogue were probably related to the conflicts within the family, especially between the mother and father, which led to their separation for a 2-year period. The team, although it tolerated considerable uncertainty, did not manage to initiate deliberating dialogue before Seppo and his father were hospitalized. Reflective, open discussion only became possible after half a year's treatment. It proved important to take into account all the family issues, not only Seppo's problems.

Sharing Emotions Generates Dialogue

A crisis can be seen as a monological impasse, in which both the individual and the family are understandably fearful of the inherent confusion and seek solutions for themselves. The family—but the patient as well—are all searching for monological answers to their suffering. "What to do?" and "What is wrong with our son?" are questions that represent the legitimate needs of our clients. But these questions can be answered in many ways. One possibility is to give monological answers. By doing so, however, there is increased risk of interrupting the process, which begins to create new meanings for the family. By giving such monological answers as, "We are going to hospitalize your son, and medication is needed because it is a question of schizo-

phrenia," therapists can think of themselves as easing the crisis, but what they are actually doing is making the client more dependent on a treatment system that presumably has knowledge the family does not.

The dialogical approach aims at a different process in which the potential resources of the patient and those nearest to him or her start to play a central role in determining how to proceed. As Anderson (2002) points out, referring to Harry Goolishian, the monological language of the psychotic patient forms a trap. The patient's comments are often responded to with silence or neglect, which increases the risk of isolation and of difficulties that arise from not understanding what he or she is trying to say. The aim of treatment should be to reduce the patient's isolation in any way possible. This is done by focusing on the dialogue itself. The task is to create a language in which all voices can be heard, both the patient's and those nearest the patient, at the same time. In a severe crisis this is not an easy task for the team. It is not only the team that has the power to become the agent in the dialogue; the team's agency is always applied in the presence of the family. Perhaps the (only) thing team members should focus on in the very first meetings in psychotic and other crises is working toward creating a dialogical exchange of utterances: how to listen, how to hear, what is most important, how to answer each utterance of the clients. Answering comes first. After answering what the clients say, the team can learn, but only if they hear and understand correctly.

The aim of listening attentively is to hear what clients are saying. What is heard is witnessed in answering with words the clients can listen to. The team does not plan its next questions in advance, or even the interview as a whole, but instead creates subsequent questions based on what clients say. In this process, everyone, even the patient with psychotic ideas, can experience how to become an agent in creating the new story of their suffering.

To facilitate this aim, some guidelines are helpful. In most severe crises—not only psychotic crises—it is important always to work as a team. The optimal number of team members is three. If only two are present, they can be trapped in the family's monological need, but if a third is present, one member is always listening, attentive to the inner dialogue in ways that create a different perspective on the problem. The second recommendation is, in every case, to include those nearest the patient in the first meeting. This guarantees opportunities to begin constructing a joint language. Accordingly, when the patient speaks about "not understandable" experiences, the people to whose lives he or she is referring are present to participate in this multivocal reality (Seikkula, Alakare, & Aaltonen, 2001a, 2001b).

In the early phase of developing OD some foundations of network therapy became relevant. They were helpful to team members in emphasizing the importance of focusing on the patient's contemporary social context rather than on "reasons" in the individual's or the family's past. What the team learned, as well, was the value of accepting strong emotions—a policy that has continued in treatment meetings. Although the team does not aim at the "depression phase," as is done in the spiral process of network meetings (Speck & Attneave, 1973; Trimble, 2002), the dialogue in OD meetings frequently becomes very emotional. This does not necessarily mean expressing dramatic emotion during a meeting but letting, for instance, the sadness have space in the room.

When I started my career as a systemic family therapist, this was rather confusing. At that time, I thought the idea of "neutrality" meant being neutral without becoming emotionally involved in the issue being discussed. Now I realize that in practicing Open Dialogue the themes of dialogue often move me as a therapist. Dialogue is embodied in the intensely emotional experiences of everyone who sits in a meeting and listens to their clients' suffering. Actually, therapists cannot be involved in a dialogue without emotionally sharing the very same emotions their clients express. In constructing a dialogue, therapists create a new reality among everyone who participates in the meeting. In new, shared relationships that reflect everyone's emotional experiences, new and helpful narratives can be created.

Conclusion

Dialogue is a powerful "intervention" in and of itself, especially when helpers understand and accept the shared emotional experience created between participants. It becomes both a prerequisite and a forum for handling experiences. Dialogue can be generated in many ways, for example, in a series of treatment meetings, in art therapy, or in individual psychotherapy. In serious crises, even though Open Dialogue involves a great deal of work, it also makes the task simpler.

References

Aaltonen, J., Seikkula, J., Alakare, B., Haarakangas, K., Keränen, J., & Sutela, M. (1997, October). Western Lapland project: A comprehensive family- and network-centered community psychiatric project. *ISPS, Abstracts and Lectures 12–16*, 124.

Alanen, Y. O. (1997). *Schizophrenia: Its origins and need-adapted-treatment*. London: Karnac Books.

Alanen, Y. O, Lehtinen, K., Räkköläinen, V., & Aaltonen, J. (1991). Need-adapted treatment of new schizophrenic patients: Experiences and results of the Turku Project. *Acta Psychiatrica Scandinavica, 83*, 363–372.

Andersen, T. (1995). Reflecting processes. Acts of informing and forming. In S. Friedman (Ed.), *The reflective team in action* (pp. 11–37). New York: Guilford.

Anderson, C., Hogarty, G., & Reiss, D. (1980). Family treatment of adult schizophrenic patients: A psycho-educational approach. *Schizophrenia Bulletin, 6*, 490–505.

Anderson, H. (1997). *Conversation, language, and possibilities*. New York: Basic Books.

Anderson, H. (2002). In the space between people: Seikkula's Open Dialogue approach. *Journal of Marital and Family Therapy, 28*, 275–279.

Anderson, H., & Goolishian, H. (1988). Human systems as linguistic systems: Preliminary and evolving ideas about the implications for clinical theory. *Family Process, 27*, 371–393.

Bakhtin, M. (1984). *Problems of Dostoyevski's poetics*. Manchester, UK: Manchester University Press.

Boscolo, L., & Bertrando, P. (1993). *Times of time*. New York: Norton.

Falloon, I. (1996). Early detection and intervention for initial episodes of schizophrenia. *Schizophrenia Bulletin, 22*, 271–283.

Falloon, I., Boyd, J., & McGill, C. (1984). *Family care of schizophrenia*. New York: Guilford.

Friedman, S. (Ed.). (1995). *The reflecting team in action*. New York: Guilford.

Gergen, K. (1994). *Realities and relationships: Soundings in social construction*. Cambridge, MA: Harvard University Press.Gergen, K. (1999). *An invitation to social construction*. London: Sage.

Gergen, K., & McNamee, S. (2000). From disordering discourse to transformative dialogue. In R. Neimeyer & J. Raskin (Eds.), *Constructions of disorders* (pp. 333–349). Washington, DC: American Psychological Association.

Gleeson, J., Jackson, H., Stavely, H., & Burnett, P. (1999). Family intervention in early psychosis. In P. McGorry & H. Jackson (Eds.), *The recognition and management of early psychosis* (pp. 380–415). Cambridge: Cambridge University Press.

Goldstein, M. (1996). Psycho-education and family treatment related to the phase of a psychotic disorder. *Clinical Psychopharmacology, 11*(Suppl. 18), 77–83.

Goodman, L., Rosenberg, S., Mueser, K., & Drake, R. (1997). Physical and sexual assault history in women with serious mental illness: Prevalence, correlates, treatment, and future research directions. *Schizophrenia Bulletin, 23*, 685–696.

Holma, J., & Aaltonen, J. (1997). The sense of agency and the search for a narrative in acute psychosis. *Contemporary Family Therapy, 19*, 463–477.

Karon, B. (1999). The tragedy of schizophrenia. *General Psychologist, 32*, 3–14.

Kemenoff, S., Jachimczyk, J., & Fussner, A. (1999). Structural family therapy. In D. Lawson & F. Prevatt (Eds.), *Casebook in family therapy* (pp. 111–145). Toronto: Brooks/Cole Wadsworth.

Keränen, J. (1992). The choice between outpatient and inpatient treatment in a family-centred psychiatric treatment system. English summary. *Jyväskylä Studies in Education, Psychology and Social Research.*

Leiman, M., & Stiles, W. (2001). Dialogical sequence analysis and the zone of proximal development and conceptual enhancements to the assimilation model: The case of Jan revisited. *Psychotherapy Research, 11*, 311–330.

McGorry, P., Edwards, J., Mihalopoulos, C., Harrigan, S., & Jackson, H. (1996). EPPIC: An evolving system of early detection and optimal management. *Schizophrenia Bulletin, 22*, 305–325.

Penn, P. (1998). Rape flashbacks: Constructing a new narrative. *Family Process, 37*, 299–310.

Penn, P., & Frankfurt, M. (1994). Creating a participant text: Writing, multiple voices, narrative multiplicity. *Family Process, 33*, 217–231.

Ricoeur, P. (1992). *Oneself as another.* Chicago: University of Chicago Press.

Seikkula, J. (1991). Family-hospital boundary system in the social network. English summary. *Jyväskylä Studies in Education, Psychology and Social Research.*

Seikkula, J. (1994). When the boundary opens: Family and hospital in co-evolution. *Journal of Family Therapy, 16*, 401–414.

Seikkula, J. (2002). Open dialogues with good and poor outcomes for psychotic crises: Examples from families with violence. *Journal of Marital and Family Therapy, 28*, 263–274.

Seikkula, J., Aaltonen, J., Alakare, B., Haarakangas, K., Keränen, J., & Sutela, M. (1995). Treating psychosis by means of open dialogue. In S. Friedman (Ed.), *The reflective team in action* (pp. 62–80). New York: Guilford.

Seikkula, J., Alakare, B., & Aaltonen, J. (1999). Potilaat sosiaalisissa verkostoissaan: Kahden vuoden seurantatutkimus akuutin psykoosin kotihoidosta. In K. Haarakangas & J. Seikkula (Eds.), *Psykoosiuuteen hoitokäytäntöön* (pp. 107–122). Helsinki: Kirjayhtymä.

Seikkula, J., Alakare, B., & Aaltonen, J. (2000). A two-year follow-up on open dialogue treatment in first-episode psychosis: Need for hospitalization and neuroleptic medication decreases. [Published in Russian, English manuscript from the authors.] *Social and Clinical Psychiatry, 10*, 20–29.

Seikkula, J., Alakare, B., & Aaltonen, J. (2001a). Open dialogue in psychosis I: An introduction and case illustration. *Journal of Constructivist Psychology, 14*, 247–265.

Seikkula, J., Alakare, B., & Aaltonen, J. (2001b). Open dialogue in first-episode psychosis II: A comparison of good and poor outcome cases. *Journal of Constructivist Psychology, 14*, 267–284.

Selvini-Palazzoli, M., Boscolo, L., Cecchin, C., & Prata, G. (1978). *Paradox and counterparadox.* New York: Jason Aronson.

Shotter, J. (1993a). *Conversational realities: Constructing life through language.* London: Sage.

Shotter, J. (1993b). *Cultural politics of everyday life.* Buckingham, UK: Open University Press.Shotter, J. (1998). Life inside the dialogically structured mind: Bakhtin's and Voloshinov's account of mind as out in the world between us. In J. Rowan & M. Cooper (Eds.), *The plural self: Multiplicity in everyday life* (pp. 71–92). London: Sage.

Smith, C. (1997). Introduction: Comparing traditional therapies with narrative approaches. In C. Smith & D. Nylund (Eds.), *Narrative therapies with children and adolescents* (pp. 1–52). New York: Guilford.

Speck, R., & Attneave, C. (1973). *Family Networks.* New York: Pantheon.

Stern, S., Doolan, M., Stables, E., Szmukler, G. L., & Eisler, I. (1999). Disruption and reconstruction: Narrative insights into the experience of family members caring for a relative diagnosed with serious mental illness. *Family Process, 38*, 353–369.

Trimble, D. (2000). Emotion and voice in network therapy. *Netletter, 7*(1), 11–16.

Trimble, D. (2002). Listening with integrity: The dialogical stance of Jaakko Seikkula. *Journal of Marital and Family Therapy, 28,* 220–282.

Tuori, T. (1994). *Skitsofrenian hoito kannattaa. Raportti skitsofrenian, tutkimuksen, hoidon ja kuntoutuksen valtakunnallisen kehittämisohjelman 10-vuotisarvioinnista.* Helsinki: STAKES raportteja, 143.

van der Kolk, B., & Fisher, R. (1995). Dissociation and the fragmentary nature of traumatic memories: Overview and exploratory study. *Journal of Traumatic Stress, 8,* 505–525.

Voloshinov, V. (1996). *Marxism and the philosophy of language.* Cambridge, MA: Harvard University Press.

Vygotsky, L. (1970). *Thought and language.* Cambridge, MA: MIT Press.

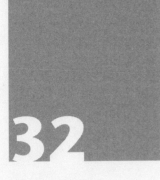

Ellen Pulleyblank-Coffey, James Griffith,

and Jusuf Ulaj

Gjakova
The First Community Mental Health Center in Kosova

This chapter describes the first community mental health center opened in Gjakova, Kosovo[2] in 2001, following 10 years of conflict in the region from 1989 to 1999. The design and training for the services at the Gjakova Center for Mental Health grew out of an ongoing collaboration between U.S. and Kosovar mental health professionals known as the Kosovar Family Professional Education Collaboration (KFPEC).[1] Since 1999 the work of the KFPEC has supported the development of a family-focused community mental health system in Kosova, the center in Gjakova being the first of seven planned community mental health centers.

This chapter[3] does not address the theoretical assumptions underlying the wider project (see Weine, Agani, & Rolland, in preparation; Griffith & the Kosovar Family Professional Education Collaborative, 2002; Weine, Agani, & Rolland, 2001) or try to come to general conclusions about cross-cultural collaboration. Instead, it offers a richly textured description of the development of one mental health center by a cross-cultural mental health team.

In Kosova, the nurturing of children and the integrity of families and family relationships are core values. Family loyalty in Kosova takes priority over individual life choices that more often typify Western societies. Many Kosovars believe that this family loyalty has enabled their survival through centuries of oppression. Due to these values, according to Dr. Ferid Agani, cofounder of the KFPEC and the director of health services in Kosova, new mental health services, rather than focusing only on patients, are being designed to respond to families' needs and to engage families' strengths in the care of mentally ill, medically ill, and war-traumatized individuals. This chapter describes the development of such family-focused community services for the chronically mentally ill and their families in Gjakova. Hopefully, this multilayered description will provide a picture that points to the many aspects of culture and society that impinge on the development of mental health services in other contexts.

History of the Region

Kosova is a region approximately the size of Kentucky, with a population of 2 million people. Its status as an independent country or as a province of Serbia is still under debate. Currently it is a protectorate of the United Nations, and NATO troops maintain the peace between ethnic Albanians (Kosovars) and Serbs in the region. Before 1998, the Kosova population was approximately 90% ethnic Albanians (Kosovars) and 10% Serbian and other ethnic groups. It is now 95% ethnic Albanian and 5% ethnic Serbians and others. All the Kosovars whom we have met desperately want to become citizens of an independent nation, and in that direction they have recently elected their first president and congress. Serwer (2001) has summarized the current political situation:

> As much as the Kosovars want independence, the Serbs want Kosovo to remain part of Serbia. Only a new UN Security Council resolution can decide final status. A new Security Council resolution can pass only if the Chinese and Russians are prepared to allow it. They have their own reasons for not wanting Kosovo to gain independence—namely the potential repercussions in Tibet and in Chechnya. China and Russia will allow Kosovo's final status to be decided in the Security Council only if the Serbian government located in Belgrade insists that they do so and at this point they do not wish to do so.
>
> Regardless of the final status of Kosovo, it is essential for there to be good relations between the Serbs and the Kosovars. For an independent Kosovo, like it or not, Serbia is still Kosovo's most important neighbor, its largest potential market, its largest potential supplier, and its greatest security threat. Independent Kosovo will never be able to defend itself with its own means from a hostile Serbia. (p. 2)

This view may make a great deal of sense when seen from the West. From within Kosova, however, Kosovars and Serbs have a long way to go before they will be ready to forge such a collaborative relationship. By the uncertainty that it creates, this instability has enormous economic, political, and social consequences at a time when the country is trying to rebuild itself and acts as an obstacle to the development of all aspects of the country's infrastructure.

The recovery from the war is difficult due to the atrocities committed against Kosovar Albanians by Serbian police, military, and paramilitary forces. These atrocities represented a planned effort to drive ethnic Albanians from Kosova and to destroy their society and culture to such an extent that it could never be reconstituted in the future, and to

then repopulate the country with displaced Serbs from the Bosnian and Croatian wars. The first step was to impose apartheid upon the Kosovar Albanian population during the interval between the accession of Slobodan Milosevic in 1987 and the onset of the 1992 war in Bosnia (Griffith, Blyta, Ukshini, Kallaba, & Weine, 2001). The following list of events summarizes how isolation and undermining of the Kosovar Albanians was accomplished:

- The Serbian language was imposed upon Albanian society, with suppression of Albanian-language publications, changing of local place-names, and destruction of Albanian cultural institutions and seizure of Albanian cultural and historical artifacts.
- Arbitrary arrests, raids on private dwellings, and police violence were inflicted upon ethnic Albanians.
- Ethnic Albanian government workers, including school and university teachers, were dismissed from their jobs.
- Ethnic Albanian children were excluded from public schools.
- Ethnic Albanian doctors and other health workers were dismissed from employment, leading to deteriorating public health.
- Ethnic Albanian medical students and resident physicians-in-training were excluded from the medical educational systems, further depleting the health care system.

Sporadic violence by Serbian soldiers, paramilitary forces, and police escalated into a systematic and organized program of state terrorism. Methods were used that would decimate or physically displace families, terrorize and demoralize the family members, and impose concrete obstacles to any future reconstitution of Albanian Kosovar society. Malcolm (1998) listed the following practices as examples of the escalation of terror and attempted genocide:

- Murder of male family members: Traditional Kosovar society is patrilineal, with a well-defined hierarchy of authority and clearly specified roles according to gender and age. The head of the family is a male role. When both adult and child male family members are killed, the traditional organization and the transmission of culture was disrupted. The goal was to render the culture inoperable, in both present and future generations.

- Rape of women: Women hold an honored and protected position in Kosovar culture. Sexual assaults upon women humiliate both the women and the men who were unable to protect them. A mantle of shame overshadowed their families, and marital intimacy, the core to family life, was profoundly disrupted.
- Burning family homes and toppling their chimneys: The family home is the most important physical attachment for Kosovar families in the villages and countryside. Burning the family home and toppling its chimney instilled despair about the possibility of ever reconstituting family life and the family dwelling.
- Forced migration: Terrorizing families forced a panicked flight from rural homes and villages to cities in or outside the country. Property records and other documents of identity were seized and destroyed by government forces to prevent a return in the future.

As a result of these acts of oppression and violence, an estimated 850,000 Kosovars were physically displaced; approximately 250,000 families have suffered directly from violence and/or dislocation. During the war, 62% of the population had a near encounter with death, and an estimated 17% subsequently suffered symptoms of post-traumatic stress disorder (Cardoza, Vergara, Agani, & Gotway, 2000). After the war, as Kosova began to recover from the violence, the region had a total of 20 psychiatrists, 5 psychologists, and no formally trained social workers to deal with this level of distress. Many of these professionals suffered trauma and loss in their own families. It is in this context that a collaboration project for the development of professional education, between Kosovar and U.S. mental health professionals, the KFPEC, was formed (Griffith et al., 2001).

The Kosovar Family Professional Education Collaboration and Services Based Training

The KFPEC began in 1999 as a university-to-university collaboration between the Department of

Neuropsychiatry at the University of Prishtina; the Institute on Genocide, Psychiatry, and Witnessing at the University of Illinois at Chicago; the Chicago Center for Family Health at the University of Chicago; and the American Family Therapy Academy, a professional organization of family therapy teachers and researchers (Weine, Agani, & Rolland, in preparation). Initially, the KFPEC included 36 Kosovar mental health professionals (psychiatrists, psychiatric residents, a psychologist, social service workers, and nurses) and 15 U.S. family therapists (psychiatrists, psychologists, social workers, and psychiatric nurses), members of the American Family Therapy Academy.

One of the initial goals of the project was to design and implement a family-focused training program for Kosovar mental health professionals. The project sought to develop a model of treatment that would respond to the current needs of Kosovar families in a culturally attuned way. It also offered an opportunity for the development of a core professional mental health community that would share a common language and perspective on mental health. This initial phase took place over an 18-month period.

Although this early work of the project demonstrated that Kosovar clinicians could rapidly acquire skills needed for family-focused mental health treatment, this achievement would have little societal impact without the concomitant development of systems of community-based, outpatient mental health services. Moreover, among mental health leaders in Kosova, there was increasing specific concern about the chronically mentally ill, many of whom suffered from a lack of adequate hospital and outpatient services, and overburdened their families and meager community resources. The direction of the project thus shifted to integrate training of professionals and the development of community mental health services, with a primary focus on the chronically mentally ill.

In 2001, the KFPEC initiated this second phase of its project, named Services-Based Training (SBT) for Kosovar Community Mental Health and Prevention, in conjunction with the development of mental health centers in the region[4] (Weine & Agani, 2001; Weine, Agani, Griffith, Ukshiivi, Pulleyblank-Coffey, & Ulaj, in preparation).

Development of services for the chronically mentally ill and their families was planned first for two regional cities, Gjakova and Ferizaj. Community nursing teams were developed in each of these sites for family assessment, family psychoeducation, in-home crisis intervention, and medication monitoring. These teams were supervised by two psychiatric residents and a nurse from the University of Prishtina who had participated in the original KFPEC trainings. This Prishtina SBT, in turn, was supervised by the chief of psychiatry and the head family therapist at the Department of Neurology and Psychiatry at the University of Prishtina. U.S. participation consisted of regular two-person team visits that discussed planning and implementation with the Kosovar mental health leadership and consulted with the SBT teams in their teaching and supervision of the community mental health nursing teams.

Initially, 30 chronically mentally ill patients in Gjakova and Ferizaj were chosen to receive the new services. Some of these patients were living with their families, though often with frequent hospitalizations. Some patients, though living with their families, were isolated from them. In all cases, families of these patients were interested in finding ways to maintain patients at home with the support of the new outpatient mental health services. Currently, the SBT program is being expanded in these two cities to include more patients and their families and will be extended subsequently to five additional centers for mental health in other cities.

Gjakova: The First Community Mental Health Center

The Region of Gjakova

Gjakova is a major city in northwestern Kosova with a mostly homogeneous population of 60,000 Kosovar Albanians. Gjakovars are known within Kosova as a particularly proud, insular group, in which there is much pressure on young people to marry within the city's population. Because of their hometown allegiance, Gjakovars are particularly close-knit and often view outsiders with suspicion.

During the 1999 war, Gjakova experienced extreme damage to property and proportionally more deaths than in other regions. The city was chosen for the site of the first mental health center because of these devastating effects of the war and also due to the existence of a large population of mentally ill patients with few available services. At the same time, it happened that there was a local psychiatrist who was a community leader and had worked with many of the local chronically mentally ill and their families. He strongly advocated for the opening of this first community mental health center in Gjakova.

The Gjakova Center for Mental Health

In March 2001, the new Gjakova Center for Mental Health was built with funds donated by the Japanese government. Administered through the Kosovar Department of Mental Health in the Department of Health, it was designed to serve a catchment area of 300,000 people. In addition to this support from Japan, its nurses received training from Italian mental health teams in Trieste, Italy, and other nongovernmental organizations from numerous other countries. Our SBT project joined this group of supporters.

Referrals to the Center for Mental Health originate from hospital staff, local doctors, social service agencies, families, and self-referrals. Though the SBT project has focused on the chronically mentally ill, the center also provides services for people suffering from extreme distress and isolation due to family disruptions following the war, drug and alcohol problems, and acute episodes of mental illness. Two to three new chronically mentally ill patients per day are currently referred to the programs of the center. Many of these patients have had long-term hospitalizations or frequent intermittent hospitalizations.

In most households in Gjakova, multiple generations live together. When a woman marries, she moves into the household of her husband. Even if he dies, as many men did in the war, she is expected to continue to live in her husband's family household. Due to the deaths of many of the men, many families have had to reconfigure roles and responsibilities, as well as to establish new in-law relationships. In families where in addition to the effects of trauma and loss there is a mentally ill family member or, in some cases, members (some ill from before the war, some as a result of the war), the SBT project offers an opportunity to the family to rebuild its resources in order to maintain an ill family member at home receiving treatment in their homes and in the center's less restrictive environment. As family members learned new ways of coping with their disabled family member, they also increased their sense of competence as a family in other areas of their lives, such as refocusing their efforts to care for their children. Traditionally, the extended family had enough resources to care for itself. With the effects of war, many families could not care for themselves and have had to look outside the family for help. Reaching out beyond the extended family is not syntonic with Kosovar cultural values. As the Center for Mental Health developed its identity as a community resource for patients and their families, it offered a bridge to available help in the community. The homogeneity of the staff with the surrounding community strengthened the likelihood of the success of this bridge in Gjakova.

This new approach presented some difficulties for patients, families, and staff. Everyone in the treating system was used to, and comfortable with, depending on a hospital setting for treatment of the chronically mentally ill, especially in times of crisis. The staff at the center was apprehensive about how these patients would adjust to the center's less restrictive environment. Up until this time, the main model of treatment was a medical model in which the use of medication was emphasized. Since the SBT project focused on family psychoeducation along with medication, family interventions in the home and at the center, and socialization at the center, patients would now have more choices about their treatment. The results were far more successful than expected. Patients, families, and staff adjusted remarkably well to the new services. The greater freedom in the environment, as well as the additional services, led to a tighter collaboration between patients, families, and staff. Since family members were invited to participate with patients at the center, and the nursing teams visited them in their homes, the focus of treatment shifted from the individual to the individual in his or her family context. This shift led to families developing strategies that better supported patients in ways that helped them continue to live at home and to stay out of crisis.

Services, Staffing, and Training in Gjakova

The SBT project developed its services as part of the collaboration between Kosovar and U.S. professionals. The Kosovars defined the goals of programs that they wished to develop. In the case of the SBT project, their priority was to develop out-patient community mental health services for the chronically mentally ill and their families. The U.S. team proposed a general framework for services to meet these goals, and in response to the Kosovars' requests, U.S consultants taught such relevant topics as differential diagnosis, contracting with families, family interviewing techniques, network theory, psychoeducation, and wraparound models of community support (Clarke, 1992). These training sessions built upon the initial KFPEC family systems training, with an emphasis on resilience in families (Walsh, 1998). The Kosovars then adapted these materials to their circumstances and have begun to manualize their work. Gjakova, as the first center, became a pilot project. There is an initial evaluation in place that will measure how effective these services are after a 2-year trial period

The following is a summary of how the services are currently provided in Gjakova for chronically mentally ill patients and their families:

Family assessment: The SBT team from Prishtina initially selected 15 patients and their families to participate in the project. Each patient and his or her family had to meet the criteria (see criteria listed later in this chapter) for inclusion. Currently 10 more families are being added to the program.

Home visits: Once identified as meeting the criteria, patients and their families are visited at home every other week for 1 hour by a two-member nursing team from the local center. During these visits, the nurses give medication when prescribed, check to see that other medications are being taken appropriately, and discuss with the family their concerns about the patient and other aspects of their lives. These visits also provide opportunities for nurses to assess incipient crises and review with families some of the ideas presented in the psychoeducation workshops given at the center.

When a family member meets the criteria but is reluctant to join the program, the chief psychiatrist often visits them to encourage their participation. If a family is in crisis, the nursing team visits more frequently and for longer periods of time, until the crisis has passed.

Psychoeducation: At least one member of

each family attends a series of seven lectures about the nature of mental illness, held at the Community Mental Health Center. After the lectures there is a small-group discussion and question-and-answer period. During these sessions families share strategies for helping patients to maintain medication schedules, become more active in the family and in the community, and learn how to avert crises. Following this first set of lectures, multifamily problem-solving groups are formed and are ongoing.

Day Treatment: Patients are encouraged to come to the center as often as possible to participate in social and vocational activities that are offered daily.

Community Resource Network: The goal of this part of the program is to bring more resources from the community to each family and to build a network of community resources for referrals and services.

The center is staffed by two psychiatrists and a group of nurses, all of whom participate in the SBT project alongside other clinical programs for less acute outpatient services. The center has been organized administratively and clinically to operate in a manner that mirrors the strongly hierarchical Kosovar families and the structure of already existing mental health programs. In the SBT program, however, doctors and nurses are expected to collaborate and work together on nonhierarchical teams. It has been a challenge for Kosovar clinicians to learn to work within an interdisciplinary model utilizing team decision making. This approach was initially developed during the first stage of the project when Kosovar and U.S. professionals worked together to link family systems theory and practice with the goals of the Kosovars' developing mental health system. Kosovar professional leaders participated fully in this initial training and modeled collaboration for their colleagues. This approach of team building seemed to fit their needs due to extremely limited resources. In addition, the loss and trauma of war had affected everyone, and this shared experience may have softened the traditional rigid hierarchy. In Gjakova, the staff has succeeded in achieving this collaboration through deliberate discussions that clarify roles according to the different clinical disciplines and at the same time through expressions of mutual respect and acknowledgment of the value of each role. This has been modeled by the chief psychiatrist, who works in this way with both nurses and doctors.

Four pairs of nurses work with 15 families who have a chronically mentally ill member. Two mental health technicians serve as case managers to help families stay engaged in the project and to connect them with community resources. When a new client and his or her family members first come to the center, they meet with one of the nurses. Following this initial meeting, the nurse consults with the psychiatrist, who often interviews the client and his or her family members as part of the intake process. This same nurse will then plan to follow this client. However, all clients are told that everyone at the center works as a team, so that if the assigned nurse is not present when they come to the center, other team members will step in. This initial visit is followed up with a home visit by the nurses and the SBT team from Prishtina. If a family is reluctant to join the program, one of the options the team has available is to request that the chief psychiatrist travel with the team to the home. When the project began in the community, these home visits by the psychiatrist (who was at that time the director of the center) were particularly significant in engaging families' participation, since this psychiatrist was well known and respected by all patients and families in the community. His visits to their homes were considered an honor and a signal of his support for their seeking mental health services for themselves and their ill family member.

The center's nursing teams and psychiatrist spend an hour each day in formal meetings at the center in which all cases are discussed with the psychiatrist. These meetings are preceded by an informal coffee gathering at the start of each day where personal and professional concerns are discussed. In addition to this day-to-day supervision, the staff participates in training sessions during the monthly visits of the team leaders from Prishtina, following an apprenticeship model of training by observing work with families by the Prishtina SBT team or by the U.S. team when in Kosova.

As a result, nurses and psychiatrists from the project are developing a view of mental illnesses that emphasizes the contexts of family and community, with medication only a part of the treatment offered. Because family life is central to Kosovar culture, this approach also supports and even supplements the extended family structure that has been disrupted by the war.

Family Assessments

To complete assessments of new referrals to the SBT project, two SBT team members come from Prishtina and join with two community nurses each week to interview patients and families in their homes. These teams assess families to ensure that they meet the inclusion criteria for the project. These criteria were developed so as to identify the population served as part of the outcome evaluation research. In addition to the diagnosis of a severe and persistent mental illness, these criteria include the following:

1. The mentally ill family member is either living in isolation apart from the family home or living only intermittently with the family due to length or frequency of hospitalizations; or
2. The mentally ill family member is at heightened risk for rehospitalization due to one of the following: inconsistent or no access to mental health services; inconsistent or no access to medication; or living in isolated physical space and excluded from participation with other family members; or
3. There is a high risk of harm to other family members due to the presence of one of the following: family violence; disrupted care of children; or more than one mentally ill family member living in the household.

Developing these criteria taught us a great deal about the process of collaboration. Initially the criteria for inclusion proposed by the U.S. team made no sense to the Kosovars. Because a small stipend was offered to families who participated in the project, the Kosovars thought that economic hardship should be the primary criterion for a family's inclusion. This stipend would only be sustained for the first 18 months of the project, however, and thus the U.S. team did not see it as central to the development of services that would ultimately be provided without a stipend. The U.S. criteria also initially focused on the chronically mentally ill who were not living with their families but were either homeless or living in a nonfamily setting. In Gjakova there were in fact no such patients, since all patients were either in the hospital or in their family homes. Both teams felt a sense of accomplishment

when criteria were finally developed that both met the design of the project and matched the realities of patients' and families' lives.

Initial Home Visit in Gjakova

The following vignette describes how a family, referred to the center, was evaluated for inclusion in the project. Two U.S. team members, three members of the Prishtina SBT team, and two members of the Gjakova SBT team met the family in their home. This family, like most of those we visited in Kosova, welcomed the team, expressing particular appreciation for the visit by the U.S. team members. (Most Kosovars whom we have met continue to be grateful to the United States for supporting NATO's intervention on their behalf in 1999.) This was a second meeting with the family. The team was still in the process of deciding whether or not they met the criteria for inclusion in the project. The goals for the session, decided on by team before the session, were to continue an assessment for inclusion in the project; to begin introducing some suggestions to the parents of how they and the center might help their adult children; to challenge some of their beliefs that mental illness is a curse; and to foster connection with and confidence in the CMH team.

Family Vignette

This family interview included a mother and father who are elderly and have three children. A son and a daughter in their 30s are both mentally ill with poorly managed psychoses. Their third child, a younger son, who is healthy, did not attend. Also attending the session was one of the brothers of the mother, who said that he was there to support the family but spoke little. The Gjakova team among themselves, before the session, expressed empathetic concern for the youngest son; they thought he might be worried and burdened because the responsibility for his ill siblings will fall to him as his parents continue to age and ultimately die. The family was encouraged to invite him to attend the next family session.

The family lived in a comfortable, very wellkept house. At all Kosovar family visits drinks are served, but in this household the mother also served us baklava, possibly as an indication of their economic well-being. Before the meeting, the team told us that the son was doing better than the daughter, as he was already connected to the center and participated actively when he was there and took his medication regularly. The parents acknowledged early in the session the difference between their children. They spoke about their son who was doing better now and had past successes in school and in the army, whereas their daughter was highly disturbed and disruptive in the family and did not take her medication consistently. From their description, it appeared that she had been suffering in this way for many years. In the session, the daughter spoke almost continuously in a disorganized manner. She frequently went in and out of the room. She only quieted when her father asked her to do so. The parents appeared poorly informed about the mental illness of their offspring and what might be reasonable expectations for their future. The father said that he wished either for a cure or that God would take them.

The team acknowledged the strengths of the family and clarified what was working well, such as the parents acting quickly and calmly to place limits, and speaking about positive aspects of their children's lives—what they are proud of, rather than only relating to the illness. The family therapist on the team explored the different relationships in the family. It seemed to her that the mother was more allied with her son, and the father with his daughter. There was a significant conflict between the father and son during the session. When the father focused his concern on his daughter, the son left the room saying, "What about me?" The father followed him and then returned, crying. He said that he believed someone was behind his son's angry outbursts toward him, that this "someone" had malevolently turned his son against him. The team attempted to put the outbursts in the context of the illness. The father listened to their explanation but seemed unconvinced. The mother spoke positively about her son and thought it would help if he was sent somewhere out of the family. She said that her son had been a technic (a male nurse) for 13 years and had been in the army and became sick when he returned in 1998. She then began to cry and left the room. The father spoke about his daughter. He said that she was a good student in secondary school but became ill during that time. Now, he said, she is distressed much of the time, and they worried for her safety. Not long before the session, she had disappeared for several days, and they did not know her whereabouts. She only appears connected to another uncle. The team thought that inviting this uncle and other extended family members to support and help this family would continue to be an important resource. By the end of the session, the family was clearly interested in continuing their relationship with the CMH team.

The patients and their family meet the criteria for inclusion in the project, namely, (1) severe and persistent mental illness of a family member, (2) patient living sporadically with family (the daughter had run away from the family home a number of times), (3) sporadic use of medication, and (4) more than one mentally ill family member living in the home.

Home Visits

Following the assessment phase, families that meet the criteria are visited at least every other week by community nurses helping them to maintain medication schedules of the patients; make links between the family, the patient, and programs at the mental health center, including psychoeducation groups and day treatment; conduct ongoing assessments for incipient crises; and provide overall support and encouragement for families and patients. There is a range of responses to this help as some families join with the center and the team easily, and others find this much more difficult. Though this has not been studied in a systematic way, it is our impression that the more isolated families are and the greater their amount of ongoing stress (such as in the family described here, with aging parents and two mentally ill family members), the longer it takes for a family to engage with the center and the team.

Though the nurses continue to be supervised by one of the psychiatrists at the center and at biweekly meetings with the visiting Prishtina SBT team, they were concerned about their ability to work with families, especially those initially resistant to their interventions. In the early stages of the project, they were encouraged to pay attention to small steps that family members took as evidence of their success. For example, they spoke of working with one family with four psychotic members. Even though well family members refused to come to the CMH due to fears of stigma, their first success came when the two psychotic brothers chose to walk home from the Center for Mental Health, something they had never done before. The second step occurred when the mother left the house for the first time in 5 years to go to an appointment at the CMH. These were successful small steps taken by the family.

As the project continues and with ongoing supervision, the nurses at the center are growing more confident about their work with families. The following is a list of services they see themselves offering to families:

- A bridge to the center: Patients who had been isolated in their homes are brought to the center. When necessary, nurses will go and either walk with or drive patients to the center.
- Medication follow-up: At each home visit, nurses assess with patient and family medication compliance.
- Psychoeducation information: During family visits and during psychoeducation workshops at the center, nurses provide information and answer questions that patients and their families are often reluctant to ask of others.
- Persistence: Whether or not patients and their families come to the center, nurses make home visits regularly, once a week when families are in crisis and biweekly in all other circumstances. They bring to these visits the ability to set goals for each family visit, build positive relationships with family members, witness family difficulties without judgment, and reengage disengaged family members.
- Hope by believing in the families: Nurses have learned to focus on the strengths and capacities in families. They communicate their belief in the strengths of families and help them recognize their competencies by pointing out positive changes.
- Regulation of the emotional temperature in the families to achieve a family climate of low expressed emotion: Nurses encourage families to observe instances in which strong emotions are expressed by family members. They talk to family members about these experiences and brainstorm with them ways of avoiding situations in which emotions are intensified.
- Avoiding crises: Nurses communicate with family members about changes, both positive and negative, that they observe but that family members may not have noticed. They encourage family members to watch for signs of an impending crisis (e.g., increased stress in the household, patient not taking medication).

In support of the Gjakova Mental Health Center's programs there are plans to build a 10-bed apartment for respite and out-of-home care for patients who do not have families, either following hospitalization or when an in-home situation is not viable. This will add another level to the continuum of care available in Gjakova.

Reaching Out Across Stigma

Stigma, a constraint that influences negatively the use of mental health resources throughout Kosova, has a particular tenor in Gjakova. In a recent interview, a Gjakova psychiatrist emphasized the loyalty of Gjakovars for their city above all others. He illustrated this with a song about their city. He said that Gjakovars, as he referred to them, believe that their traditions and loyalty to each other have made their city unique even in the face of disaster. Other conversations indicated that social stratification of families is particularly delineated in Gjakova and is measured at the time of death of any family member. People pay particularly close attention to how many visitors come to visit the family as a show of respect for the significance of the family. This pride has helped Gjakovars survive terror and torture, but it has also exacerbated the effects of stigma when a family member is mentally ill. This stigma has been identified by the Gjakova community nurses as their greatest concern for the future of the project. Also unique to Gjakova is that most marriages occur from within the Gjakova community. As a result, everyone not only knows everyone else but also knows the history of each family. And there is extreme concern that a family pedigree might be labeled as having "bad genes" due to mental illness. Because marriage and the family are so central for the Kosovar society, community awareness that there are "bad genes" in a family can mean that all the siblings in that family will be unable to marry. This concern may keep mentally ill members, especially daughters, hidden away rather than brought to a center for treatment.

Although home visits are accepted, families may not wish to be seen coming to the Gjakova

Center for Mental Health, known locally as a place for "crazy people." Stigma is not attached to a particular diagnostic category but arises whenever someone is observed going into the Center for Mental Health. Lack of accurate information about mental illness and superstitious convictions abound, including an attribution of black magic as causative.

Different staff members approach the problem of stigma on the basis of their understanding of traditions. The psychiatrist interviewed believes that families need to be protected from the prying eyes of their neighbors and suggests that the identification sign on the car from the center be removed, and that mental health workers park away from the house that they are visiting. Another leading psychiatrist believes that the center needs to confront stigma more directly. His approach is to use his own status in the community. He says that since it is an honor for the doctor to visit a family at home, he openly visits the family homes of all new patients. In this way, he believes that he signals his support and recognition of their needs and encourages other community members to do the same.

Staff members use many creative ways of making contact with families who are reluctant to be seen at the center. One nurse who knew a referred family as a friend visited them for a number of times before mentioning the services of the center. Another nurse visited a client who lived behind his family compound and had been hidden from view for a long time. Little by little, the nurse developed a relationship with the patient and his family just by returning to the house and listening to all their concerns. Over time he was able to bring this patient out of his isolation and into the center.

As relationships develop between families and nurses, it is not unusual for staff members to visit families on days that they think might be particularly stressful for them, or on a holiday to greet family members and offer their support. Nurses are also willing to pick up reluctant clients (the center owns two vans) and drive them to the center. As a way of introducing patients and their families to the center, nurses sometimes begin a relationship by offering basic medical services like blood pressure measures before introducing mental health services. Clearly, the effects of stigma require that the mental health staff understand its impact and develop creative solutions to overcome its effects.

Psychoeducation

Patients and their families are offered an educational program about psychotic illnesses that includes the following topics: acknowledgment of the burden that severe psychiatric disorders place on the patient and the family; the biological basis for the illness; course, symptoms, and risk factors for relapse; need for medications and monitoring of side effects; common family difficulties; and ways families can help each other and their ill family member. Because families with mentally ill family members are isolated not only from the center but also from other families struggling with similar problems, the project emphasizes the value of connecting families with each other through structured multifamily groups to melt isolation, share wisdom, form community, and address stigma, following the family guidelines developed by McFarlane (2002) for multifamily psychoeducation groups. McFarlane's model was chosen because those of us on the U.S. team had extensive experience with his work. Following the lecture series on the psychoeducation topics, ongoing multifamily problem-solving groups are formed as part of the services offered by the SBT team at the center.

In the psychoeducation lecture series, efforts have been made to connect information to the families' actual experiences and to specific attributes of psychotic disorders (impairment of communication processing, affect dysregulation, intrusive and irrational thoughts). Illustrations with concrete examples are drawn from their own lives.

In teaching this model to the community nurses and SBT teams, we have used the same steps of the group problem-solving process that they use in their psychoeducation groups. The fact that each step of this process requires each person in the group to speak has challenged cultural expectations that either training or psychoeducation should occur only in a lecture format. Traditionally, discussions would be dominated by the psychiatrists or male nurses (technics), but the group problem-solving format requires that everyone has equal say. A great deal of leadership is required from the team leader to keep reminding everyone of the ground rules and to continue to make room for full participation of all team members.

As with all the models that we have presented, significant time was spent discussing the relevance of this process in the Kosova context. The team noted how different it is from their usual cultural expectations about a learning environment. However, due to their desire to work together as a team, they decided that they would develop this method further.

Their psychoeducation program was planned in the following way:

- The program begins with socializing, including the patients.
- Patients then have a social group of their own.
- Families meet together for a brief lecture given by one of the SBT psychiatrists or residents, who introduces the principles of psychoeducation.
- Large family group then splits into two small groups facilitated by a psychiatrist or psychiatry resident and a nurse from the SBT team and observed by the community nursing teams. In these small groups, families are encouraged to ask questions about the lectures and share their knowledge with each other.
- Everyone meets back together again and socializes briefly before leaving.

Community Networks

One of the goals of the project is to support the work of the Center for Mental Health by reaching out to individuals and services that offer additional resources in the community. During the initial year of the program, the center has barely begun to work with other local agencies, though it does receive some referrals from schools, police, and religious leaders. There are plans to work more closely with family medical doctors, the schools, and the criminal justice system.

One of the ways in which the center's staff have been able to establish links with other community services is by inviting representatives of different agencies to meetings with them at the Center for Mental Health when the U.S. consultants visit. Participants in these meetings have included the principal of the high school, family medical doctors, the principal of the elementary school, social workers from social welfare agencies, religious leaders from the local mosque, policemen, representatives of the judicial system, and local media from television and newspapers. The goals of these meetings are to in-

form community leaders about the services offered by the Center for Mental Health, to develop a shared understanding about mental illness, and to begin to discuss ways they can work together to set up resource networks, initially for the families in the SBT project. These meetings have been met with a great deal of enthusiasm.

Participants have given examples of how they see their work connecting with the center, such as the following:

- A social worker was asked to work with a couple on the verge of divorce. In the initial interview, he discovered that they have a daughter suffering from a serious mental illness whom they have been trying to hide. This has put a great strain on their relationship. The social worker connected the couple to the center, and this de-escalated their conflict.
- A representative of the court spoke of a man who was now in custody. He believes that this man is not a criminal but mentally ill. The family of this man prefers that he be in jail, since this is less shameful than having a mental illness. The dilemma for the court representative is that the procedures of the court do not include psychiatric referrals.
- A principal at an elementary school commented on how parents need information about what are normal developmental stages and what are signs of serious illness, with special emphasis on the effects of trauma and loss.

Evaluation After 1 Year

The new director was interviewed for a trip report after 9 months with the project. The following quotations express his beliefs about the successful aspects of the program:

- "Families are very responsive and interested to participate in the project, including those who previously had not been engaged in mental health services."
- "Families are asking about the nature of their family member's illness and how they should behave toward him or her."
- "Medication is being used more regularly."
- "Patients who used to come when in crisis, usually brought by the police due to aggres-

sive behavior, are getting to the center much earlier."

- "The center is becoming more connected with social welfare and is therefore developing a positive identity in the community."

He described a case in which a mother (whose daughter had been paranoid and housebound for many years) joined the project. The nurses worked with her and the family, and the family members now understand more clearly about the daughter's illness. They are helping her to take her medications. She is receiving better personal care, including care of her teeth, which were in bad condition, and she has begun to walk in the village and visit the center. In another case, the nursing team has been more successful staying in contact with a psychotic man who now consents to intramuscular antipsychotic medications. A year ago this man had nearly killed his wife in a bout of pathological jealousy.

When interviewed, the community nursing team expressed confidence in the success of the program. They evaluated the first 15 families who participated in the project. As an example of a successful case, the Gjakova nurses described a family for whom the team had used community resources to alleviate family stresses hindering participation in the project. When they first contacted this family, the client was unwilling to join the project at the center. He was focused on two family issues that were unresolved: his inability as a father to provide support for the family, and the refusal of his 16-year-old daughter to go to school because other children were teasing her about his illness. The nursing team worked on these problems with the family. They began by contacting the principal of the elementary school who had attended the community resource meetings. With his help they found a solution for the daughter. After they realized that the mother's family was from a neighboring town, they located an appropriate school for the daughter there, where she willingly began attending school. The father, who had been agitated by his daughter's problem, became more accessible to the team.

The team was also able to help the family improve its economic condition by mediating a family dispute about finishing and renting two small shops owned by the family. Before long, the shops were rented, some family income was generated, and the family began participating regularly at the Center for Mental Health.

The nurses provided another example of a successful case, that of a family in which the mother completed the basic seven-session family psychoeducation series and will continue regular participation in programs of the Center for Mental Health. When the nursing team first contacted this family, the children were leaving the home to avoid the father, a rather disorganized, noncompliant schizophrenic. Since the nurses engaged with the family, the patient began accepting the medications. The team attributed his improved adherence to his wife coming to understand his illness differently and blaming him less after attending family psychoeducation groups. At the last meeting, she had commented, "In the beginning, I thought he did these things because he wanted to do them. Now I understand they are symptoms of his illness."

The mother also shared her new understanding of the father's illness with the children. Progressively the children's behavior toward their father changed as they became more accepting of him. In fact, initially the daughter had refused to meet with the nursing team during home visits, and now she greets them at the door and welcomes them.

A case brought for consultation because of its difficulties involved a 48-year-old chronically psychotic man who lives in a building adjacent to the one where his brother's family lives. He has been cared for by this family, who pay for his electricity and meals. This patient also has had close ties with two sisters, one of them living in Gjakova. The brother and that sister met with the SBT team. Initially, the family eagerly engaged in the program, with the mentally ill family member coming to the center, and the family members participating in psychoeducation. However, after the brother's 11-year-old daughter, with whom the client had a close relationship, died in a drowning accident, the family has since withdrawn from the project, and the client's symptoms are increasing. The sister, who was helping her sick brother by cleaning his home, stopped doing it, arguing that she had too many other obligations. The man refused to do it on his own. The U.S. consultants suggested that the team consider meeting with the whole family in a session focused on grief for their daughter before trying to actively reengage them in the center's ongoing program.

The nursing teams discussed their difficulties

in responding to crises, both in anticipating that a particular event would lead to a crisis and how to develop a social support network, including the involvement of extended family members not directly involved in psychoeducation. They also requested training in family grief and in crisis intervention.

Conclusion

In a project such as this, many lessons are learned about working in collaboration across cultural differences. This chapter addresses some of those lessons learned from our work in Gjakova. A challenge was the extremely insular nature of this community within which a new mental health center was being developed, part, in fact, of a new mental health system. Strong boundaries around families and the community made it particularly difficult for any outsiders to be welcomed in, regardless of how necessary the services they offered. It has proved essential that many of the nurses and doctors on the CMH teams were natives from that town, and their families well-known. However, the stigma attached to mental illness made some families unwilling to open up even to those well-known providers.

The U.S. team's support has helped to solidify a process that the SBT team and the community nurses have taken upon themselves to develop, with increasing independence. Within 12 months, they successfully engaged families that met the project criteria for participation, created family psychoeducation groups, began a community resource network, and created a program of ongoing home visits for patients and families.

Working in Gjakova alerted us to the nuances of differences within a homogeneous population. Because it is a culture within a culture, we had to question the assumptions we held about the culture at large. For example, many Western influences in the country are having a significant impact on the traditional family. This is much less true in Gjakova. One way to conceptualize this is to think of Gjakova as being on the traditional end of a family continuum from traditional to Westernized beliefs and practices. This means that services that might develop easily in Prishtina, a major city, or even in Ferizaj, a less traditional city, take much longer in Gjakova and actually have a different character due to the power of stigma on this group.

Gjakovars value the social and religious networks that have long existed to support them. This pride has extended to the development of the first mental health center in the country and the desire of the community for its success. In spite of meager salaries and often unreasonable expectations for long hours, the staff at the center are extremely motivated. Recently, when their head nurse, who had been an important source of support, was killed in an automobile accident, the staff mobilized around her death, working with patients to create a memorial for her that filled the center's walls with drawings in her memory. In good times and in bad, they are committed to each other and to the purposes of the center.

The tension between strengths and obstacles, along with economic pressures and an uncertain political future, presents serious challenges to the longevity of the project once the U.S. team finishes its 3-year presence. The Kosovars are well aware of these pressures and are working toward integrating these innovative services into their developing infrastructure. The commitment of the U.S. team is to continue as consultants and witnesses to this development. We are learning many lessons from the Kosovars, particularly how, in the face of grave difficulties, resilience exists not only in clients and families but also in the mental health teams who work against great odds to bring services to their community.

Notes

1. This chapter could not have been written without the support of the Joint Distribution Committee, the American Family Therapy Academy, and all the American and Kosovar KFPEC team members. A number of internal reports, available from the author, further describe the project, including C. Becker & J. Griffith, Internal Report for the SBT Project (2002); J. Griffith & E. Pulleyblank Coffey, Internal Report for SBT Project (October 2002); E. Pulleyblank Coffey & M. Elliot, Internal Report for the SBT Project (May 2002); S Weine & F. Agani, The Kosovar Family Professional Education Collaborative, grant proposal to the Emergency Jewish Fund for Kosovo (May 2000).

2. The Kosovars use the spelling "Kosova," though others, including the Serbs, often use the spelling "Kosovo." Because this chapter describes the Kosovars' work, we will use their spelling.

3. Some material for this chapter was gathered

through interviews of staff at the Gjakova Mental Health Center. See Appendix.

4. The SBT program was designed by Weine and Agani and funded through the Emergency Fund for Kosova and the Jewish Joint Distribution Committee.

Appendix: Gjakova Interview for Case Study, KFPEC, May 2002

History and Social Context

History of Gjakova particularly relevant to its selection as the first community mental health site.

Special characteristics of the city. Population, area, economics, cultural history and practices.

Participants in the Program

Who is served? What diagnostic categories are represented in your patient population?

From whom are they referred?

What do you think of the current inclusion criteria?

Numbers of patients seen.

Numbers of family members/children seen?

Services

What are the different components of the program at your center? Describe how the SBT program works at its best. Give a case example.

In general, how long do patients wait for services? How often are they seen once they are in the program? How long do they remain in the program? At the end of the program are they referred somewhere else?

What clinical practices are included in treatment?

What common challenges do you face on a clinical level?

Who coordinates the assessment, planning and treatment?

How is medication used in treatment? Primary, Supportive, Both/and.

What are the components of the current psycho-education program? Who attends? How often?

How often are family members seen in family sessions? Who conducts those sessions? Do you do family sessions in peoples' homes or at the center?

Training

Describe the SBT Training. Who participates in training? How often? How would you change or add to the training?

Funding

What are your sources of funding?

How much of this budget goes into this program?

How reliable is your funding?

Have there been significant changes in funding over time?

What does the program cost per family unit?

If funding were not an issue, what would you do differently?

Service Coordination with the Community

How important is it to work with other groups in the community?

How are you training staff to work with other agencies?

How successful are you in involving community people. Give an example of a case in which other community agencies or individuals participated with the mental health team.

What obstacles exist in coordination with other services and community helpers?

Staff

How many staff members are involved in the program?

Describe your staff in terms of education and experience.

Does your staff work in teams? How often do they meet?

What kinds of supervision and learning opportunities are available?

What is an average length of employment?

What are the incentives for remaining at the center? Or, what else provides support to clinicians/case managers in helping them do what they do?

Family Involvement in the Center

Do the people you serve provide feedback about how the program is helping or not helping them?

Are the people you serve involved in other ways with the center?

Conclusion

Are there other obstacles you haven't yet mentioned that make it difficult to accomplish everything you set out to accomplish?

If you were designing the project now, what would you do differently?

What advice do you have for us?

Are there other questions we should have asked but didn't?

References

Cardoza, B., Vergara, A., Agani, F., & Gotway, C. A. (2000). Mental health, social functioning, and attitudes of Kosovar Albanians following the war in Kosovo. *JAMA, 284,* 569–577.

Clarke, R. (1992). Wrapping community based mental health services around children with severe behavior disorders: An evaluation of Project Wraparound. *Journal of Child and Family Studies, 1,* 241–261.

Griffith, J. L., Blyta, A., Ukshini, S., Kallaba, M., & Weine, S. (2001, July). *Promoting family resistance to effects of culturecide: The Kosovar Professional Educational Collaborative.* Presented at "Cultures of Violence, Cultures of Peace," the 24th Annual Scientific Meeting of the International Society of Political Psychology, Cuernavaca, Morelos, Mexico.

Griffith, J. L., & the Kosovar Family Professional Educational Collaborative. (2002, July). *Promoting mental health after ethnic violence through family-centered interventions in Kosovo.* Presented at the 25th Annual Scientific Meeting of the International Society for Political Psychology, Berlin, Germany.

Malcolm, N. (1998). *Kosovo: A short history.* New York: New York University Press.

McFarlane, W. (2002). *Multifamily groups and treatment of severe psychiatric disorders.* New York: Guilford.

Serwer, D. (2001). United States Institute of Peace. "Albanian Forum" at the Albanian Institute for International Studies, Tirana.

Walsh, F. (1998). *Strengthening family resilience.* New York: Guilford.

Weine, S., & Agani, F. (2001). Services Based Training Teams for Kosova Community Mental Health and Prevention. Grant Proposal to the Joint Distribution Committee.

Weine, S., Agani, F., Griffith, J., Ukshini, S., Pulleyblank-Coffey, E., & Ulaj, J. (in preparation). *Services-based training teams for Kosova community mental health and prevention.* Manuscript in preparation.

Weine, S., Agani, F., & Rolland, J. (2001, December). *The Kosovar Family Professional Education Collaborative.* Paper presented at the International Society for Traumatic Stress Studies, San Antonio, TX.

Weine, S., Agani, F., & Rolland, J. (in preparation). *The Kosovar Family Professional Education Collaborative.* Manuscript in preparation.

33

Joshua Miller

Critical Incident Debriefings and Community-Based Clinical Care

Community-based clinical practice covers the spectrum of clinical interventions, from crisis intervention to long-term care of people with chronic conditions. In any community there will be disasters: a car crash that kills and injures high school students after a prom, the suicide of a psychiatrist at a local mental health center, a fire that consumes a sleeping child. Disasters can be due to "natural" causes (e.g., a hurricane, earthquake, flood) or caused by humans (e.g., murder, hijacking, sexual assault, police brutality). There are differences in the scale of disasters, with some affecting large groups of people, such as a tornado inflicting damage on a street or in a neighborhood. Some disasters affect the entire community (e.g., the murder of a mayor or city councillor) or even an entire country (e.g., the Columbine school shootings, the Oklahoma City bombing), or in some instances, the world (e.g., the attacks of September 11, 2001).

Critical Incident Stress Debriefing (CISD) has emerged as an intervention in response to disasters. It is a structured group process for survivors and victims of disasters and other trauma-inducing events (Everly & Mitchell, 2000; Miller, 2000). Debriefings are usually considered part of a larger system of crisis responses to "critical incidents" known as Critical Incident Stress Management (CISM; Ev-

erly & Mitchell, 2000), which include more immediate responses known as "defusings," briefings for management, and individual crisis intervention. CISD and CISM are community-based interventions and often rely on a peer or volunteer model of responders and facilitators.

In this chapter I will focus on debriefings, the most widely used crisis intervention service in response to disasters. I will describe what debriefings are, summarize research about their effectiveness, and consider how they are an essential component of a community-based system of clinical care.

Debriefings

Debriefings were originally developed for soldiers and emergency workers; expanded to disaster relief workers, uniformed personnel (firefighters, ambulance drivers, and emergency medical technicians [EMT]), and law enforcement officers; and eventually adapted for use with survivors of direct trauma (Armstrong, O'Callahan, & Marmar, 1991; Dyregrov, 1997; Mitchell, 1983). Debriefings are offered by national disaster relief organizations (e.g., Red Cross), community-based volunteer groups, professional responders, and agency-based teams, all of which utilize the services of mental health clinicians in partnership with trained volunteers and peer responders. A debriefing has a clear goal: to help participants to sufficiently process the consequences of a disaster and the consequent crisis-induced stress, and to enable them to continue with their jobs and remain engaged with their families and communities (Pueler, 1988; Raphael, 1986). One notable aspect of a disaster is that it affects more than one person. Therefore, debriefings are designed to work with groups of people to process the critical event and resultant stress and to collectively provide mutual support, healing, and self-help.

Debriefings are led by a facilitator or a small team of facilitators, who guide the group through a semistructured set of questions. The typical format for a debriefing involves reviewing accounts of what occurred; reflections about cognitive, emotional, and physical reactions; psychoeducational teaching about typical stress responses and useful coping mechanisms; and eliciting ideas and plans for healing, self-care, and mutual aid and support (Miller, 2000). Individual participants may be referred for further assistance and treatment.

Although debriefings are provided by a variety of organizations to different target groups in varied situations, the similarities between models of debriefings outweigh their differences. Warheit (1988) notes seven key components that are found in most models of debriefings:

1. The impact of the critical incident on survivors and response personnel is assessed;
2. Critical issues surrounding the problem, particularly relating to safety and security, are identified;
3. Ventilation of thoughts, emotions, and experiences occurs, and reactions are validated;
4. Future reactions and responses are anticipated and predicted;
5. The event and the response to it are thoroughly explored and reviewed;
6. There is an attempt to bring closure to the event and to connect people to community resources; and
7. The debriefing assists people with making a reentry back to their community or workplace.

It is interesting to note the common properties of debriefings because they are frequently marketed in different ways. One of the biggest differences is whether or not the debriefing is presented as a clinical intervention. Some are called "psychological" debriefings and are clearly seen as clinical interventions (Dyregrov, 1997; Raphael, 1986). However, when offered to uniformed personnel, the clinical aspects of debriefings are de-emphasized, perhaps due to the cultures of hardiness that are part of being a police officer or firefighter, and the accompanying stigma of receiving mental health services, which can be seen as a sign of weakness. With uniformed personnel, the aspects of debriefings that are stressed are the importance of talking with peers, who understand what the job is like, the need for self-care, and the importance of mutual support. When beginning a debriefing with uniformed personnel, the facilitator will often stress, "this is not therapy." Yet the actual process and phases of debriefings offered by different organizations to different target groups are remarkably similar

Table 33-1 compares five different debriefing prototypes. Mitchell's (1983) model was developed initially for use with emergency response personnel, while the National Organization of Victim Assistance (NOVA; Young, 1997) and the American Red Cross (1995) respond to a wide range of disasters and traumatic events. The community team model is based on the model used by the Community Crisis Response Team of Western Massachusetts (Miller, 2000), which offers debriefings to schools, local communities, and various formal and informal groups. Raphael's (1986) psychological debriefings were also developed for workers and helpers responding to disasters. Although the name for a given phase may differ slightly and the amount of time spent processing that phase may also vary, the actual sequence of phases is very similar, moving from introductions, ground rules, and information about what happened to describing thoughts, feelings, and reactions. All models close with a focus on self-care, mutual support, and reintegration into the community and one's life commitments and routines. This is called a "wave model," moving from information and thoughts through feelings and eventually to self-care and normalization (Everly & Mitchell, 2000).

I have had direct experience with three models in my work with three volunteer teams: the Mitchell model, American Red Cross model, and the community team model. I have also used aspects of the NOVA model in my work for managed care

Table 33-1. Comparison of Debriefing Models

Mitchell Critical Incident Stress Debriefing	National Organization of Victim Response Debriefing	American Red Cross Debriefing	Community Team Model	Raphael's Psychological Debriefing
1. Introductions and ground rules	1. Introductions and ground rules	1. Groundwork	1. Introductions and ground rules	1. Initiation into disaster role
2. Fact Phase	2. Cognitive level of experience.	2. Disclosure of events	2. Cognitive Phase	2. Workers own experience of disaster
3. Thought Phase	3. Sensory experience.	3. Feelings and reactions	3. Reaction phase.	3. Review of negative aspects and feelings
4. Feeling Phase	4. Emotions	4. Coping strategies	4. Self-care strategies	4. Review of positive aspects and feelings
5. Reaction Phase	5. What has happened since the event	5. Termination	5. Closing, rituals, follow-up	5. Relationships with workers and family
6. Normalizing, teaching phase.	6. Normalizing the experience			6. Empathy with others
7. Re-entry	7. Closure			7. Disengagement from disaster role
				8. Integration of disaster experience
Armstrong, et al., 1991; Mitchell, 1983	Young, 1997	Armstrong, et al., 1991; American Red Cross, 1995	Miller, 2000	Raphael, 1986

companies. I have found that the Mitchell and Red Cross models' emphasis on creating a narrative is a very important place to begin. Much of this work, like therapy, is helping participants articulate their story of a disaster and its negative consequences and to then reconstruct a narrative of healing and efficacy. As part of this process, it is useful to help participants to get in touch with their thoughts and feelings. After disclosing the facts, it is helpful for participants to describe their cognitive reactions: thoughts at the time of the critical incident, as well as their present thinking about the event. Feelings are also important to reveal and process *only if there is sufficient time!* It is not helpful to encourage people to open themselves up if there is not enough time to process this or to move on to coping and self-care strategies. All the models that I have used place an emphasis on empowerment types of activities—normalizing and depathologizing typical stress responses, emphasizing self-care activities, and encouraging mutual support from group members.

The use of a particular model depends on the organization that is sponsoring the debriefings, the culture of the participants, and the nature of the critical incident. Emergency medical service teams respond to uniformed (fire, police, ambulance) personnel and usually subscribe to the Mitchell model. In my experience, such teams emphasize sticking to the format quite rigidly. In contrast, my work with a community team has involved taking a more flexible approach, adapting the debriefing to the audience and setting. Uniformed personnel regularly face harrowing situations and have developed cultures of strength and self-reliance. Weakness is something to be feared. When conducting debriefings with such groups, facilitators are encouraged to not ask "How did you feel?" but rather "What was the hardest part for you?" This is very different from conducting a debriefing with college counselors after a student commits suicide, where exploration of feelings is culturally compatible and indeed expected.

I once conducted a debriefing on behalf of a community team for a group of friends of a person who had been murdered. The debriefing focused a great deal on feelings and ended with a ritual suggested by the group that involved a group hug and a great deal of emotional expression. This would not have been appropriate with a group of firefighters or possibly even employees who had survived the attack on the World Trade Center.

The nature of the critical incident also influences the process and emphasis of a debriefing. When I was working with survivors of the attack on the World Trade Center in New York, counselors would usually check in with people about their sensory impressions at the time of the disaster. Almost all participants had vivid sensations such as the smell of burning airplane fuel, the sound of the planes before they hit the building, the images of smoke and debris, the sound of elevators crashing in their shafts. These were powerful, deeply embedded images that were easily triggered by everyday city sights, sounds, and smells. People described breaking into a cold sweat upon hearing a siren or an airplane without realizing what the precipitating stimulus was. In contrast, when debriefing teachers and students at a driving school after two students died in a car accident, the sensory stimuli were not essential, but it was important to spend a great deal of time on the participants' memories of the victims and their feelings of guilt for not having prevented the incident.

Ultimately, all the models follow the same ripple of the wave but have different points of emphasis, varying ways of phrasing questions, and different philosophies about how flexible or rigid the protocols should be. It is ultimately up to the facilitators and the organization they represent to try to offer a debriefing process that best fits the group of people requiring this form of crisis response.

Debriefings and Community-Based Clinical Care

Debriefings respond to vulnerable populations in immediate need of services, possibly preventing serious negative mental health and social consequences, and referring individuals to needed resources. Debriefings stress coping skills, social support, and interpersonal connections. They offer a place where individuals can create narratives about what happened and their own personal reactions. Often people find that there are others who have had similar experiences. They can also learn from those with different reactions. Ultimately, a group narrative is created that binds people together and creates a sense of shared experience.

The combination of peers working alongside clinicians as facilitators exemplifies community-based clinical practice. The presence of peers em-

powers participants as they see people like them (fellow firefighters, construction workers, residents of their community) with the skills and understanding to help them to cope with their grief and trauma. This demystifies and de-professionalizes the process, reducing the social distance between the helper and the helped, rendering the process more accessible and supporting the notion that participants' reactions are normal responses to abnormal events. It is also empowering to peers to be able to help their colleagues, neighbors, and friends. And yet a debriefing conducted after events like Columbine, Oklahoma City, and September 11, 2001, requires clinical skill and judgment. Participants often have powerful, vivid recollections of the disasters, accompanied by strong, powerful affect. Other participants are dazed and numb and need help with getting in touch with their reactions through gentle probing or skillful group facilitation. Some participants have developed functional defense mechanisms, which a skilled clinician can discern and respect. There is also a need to assess during a debriefing who might be at risk of depression, chemical abuse, or self-destructive behavior; these participants might well require referrals for further treatment and clinical interventions.

Like other forms of community-based clinical practice, debriefings place a high value on client empowerment and emphasize assets, social support, mutual aid, and networking, and are consistent with resiliency and strengths-based approaches (Miller, 2003). Some models of debriefing also emphasize cultural competency (Young, 1997), which is a central tenet of all good community-based clinical practice.

Debriefings are offered to groups. This helps to bring people together and to create opportunities for learning from others and for mutual aid and support. Therefore, clinical group-work skills, such as listening skills and empathic capacity, enhance debriefings (Dyregrov, 1997). Additional clinical skills that enhance the effectiveness of debriefings are understanding how to pace a group, being able to tolerate silences, affirming and validating experiences, fostering interaction between group members, tracking affect and mediating, and resolving conflict.

Most debriefings are nested in a community context, whether the community is residential, professional, or one of intimate relationships, such as circles of friends. The death of a high school student can result in debriefings within the high school community for teachers, administrators, and students or within the deceased's residential community for relatives, friends, neighbors, and other affected families and individuals. The murder of a man by police in a synagogue can bring together communities of friends or members of the congregation. Therefore, it is important that debriefings are offered through a variety of services: community-based mental health teams, agency-based crisis intervention units, and local and national volunteer disaster response teams (Miller, 2000).

Using Principles of Community-Based Clinical Practice to Enhance Critical Incident Stress Debriefings

Although CISD is a community-based intervention, more consciously employing principles of community-based clinical practice (CBCP) can strengthen their efficacy. Principles of CBCP can be applied to debriefings in a number of ways:

1. Constructing debriefings ecologically;
2. Valuing strengths, resiliency, and group and community connectedness;
3. Conceptualizing debriefings with narrative theory;
4. Thoughtfulness about group process; and
5. Ensuring equal access for all members of a community.

Ecologically Constructed Debriefings

Theoretically, debriefings conceptualize the person in their environment, working with natural groups and systems, encouraging mutual aid and support, and taking a strengths perspective. Employing an ecological perspective (Germain, 1979; Germain & Gitterman, 1980, 1995) can further enhance the theoretical basis of debriefings. According to the ecological perspective, "both person and environment can be fully understood only in terms of their relationship, in which each continually influences the other within a particular context" (Germain & Gitterman, 1995, p. 816). While this is implicit in debriefing philosophy, it is useful to explicitly conceptualize debriefings through an ecological lens. The framework focuses on the *fit* between the per-

son and environment (or group of people and the environment) and considers *life stressors* as well as stress. Ecological theory uses terms and concepts such as "relatedness," "adaptations," "competence," "self-direction," and "habitat and niche," the last of which refers to a person's physical and social environment (Germain & Gitterman, 1995). An ecological perspective provides concepts often missing from debriefing literature, such as types and manifestations of power, different aspects of time (individual, historical, and social), and the notion of a person having a "life course" (Germain & Gitterman, 1995). This conceptualization places disasters and debriefings in a larger ecological and historical context, offering a more nuanced view of human behavior. Debriefings become part of a larger social web, situated in a continuum of time that began before the disaster and will continue after the debriefing. Zinner and Williams (1999) conceptualize this as a contextualized timeline for group survivorship and community recovery with the following periods: pretrauma, trauma, primary intervention period, secondary adjustment period, and posttrauma period.

The events of September 11 offer a good example of how a more ecological approach to debriefings might be valuable. Many people who escaped from the World Trade Center received debriefings offered by clinicians hired by managed care corporations and offered through employee assistance programs. This was both valuable and problematic. It was important for employees to receive services, and many of them did as a result of this service delivery model. It also fostered mutual support among colleagues. However, there was also an emphasis on getting back to work, and supervisors offered mixed messages about wanting their employees to take care of themselves while also wanting them to contribute to the corporation. Participants were also wary about revealing too much in front of their colleagues. This tension is structured into debriefings being offered by an employer, however well intended. However, workers inside the World Trade Center and people passing by who did not work for large corporations might not have received debriefings. An ecological model and systems of care approach would assess all the potential people directly affected by the World Trade Center disaster and try to map out different ways to reach and serve individuals, families, groups, and subgroups. It would consider conflicts of interest arising from employer-generated services and consider various ways of reaching people— through neighborhoods, religious organizations, trade unions, and other formal and informal groups and systems. This does not negate the need for employer-offered services but rather offers a complementary, more varied and flexible service delivery system.

Strengths, Resiliency, and Group and Community Connectedness

The contextualized, developmental framework of an ecological approach fits well with the CBCP emphasis on strengths and resiliency (Saleeby, 1996; Weick, Rapp, Sullivan, & Kisthardt, 1989). A debriefing is a way of helping people move from a narrative of victim to one of survivor. A major function of debriefings, and perhaps a more important one than the ability to prevent posttraumatic stress, is to connect participants with one another. Palmer (1999), using a case-based research method, has concluded that the most important variable in resiliency is "human relatedness" with other individuals, families, community networks, and social support groups. Debriefings are exercises in human relatedness; an explicit goal is to create a group narrative of disaster and healing and to foster group cohesion and mutual support.

Gilgun (1999) has developed a model of assessing client risks and strengths, the Clinical Assessment Package for Assessing Client Risks and Strengths (CAPACRS), which uses a number of scales to assess risk and resiliency in children and families: emotional expressiveness, family relationships, family embeddedness in community, and peer relationships. While CISD encourages emotional expressiveness and utilizes peer relationships, more could be done to work with family groups and to understand how families and communities are intricately and mutually embedded (Miller, 2001).

Since connectedness with family and community is so important, debriefings could actively bring family and/or community members together for debriefings even when they have not directly experienced critical incidents. This process views the effects of critical incidents more systemically: even those not directly victimized by a disaster can experience forms of secondary trauma. Such debriefings would allow families to understand the

reactions that some of their members are experiencing while also fostering support and help from those less triggered and destabilized by critical incidents. Family debriefings respond to one of the problems with debriefing people solely by virtue of their shared exposure to critical incidents: while this group may have a special, shared understanding of the critical incident and its impact, they then have to adjust to being with family, friends, and colleagues who do not have this shared experience, and reentry problems can occur (American Red Cross, 1995). For example, spouses and children of those who survived the World Trade Center collapse were certainly affected by this event, yet they were not present for debriefings offered via employee assistance programs for the family member who directly escaped the disaster. Individuals who directly experience disaster frequently comment that their loved ones do not truly grasp or understand what they went through (Miller, 2002a), while relatives of the victim may be baffled and confused by the victim's withdrawal and alienation. If a survivor is drinking heavily or isolating him- or herself, what is a spouse, partner, or child to make of this? This behavior can have recursive effects within the family as potential supports are withdrawn or even become antagonistic. Debriefing families together could mitigate such recursive effects. There may be a need to conduct debriefings with individuals who directly experienced the disaster, such as a work group that survived 9/11, and subsequently offer family debriefings as a follow-up.

The same is true of bringing together friends and other relevant members of the community who can support the victim and his or her family. Clinicians conducting debriefings could map out natural community groups, networks, and relationships *before* conducting debriefings as part of a pre-debriefing assessment process. Intentionally bringing a heterogeneous group of people together, including those who directly experienced the event and those who can offer support, could buffer and help contain the traumatic effect of the critical incident, while strengthening bonds between those directly and indirectly impacted by the tragedy. The guiding principal would be less about who experienced a critical incident and more about who can be supportive and helpful. It is also worthwhile to foster debriefing groups with potential for developing relationships that can continue after the crisis. A strengths-based and resiliency approach suggests that there is value in bringing together people with differential exposure to crisis and disaster; they can learn from one another and as a group offer balance between hope and despair, optimism and pessimism.

For example, when there has been domestic violence in a community leading to murder, many different systems and groups of people are affected—people who knew the victim, social service and law enforcement personnel who tried to save the victim, teachers of the victim's children, members of the church that the victim attended, and many more. Not only groups within the community but also the community itself may be affected by the event. If there had been previous domestic fatalities, this can become part of an ongoing community narrative about domestic violence. While it is certainly important to offer debriefings to people within a formal or informal group, say the teachers at the school the children attended, it might also be helpful to offer community debriefings that may bring together people who were more directly involved with people who are concerned and affected but less directly triggered by the tragedy. This could be done by holding open community meetings where debriefings are offered or by consciously inviting members from different groups and constituencies to expand and open the debriefing process. This would integrate the group-based process that debriefings traditionally follow with a community-oriented approach that taps and builds on community assets and resources.

Strengths- and relationship-based community practice also has implications for the role of the debriefing facilitators. An empowerment and strengths-based approach works best when there is minimal social distance between facilitators and those receiving help (Saleeby, 1996). Polio, McDonald, and North (1996) have developed a set of "practice principles" to guide strengths-based practice (that also incorporates the values of feminism) with "street" populations. One is that workers are sensitive to their professional privilege and the barriers that accrue from this; a second is that workers participate as group members rather than as leaders. Many debriefings are facilitated by trained professionals and offered by national organizations such as the Red Cross and the National Organization of Victim Assistance. Other organizations, such as the emergency medical services network, utilize a mixture of trained peers with a professional clinician as consultant. To further a strengths-based orientation, there should perhaps be a greater emphasis on the use of community-based teams of volunteers (Miller, 2000) or on a trainer-of-trainers model, where professional clinicians would have more of a training and consultation role with lay facilitators, rather than leading the debriefings. In my experience the ideal combination is to have a team of facilitators composed of peers and/or community volunteers with at least one professional clinician. This amalgamation both lessens social distance and stigma and also adds the skills of a professional responder to work with complex group dynamics and to assess for severe and unresolved stress reactions.

Whatever the mixture of facilitators, it is always helpful for this group to process their work together afterward and, ideally, to be debriefed by an outside facilitator. This follow-up is essential to understanding complex group dynamics and untangling knots that may have occurred within the facilitation team. It also presents the opportunity for facilitators to learn from one another. Perhaps most important, it aids facilitators with processing their own feelings and reactions and helps to prevent or at least respond to secondary traumatic stress. I have found that the potential for absorbing secondary trauma is always present, as it is in any clinical work. This is more likely to occur when the debriefing facilitator has a personal connection to the incident or the group being debriefed, or has personal analogues that are triggered by the critical incident or the stories of the debriefing participants. While firefighters conducting a debriefing can be more empathetic toward their colleagues, they may also be more prone to overidentifying with their guilt. If a clinician conducting a debriefing after a domestic murder and suicide experienced this with a client in the past, then any unresolved feelings from that earlier trauma might be reactivated. One of the paradoxes of 9/11 is that no one was immune from the trauma of the event, including the debriefing facilitators.

Conceptualizing Debriefings as Narratives

CISD is in essence the creation of individual and group narratives to understand, experience, explain, reconstruct, and transform traumatic incidents. Much has been written about the use of narratives for healing purposes (Chambon, 1994; Laird, 1993; Riessman, 1993; White & Epston, 1990). Narrative theory encourages clinicians to pay attention to the structure of narratives and the metaphors that are used, which raises important questions when viewing debriefings as a narrative intervention and applying the principles of CBCP. Are the structures and sequences of debriefing narrative construction the most helpful? For example, do individual narratives find adequate expression and validation within the context of group debriefing frameworks? Are the metaphors employed in the psychoeducational sections of debriefings ones that foster empowerment and resiliency, or do they reflect a medical model or pathology-oriented vision of crisis and trauma (Stuhlmiller & Dunning, 2000)? Do the normalization and self-care responses, presented as psychoeducational guidelines in most debriefing models, permit enough space for the diversity and complexity of individual narratives of responses to trauma?

Exploring these questions and utilizing the lens of narrative theory may lead to critical assessments and revisions of the debriefing narrative process. A narrative conceptualization lends itself to continuing the healing and restorying well after the formal debriefing process. An example would be to suggest follow-up activities, such as directed journaling, which evolve from debriefings and continue the work of self-growth and healing. This raises the question of what would happen to the homework. Would there be a follow-up session (or sessions) to compare responses, or would the group be encouraged to share their reactions in self-led follow-up sessions? Or would journaling be viewed as a personal and individual process of healing? I do not have answers to these questions; rather, I suggest them for consideration as part of enhancing the efficacy of the debriefing process.

Group Process Considerations

Many community-based clinical practitioners are trained in group work and recognize the importance of careful attention to group process. In this section I will consider the tensions between the individual and group in debriefings, examine group structure, sequence, and timing, and explore the balance between a structured versus spontaneous group process.

Balancing the Needs of Individuals and Groups

The balance between individuals and groups is one that all group workers grapple with. Individuals seek both inclusion and differentiation (Brewer, 2001). The balance between the unique experiences and needs of individuals and the collective good of a group is implicit in debriefings and is built into most debriefing models. Debriefings involve the goal of helping and supporting individuals experiencing reactions to critical incidents, but debriefings also can have organizational goals, such as helping a group of workers regain their capacity to carry out their work responsibilities. Although these goals may correspond, at times they diverge, and clinicians should be mindful of potential conflicts of purpose. Confidentiality, although a stated rule for all debriefings, is also a contingent notion. When a work group is debriefed, there may be concerns about manifesting weakness or acknowledging that one is dealing with trauma by drinking excessively.

In an effort to respond to these tensions, there are often "support" facilitators who focus on individuals who may be particularly triggered or experiencing post–traumatic stress disorder (PTSD) and who assist with referrals for therapy and counseling, while "lead" and "assist" facilitators concentrate more on the group process (Miller, 2000). However, scanning for individual distress relies on picking up overt, observable cues. Allowing participants to self-identify unresolved issues or pressing needs, perhaps through offering exit interviews or having counselors available immediately after debriefings, would help individuals whose needs were not met by a group debriefing. Community-based clinicians are cognizant of the importance of easy access, removal of roadblocks, and follow-up when people are seeking mental health services and could help debriefing facilitators and organizations strengthen this aspect of their intervention model.

Conflicts and splits within groups can affect feelings of safety and security by individual group members. If such fissures occur during debriefings, then models of conflict resolution and options for breaking into subgroups might enhance the debriefing process. Community-based clinicians know that one size does not fit all and that some occasions require creativity and flexibility.

Consideration of Structure, Sequence, and Timing

Historically, debriefings have primarily been single events and conducted with groups. Debriefings are now seen as one aspect of a continuum of crisis intervention services ranging from predisaster preparations to follow-up activities, including referrals for clinical services (Everly & Mitchell, 2000). The structure and sequence of debriefings has been remarkably similar for most debriefing models (see table 33-1), and yet it would be surprising if one model fit all groups at all times for all types of critical incidents. Are the current structure and sequence of debriefing the most effective for all groups at all times, or can different modules be developed that expand certain sections of the process and de-emphasize or eliminate others? Should the sequence always remain the same? When should debriefings optimally be offered?

Is there any reason that a group should be exposed to only one debriefing? Could debriefings take place at different intervals with different areas of emphasis? Why not have multiple debriefings that build on one another? Initial debriefings could focus on the crisis nature of the critical incident and follow the traditional debriefing structure. But subsequent debriefings might focus more on medium- and long-term effects of the critical incident, as well as evaluate the effectiveness of earlier interventions, leading to new support networks and coping strategies. Social workers in agencies with ongoing access to consumers could develop and evaluate a more sequential, developmental model of debriefings. Follow-up debriefings could be scheduled in advance or offered on an as-needed basis.

Fine-Tuning the Balance Between Formula and Spontaneity

Models of debriefings have for the most part followed a fairly scripted and formulaic structure (see figure 33-1), although Dyregrov (2000) has advocated for achieving a balance between following a predetermined format and spontaneity. Because paraprofessionals and peers are used in so many debriefing programs, and also in an effort to ensure the greatest benefit and the least amount of harm, there has been a tendency to present debriefings in a tightly structured, nearly invariant fashion (Miller, 2000). Although consistency is important, rigidity can limit effectiveness. There is a difficult balance to achieve between consistency and predictability with flexibility and creativity. Debriefings work well when there is a format and structure, but any group process that is responding to disaster and emotional distress must remain fresh and vital.

Ensuring Equal Access and Equitable Treatment

Another question deserving attention is who receives debriefings and who does not? Social exclusion and such forces as racism, sexism, homophobia, and many other forms of oppression isolate populations within communities. Differential opportunity structures limit access by some to employment, neighborhoods, health care, resources, and services. What barriers exist for marginalized populations who have experienced critical incidents to receiving debriefings, and how can they be overcome? For example, employees of large corporations located in the World Trade Center were more likely to receive CISM services than those working for small firms (Miller, 2002a, 2002b). Within the structure of debriefings themselves, what dynamics of power, privilege, and oppression are manifested, and how can they be confronted?

CBCP appreciates the power of societal inequities, differential privilege and access to services and resources, and institutionalized societal oppression. Such structural inequities do not disappear when disaster strikes. There has been surprisingly little written about this issue in the debriefing literature. Who receives debriefings, and who does not? Which facilitators and organizations offer debriefings? Are there cultural biases built into debriefing models? Are social inequities and/or intergroup conflicts enacted in the actual debriefings? It is important to examine how durable relationships of power and powerlessness affect people, families, and communities before, during, and after a crisis.

Do Debriefings Help?

There has been disagreement and controversy over the effectiveness of debriefings. The research evidence thus far is inconclusive, incomplete, and at times flawed (Bisson, McFarlane, & Rose, 2000; Deahl, 2000; Everly & Mitchell, 2000; Miller, 2003; Raphael, 2000; Raphael, Meldrum, & McFarlane, 1995). Researchers and practitioners have differed over what to study, how to conduct the research, and the meaning of results, all of which reflect theoretical differences over how to conduct meaningful research, disagreement over what debriefings can realistically accomplish, and competition and turf wars. Deahl (2000) describes this as both a political and a professional issue:

> The effectiveness of acute interventions to prevent PTSD or other long-term psychological sequelae has become increasingly politicized and more than a matter of science. The interpretation of a number of recent randomized controlled trials (RCTs) is keenly contested. Many workers in the field of psychological trauma clearly have powerful vested interests in promoting the efficacy of interventions, such as PD [psychological debriefing], that often they themselves have developed. (p. 931)

One issue of contention is whether research should focus on the ability of debriefings to prevent future occurrences of PTSD or whether a different evaluative measure, such as reducing stress or helping people to make meaning from a crisis, should be used (Deahl, 2000). In part this stems from the overuse of the term PTSD, when often people are suffering from acute stress disorder, chronic stress, secondary trauma that does not reach the level of PTSD, or nonspecific stress disorders (Miller, 2002b; Perrin-Klingler, 2000). Everly and Mitchell (2000) and Deahl (2000) caution against using inoculation against future PTSD as the standard for evaluation. Another area of disagreement is whether randomized controlled trials are the "gold standard" for evaluating debriefings (Bisson et al. 2000; Raphael et al., 1995) or whether there are other ways to study debriefings, such as observational or case studies (Deahl, 2000).

A range of methodological problems have occurred in efforts to evaluate the effectiveness of debriefings: (1) different types of critical incidents (ranging from sexual assault to traffic accidents) have been compared; (2) there has been no standardized agreement about what constitutes a debriefing; (3) debriefings being researched were offered at different time intervals after a critical incident; (4) different recipient groups (emergency responders, soldiers, gravediggers, motorists, etc.) were compared; (5) there has been a lack of standard evaluative instruments and research methodologies; and (6) many evaluations have lacked randomly assigned control groups (Armstrong et al., 1998; Bisson et al., 2000; Chemtob, Tomas, Law, & Cremniter, 1997; Deahl, 2000; Everly & Mitchell, 2000; Raphael et al., 1995; Raphael, 2000). Studies have also neglected to adequately consider other variables, such as aspects of strength and resiliency, which are often independent of the debriefing although possibly more significant for future mental health (Gist & Woodall, 2000). People have differential responses to critical incidents depending on the nature of the catastrophe, their proximity and relationship to the disaster, history, strengths, and vulnerabilities, interpersonal and community supports, and the meaning they make of the event (Miller, 2002b), all of which make it difficult to measure the "success" of a debriefing. There have also been ethical concerns about forming control groups that do not receive treatment after a critical incident if there is a possibility that debriefings help (Deahl, 2000). Despite these inconsistencies, there does seem to be agreement by those who have reviewed the literature on two key points: (1) there is no conclusive evidence that debriefings help prevent future PTSD for those exposed to severe critical incidents, and (2) many of those who receive debriefings report finding that they are helpful (Bisson et al., 2000; Carlier & Gersons, 2000; Chemtob et al., 1997; Deahl, 2000; Everly & Mitchell, 2000; Miller, 2003; Raphael, 2000).

The controversy over the efficacy of debriefings is not unlike that surrounding the utility of other forms of psychotherapy. Both those who provide and those who receive debriefings report finding them to be helpful, but it has been less easy to conduct research clearly demonstrating that debriefings lead to measurable positive outcomes.

Suggestions for Future Research and Dissemination

Most research conducted about debriefings has been evaluative, outcome oriented, focusing on consumer satisfaction, job performance, and reduction of traumatic symptoms (Armstrong et al., 1998; Bisson et al., 2000; Chemtob et al., 1997;

Deahl, 2000; Everly & Mitchell, 2000; Raphael et al., 1995; Raphael, 2000; Walker, 1990). This approach is valuable and should continue. Community-based clinical practitioners can contribute to this research and design and implement experimental studies that utilize randomized control groups, which for some will always remain the "gold standard." However, a number of qualitative research methodologies would also be applicable to debriefings and consistent with the principles of CBCP: phenomenological (Seidman, 1991), narrative (Riessman, 1993), and action (Urehara et al., 1996).

It is not only the outcome of debriefings that should be evaluated but also the process itself. Debriefings are acts of constructing and reconstructing a group narrative of tragedy and disaster, so *how* this occurs and *why* these are important topics for research in addition to evaluating debriefing outcomes. How do participants experience debriefings, and what is it about the process that they find helpful? This has implications both for the method and for how to improve outcomes. Phenomenological research seeks to understand the experience and meaning of participants: What led up to the debriefing, what was their experience of the debriefing, and what meaning do they make of the debriefing (Seidman, 1991). These questions could be explored, perhaps, through post-debriefing interviews.

Narrative research relies on a textual analysis, which could result from a transcription from a debriefing. This would contribute to a better understanding of the construction of disaster narratives and the reconstruction of healing narratives. Case studies would be valuable for this enterprise (Deahl, 2000), although issues of confidentiality would need to be carefully considered.

Deahl (2000) raised the important question of the ethics of having control groups that do not receive debriefings if the intervention might be helpful. This problem is in some ways addressed by the tradition of action research, which conceptualizes research as a collaborative process that empowers people, with clear positioning of the researcher, who works toward a social goal (Reason, 1994). In this paradigm the researcher would be embedded in the group, and research would be conducted in collaboration with participants, not by an outside, "objective" researcher.

Empowerment-based practice involves less hierarchy between those who are being helped and those who do the helping, and the same should hold true for research. Community-based clinical practitioners can both conduct research and train others in how to conduct their own research. Observing, recording, tracking, coding, interviewing, analyzing, and understanding the experience and meaning of debriefings for both consumers and facilitators are all research activities that clinicians can employ during and after debriefings to better understand the process and to guide future development. They are also activities that community volunteers and disaster relief workers can be trained to do.

Conclusion

This chapter has considered debriefings from the perspective of CBCP. Clinical disaster relief work brings together citizens, volunteers, relief workers, and a myriad of professionals in the service of the community. Communities are best served when debriefings and other disaster relief services respect the natural relationships and connections that existed before the crisis and there is an appreciation of community assets and the human capacity to heal and prosper when confronted with adversity.

Community-based clinical practitioners recognize that clinical services occur in the context of communities and organizations. Critical incident stress debriefings are interventions that are founded on empowerment and resiliency and that utilize peer and lay facilitators, as well as community-based clinicians. They exist on the interstice of clinical interventions and mutual aid groups and embody the values and intentions of community-based clinical practice.

References

American Red Cross. (1995). Disaster mental health services I. Washington, DC: Author.

Armstrong, K., O'Callahan, W., & Marmar, C. R. (1991). Debriefing Red Cross disaster personnel: The multiple stressor debriefing model. *Journal of Traumatic Stress, 4,* 581–593.

Armstrong, K., Zatzick, D., Metzler, T., Weiss, D. S., Marmar, C. R., Garma, S., Ronfeldt, H., & Roepke, L. (1998). Debriefing of American Red Cross personnel: A pilot study on participants' evaluations and case examples from the 1994 Los Angeles earthquake relief operation. *Social Work in Health Care, 27*, 33–50.

Bisson, J. I., McFarlane, A. C., & Rose, S. (2000). Psychological debriefing. In E. B. Foa, T. M. Keane, & M. J. Friedman (Eds.), *Effective treatments for PTSD: Practice guidelines from the International Society for Traumatic Stress Studies* (pp. 39–59). New York: Guilford.

Brewer, M. B. (2001). Ingroup identification and intergroup conflict: When does ingroup love become outgroup hate? In R. D. Ashmore, L. Jussim, & D. Wilder (Eds.), *Social identity, intergroup conflict and conflict reduction* (pp. 17–41). New York: Oxford University Press.

Carlier, I. V. E., & Gersons, B. P. R. (2000). Brief intervention programs after trauma. In J. M. Violanti, D. Paton, & C. Dunning (Eds.), *Posttraumatic stress intervention: Challenges, issues, perspectives* (pp. 65–80). Springfield, IL: Thomas.

Chambon, A. S. (1994). The dialogical analysis of case materials. In E. S. Sherman & W. J. Reid (Eds.), *Qualitative analysis in social work* (pp. 205–215). New York: Columbia University Press.

Chemtob, C. M., Tomas, S., Law, W., & Cremniter, D. (1997). Postdisaster psychosocial intervention: A field study of the impact of debriefing on psychological stress. *American Journal of Psychiatry, 154*, 415–417.

Deahl, M. (2000). Psychological debriefing: Controversy and challenge. *Australian and New Zealand Journal of Psychiatry, 34*, 929–939.

Dyregrov, A. (1997). The process in psychological debriefings. *Journal of Traumatic Stress, 10*, 589–605.

Dyregrov, A. (2000). Helpful and hurtful aspects of psychological debriefing groups. In G. S. Everly Jr. & J. T. Mitchell (Eds.), *Critical incident stress management: Advanced group crisis interventions: A workbook* (pp. 47–56). Ellicott City, MD: International Critical Incident Stress Foundation.

Everly, G. S., Jr., & Mitchell, J. T. (Eds.). (2000). *Critical incident stress management: Advanced group crisis interventions: A workbook.* Ellicott City, MD: International Critical Incident Stress Foundation.

Germain, C. B. (Ed.) (1979). *Social work practice: People and environments.* New York: Columbia University Press.

Germain, C. B., & Gitterman, A. (1980). *The life model of social work practice.* New York: Columbia University Press.

Germain, C. B., & Gitterman, A. (1995). Ecological perspective. In *Encyclopedia of Social Work* (19th ed., pp. 816–824). Washington, DC: NASW Press.

Gilgun, J. F. (1994). Hand in glove: The grounded theory approach and social work practice research. In E. Sherman & W. J. Reid (Eds.), *Qualitative research in social work* (pp. 115–125). New York: Columbia University Press.

Gilgun, J. (1999). CASPARS: New tools for assessing client risks and strengths. *Families in Society, 80*, 450–459.

Gist, R., & Woodall, R. (2000). There are no simple solutions to complex problems. In J. M. Violanti, D. Paton, & C. Dunning (Eds.), *Posttraumatic stress intervention: Challenges, issues, perspectives* (pp. 81–96). Springfield, IL: Thomas.

Laird, J. (Ed.). (1993) *Revisioning social work education: A social constructionist approach.* Binghamton, NY: Haworth.

Miller, J. (2000). The use of debriefings in response to disasters and traumatic events. *Professional Development: The International Journal of Continuing Social Work Education, 3*(2), 24–31.

Miller, J. (2001). Family and community integrity. *Journal of Sociology and Social Welfare, 28*(4), 23–44.

Miller, J. (2002a). Affirming flames: Debriefing survivors of the World Trade Center attacks. *Brief Treatment and Crisis Intervention, 2*, 85–94.

Miller, J. (2002b). Reflections on 9/11: Vulnerability and strength in the "New World Order." *Smith Studies in Social Work, 73*, 73–82.

Miller, J. (2003). Critical stress debriefing and social work: Expanding the frame. *Journal of Social Service Research.*

Mitchell, J. T. (1983). When disaster strikes: The critical incident stress debriefing process. *Journal of Emergency Medical Services, 8*, 36–39.

Palmer, N. (1999). Fostering resiliency in children: Lessons learned in transcending adversity. *Social Thought, 19*, 69–87.

Perrin-Klinger, G. (2000). The integration of traumatic experiences: Culture and resources. In J. M. Violanti, D. Patton, & C. Dunning (Eds.), *Posttraumatic stress intervention* (pp. 43–64). Springfield, IL: Charles Thomas.

Polio, D., McDonald, S. M., & North, C. S. (1996). Combining a strengths-based approach and feminist theory in group work with persons "on the streets." *Social Work with Groups, 19*(3/4), 5–20.

Pueler, J. N. (1988). Community outreach after emergencies. In M. Lystad (Ed.), *Mental health response to mass emergencies: Theory and practice* (pp. 239–261). New York: Brunner/Mazel.

Raphael, B. (1986). *When disaster strikes: How individuals and communities cope with catastrophe.* New York: Basic Books.

Raphael, B. (2000). Conclusion: Debriefing—science, belief and wisdom. In B. Raphael & J. Wilson (Eds.), *Psychological debriefing: Theory, practice and evidence* (pp. 351–359). Cambridge: Cambridge University Press.

Raphael, B., Meldrum, L., & McFarlane, A.C. (1995). Does debriefing after psychological trauma work? *British Medical Journal, 310,* 1479–1480.

Reason, P. (1994). Three approaches to participative inquiry. In N. K. Denzin & Y. S. Lincoln (Eds.), *Handbook of qualitative research* (pp. 306–323). Thousand Oaks, CA: Sage.

Riessman, C. K. (1993). *Narrative analysis.* Newbury Park, CA: Sage.

Saleeby, D. (1996). The strengths perspective in social work practice: Extensions and cautions. *Social Work, 41,* 296–305.

Seidman, I. E. (1991). *Interviewing as qualitative research: A guide for researchers in education and the social services.* New York: Teachers College Press.

Stuhlmiller, C., & Dunning, C. (2000). Challenging the mainstream: From pathogenic to salutogenic models of posttrauma intervention. In J. M. Violanti, D. Paton, & C. Dunning (Eds.), *Posttraumatic stress intervention: Challenges, issues, perspectives* (pp. 10–42). Springfield, IL: Thomas.

Urehara, E. S., Sohng, S. L. S., Bending, R. L., Seyfried, S., Richey, C. A., Morelli, P., Spencer, M., Ortega, D., Keenan, L., & Kanuha, V. (1996). Towards a values-based approach to multicultural social work research. *Social Work, 41,* 613–621.

Walker, G. (1990). Crisis-care in critical incident debriefing. *Death Studies, 14,* 121–133.

Warheit, G. J. (1988). Disasters and their mental health consequences: Issues, findings and future trends. In M. Lystad (Ed.), *Mental health response to mass emergencies: Theory and practice* (pp. 3–21). New York: Brunner/Mazel.

Weick, A., Rapp, C., Sullivan, W. P., & Kisthardt, W. (1989). A strengths perspective for social work practice. *Social Work, 34,* 350–354.

White, M., & Epston, D. (1990). *Narrative means to therapeutic ends.* New York: Norton.

Young, M. A. (1997). *The community crisis response team training manual* (2nd ed.). Washington, DC: National Organization for Victim Assistance.

Zinner, E. S., & Williams, M. B. (1999). Summary and incorporation: A reference frame for community recovery and restoration. In E. S. Zinner & M. B. Williams (Eds.), *When a community weeps: Case studies in group survivorship* (pp. 237–254). Philadelphia: Brunner/Mazel.

A patchwork, partially constructed vision may strike exactly the balance between humility and boldness that's needed in these unpredictable times . . . we may proceed best, as Mary Catherine Bateson writes, "by improvisation, discovering the shape of our creation along the way, rather than pursuing a vision already defined." So long as we stay open to new information, learning as we go, not allowing ourselves to be distracted by the search for absolute certainty, we can continue to work toward goals we can feel proud of. We can conduct what Gandhi called "experiments in truth," or as the priest who founded the Spanish Mondragon co-ops once said, "build the road as we travel" (pp. 303–304).

    —P. R. Loeb, *Soul of a citizen: Living with conviction in a cynical time.*

Index